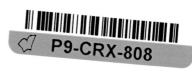

Ion Channels in the Cardiovascular System:

Function and Dysfunction

Ion Channels in the Cardiovascular System:

Function and Dysfunction

edited by

Peter M. Spooner
Arthur M. Brown
William A. Catterall
Gregory J. Kaczorowski
Harold C. Strauss

Futura Publishing Company, Inc.
Armonk, New York

Library of Congress Cataloging-in-Publication Data

Ion channels in the cardiovascular system / Peter M. Spooner . . . [et al.], editors.
    p.   cm.
   Includes bibliographical references and index.
   1. Heart—Pathophysiology. 2. Ion channels. 3. Arrhythmia.
4. Cardiac arrest. 5. Heart conduction system. I. Spooner, Peter M.
   [DNLM: 1. Ion Channels—physiology. 2. Cardiovascular System—
physiology. 3. Arrhythmia—physiopathology. 4. Death, Sudden,
Cardiac—pathology. WG 102 I64 1993]
   RC682.9.I584 1993
   616.1'207—dc20
   DNLM/DLC
   for Library of Congress   93-37793
                                                        CIP

Published by
Futura Publishing Company, Inc.
135 Bedford Road
Armonk, NY 10504-0418

LC #: 93-37793
ISBN #: 0-87993-591-X

Original cover graphics contributed by Khanh Nguyen, NHLBI, Bethesda, MD.

Table of Contents

vii

List of Contributors

Peter H. Backx, Division of Cardiology, Department of Medicine, The Johns Hopkins University, Baltimore, MD

Joel C. Barrish, Bristol-Myers Squibb, Pharmaceutical Research Institute, New York, NY

Kurt Beam, Department of Physiology, Colorado State University, Ft. Collins, CO

Bruce Bean, Department of Neurobiology, Harvard Medical School, Boston, MA

Paul B. Bennett, Departments of Pharmacology and Medicine, Vanderbilt School of Medicine, Nashville, TN

Wolfgang Berger, Institut für Biochemische Pharmakologie, University of Innsbruck, A-6020 Innsbruck, Austria

M. Biel, Institut für Pharmakologie und Toxikologie, Technische Universität Munchen, D-8000 Munich 40, Germany

Shawn C. Black, Department of Pharmacology, University of Michigan Medical School, Ann Arbor, MI

E. Bosse, Institut für Pharmakologie und Toxikologie, Technische Universität Munchen, D-8000 Munich 40 Germany

A. P. Braun, Department of Medical Physiology, University of Calgary School of Medicine, Calgary, Alberta, Canada

Arthur M. Brown,* Department of Molecular Physiology and Biophysics, Baylor College of Medicine, Houston, TX

Donald L. Campbell, Department of Pharmacology, Duke University Medical Center, Durham, NC

A. C. Campos de Carvalho, Department of Neuroscience, Albert Einstein College of Medicine, Bronx, NY, and Federal University of Rio de Janiero, Rio de Janiero, Brazil

Agustin Castellanos, Division of Cardiology, Department of Medicine, University of Miami School of Medicine and the, Miami VA Medical Center, Miami, FL

William A. Catterall,* Department of Pharmacology, University of Washington, Seattle, WA

*Member of the Research Assessment Panel.

Todd Chapman, Department of Physiology, University of Nevada School of Medicine, Reno, NV

Liguo Chi, Department of Pharmacology, University of Michigan Medical School, Ann Arbor, MI

G. J. Christ, Department of Urology, Albert Einstein College of Medicine, Bronx, NY

R. B. Clark, Department of Medical Physiology, University of Calgary School of Medicine, Calgary, Alberta, Canada

Thomas J. Colatsky, Division of Cardiovascular and Metabolic Disorders, Wyeth-Ayerst Research, Princeton, NJ

Karen K. Deal, Department of Pharmacology, Vanderbilt Medical School, Nashville, TN

Mariella De Biasi, Department of Molecular Physiology and Biophysics, Baylor College of Medicine, Houston, TX

Henry J. Duff, Department of Pharmacology, University of Washington, Seattle, WA

G. I. Fishman, Departments of Molecular Genetics and Medicine, Albert Einstein College of Medicine, Bronx, NY

V. Flockerzi, Institüt fur Pharmakologie und Toxikologie, Technische Universität Munchen, D-8000 Munich 40, Germany

David M. Floyd, Bristol-Myers Squibb, Pharmaceutical Research Institute, New York, NY

Harry A. Fozzard, Cardiac Electrophysiology Laboratories, Departments of Pharmacological & Physiological Sciences and Medicine, and University of Chicago, Chicago, IL

Gregory S. Friedrichs, Department of Pharmacology, University of Michigan Medical School, Ann Arbor, MI

Jesús García, Department of Physiology, Colorado State University, Ft. Collins, CO

Maria L. Garcia, Membrane Biochemistry and Biophysics, Merck Research Laboratories, Rahway, NJ

Alfred L. George, Jr., Departments of Pharmacology and Medicine, Vanderbilt School of Medicine, Nashville, TN

W. R. Giles, Department of Medical Physiology, University of Calgary School of Medicine, Calgary, Alberta, Canada

Hartmut Glossmann, Institut für Biochemische Pharmakologie, University of Innsbruck, A-6020 Innsbruck, Austria

Alan L. Goldin, Department of Microbiology and Molecular Genetics, University of California–Irvine, Irvine, CA

Jack Z. Gougoutas, Bristol-Myers Squibb, Pharmaceutical Research Institute, New York, NY

Pádraig J. Hart, Department of Physiology, University of Nevada School of Medicine, Reno, NV

Steffen Hering, Insitut für Biochemische Pharmakologie, University of Innsbruck, A-6020 Innsbruck, Austria

Peter Hess, Department of Cellular and Molecular Physiology, Program in Neuroscience, Harvard Medical School, Boston, MA

F. Hofman, Institut für Pharmakologie und Toxikologie, Technische Universität Munchen, D-8000 Munich 40, Germany

Burton Horowitz, Department of Physiology, University of Nevada School of Medicine, Reno, NV

Melissa H. House, Department of Molecular Physiology and Biophysics, Vanderbilt Medical School, Nashville, TN

Joseph R. Hume, Department of Physiology, University of Nevada School of Medicine, Reno, NV

John T. Hunt, Bristol-Myers Squibb, Pharmaceutical Research Institute, New York, NY

N. K. Jurkiewicz, Department of Pharmacology, Merck Research Laboratories, West Point, PA

Gregory J. Kaczorowski, * Membrane Biochemistry and Biophysics, Merck Research Laboratories, Rahway, NJ

Robert S. Kass, Department of Physiology, University of Rochester School of Medicine and Dentistry, Rochester, NY

Arnold M. Katz, * Cardiology Division, Department of Medicine, University of Connecticut, Farmington, CT

Kenneth M. Kessler, Division of Cardiology, Department of Medicine, University of Miami School of Medicine and the Miami VA Medical Center, Miami, FL

S. David Kimball, Bristol-Myers Squibb, Pharmaceutical Research Institute, New York, NY

Timothy J. Knittle, Department of Molecular Physiology and Biophysics, Vanderbilt Medical School, Nashville, TN

Wan F. Lau, Bristol-Myers Squibb, Pharmaceutical Research Institute, New York, NY

John H. Lawrence, Division of Cardiology, Department of Medicine, The Johns Hopkins University, Baltimore, MD

Paul C. Levesque, Department of Physiology, University of Nevada School of Medicine, Reno, NV

Benedict R. Lucchesi, Department of Pharmacology, University of Michigan Medical School, Ann Arbor, MI

William C. Lumma, Jr., Merck Research Laboratories, West Point, PA

Peter J. Manley, Department of Pharmacology, University of Michigan Medical School, Ann Arbor, MI

Eduardo Marban, Division of Cardiology, Department of Medicine, The Johns Hopkins University, Baltimore, MD

Rafael Mejía-Alvarez, Division of Cardiology, Department of Medicine, The Johns Hopkins University, Baltimore, MD

A. P. Moreno, Department of Neuroscience, Albert Einstein College of Medicine, Bronx, NY

Issam F. Moubarak, Division of Cardiovascular and Metabolic Disorders, Wyeth-Ayerst Research, Princeton, NJ

Robert J. Myerburg, Division of Cardiology, Department of Medicine, University of Miami School of Medicine, and the Miami VA Medical Center, Miami, FL

Randal Numann, Department of Pharmacology, University of Washington, Seattle, WA

H. Bradley Nuss, Division of Cardiology, Department of Medicine, The Johns Hopkins University, Baltimore, MD

Jeanne Y. Oh, Department of Pharmacology, University of Michigan Medical School, Ann Arbor, MI

Brian O'Rourke, Division of Cardiology, Department of Medicine, The Johns Hopkins University, Baltimore, MD

L. A. Pardo, Max-Planck-Institut für Experimentelle Medizin, D-3400 Gottingen, FRG

D. Earl Patton, Department of Microbiology and Molecular Genetics, University of California–Irvine, Irvine, CA

Sunny Po, Department of Pharmacology, Vanderbilt School of Medicine, Nashville, TN

Yusheng Qu, Department of Pharmacology, Duke University Medical Center, Durham, NC

Randall L. Rasmusson, Department of Biomedical Engineering, Duke University Medical Center, Durham, NC

Steven L. Roberds, Department of Pharmacology, Vanderbilt School of Medicine, Nashville, TN

M. B. Rook, Department of Neuroscience, Albert Einstein College of Medicine, Bronx, NY

P. Ruth, Institut für Pharmakologie und Toxikologie, Technische Universität Munchen, D-8000 Munich 40, Germany

J. C. Sáez, Department of Neuroscience, Albert Einstein College of Medicine, Bronx, NY

M. C. Sanguinetti, Department of Pharmacology , Merck Research Laboratories, West Point, PA

Todd Scheuer, Department of Pharmacology, University of Washington, Seattle, WA

Peter J. Schwartz, Department of Medicine, University of Pavia , Pavia, Italy, and Istituto di Clinica Medica II, University of Milan, Milan, Italy

Robert S. Slaughter, Membrane Biochemistry and Biophysics, Merck Research Laboratories, Rahway, NJ

Thomas W. Smith,* Cardiovascular Division, Department of Medicine, Brigham and Women's Hospital, Boston, MA

Dirk J. Snyders, Departments of Pharmacology and Medicine, Vanderbilt School of Medicine, Nashville, TN

Walter Spinelli, Division of Cardiovascular and Metabolic Disorders, Wyeth-Ayerst Research, Princeton, NJ

Peter M. Spooner,* Cardiac Functions Branch, Division of Heart and Vascular Diseases, National Heart, Lung, and Blood Institute, National Institutes of Health, Bethesda, MD

David C. Spray, Department of Neuroscience, Albert Einstein College of Medicine, Bronx, NY

Harold C. Strauss,* Departments of Pharmacology and Medicine, Duke University Medical Center, Durham, NC

Jörg Striessnig, Institut fur Biochemische Pharmakologie, University of Innsbruck, A-6020 Innsbruck, Austria

W. Stühmer, Max-Planck-Institut für Experimentelle Medizin, D-3400 Gottingen, FRG

Michael M. Tamkun, Departments of Pharmacology, and Molecular Physiology and Biophysics, Vanderbilt Medical School, Nashville, TN

Gordon Tomaselli, Division of Cardiology, Department of Medicine, The Johns Hopkins University, Baltimore, MD

Stephen S. Tsung, Department of Physiology, University of Nevada School of Medicine, Reno, NV

Jan Tytgat, Department of Cellular and Molecular Physiology, Program in Neuroscience, Harvard Medical School, Boston, MA

Andrew C. G. Uprichard, Department of Pharmacology, University of Michigan Medical School, Ann Arbor, MI

Carol A. Vandenberg, Department of Biological Sciences and Neuroscience Research Institute, University of California—Santa Barbara, Santa Barbara, CA

M. P. Walsh, Department of Medical Biochemistry, University of Calgary School of Medicine, Calgary, Alberta, Canada

August M. Watanabe,* Lilly Research Laboratories, Eli Lilly & Company, Indianapolis, IN

A. Welling, Institut für Pharmakologie und Toxikologie, Technische Universität Munchen, D-8000 Munich 40, Germany

James W. West, Department of Pharmacology, University of Washington, Seattle, WA

Douglas P. Zipes, Department of Medicine, Krannert Insitute of Cardiology, Indiana University School of Medicine and, Roudebush VA Medical Center, Indianapolis, IN

PREFACE

Ion Channels in the Cardiovascular System: Function and Dysfunction

This volume summarizes new, exciting research on the structure, function and regulation of ion channels in the cardiovascular system. Ion channels of major interest in these tissues are members of related families of complex glycoproteins which mediate the transport of sodium (Na^+), potassium (K^+), calcium (Ca^{++}), or chloride (Cl^-) ions across cell membranes. Because of the critical importance of these ions in generating conducting signals and action potentials which elicit the physiologically essential function of contraction in cardiac and vascular muscle, the focus of interest is on the nature of those channels responsible for control on the cell's active electrical state. From this perspective ion channels in cardiovascular cells represent both the foundation for normal contractile function and, it is becoming increasingly apparent, an important contributor to disorders of electrical signalling and communication.

Over recent years research on ion channels has become a topic of great importance in efforts to understand the causes and consequences of cardiovascular disease and in devising effective strategies for its alleviation. This volume deals with both the fundamental biology and clinical implications of the function and dysfunction of major ion channel types. Particular focus is given to channels in the heart. There, a repetitive, precisely choreographed sequence of currents through families of Na^+, Ca^{++}, K^+, and Cl^- channels is responsible for generating the normal sinus rhythm of pacing potentials, the transmission of these signals through specialized conducting pathways and, cardiac action potentials which trigger the process of "excitation-contraction" coupling. This latter series of events, in turn depends on the function of yet different sets of ion channels, and results in the release of intracellular Ca^{2+} which initiates physical interactions between actin and myosin resulting in contraction.

A major purpose of this volume is to focus attention on the molecular events responsible for alterations in the flow of different ions through their appropriate channels, as each channel type is opened and closed in response to specific chemical or electrical signals. Such "gating" from a closed to an open channel state results usually in a movement of charge with great rapidity and ionic specificity, as individual ions flow through open channel "pores". This sudden onset of passive charge flow down preestablished electrochemical gradients that characterizes channel-mediated transport, is in marked contrast to the slower, more regular "active" movement of ions powered by membrane transport enzymes, such as the well characterized Ca^{2+} or Na^+-K^+ ATPases. As presently envisioned, flow through each individual ion channel is a stochastic process, occurring in an "all or none" manner, as each molecule is "gated" open from a closed configuration. Gating occurs in response to either specific chemical signals (eg. acetylcholine, epinephrine, dopamine), or in the case of voltage modulated channels, to local changes in membrane electrical field.

Many of the chapters in this volume deal with mechanisms by which changes in channel conductance occur or with their consequences or causes in different physiological situations. This includes changes seem under "normal" functional states as well as "dysfunctional" or pathological changes occurring as a result, or cause of disease. Many also emphasize the response of different channels to drugs and other potentially useful therapies which could be used to delineate function or remedy disease. This information especially is of considerable importance not only in expanding our knowledge of channel biology, but is also of potentially great practical health consequence because of the known involvement of channel pathology in many types of disabling and life threatening arrhythmias, cardiac hypertrophy and sudden cardiac death; health problems that play a role in more than 300,000 cardiovascular deaths in the United States alone each year.

Knowledge of the nature of channel proteins and their role in disease etiology has increased exponentially over the past several years as a result of two innovations detailed extensively throughout the chapters which follow. One is the acquisition of an increasingly detailed molecular description of the organization, composition and expression of many different types of channel proteins. The other is the enormous progress in functional electrical analyses of individual ion currents afforded by developments in electrophysiology, exemplified by the acclaimed work of Drs. Erwin Nehrer and Bert Sakmann, recognized by their 1992 Nobel prize in Physiology and Medicine.

Documenting progress achieved in applying these powerful new tools to cardiac and vascular cells and developing a better understanding of their clinical implications is the primary purpose of this book, one of a number of effects in a program on basic aspects of arrhythmias suggested by the National Heart Lung and Blood Institute, National Institutes of Health at Bethesda Md. The chapters presented were selected and edited by an outstanding group of research leaders with many years experience in the fields of channel biology from basic, clinical and pharmaceutical environments. Each also has been involved with Institute efforts in developing more effective approaches to antiarrhythmic therapies over many years having participated in other educational efforts, conferences and Institute supported clinical trials directed at the problem. Each has a unique perspective, and all share a great appreciation of the clinical dilemma posed by the pathobiology of dysfunctional cell ion transport systems. The authors whose work is included represent an even more diverse group of scientists from academic, clinical and pharmaceutical laboratories across the world. Their work addresses fundamental issues important in developing efficacious, cost-effective alternatives to prevailing more dangerous surgical and implantation approaches to arrhythmia control. Each summarizes work from a leading research laboratory on topics fundamental to the broad issue of developing better channel-directed cardiovascular therapies.

Intellectually, this volume follows from an earlier Institute supported Conference on "Ion Channel Function" held at Chantilly Virginia in 1992 and an earlier American Heart Association conference on the "Structure and Function of Ion Channels in the Heart and Vascular System" organized by Drs. Harry Fozzard and Peter Davies at the University of Chicago in 1990 which dealt with characterizing Na^+, K^+, and Ca^{2+} channels that contribute to the cardiac action potential. Both meetings also touched to some extent on channels in vascular smooth muscle, a topic largely ignored here because it has expanded to a size sufficient to require a separate volume on its own. Additional insight on a number of relevant issues in channel function has also emerged during several other formal discussions since that time, notably the Spring 1992 Gordon Research Ion Channels Conference. Documentation of progress achieved to date however, has not been forthcoming for a variety of reasons, and thus, it was felt important to try to capture and summarize recent knowledge with the solicitation and publication of the contributions presented here.

The six Sections of this book are organized on the basic themes which have emerged over recent years. They cover: "Ion Channels and Cardiac Disease"; "Ion Channels and Cardiovascular Function"; "Channel Modulation and Autonomic Control"; Structure-Function of Ion Channels"; Molecular Pharmacology"; and "Drug Discovery". Each Section is preceded by a short Foreword intended to highlight important findings in the chapters, and to editorialize on their significance. As is the case with all such efforts, not every approach or topic important to the field is as fully or fairly represented as desirable, a reflection not just of the editor's bias, but of realistic practical limitations despite a volume of this size. Nevertheless, all of those involved believe without apology that the papers presented provide valuable insights into current problems in the field and will help extend our knowledge of the function and dysfunction of cardiovascular channels. It is all our hope's that the publication of the exciting work contained herein will also result in an increasing understanding of channel biology and a greater awareness of its potential to contribute to treating cardiovascular disease.

Peter M. Spooner

ACKNOWLEDGMENTS

Ion Channels in the Cardiovascular System: Function and Dysfunction

Organizing a volume of this nature required the assistance, good will and talent of a great many colleagues, friends and author-investigators, along with the support of organizations committed to applying advances in basic science to important problems in cardiovascular health.

Programmatic assistance from the National Heart Lung and Blood Institute (NHLBI) to efforts directed at cardiac arrhythmias and sudden cardiac death has, over the years, has been critical and generous. Production of this compendium volume was likewise supported by the Institute in multiple ways and we would therefore like to thank its Director, Dr. Claude Lenfant and Dr. Eugene Passamani, Director of Heart and Vascular Diseases for their interest in producing this work. The Division's early financial contributions to the idea of assessing and publishing a state of the art research volume exploring the role of ion channels in arrhythmic diseases was essential in securing a successful result. Also essential in concept development was the contribution of Dr. Robin Yeaton Woo, then with the American Association for the Advancement of Science. The staff of the now defunct AAAS Press also provided much help in organizing the work and in its production. Steve Korn and his colleagues at Futura Publishing have earned our sincere appreciation for ensuring its successful completion. The combined skill of this group in ensuring a timely, effective, well organized volume will be appreciated by many in years to come.

From inception, the editors of this volume believed the goal of developing effective channel directed therapies for cardiovascular disease can best be facilitated by integrating the complementary abilities and insights of basic scientists, academic clinicians and scientists working on drug discovery in pharmaceutical and biotechnology laboratories. Consequently, we believed it essential to include here contributions from all three perspectives. To achieve this goal a similarly diverse Scientific Organizing Committee was asked to solicit contributions from a full range of the different disciplines involved. This group, consisting of Dr.s Arnold M. Katz, University of Connecticut; Thomas W. Smith, Brigham and Woman's Hospital; Harold C. Strauss, Duke University; August Watanabe, Eli Lily; Greg J. Kaczorowski, Merck Sharpe & Dohme along with NHLBI staff was led by Co-chairs, Dr.s Arthur M. Brown, Baylor University and William A. Catterall, University of Washington. The committee was responsible for the selection of the chapters contained herein and with their scientific editing. The same group not only has had extensive research experience in the ion channel/arrhythmia field, but most have also had considerable experience with NHLBI efforts in antiarrhythmic programs over many years. Many of this same group for example, had served on a Research Assessment Panel for a related NHLBI conference on Ion Channels held in Chantilly, Virginia in the Fall of 1992. Because of its obvious importance to the contributions in this volume and its intended readership, their report, which highlights research support needs for the future of the field, is appended as the final chapter of the book. We are grateful for their considerable efforts and for agreeing to letting us include the report here.

We'd like to specially acknowledge several essential individual contributions. Critically important has been the generous contributions of time and effort from Dr. Arthur "Buzz" Brown, one of the real pioneers of an interdisciplinary approach to the cardiac ion channels field and one of its leaders for many years. "Buzz's" perspective, that antiarrhythmic efforts could be greatly improved through better utilization of progress in basic science, was a significant factor in catalyzing this effort. His is also the primarily scientific voice in producing the "Forewords" which precede each Section of the book, and which act to unite different topics and assist in the interpretation of the individual papers. He, along with Bill Catterall, working with the full Committee, were the major arbiters in providing a well balanced and scientifically diverse group of papers. "Buzz" also helped enormously with their consolidation into the different topical Sections. His and the whole editorial committee's efforts were characterized by skill, diplomacy and an insistence on a level of quality and clarity which help greatly in conveying the different research findings of each of the thirty different authors represented. The other individual who helped enormously in conceptually organizing the project was Dr. Arnold Katz. His insistence on integrating topics relevant to both basic and clinical science and his understanding of the role of ion channels in the cardiovascular system have resulted in a real interdisciplinary integration and a research compendium which should provide an important resource to members of the many diverse groups represented here. Arnie has been a pioneer in developing an appreciation of a real molecular cardiology in this country. His contributions in helping with this project, and in providing the first chapter which presents a unique and cogent summary of the problem, add a valuable dimension that distinguishes this effort from a more traditional academic treatment.

Lastly, we thank all those scientists, physicians and support staff who contributed their time, interest and talent by participating in this effort. In the end it really is their many accomplishments, dedication and willingness to share their hard won results to achieve important goals, which assured the efforts represented by this book were a real success.

Peter M. Spooner

Introduction: Ion Channels and Cardiology—The Need for Bridges Across a Widening Boundary

Arnold M. Katz

Basic and clinical electrophysiology are advancing along diverging trajectories. Whereas basic research is focusing on the molecular control of electrogenic ion fluxes across cardiac membranes, clinical efforts to prevent sudden death are relying to an increasing extent on ablation therapy and devices such as implantable defibrillators. Realization that antiarrhythmic drugs, once thought to be of value in preventing sudden death, exert proarrhythmic effects that can outweigh their beneficial actions (1) has led cardiologists to turn away from pharmacological therapy in patients at risk for a lethal arrhythmia. The result has been a weakening of the link between the biomedical scientist and the clinical cardiologist, which comes at a time when the opportunity for collaborations to improve patient management has never been greater.

Widening of the boundary between basic and clinical electrophysiology also reflects the rapid growth of knowledge in these fields, which is making it increasingly difficult for these two groups of scientists to speak to each other. Practicing physicians tend to view the heart as an organ that pumps blood; although the intricacy of the heart's machinery is generally appreciated by the clinician, the vast body of new molecular data is overwhelming in both volume and complexity. Basic scientists, on the other hand, although able to relate specific aspects of the heart's performance to precisely characterized features of specific molecules within myocardial cells, are usually not trained to deal with the challenges of diseased patients.

This introduction examines the evolution of our understanding of the electrical activity of the heart to provide a historical perspective that may help address the central challenge of this text: unification of the diverging interests of the basic scientist who studies the molecular basis of cardiac excitation, and the clinician who must deal with the challenge of the patient at risk for a serious arrhythmia or sudden cardiac death.

Three Paradigms in the Search for Understanding of the Electrical Activity of the Heart

The development of our understanding of cardiovascular physiology and pathophysiology can be viewed in terms of a succession of paradigms, which T. S. Kuhn (2) has described as "models from which spring particular coherent traditions of scientific research." The shifting focus of our efforts to understand the function and control of the heart is readily understood if we examine the application of three paradigms used to explain the regulation of the heart's performance (Table 1), where the focus has shifted from *organ physiology* to *cell biochemistry and biophysics,* and most recently to altered *gene expression* (3).

The first of these paradigms, applied to cardiac regulation at the beginning of this century, described the influence of diastolic volume on the work of the heart. This is, of course, Starling's Law of the Heart, which represents control at the *organ* level. By the 1960s, regulation of cardiac work was viewed in terms of changes in myocardial contractility, which are brought about mainly by alterations in the calcium fluxes that effect excitation-contraction coupling and relaxation of the cardiac cell (4). Over the past decade, it has become clear that cardiac performance is also influenced by a third paradigm, altered gene expression, which mediates long-term adjustments of cardiac function to such chronic conditions as aging, endocrinopathies, and heart failure (3, 4).

Evolution of Mechanisms of Cardiovascular Regulation

As the focus of scientific inquiry has moved from the first to the second, and now to the third of these paradigms, we encounter regulatory mechanisms of increasing levels of complexity. This almost certainly reflects the fact that these paradigm shifts reveal a sequence of regulatory mechanisms that, in reverse order, recapitulate the evolution of biological control. Regulation by altered organ function must have appeared most recently,

Table 1. Three paradigms in cardiovascular physiology and pathophysiology

Paradigm	Regulation of Cardiac Work	Heart Failure	Electrophysiology
Organ physiology	Changing end-diastolic fiber length (Starling's Law of the Heart)	Reduced cardiac pumping, salt and water retention, and vasoconstriction	Bradyarrhythmias, tachyarrhythmias, and disorganized impulse conduction
Cell biochemistry	Changing myocardial contractility; Ca fluxes	Impaired myocardial contractility and relaxation	Abnormal ionic currents; altered channel function
Gene expression	Altered synthesis of myocardial proteins	Myocardial alterations; cardiomyopathy of overload	Altered ion channel synthesis and assembly

about 600 million years ago, because this mechanism could operate only after the evolution of multicellular life forms. Regulation by changing intracellular composition became possible earlier in evolution, perhaps 1.4 billion years ago, when cells had developed membranes of sufficient complexity to control their internal environment. The ability to respond to changing environment by synthesis of altered gene products probably appeared at the dawn of life, more than 3 billion years ago, when simple life forms had not yet evolved means to stabilize the environment surrounding their genetic material. Thus, this third paradigm likely represents the oldest mechanism that allowed our earliest ancestors to adapt to a changing environment; having had the longest time to evolve, it is not surprising regulation by altered gene expression is turning out to be the most complex of the paradigms listed in Table 1.

Three Paradigms in the Search for Understanding of Cardiac Electrophysiology

Our efforts to understand normal and abnormal cardiac electrophysiology can also be traced through the three paradigms previously discussed (5). Evaluation of clinical disorders of cardiac electrical function was made possible by the development of the string galvanometer at the beginning of this century, which allowed high-fidelity recording of electrical signals from the human heart. The advent of clinical electrocardiography led to several decades of clinical and animal research that, using the paradigm of *organ physiology*, focused on the mechanisms of arrhythmias, as related to abnormal propagation of the wave of depolarization in normal and diseased hearts (Fig. 1). By the middle of this century, recordings from microelectrodes inserted into living cardiac cell made it possible to study the cellular basis of the heart's electrical activity. Work in the second paradigm of *cell biochemistry and biophysics* advanced rapidly, with characterization of the ionic currents responsible for the waves seen in the clinical electrocardiogram. This second paradigm views cardiac arrhythmias as arising from abnormalities in the cellular mechanisms that control the waxing, waning, inactivation, and reactivation of specific ion currents. Antiarrhythmic drug therapy uses the paradigm of cell biochemistry and biophysics to analyze drug actions in terms of effects on ionic currents, rather than modification of such variables as conduction velocity, and the pathways of impulse propagation. It is only recently that a third paradigm, altered *gene expression,* has been recognized as a possible factor in the genesis of arrhythmias and the pathogenesis of sudden cardiac death. This third paradigm promises to provide an understanding of how synthesis and assembly of abnormal ion channel structures can disorganize conduction in the diseased heart.

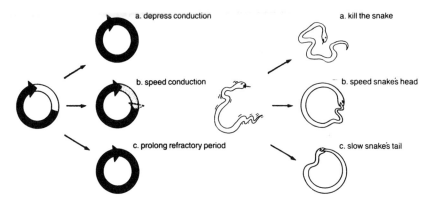

Figure 1. Three ways of abolishing a reentrant arrhythmia, viewed as a circus movement in a ring of excitable tissue. **(Left:)** The circus movement can be stopped if conduction is completely blocked **(a);** if conduction is accelerated so that the front of the impulse reaches the previously depolarized tissue **(b);** or if the refractory period is prolonged so the front of the impulse encounters tissue that can no longer be excited **(c). (Right:)** These mechanisms can be viewed as a snake traveling in a circle. The snake stops if it is killed **(a),** if it reaches ahead so as to bite its tail **(b),** or if its tail lags behind so as to be bitten by the advancing head **(c).** [Adapted from (4).]

Ion Channel Structure

Ion channels are tetrameric structures that contain four domains, each consisting of a polypeptide chain that includes six transmembrane segments (6). In sodium and calcium channels, the four domains are covalently linked, whereas potassium channels are made up of four independently synthesized domains. Plasmalemmal ion channels are members of a family of proteins that, early during evolution of the eukaryotes, gave rise to two classes of voltage-dependent ion channels (Fig. 2).

Noncovalently Linked Channels

Potassium channels, along with the monomeric cyclic nucleotide gated channels, are considered to be the most primitive of the voltage-dependent ion channels. This is because they are made up of four noncovalently linked monomers, each of which resembles the putative ancestral channel subunit. The ability to combine different monomers in assembling the tetrameric channels allows considerable diversity in potassium channel structure (7).

Duplication and divergence of the gene encoding the primitive channel protein gave rise to a second, less variable, class of channels in which the four products of gene duplication and divergence remain covalently linked.

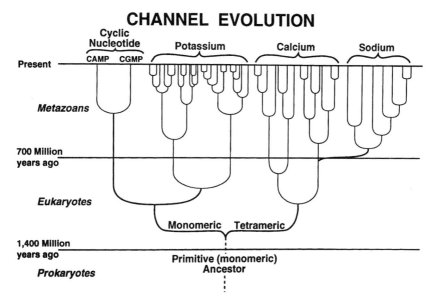

Figure 2. Evolution of the family of channel proteins. Near the end of the Archeozoic or early during the pre-Cambrian period, when eukaryotes evolved from the prokaryotes, a primitive monomeric channel protein is believed to have given rise to the noncovalently linked subunits of potassium and cyclic nucleotide-gated channels, and to tetrameric calcium channels. Later, at about the time of the rapid evolution of complex metazoan phyla early during the Cambrian period, tetrameric sodium channels evolved from the calcium channels. There appear to be many more potassium channel subtypes than subtypes of the calcium channel; evidence that there are even fewer sodium channel subtypes is consistent with their more recent evolution.

Covalently Linked Channels

The most primitive of the covalently linked tetrameric channels are calcium selective; these calcium channels, along with potassium channels, were probably present in the common ancestor of protozoa, green algae, and green plants. Today, both are found in simple animal phyla such as protozoa, coelenterates, and ctenophores (8, 9).

At around the beginning of the Cambrian period, the tetrameric calcium channels appear to have given rise to a new class of channels that rectify sodium rather than calcium transport. Because sodium is much less toxic to the cell interior than calcium, sodium channels can generate large, rapidly rising action potentials that conduct more rapidly than most calcium-dependent action potentials. Success of the variety of multicellular life forms that arose during the Cambrian explosion (10) may have been stimulated by the evolution of sodium channels. It is no surprise that today sodium channels are found almost exclusively in elaborate multicellular organisms that depend on speedy communication between different regions of their bodies.

Three Paradigms in the Regulation of the Electrical Activity of the Heart

Evolutionary considerations help provide a basis to understand how the paradigms listed in Table 1 describe three quite different mechanisms that control the electrical activity of cells. The most primitive means to alter electrophysiologic behavior is to vary *gene expression*. This occurs in prokaryotes, whose capacity for rapid multiplication and diversification allows these simple species to survive environmental change by producing progeny able to synthesize a more successfully adaptive gene product. The metabolic control made possible by alterations in *cell biochemistry and biophysics,* such as initiated by channel phosphorylation, evolved later and provided increasingly more precise controls of cellular function in eukaryotes. Regulation by altered conduction through the heart itself makes possible the integrated circuits involving specialized cells seen in the human heart, which include atrioventricular nodal cells and the His-Purkinje fibers. These cells, which are specialized for slow and fast conduction, respectively, optimize the timing of atrial and ventricular contraction and ensure the synchronous contraction of the ventricles (4). Such specializations are, of course, manifestations of the third paradigm of *organ physiology*.

One can even follow these three paradigms, as each, in turn, has been used by clinicians to guide the approach to therapy in the cardiac patient. The paradigm of *organ* physiology provided the rationale for the Cardiac Arrythmia Suppression Trial mentioned earlier in this introduction, which based therapy on reduction in the number of ectopic beats generated in the diseased human heart. This study yielded what to many was a paradoxical clinical result: drugs that reduce nonlethal arrhythmias can increase the likelihood of a lethal arrhythmia (1). But as illustrated in Fig. 3, this

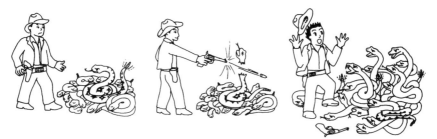

Figure 3. The attempt to survive in a snake pit **(left)** by shooting one threatening snake **(center)** can fail when the shot awakens a large number of previously dormant serpents. This result is reminiscent of the Cardiac Arrhythmia Suppression Trial, where a drug that abolished nonlethal premature systoles, which identify risk for lethal arrhythmias, was found to increase the hazard of sudden cardiac death.

result may not, in fact, be counterintuitive! Efforts are now being made to use the second paradigm to design drugs to interact with one or another ion current; the clinical value of this *cellular* approach to the management of arrhythmias, however, remains to be demonstrated. Today, an even more exciting theme can be faintly perceived in cardiac electrophysiology: the possibility that clinicians might be able to modify channel function in a diseased heart by redirecting expression of *genes* that encode abnormal ion channels. Although practical applications of this paradigm lie in the future, this exciting approach should stimulate the clinically oriented reader to seek bridges linking arrhythmias in the cardiac patient to the basic biology of ion channels. Conversely, the clinical problems faced by the cardiologist who treats the patient at risk for a lethal arrhythmia should encourage the basic scientist to try to build bridges connecting basic research to the many unanswered questions posed by human disease. As has occurred so often in the past, such interdisciplinary bridges not only have the potential to address human tragedy—disease—but also allow us to visualize some of nature's most fascinating challenges (10).

Acknowledgment

This study was supported in part by the National Heart, Lung, and Blood Institute Program Grant HL-33026.

References

1. CAST Investigators (The Cardiac Arrhythmia Suppression Trial Investigators). (1989). Preliminary report: Effect of encaininde and flecainide on mortality in a randomized trial of arrhythmia suppression after myocardial infarction. *N. Engl. J. Med.* **321**:406–412.
2. Kuhn, T.S. (1970). *The Structure of Scientific Revolutions* (The University of Chicago Press, Chicago, IL), 2nd ed., p. 92.
3. Katz, A.M. (1988). Molecular biology in cardiology, a paradigmatic shift. *J. Mol. Cell Cardiol.* **20**:355–366.
4. Katz, A.M. (1992). *Physiology of the Heart* (Raven Press, New York), 2nd ed.
5. Katz, A.M. (1992). T wave "memory": Possible causal relationship to stress-induced changes in cardiac ion channels? *J. Cardiovasc. Electrophys.* **3**:101–110.
6. Catterall, W.A. (1988). Structure and function of voltage-sensitive ion channels. *Science* **242**:50–61.
7. Aldrich, R.W. (1990). Potassium channels. Mixing and matching. *Nature* **345**:475–476.
8. Hille, B. (1992). *Ionic Channels of Excitable Membranes* (Sinauaer, Sunderland, MA), 2nd ed.
9. Gould, S.J. (1989). *A Wonderful Life. The Burgess Shales and the Nature of History* (W.W. Norton Co., New York).
10. Katz, A.M. (1987). Role of the basic sciences in the practice of cardiology, *J. Mol. Cell Cardiol.* **19**:3–17.

PART ONE

Ion Channels and Cardiac Disease: Dimensions of the Problem

Dr. Katz's comments in the Introduction pose this paradox: at the present time our knowledge of the molecular basis of cardiac electrical activity is *increasing* by leaps and bounds thanks to recombinant DNA technology and patch clamp electrophysiology, but **application** of this information to the development of effective new therapies for cardiac arrhythmias is *decreasing*. The dilemma arises from numerous factors, two of the most important being the complexity of electrical dysfunction in the intact heart and the disappointment to date of preventative therapy for patients at risk from cardiac arrhythmias.

The initial four chapters comprising the first part of this book provide an appreciation of the clinical dimensions of the problem and identify those aspects of regulatory and integrative physiology important to understanding the scientific issues underlying sudden cardiac death and other life-threatening arrhythmias. This part highlights conceptual difficulties inherent in a pharmacological approach and provides a comprehensive introduction to the problem of identifying patients at risk. Dr. Myerburg and colleagues survey, in Chapter 1, recent epidemiological studies of sudden cardiac death in the United States. Here cardiovascular disease remains the most prevalent cause of death, with electrical instabilities causally related to about 300,000 deaths per year. The analysis considers static and dynamic variables and emphasizes the contribution of both ischemia and alterations in tissue integrity as determinants of susceptibility. While the standard cardiovascular risk factors are obviously important in identifying susceptibility, it becomes clear that the highest risk groups for sudden death within this population cannot be identified with the usual clinical predictors (i.e., low ejection fraction, ischemic disease, etc). This raises the unresolved problem of identifying factors contributing to susceptibility in individual patients and intensifies the search for autonomic and other neural clues as triggering mechanisms. These issues are amplified in the succeeding two chapters.

Chapter 2 by Dr. Zipes, introduces the role of autonomic modulatory pathways and the potentially important cellular mechanisms that are likely to be involved. This leads to a detailed consideration of risk identification by autonomic evaluation in Chapter 3 by Dr. Schwartz. Dr. Zipes provides an appreciation of how the release of metabolites, such as ATP and other adenine nucleotides, are linked to insults like ischemia and how changes in neurochemical outflow of the transmitter acetylcholine directly influence ionic currents and transport pathways. Dr. Schwartz's tenet that autonomic pathways may be initiators of instability in animal models and patients provides the basis for insights on prognostic indicators. Some of these are currently being evaluated in the International Autonomic Tone and Reflexes after Myocardial Infarction (ATRAMI) clinical trial.

The concluding chapter in this section by Dr. Strauss underscores a major motivation for holding the Chantilly conference from which this volume has emerged, namely that development of effective drug therapy for the prevention of arrhythmias has been marked with more disappointment than success. He expands on the underlying reasons for the conundrum posed earlier by Dr. Katz: ". . .the counterintuitive finding that (pharmacologic) agents developed to prevent non-lethal arrhythmias can increase the risk of sudden death"! Dr. Strauss traces the evolution of this assertion through a recent history of clinical trials undertaken to explore antiarrhythmic therapy culminating in the NHLBI Cardiac Arrhythmia Suppression Trial (CAST). He identifies the problems involved in selecting appropriate drug targets and developing effective new therapeutic compounds, a theme dealt with in great detail in Chapters 24–27. He also provides an excellent introduction to topics developed in the following parts; the nature, type and organization of ion channel proteins important in generating membrane currents.

Peter M. Spooner & Arthur M. Brown

Antiarrhythmic Implications from the CAST Trial: Impetus for New Directions

Harold C. Strauss

Negative outcomes from clinical trials generally do not generate much interest. However, the outcome from the Cardiac Arrhythmia Suppression Trial (CAST)—a landmark, long-term, multicenter, multidrug, placebo-controlled trial of the safety and efficacy of antiarrhythmic drug therapy in reducing the risk of sudden cardiac death—has had a profound influence on the field of cardiac arrhythmias. As a result of CAST, the therapeutic implications of antiarrhythmic drug use in the management of cardiac arrhythmias, as well as the implications for regulatory authorities and the pharmaceutical industry, have been widely discussed (1, 2). In fact, CAST was the catalyst for this conference, "Ion Channels in the Cardiovascular System: Function and Dysfunction."

In many ways research in this field has come full circle, proceeding initially with much optimism, from bench to bedside, as many of the hypotheses generated in the laboratory about the adverse consequences of ventricular premature depolarizations appeared to be confirmed in man. Now it is widely recognized that the next major step forward in this field must come from the introduction of new and more effective drugs into the clinic and that antiarrhythmic drug development must evolve from discoveries being made in the laboratory. As a result of regulatory guidelines for new drug development, the cost of bringing new drugs into the clinic appears prohibitive to the pharmaceutical industry, discouraging many from seeking solutions to the problems of how to treat cardiac arrhythmias and reduce the incidence of sudden cardiac death. However, recent breakthroughs in research on cardiac electrophysiology have enabled us to focus on individual ion channel proteins, the molecules that generate excitatory and repolarizing currents in normal and diseased myocardial cells. Increased understanding of drug-channel protein interactions will ultimately allow us to develop newer and more effective drugs to deal with this enormous public health problem. This chapter will review the background that led to CAST and will discuss those factors that may have been responsible for its adverse outcome and the limitations of current antiarrhythmic drugs.

In the mid-1970s, sudden cardiac death due to serious arrhythmias in patients with arteriosclerotic heart disease was widely recognized as a public health challenge of great magnitude and importance (3, 4). Attempts to deal with this problem were thwarted by the lack of effective antiarrhythmic drugs with acceptable side effects. Because of this limitation and the importance of the sympathetic nervous system as a risk factor in arteriosclerotic heart disease (5, 6), the National Heart, Lung, and Blood Institute (NHLBI) initiated the Beta-Blocker Heart Attack Trial (BHAT) in 1977 to determine whether the regular, chronic administration of propranolol to patients who had recently recovered from at least one documented myocardial infarction would significantly reduce mortality from all causes: cardiovascular mortality, sudden cardiac death, and nonfatal myocardial infarction during the follow-up period. Although propranolol was recognized to have indirect antiarrhythmic properties, there was little evidence supporting a direct antiarrhythmic effect. The prevailing view in the mid-1970s was that there were no drugs available that were suitable for inclusion in such a trial (4, 7). Hence, it was deemed necessary to also evaluate propranolol's effectiveness in reducing mortality due to sudden cardiac death in patients with prior myocardial infarction and complex ventricular arrhythmias.

Although BHAT demonstrated that propranolol reduced total mortality, cardiovascular mortality, and sudden cardiac death (8), the outcome of the trial was not entirely consistent with the effects that would have been predicted for a drug that exerted its effects solely via arrhythmia suppression. Specifically, propranolol's protective effect was dependent on the absence or the presence and type of complications manifest early during the course of myocardial infarction (9). The fact that propranolol's protective effect was minimal in the subgroup of patients without complications and greatest in those with electrical complications is consistent with an arrhythmia suppression hypothesis. However, the drug also exerted a protective effect in those patients with mechanical complications, which is not entirely consistent with this hypothesis. More importantly, the secondary hypothesis, that sudden death would be preferentially reduced by propranolol in patients with complex ventricular arrhythmias, as opposed to those patients without such arrhythmias, could not be confirmed (10).

In an attempt to characterize the risk factors better for sudden cardiac death, concurrent clinical studies proceeded on postinfarction patients (11–20). These studies demonstrated the importance of ventricular arrhythmias documented ~10 days after myocardial infarction as an independent risk factor. Further, a sigmoidal relationship between mortality rate and ventricular premature depolarization (VPD) frequency was demonstrated, with the steep portion of the curve falling between 1 and 10 VPDs/hr (12, 15, 16). Finally, repetitive VPDs were demonstrated to be associated with increased risk of death, independent of VPD frequency (15, 16, 19). These findings provided the rationale for treating certain postinfarction ventricular arrhythmias and suggested entry criteria for ventricular arrhythmias, such as frequency and repetitiveness, that would be ideal for patient recruitment into any prospective clinical trial. Although both basic and clinical research suggest that there is an interaction between substrate (damaged tissue), trigger factors (ventricular arrhythmia), autonomic tone, and disease state (ischemia), the relative importance of each of these variables could not be discerned from these clinical studies (6, 21). Another consideration is the relationship between VPDs and the more serious ventricular arrhythmias that sometime occur in these patients (1, 6). Are these VPDs elicited by the same arrhythmogenic mechanisms responsible for the more serious ventricular arrhythmias, or do they merely represent electrical triggers leading to the initiation of more serious arrhythmias via other mechanisms? These questions could not be addressed by these clinical studies.

Although propranolol was shown to decrease cardiac mortality and sudden cardiac death after myocardial infarction, this drug belongs to a class of drugs that is less than ideal for testing the hypothesis that suppression of postinfarction ventricular arrhythmias reduces cardiac mortality and sudden cardiac death. The shortcomings of drugs in this class include their limited efficacy as antiarrhythmic agents, negative inotropic effects, and additional nonantiarrhythmic actions (21–23). As a result, the BHAT data did not identify the mechanism underlying propranolol's action and did not answer the question of whether drugs that suppress nonsymptomatic ventricular arrhythmias can confer additional therapeutic benefits either by forestalling the sequence of events leading to a lethal arrhythmia or by direct suppression of the lethal arrhythmia. Therefore, a large-scale, antiarrhythmic drug clinical trial was initiated by the NHLBI to determine whether arrhythmia suppression in the postinfarction patient would be beneficial, as predicted by the VPD suppression hypothesis.

In designing an optimal clinical trial to examine the effects of spontaneous arrhythmia suppression, the following considerations were taken into account. First, only patients with suitable spontaneous ventricular arrhythmias after acute myocardial infarction would be selected (24, 25). Therefore, entry criteria were based on VPD frequency and characteristics, arrhythmia variability after a myocardial infarction, and the appropriate time after the infarct. Second, flexible dosing strategies were required, because ventricular arrhythmias must be reduced substantially in most trial participants. Third, because the arrhythmias must be suppressed for 1 to 2 years, it was necessary to select drugs with minimal side effects to maximize compliance and minimize drop-out rate. Fourth, the trial must have sufficient power (i.e., adequate sample size) to identify a 20 to 25% reduction in mortality. Fifth, proarrhythmic and other adverse effects must be detected and managed. Finally, cause-specific mortality (e.g., sudden or arrhythmic death) should be used as an endpoint in addition to total mortality.

The Cardiac Arrhythmia Pilot Study (CAPS) was designed to determine the feasibility of the subsequent, larger scale, clinical trial to answer the question, "Does treatment with antiarrhythmic therapy reduce mortality in patients with coronary heart disease and ventricular ectopy?" (25). CAPS also addressed a number of key issues, such as whether recruitment goals could be met, how arrhythmia variability would impact on assessment of drug efficacy, and whether the logistics of dose adjustment could be worked out for a large-scale, multicenter trial. In addition, the proarrhythmic effects of the drugs selected had to be assessed, along with their efficacy and toxicity over a relatively long period of observation.

For this pilot study, the rationale was to use drugs that were very effective in suppressing VPDs (encainide and flecainide), as well as to use promising drugs with different electrophysiologic properties (moricizine and imipramine) (24). This rationale for drug selection was intended to complement existing information about procainamide and quinidine and to maximize the choices for the subsequent trial. These drugs are class I antiarrhythmic agents, which reduce the upstroke velocity of the transmembrane action potential via sodium channel blockade, and, as a result, they decrease conduction velocity in the heart. Encainide and flecainide were much more efficacious in suppressing single and repetitive VPDs than imipramine, moricizine, or placebo. At the completion of dose titration, there was no significant difference between any of the five treatments in the prevalence of serious adverse cardiac effects confirmed by drug washout, such as proarrhythmic effects or disqualifying events. Thus, CAPS demonstrated the relatively high efficacy of encainide and flecainide in suppressing ventricular arrhythmias in postinfarction patients and showed that these compounds were well tolerated in the year after infarction. These data also indicated that large-scale clinical trials to evaluate the effect of arrhythmia suppression with antiarrhythmic drugs on mortality were feasible.

This evolution in information, coupled with the introduction of new antiarrhythmic drugs, led to the initiation of CAST (26, 27). This multicenter, randomized, placebo-controlled study was designed to test whether suppression of spontaneous ventricular arrhythmias with class I antiarrhythmic drugs after myocardial infarction would reduce death rate from arrhythmias. Encainide, flecainide, and moricizine were evaluated in patients who had experienced a myocardial infarction and who had asymptomatic or mildly symptomatic ventricular arrhythmias. Patients initially underwent an open-label titration, during which up to three drugs at two doses were each evaluated. The titration was stopped as soon as a drug and dose were found that suppressed the arrhythmias. The criteria for identification of a successful drug were 80% or greater reduction of VPDs and 90% reduction of runs of unsustained ventricular tachycardia. Patients who tolerated the successful drug were randomized to the drug or a corresponding placebo for the main study. Patients whose arrhythmias were only partially suppressed were enrolled in a substudy. The only patients who were not treated long-term were those who died, who showed intolerance to all drugs, or who showed no suppression or an increase of arrhythmias during open-label titration.

Approximately 22 months after initiation of CAST, the Data Safety and Monitoring Board reviewed the data on 1,727 patients and recommended that encainide and flecainide be discontinued, and that a modified trial be continued with moricizine (1, 26–29). As a result, the first part of the trial was designated as CAST, and the remaining part that was continued was designated as CAST-II.

CAST data showed that treatment with encainide or flecainide was associated with a worse outcome, whether the endpoint was death due to arrhythmia, death due to any cardiac cause, or death due to any cause (26, 27). The relative risk of death or cardiac arrest due to arrhythmia was 2.64 (95% confidence interval, 1.60–4.36) in the treated group versus the placebo group. The randomization produced excellent balance for all of the important baseline variables, excluding any identifiable confounding factors that could explain the marked difference in mortality rates between the active drug and placebo groups. The adverse outcome in patients treated with encainide or flecainide was attributed primarily to unforeseen death or cardiac arrest due to arrhythmia caused by the study drugs, although surprisingly, there was no higher incidence of nonlethal arrhythmic events in the treated group.

Because moricizine demonstrated an insignificant but favorable trend in mortality, the trial was continued as CAST-II with moricizine alone (28, 29). Modifications in CAST-II also included the identification of higher risk patients and assessment of the effects of drug treatment during the titration phase of the trial. The latter was introduced, because the number of deaths during titration in the main trial was unexpectedly high. As a result, entry criteria were modified, and CAST-II began with a 2-week controlled trial that assessed the early effects of low-dose moricizine.

The Data and Safety Monitoring Board recommended early termination of CAST-II for two reasons (29). First, the 2-week trial evaluating the early effects of moricizine revealed increased mortality among treated patients as compared with patients given placebo. The relative risk was 5.6 (95% confidence interval, 1.7–19.1). Seventy percent of the patients who were treated with low-dose moricizine and who died or had a cardiac arrest did so during the first week of titration, and the remainder during the second week. The survival curve demonstrated an adverse effect early after starting treatment, which is consistent with the proarrhythmic effect of the drug (30). Second, analysis of long-term therapy in patients with adequate suppression of ectopic beats demonstrated no significant difference between groups in the number of deaths or cardiac arrests due to arrhythmias, and continuation of the trial was unlikely to produce a favorable outcome.

CAST and CAST-II were important studies for several reasons. Convincing data were provided about antiarrhythmic therapy with class I agents during the postinfarction period. Two class I–C antiarrhythmic agents that demonstrated marked potency and VPD suppression (encainide and flecainide) adversely impacted on outcome during the follow-up period. Another class I agent, moricizine, whose properties fall somewhere between class IA and IB drugs, adversely affected outcome shortly after onset of therapy.

The inescapable conclusion of CAST was that class I agents are harmful to patients. However, the relatively low mortality rate in the placebo group, as well as other factors in the encainide and flecainide treatment group, have been identified as possible confounding variables (1). Briefly, these were first, changes in the therapy of patients with coronary artery disease may have modified the arrhythmogenic substrate in these patients sufficiently to invalidate the original VPD suppression hypothesis. Second, the number of deaths during the drug titration phase of CAST were unexpectedly high and may have eliminated a relatively high risk group before randomization. Third, suppression of ventricular arrhythmias by therapy may define a group with better prognosis, even in the absence of therapy. Fourth, the prevalence of high-risk patients with repetitive VPDs or episodes of nonsustained ventricular tachycardia was low (~20%), predicting a lower risk. Finally, the distribution of ejection fraction [0.40 ± 0.10 (mean ± SD) in the encainide-flecainide group and 0.39 ± 0.09 in the placebo group] predicted a low mortality.

Conversely, a variety of explanations have been proposed for the unexpected results of CAST, where 4.5% in the encainide-flecainide group had a nonfatal cardiac arrest or sudden death, compared with 1.2% in the placebo group (1). Whether or not these untoward events can be ascribed to proarrhythmic effects is unclear. Proarrhythmia in the traditional sense is a term applied when existing arrhythmias are aggravated or new arrhythmias commonly attributed to antiarrhythmic agents appear (30). The prevailing view is that proarrhythmic effects are usually observed early following onset of treatment (30). However, during the long-term follow-up phase of CAST, there was no higher incidence of nonlethal arrhythmias, as might be expected if these drugs were demonstrating a proarrhythmic effect. Surprisingly, the deaths in the active treatment groups were equally distributed throughout the period of drug treatment, perhaps reflecting a change in the clinical setting (e.g., progression of myocardial ischemia, change in electrolyte balance, or autonomic tone) (1, 2, 6, 30, 31). For example, in a longitudinal study that evaluated the effects of flecainide on supraventricular arrhythmias, a much lower mortality was observed than was seen in CAST (32), suggesting that infarct-related arrhythmogenic substrates or other manifestations of myocardial ischemia enhance the arrhythmogenic properties of these drugs (31, 33).

Let us examine the potential complexities underlying ventricular arrhythmias. Reentry is believed to represent an important mechanism underlying ventricular arrhythmias in patients with prior myocardial infarction, wherein the infarct creates regions with altered propagation, refractory, and excitability characteristics (2). Therapeutic strategies designed to interrupt this circular path are aimed at slowing conduction or prolonging repolarization (and, as a result, refractoriness), and they are dictated in part by the relationship between circuit time and the duration of repolarization (2). Although depression of conduction may be the more effective approach in some, prolongation of repolarization may be more appropriate in other instances to interrupt a reentrant ventricular arrhythmia. Sodium channels in the former and potassium channels in the latter instance represent the targets for antiarrhythmic drug action (2). Unfortunately, determination of the optimal approach in patients is primarily empirical, and, even in those patients who undergo electrophysiologic study, it may not always be possible to establish the mechanism through which antiarrhythmic drugs exert their effects. In part, this is due to the inability to measure the electrophysiologic effects of antiarrhythmic drugs at the vulnerable or target site, as well as the absence of specificity of ion channel blockade by antiarrhythmic drugs (2). Hence, deducing optimal therapeutic strategies is limited with the current antiarrhythmic drug selection. Further, as the clinical setting changes, the changes in metabolic state may alter regulatory enzymes and second messengers, leading to an alteration in the mechanism underlying the arrhythmia and possibly rendering the antiarrhythmic drug less effective in suppressing the arrhythmia. For example, calcium overload can develop during myocardial ischemia in a patient who is concurrently receiving a class I agent to suppress a reentrant arrhythmia (21, 34–36). Calcium overload has been reported to cause calcium oscillations and activation of an inward current. This may represent another mechanism underlying ventricular arrhythmias less responsive to a specific drug in abolishing a reentrant ventricular arrhythmia (37). Further, potentiation of the depressant action of antiarrhythmic drugs in this setting could account for the increased mortality in CAST.

Hence, the role of VPDs in initiation of lethal or malignant ventricular arrhythmias remains unclear (1). The chronic VPD may be an "innocent bystander" totally unrelated to the tachyarrhythmia; its suppression would therefore be of no benefit. Second, a VPD of one mechanism may initiate a ventricular tachyarrhythmia of another mechanism. Suppression of VPDs that play a contributing, but nonessential, role in the initiation of ventricular tachyarrhythmia might be beneficial, but only if the drug has no harmful effect on the mechanism of the sustained tachyarrhythmia. Third, the VPD may be caused by the same mechanism responsible for the sustained tachyarrhythmia. When the VPD is caused by the same mechanism responsible for the sustained tachyarrhythmia, its suppression should be beneficial. Finally, because of the complex interaction between the drug and the arrhythmogenic substrate, it is recognized that an antiarrhythmic drug that may suppress one type of ventricular arrhythmia under certain conditions may actually promote another type of ventricular arrhythmia under different conditions.

Although the relative toxicity of the drugs chosen for CAST as compared with other antiarrhythmic drugs is unknown, the results of CAST and CAST-II are consistent with other studies of class I antiarrhythmic agents, which report an increased mortality rate in patients after myocardial infarction. A recent meta-analysis has suggested an increased risk of mortality among patients with ventricular arrhythmias treated with quinidine (38). Similar but less conclusive findings were observed with mexiletine (39). Analysis of other antiarrhythmic drug studies also suggests they offer no benefit for patients whose clinical characteristics resemble those treated in CAST (40, 41). Small studies of amiodarone (class III agent) after myocardial infarction suggest an improvement in survival (42, 43). Other larger studies of amiodarone are under way. A controlled trial of implantable cardiac defibrillators versus medical antiarrhythmic drug therapy has been implemented by the NHLBI. The study will determine whether a treatment strategy based on initial placement of an implantable cardiac defibrillator or one based on antiarrhythmic drug therapy using amiodarone or sotalol results in longer survival.

Proarrhythmic effects of antiarrhythmic drugs are difficult to evaluate because of the influence of a multitude of clinical factors (e.g., autonomic tone, electrolytes, and pH) on drug toxicity (2, 33), possible changes in gene expression of ion channels associated with different clinical states (44, 45), differences in contribution of specific ion channel currents to repolarization in different patients, the lack of ion channel specificity in antiarrhythmic drug action, and the limited information on the ideal kinetics of drug-channel interactions to minimize proarrhythmic effects. For example, repolarization represents a balance between at least seven different inward and outward currents (2, 46). Depending on the relative current densities of each of the different potassium currents, blockade of one type of potassium current by a drug may contribute to repetitive depolarizations in one patient and not in another. Hence, clinical answers to questions about drug safety, efficacy, and underlying mechanisms will be optimally provided through use of specific ion channel blocking drugs evaluated in patients with ventricular arrhythmias. Advances in our understanding of the structure of ion channel proteins and of antiarrhythmic drug binding sites and increased knowledge of drug-channel interactions will also help accelerate progress in this area. Until then, the empirical approach will be necessary, but it will likely prove much slower in yielding answers to these critical questions.

Although the therapeutic implications of CAST and CAST-II are still being debated, sudden cardiac death remains a national health problem of major significance. Even if implantable defibrillators prove to be more efficacious than medical therapy in high-risk patients, this will address only a small part of the problem, because high-risk patients constitute only a small fraction of the group of patients succumbing to sudden cardiac death (21). The search for safe and effective antiarrhythmic drugs should therefore remain one of the highest priorities for academic medicine, government, and the pharmaceutical industry.

Acknowledgment

I am indebted to Steffani H. Webb for invaluable editorial assistance.

References

1. Akhtar, M., Breithardt, G., Camm, A.J., Coumel, P., Janse, M.J., Lazzara, R., Myerburg, R.J., Schwartz, P.J., Waldo, A.L., Wellens, H.J.J., and Zipes, D.P. (1990). CAST and beyond: Implications of the cardiac arrhythmia suppression trial. *Circulation* **81**:1123–1127.

2. Bigger, J.T., Jr., Breithardt, G., Brown, A.M., Camm, J., Carmeliet, E., Fozzard, H.A., Hoffman, B.F., Janse, M.J., Lazzara, R., Mugelli, A., Myerburg, R., Roden, D.M., Rosen, M.R., Schwartz, P.J., Strauss, H.C., Woosley, R.L., and Zaza, A. (1991). The Task Force on the Working Group on Arrhythmias of the European Society of Cardiology, The Sicilian gambit: A new approach to the classification of antiarrhythmic drugs based on their actions on arrhythmogenic mechanisms. *Circulation* **84**:1831–1851.

3. Cardiac Diseases Branch, NHLBI. (1976). Workshop on Chronic Antiarrhythmic Therapy and the Prevention of Sudden Death: Summary Report (NHLBI, Bethesda, MD).

4. Byington, R.P. (1984). Beta-blocker heart attack trial: Design, methods, and baseline results. *Controlled Clin. Trials* **5**:382–437.

5. Zipes, D.P. (1992). Autonomic innervation of the heart: Role in arrhythmic development during ischemia and in the long QT syndrome, in *The Heart and Cardiovascular System* (Raven Press, New York), pp. 2095–2112.

6. Wharton, J.M., Coleman, R.E., and Strauss, H.C. (1992). The role of the autonomic nervous system in sudden cardiac death. *Trends Cardiovasc. Med.* **2**:65–71.

7. Lovell, R.R.H. (1975). Arrhythmia prophylaxis: Long-term suppressive medication. *Circulation* (Suppl. III):236–240.

8. β-Blocker Heart Attack Trial Research Group. (1982). A randomized trial of propranolol in patients with acute myocardial infarction. I. Mortality results. *J.A.M.A.* **247**:1707–1714.

9. Furberg, C.D., Hawkins, C.M., and Lichstein, E. (1984). Effect of propranolol in postinfarction patients with mechanical or electrical complications. *Circulation* **69**:761–765.

10. Friedman, L.M., Byington, R.P., Capone, R.J., Furberg, C.D., Goldstein, S., and Lichstein, E. (1986). Effect of propranolol in patients with myocardial infarction and ventricular arrhythmia. *J. Am. Coll. Cardiol.* **7**:1–8.

11. Ruberman, W., Weinblatt, E., Goldberg, J.D., Frank, C.W., and Shapiro, S. (1977). Ventricular premature beats and mortality after myocardial infarction. *N. Engl. J. Med.* **297**:750–757.

12. Multicenter Post-Infarction Research Group. (1983). Risk stratification after myocrdial infarction. *N. Engl. J. Med.* **309**:331–336.

13. Moss, A.J., Bigger, J.T., Jr., and Odoroff, C.L. (1987). Postinfarct risk stratification. *Prog. Cardiovasc. Dis.* **29**:389–412.

14. Ruberman, W.R., Weinblatt, E., Goldberg, J.D., Frank, C.W., Chaudhary, B.S., and Shapiro, S. (1981). Ventricular premature complexes and sudden death after myocardial infarction. *Circulation* **64**:297–305.

15. Bigger, J.T., Jr., Fleiss, J.L., Kleiger, R., Miller, J.P., Rolnitzky, L.M., and the Multicenter Post-Infarction Research Group. (1984). The relationships among ventricular arrhythmias, left ventricular dysfunction, and mortality in the 2 years after myocardial infarction. *Circulation* **69**:250–258.

16. Bigger, J.T., Jr., Weld, F.M., Coromilas, J., Rolnitzky, L.M., and DeTurk, W.E. (1983). Prevalence and significance of arrhythmias in 24-hour ECG recordings made within one month of acute myocardial infarction, in *The First Year After a Myocardial Infarction* (Martinus Nijhoff, Boston, MA), pp. 161–175.

17. Mukharji, J., Rude, R.E., Poole, W.K., Gustafson, N., Thomas, L.J., Strauss, H.W., Jaffe, A.S., Muller, J.E., Roberts, R., Raabe, D.S., Croft, C.H., Passamani, E., Braunwald, E., Willerson, J.T., and the MILIS Study Group. (1984). Risk factors for sudden death after acute myocardial infarction: Two-year follow-up. *Am. J. Cardiol.* **54**:31–36.

18. Moss, A.J., Davis, H.T., DeCamilla, J., and Bayer, L.W. (1979). Ventricular ectopic beats and their relation to sudden and nonsudden cardiac death after myocardial infarction. *Circulation* **60**:998–1003.

19. Bigger, J.T., Jr., and Weld, F.M. (1981). Analysis of prognostic significance of ventricular arrhythmias after myocardial infarction. Shortcomings of Lown grading system. *Br. Heart J.* **45**:717–724.

20. Bigger, J.T., Jr., Weld, F.M., and Rolnitzky, L.M. (1981). The prevalence and significance of ventricular tachycardia detected by ambulatory ECG recording in the late hospital phase of acute myocardial infarction. *Am. J. Cardiol.* **48**:815–823.

21. Myerburg, R.J., Kessler, K.M., and Castellanos, A. (1993). Epidemiology of sudden cardiac death: Population characteristics, conditioning risk factors, and dynamic risk factors, in *Ion Channels in the Cardiovascular System: Function and Dysfunction* (AAAS Press, Washington, DC, in press).

22. May, G.S., Eberlein, K.A., Furberg, C.D., Passamani, E.R., and DeMets, D.L. (1982). Secondary prevention after myocardial infarction: A review of long-term trials. *Prog. Cardiovasc. Dis.* **24**:331–352.

23. Bigger, J.T., Jr., and Hoffman, B.F. (1990). Antiarrhythmic drugs, in *The Pharmacological Basis of Therapeutics* (Pergamon Press, Elsmford, New York), pp. 840–873.

24. The Cardiac Arrhythmia Pilot Study (CAPS) Investigators. (1988). Effects of encainide, flecainide, imipramine and moricizine on ventricular arrhythmias during the year after acute myocardial infarction: The CAPS. *Am. J. Cardiol.* **61**:501–509.

25. Greene, H.L., Roden, D.M., Katz, R.J., Woosley, R.L., Salerno, D.M., Henthorn, R.W., and the CAST Investigators. (1992). The Cardiac Arrhythmia Suppression Trial: First CAST. . . Then CAST-II. *J. Am. Coll. Cardiol.* **19**:894–898.

26. The Cardiac Arrhythmia Suppression Trial (CAST) Investigators. (1989). Preliminary Report: Effect of encainide and flecainide on mortality in a randomized trial of arrhythmia suppression after myocardial infarction. *N. Engl. J. Med.* **321**:406–412.

27. Echt, D.S., Liebson, P.R., Mitchell, L.B., Peters, R.W., Obias-Manno, D., Barker, A.H., Arensberg, D., Baker, A., Friedman, L., Greene, H.L., Huther, M.L., Richardson, D.W., and the CAST Investigators. (1991). Mortality and morbidity in patients receiving encainide, flecainide, or placebo. The Cardiac Arrhythmia Suppression Trial. *N. Engl. J. Med.* **324**:781–788.

28. Ruskin, J.N. (1989). The cardiac arrhythmia suppression trial (CAST). *N. Engl. J. Med.* **321**:386–388.

29. The Cardiac Arrhythmia Suppression Trial II Investigators. (1992). Effect of the antiarrhythmic agent moricizine on survival after myocardial infarction. *N. Engl. J. Med.* **327**:227–233.

30. Zipes, D.P. (1988). Proarrhythmic events. *Am. J. Cardiol.* **61**:70A–76A.

31. Lederman, S.N., Wenger, T.L., Bolster, D.E., and Strauss, H.C. (1989). Effects of flecainide on occlusion and reperfusion in dogs. *J. Cardiovasc. Pharmacol.* **13**:541–546.

32. Pritchett, E.L.C., and Wilkinson, W.E. (1991). Mortality in patients treated with flecainide and encainide for supraventricular arrhythmias. *Am. J. Cardiol.* **67**:976–980.

33. Snyders, D.J., Bennett, P.B., and Hondeghem, L.M. (1992). Mechanisms of drug-channel interaction, in *The Heart and Cardiovascular System* (Raven Press, New York), pp. 2165–2193.

34. Jennings, R.B., Schaper, J., Hill, M.L., Steenbergen, C., Jr., and Reimer, K. (1985). Effects of reperfusion late in the phase of reversible ischemic injury: Changes in cell volume, electrolytes, metabolites, and ultrastructure. *Circ. Res.* **56**:262–278.

35. Yee, R., Brown, K.K., Bolster, D.E., and Strauss, H.C. (1988). Relationship between ion perturbations and electrophysiologic changes in a canine Purkinje fiber model of ischemia and reperfusion. *J. Clin. Invest.* **82**:228–233.

36. Kusoka, H., Porterfield, J.K., Weisman, H.F., Weisfeldt, M.L., and Marban, E. (1987). Pathophysiology and pathogenesis of stunned myocardium. Depressed Ca^{2+} activation of contraction as a consequence of reperfusion-induced cellular calcium overload in ferret hearts. *J. Clin. Invest.* **79**:950–961.

37. Wit, A.L., and Rosen, M.R. (1992). Afterdepolarizations and triggered activity: Distinction from automaticity as an arrhythmogenic mechanism, in *The Heart and Cardiovascular System* (Raven Press, New York), pp. 2113–2163.

38. Morganroth, J., and Goin, J.E. (1991). Quinidine-related mortality in the short-to-medium-term treatment of ventricular arrhythmias: A meta-analysis. *Circulation* **84**:1977–1983.

39. Impact Research Group, (1984). International mexiletine and placebo antiarrhythmic coronary trial. I. Report on arrhythmia and other findings. *J. Am. Coll. Cardiol.* **4:**1148–1163.

40. Furberg, C.D. (1983). Effect of antiarrhythmic drugs on mortality after myocardial infarction. *Am. J. Cardiol.* **52:**32C–36C.

41. U. K. Rhythmodan Multicentre Study Group. (1984). Oral disopyramide after admission to hospital with suspected acute myocardial infarction. *Postgrad. Med. J.* **60:**98–107.

42. Burkart, F., Pfisterer, M., Kiowski, W., Follath, F., and Burckhardt, D. (1990). Effect of antiarrhythmic therapy on mortality in survivors of myocardial infarction with asymptomatic complex ventricular arrhythmias: Basel Antiarrhythmic Study of Infarct Survival (BASIS). *J. Am. Coll. Cardiol.* **16:**1711–1718.

43. Cairns, J.A., Connolly, S.J., Gent, M., and Roberts, R. (1991). Post-myocardial infarction mortality in patients with ventricular premature depolarizations: Canadian Amiodarone Myocardial Infarction Arrhythmia Trial Pilot Study. *Circulation* **84:**550–557.

44. Mori, Y., Matsubara, H., and Koren, G. (1992). cAMP modulates the expression of a rat delayed rectifier K^+ channel at the pretranslational level. *J. Mol. Cell. Cardiol.* **24:**S277.

45. Duff, H.J., Offord, J., West, J., and Catterall, W.A. (1992). Class I and class IV antiarrhythmic drugs and cytosolic calcium regulate mRNA encoding the sodium channel α subunit in rat cardiac muscle. *Molec. Pharmacol.* **42:**570–575.

46. Fozzard, H.A. (1993). Cardiac electrogenesis and the sodium channel, in *Ion Channels in the Cardiovascular System: Function and Dysfunction* (AAAS Press, Washington, DC, in press).

2

Epidemiology of Sudden Cardiac Death: Population Characteristics, Conditioning Risk Factors, and Dynamic Risk Factors

Robert J. Myerburg, Kenneth M. Kessler, and
Agustin Castellanos

Fifty percent or more of all cardiovascular deaths are sudden and unexpected (1–4), when defined as death within 1 hr of the onset of an abrupt change in cardiovascular status (2). This proportion accounts for an annual incidence of >300,000 deaths/year in the United States (4, 5). Although it is likely that a decrease in the absolute number of sudden deaths has occurred in parallel with a general reduction in cardiovascular mortality in the United States in recent years (2–4), the proportion of deaths that are sudden appears to have remained constant. For an alteration in death rate to affect the specific problem of sudden cardiac death (SCD), it must produce an absolute reduction in sudden death mortality rates, which translates directly to an equivalent reduction in total cardiovascular mortality (6).

The epidemiology of SCD can be viewed from several perspectives, each of which provides important insights into the problem and no one of which exerts exclusive domain for preventive strategies (Fig. 1). These include (a) population dynamics; (b) time dependence of risk; (c) risk factors that are continuously present over time *(static)* and relate to the probability of developing conditioning or predisposing influences; (d) risk factors that are dynamic *(transient)* and can exert influences on cardiac electrophysiology at a specific point in time; and (e) "response risk," referring to specific individual susceptibility to adverse influences of conditioning and/or dynamic risk factors. Major new insights into the SCD problem will require better understanding of each of these factors, which range from classical epidemiology to membrane channel physiology.

Population Dynamics

Several epidemiological surveillance studies have provided information on the relative and absolute rates of SCD. During a 26-year follow-up

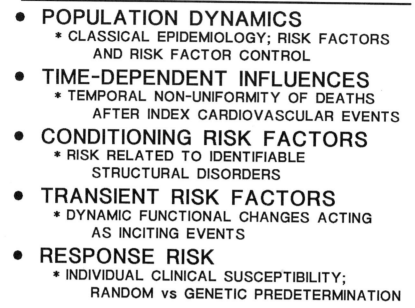

EPIDEMIOLOGY OF SUDDEN DEATH

- **POPULATION DYNAMICS**
  - * CLASSICAL EPIDEMIOLOGY; RISK FACTORS AND RISK FACTOR CONTROL

- **TIME-DEPENDENT INFLUENCES**
  - * TEMPORAL NON-UNIFORMITY OF DEATHS AFTER INDEX CARDIOVASCULAR EVENTS

- **CONDITIONING RISK FACTORS**
  - * RISK RELATED TO IDENTIFIABLE STRUCTURAL DISORDERS

- **TRANSIENT RISK FACTORS**
  - * DYNAMIC FUNCTIONAL CHANGES ACTING AS INCITING EVENTS

- **RESPONSE RISK**
  - * INDIVIDUAL CLINICAL SUSCEPTIBILITY; RANDOM vs GENETIC PREDETERMINATION

Figure 1. Epidemiology of SCD. Perspectives ranging from classical population-based epidemiology to individual susceptibility based on pathophysiological response characteristics that may be genetically determined. No one of these levels of epidemiological considerations dominates the risk profile.

of the Framingham, MA, population, 5,209 men and women—30 to 59 years of age and free of identified heart disease at baseline—SCD accounted for 46% of the coronary heart disease deaths among men and 34% among women (7). The incidence of SCD increased with age, but the proportion of coronary deaths that were sudden was greater in the younger age group. Pooled data from Albany, NY, and Framingham, MA, on 4,120 men identified SCD as the initial and terminal manifestation of coronary heart disease in more than one-half of all sudden death victims (8). In the Tecumseh, MI, study of 8,641 subjects, 46% of all coronary heart disease deaths occurred within 1 hr of onset of acute symptoms (9). In the Yugoslavian cardiovascular disease study, involving 6,614 men, age 35 to 62 and free of coronary disease at entry, 75% of all coronary deaths occurred suddenly, and two-thirds of the victims had had no documented coronary events before death (10).

When SCD is measured as the absolute number of events annually within defined subpopulations, it is clear that the highest risk clinical subgroups most frequently cited, such as patients with low ejection fractions, a history of heart failure, and survivors of out-of-hospital cardiac arrests, do *not* account for the majority of SCD events (5). Thus, subgroups with the highest case fatality rates have the lowest population attributable risk, and the larger numbers are contained within larger population pools. The magnitude of risk, expressed as incidence, is compared with the total number of events annually under six different conditions in Fig. 1. These estimates are based on published epidemiological and clinical data (4, 5, 11). When the >300,000 SCDs that occur annually among an unselected adult population in the United States is expressed as a fraction of the total adult population, the overall incidence is 0.1% to 0.2%/year. When the more easily recognized high-risk subgroups are removed from this total population base, the calculated incidence for the remaining population decreases and the identification of specific individuals at risk becomes more difficult. Based on these estimates, a preventive intervention designed for the general adult population would have to be applied to the 999/1,000 people who will not have an event during the course of a year in order to reach and potentially influence the unidentified 1/1,000th who will. A model of such limited efficiency prohibits the application of most active interventions and highlights the need for specific markers of increased risk.

The public health relevance of this point lies within the relationship between the size of the denominator in any population pool and the number of events occurring within that subgroup. For example, with escalation from high coronary risk subgroups without prior clinical events (risk = 1% to 2%/year, see Fig. 1) to those with prior coronary events (e.g., low ejection fraction and heart failure, or survival after out-of-hospital cardiac arrest), the probability of identifying individuals at higher risk becomes progressively greater, but the absolute number of individuals who can be identified for interventions decreases with each escalation (Fig. 2). Thus, the major challenge for the future resides not only simply in the need to focus on the highest risk clinical subgroups, but rather to develop methods that will identify high-risk clusters within subgroups that have lesser degrees of excess risk. Such a strategy would provide better resolution of SCD risk and greater efficiency for preventive and therapeutic interventions. To achieve this goal, the total number of SCDs within a specified population, the fraction of deaths that are sudden, and total mortality all must be known. Diagnostic or screening procedures, which are easily applied to larger populations and which have specified implications for SCD, are needed to resolve these population-based limitations. An example of current interest is clinical measures of the variability of autonomic influences on cardiac electrophysiology in groups at increased risk for SCD, such as the postmyocardial infarction patient (12, 13) or cardiac arrest survivor (14). In the postmyocardial infarction patient, emerging information suggests that data derived from various measures of heart rate variability may provide relatively easily obtained information on cardiac-autonomic interactions that influence cardiac electrophysiology (15). Added to other techniques for risk stratification, this approach may help resolve higher risk clusters within larger population bases.

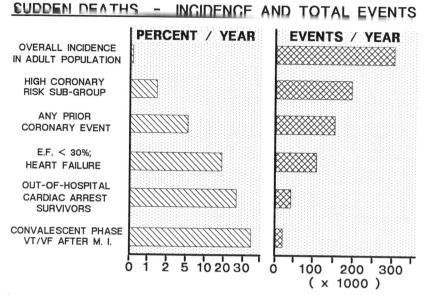

Figure 2. Relation between annual incidence and total number of SCDs among population subgroups. Approximation of incidence figures (%/year) and the total number of events/year is shown for the overall adult population in the United States and for increasingly higher risk subgroups. The overall adult population has an estimated sudden death incidence of 0.1% to 0.2%/year, totaling >300,000 sudden deaths/year. Within subgroups identified by increasingly powerful risk factors, the incidence increases progressively, but is accompanied by a progressive decrease in the total number events. There is an inverse relation between incidence and total number of events because of the progressively smaller denominator pool in the highest subgroup categories. Successful interventions among larger population subgroups will require specific markers to identify higher risk clusters within the lower risk subgroups. See text for further details. The horizontal axis for the incidence figure is nonlinear and should be interpreted accordingly. E.F., ejection fraction; M.I., myocardial infarction. [From Myerburg et al. (5).]

Time-Dependent Risk

In many clinical circumstances, the risk of death during follow-up after surviving a major change in cardiovascular status is not linear over time (16–19). Survival figures for both sudden and total cardiac mortality demonstrate that the highest secondary death rates occur during the initial 6 to 18 months after an index event. After 24 months, the slopes of the survival curves begin to approach the configuration of those describing a similar population that has remained free of interposed cardiovascular events (Fig. 3). In addition, the configuration of survival curves are likely influenced by the magnitude of increased risk after an index event. The data from the National Heart, Lung, and Blood Institute Cardiac Arrhythmia Suppression Trial (20, 21) study demonstrate linear survival curves among

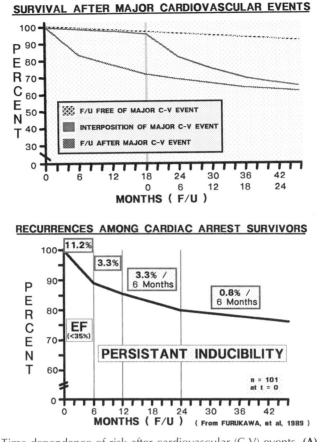

Figure 3. Time dependence of risk after cardiovascular (C-V) events. **(A)** Survival curves during follow-up (F/U) of a hypothetical population of patients with known C-V disease, but free of a major event **(top curve)** and for populations of patients who have survived major C-V events **(bottom curve).** Attrition over time is accelerated both in absolute and relative terms for the initial 6 to 24 months after the major C-V event. Subsequently, for the latter, the slope of the survival curve parallels more closely that of the lower risk population. After 24 months, the curves for the two populations may parallel each other. The **middle curve** demonstrates the dynamics of risk over time in a low-risk population, with an interposed major event. When interposed events are normalized to a point in time (e.g., 18 months), the subsequent attrition is accelerated for the next 18 to 24 months. This pattern has been observed for death or myocardial infarction among patients with stable angina pectoris who convert to unstable angina. [From Myerburg et al. (5).] **(B)** Survival curve demonstrates time dependence of risk of recurrences among survivors of cardiac arrest with coronary artery disease. Risk was highest during the first 6 months (11.2%) and then fell to 3.3%/6 months for the next three semiannual blocks. After 24 months, the rate fell to 0.8% for each 6-month block thereafter. A low ejection fraction (EF) was the most powerful predictor of death during the first 6 months. Subsequently, persistent inducibility during programmed stimulation was the most powerful predictor. [Modified from Furukawa et al. (18). Also from Myerburg et al. (5).]

the placebo population during long-term follow-up, whereas data from the multicenter postinfarction program (16, 17) demonstrate that subgrouping postmyocardial infarction patients according to increasing risk based on interactions between premature ventricular contraction (PVC) frequency and ejection fractions results in progressively higher risk as the number and power of risk factors increases. The added mortality in the higher risk subgroups tends to be expressed early. Thus, time-dependent risk within higher risk subgroups focuses the greatest opportunity for effective intervention strategies in the early period after conditioning cardiovascular events. Mortality patterns having these characteristics have been observed among survivors of out-of-hospital cardiac arrest (18), among patients with recent onset of heart failure, and those who have had high-risk markers after myocardial infarction (19). In contrast, data from one of the angiotensin-converting enzyme inhibitor trials (i.e., SAVE) suggest that the benefit of limiting cardiac enlargement on subsequent mortality, a risk factor that has a delayed onset after the conditioning myocardial infarction, is expressed late after the index event (22). Thus, time as a fimension for measuring risk must be integrated into strategies designed for population interventions. Ignoring this characteristic of the clinical epidemiology of SCD would contribute to the preselection of study groups that constitute lower risk components from a population with an overall high-risk characteristic. Specifically, studies favor enrollment of patients more than 12 to 18 months after an event to which the study is indexed would be characterized by lower than predicted event rates if late entrants are heavily represented in a study population in which the index event expresses an early mortality.

Conditioning Risk Factors

Because coronary heart disease accounts for ~80% of SCDs in Western societies (4), it is logical that most of the major studies of risk factors for SCD have focused on this single etiologic category. Data from multiple studies have demonstrated a concordance between risk factors for coronary atherosclerosis, total cardiovascular mortality, and SCD (1, 2, 11, 23, 24). In most studies, ~50% of all deaths related to coronary heart disease are sudden and unexpected, although proportions of sudden- to non-sudden deaths may vary as a function of the severity of left ventricular dysfunction and functional impairment (25). Among patients having cardiomyopathies, those in better functional classes have a lower overall death rate, but a higher fraction of the deaths are sudden. Among class IV patients, total death rate is higher, but the fraction that is sudden is lower. There is a competition of risk for sudden and non-sudden deaths, which means, among other things, that the extent to which sudden death mortality improvement will influence total mortality may be inherently limited by competing risks.

The absolute magnitude of risk relates well to the number of conventional risk factors present. In the Framingham study (7), there was a 14-fold increase of risk from the lowest risk decile to the highest risk decile. In the Yugoslavian cardiovascular disease study, the probability of SCD was 11 times higher in the top quintile than in the bottom quintile of multivariate risk distribution (10). Thus, the risk factors such as age, family history, gender, cigarette smoking, the hypertension/hypertrophy complex, hyperlipidemias, and other conventional coronary risk factors, provide easily identifiable markers for risk of SCD. The markers may be considered *static* because of their presence longitudinally over time, but they are limited in that they identify risk of the underlying disease responsible for SCD rather than for the pathophysiology of its expression. Because pathophysiological susceptibility does not necessarily equate with structural heart disease risk (see later data), the ability of these longitudinally expressed static risk factors to identify individuals who will develop disease expression is limited. There can be no argument that they can be used to identify high-risk subgroups in epidemiological terms, and it is likely that, for some of these risk factors, interventions will influence risk and significantly alter the number of events experienced among the population. However, specific active interventions are difficult to apply to large population bases. Therefore, whereas conventional risk factors have taught us much about the nature of the problem and provided important preventive opportunities, they lack the specific focus required for *efficient* strategies in individual patients.

A higher level of conditioning risk is derived from the presence of specific structural cardiac abnormalities. Once established, they constitute the substrate upon which triggering events can initiate unstable cardiac electrophysiologic disturbances (Fig. 4). Structural abnormalities are described in more detail herein.

Transient Risk Factors

The "PVC hypothesis" is an expression of the premise that PVCs serve a primary triggering function for the initiation of ventricular tachycardia or fibrillation (VT/VF), and presumes that PVC suppression would protect against SCD by eliminating the electrophysiological triggers. Despite consistent data identifying chronic PVCs as a risk factor for SCD in patients with underlying heart disease (16, 26–29), special circumstances are required to demonstrate the initiation of spontaneous life-threatening arrhythmias by PVCs. Ambulatory recordings of the spontaneous onset of cardiac arrest show a tendency to increases in sinus rate and PVC frequency before VF (30–32), likely reflecting a change in sympathetic tone or hemodynamic status as an intermediary in the PVC–VT/VF relationship. This leads to a concept that transiently active factors are the key pathophysiologic conditions for potentially fatal arrhythmias, rather than fortuitous relationships

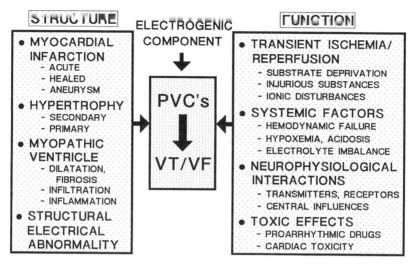

Figure 4. Pathophysiology of SCD: interaction of structure, function, and the electrogenesis of VT/VF. The four common categories of structural abnormalities, which include most specific etiologies of SCD, interact withone or more functional perturbations that cause transient destabilization. This interaction is proposed as the mechanism that converts chronic ambient arrhythmias (PVCs) into the triggering events for sustained and potentially fatal VT/VF. See text for details. [Modified from Myerburg et al. (33).]

between chronic PVCs and steady-state structural abnormalities. Transient risk factors serve to destabilize ventricular myocardium at a specific point in time, permitting the genesis of potentially fatal arrhythmias by a definable relationship between chronic abnormalities and acute pathophysiologic changes.

The relationship between structure and functional changes received little attention until recent years, despite recognition that the PVC–VT/VF relationship had a much higher probability of expression in the presence of structural heart disease than in its absence (33) (Fig. 4). Healed myocardial infarction received the greatest attention as a structural risk factor. More recently, insights are emerging into other forms of structural abnormalities, such as left ventricular hypertrophy and the myopathies. The role of left ventricular hypertrophy as a risk factor for SCD has been recognized in epidemiologic studies (34, 35), and clinical associations have been described (36, 37). New information on potentially arrhythmogenic membrane channel and electrophysiologic alterations of hypertrophied myocardium is beginning to emerge (38, 39), providing insight into mechanisms by which this specific structural abnormality may contribute to the genesis of potentially fatal arrhythmias. The fact that *regional* hypertrophy is common after healing of myocardial infarction (40, 41) carries more implications on the general role of hypertrophy-induced electrophysiologic disturbances in the generation of life-threatening arrhythmias.

After recognition that the PVC–VT/VF relationship subserves structural conditioning factors, clinical investigators and physiologists have begun to study the factors directly responsible for the initiation of fatal arrhythmias at a specific point in time. The transient nature of these events makes their prospective elucidation a difficult clinical and epidemiological problem. Thus, it was initially the development of a base of experimental information on the role of myocardial ischemia in creating an electrophysiologic risk of VT/VF that first led to the concept of an initiating or transitional event, in which PVCs could initiate VT/VF under a predictable set of circumstances (42). Subsequently, other functional perturbations received attention. Intense functional changes alone may destabilize this system in the absence of structural abnormalities, but the vast majority of cardiac arrests occur in hearts with preceding structural abnormalities. As shown in Fig. 4, the major functional influences or categories of transient risk factors may be separated into four groups: (1) ischemia/reperfusion; (2) systemic abnormalities; (3) autonomic factors; and (4) cardiotoxic factors, including the general problem of proarrhythmia.

Transient Ischemia and Reperfusion

The ischemia that occurs at the onset and during the early phase of acute myocardial infarction has a clearly established clinical and experimental association with potentially fatal arrhythmias. However, the majority of SCD victims and survivors of out-of-hospital cardiac arrest do not have acute transmural myocardial infarctions (43). Approximately 80% of SCDs due to coronary heart disease are not associated with acute myocardial infarction (44), and it is assumed that transient acute ischemia is one of the major triggering factors; however, its transient nature has precluded systematic clinical study. Unstable angina pectoris and silent ischemia also appear capable of initiating potentially fatal arrhythmias (45–48), although there is only limited clinical documentation of such mechanisms (49). Both are associated with a statistically increased risk of SCD in the presence of preexisting coronary artery disease.

Clinical and epidemiological data indicating associations between ischemia and potentially fatal arrhythmia are paralleled by experimental data that demonstrate adverse effects of ischemia, especially in the presence of a prior myocardial infarction. Such experimental data are providing insight into mechanisms responsible for these arrhythmias (42). These data range from studies in intact hearts in situ to specific channel abnormalities, and serve both as explanations for the deranged electrophysiology and as targets for treatment. Moreover, the epidemiologic impact of left ventricular hypertrophy, especially in the presence of coronary artery disease and prior myocardial infarction, is paralleled by observations of specific channel abnormalities in hypertrophied myocytes, some of which become manifest primarily during ischemia. These observations include differences in ATP-sensitive K^+ channels during ischemia in the hypertrophied myocardium compared with normal, and between endocardium and epicardium in normal hearts (50), as well as changes in Ca^{++} and K^+ currents under conditions of metabolic inhibition as a surrogate for ischemia (51). Thus, some of the epidemiologic factors that increase risk of SCD are paralleled by abnormalities at the level of membrane channels, which could serve as an explanation for increased risk. Although the interaction between epidemiology and membrane physiology is only in its infancy, their interrelationships warrant further exploration, as discussed in later chapters.

Transient ischemia enhances susceptibility to the initiation of sustained ventricular arrhythmias, and, in addition, the role of subsequent or concomitant reperfusion of ischemic muscle is beginning to be clarified. Reperfusion appears to induce a different type of electrical instability, characterized by very rapid electrical activity, which may be due to abrupt changes in refractoriness (52), as well as to generation of afterdepolarizations, the latter being experimentally sensitive to Ca^{++} blockade (53). Hypertrophied myocytes appear to be more prone to generate reperfusion-induced early afterdepolarizations and triggered activity than are normal myocytes, apparently due to depressed delayed rectifier current (I_k) in the hypertrophied myocyte (54). In situ studies of the frequency of VF during ischemia and reperfusion in previously hypertrophied hearts support the potential importance of such data (55).

Systemic Factors in Transient Risk

Acute or subacute systemic abnormalities may modulate chronic structural abnormalities, thereby influencing electrophysiologic stability and susceptibility to arrhythmias. Among the larger studies of survivors of out-of-hospital cardiac arrest, definable (but small) subgroups have had recognizable reversible systemic abnormalities that contribute to the potentially fatal arrhythmias. It is generally accepted that when such factors can be identified and controlled, no other preventive interventions against recurrences are required (44). Hypoxemia, acidosis, and electrolyte imbalances may contribute to such destabilization (56–58), and such factors are often recognizable clinically and reversible with appropriate therapy. Clues regarding mechanisms by which this type of transient risk may influence electrophysiology are beginning to evolve. For instance, in myocytes from globally hypertrophied hearts, conductance through ATP-sensitive K^+ channels may be *increased* by a reduction in pH (59). When a hypertrophied heart becomes regionally ischemic and acidotic, this characteristic may cause, or contribute to, dispersion of electrophysiological properties. Chronic electrolyte disturbances, most prominently hypokalemia associated with long-term use of diuretics, associated with increased risk of cardiovascular mortality (57). Hypokalemia as a cause of polymorphic VT and torsade de pointes is well recognized (58, 60), most notably in patients with chronically abnormal hearts, or in the presence of class I antiarrhythmic drugs.

The most common systemic factor, but one that has been difficult to identify operationally, is the role of transient hemodynamic dysfunction in patients with previously abnormal hearts. Severe acute or subacute hemodynamic deterioration may cause a secondary cardiac arrest, which has long been known to carry a very high short-term mortality rate (56, 61); but the relationship between chronically impaired left ventricular function, predisposition to VT/VF, and acute modulations in hemodynamic status are important focuses for the future. It has been shown experimentally that volume loading of isolated perfused canine left ventricles shortens refractory periods (62, 63), and regional disparity in hearts with prior myocardial infarction has been demonstrated (63). Stretch-induced modulation of membrane channels may play a role in such changes. Clinical studies to define underlying mechanisms have been limited to date.

Autonomic Fluctuations and Transient Risks

Both systemic and local cardiac neurophysiologic factors are receiving increasing attention as markers for identifying high-risk subgroups and for elucidating mechanisms of fatal arrhythmias (64). Autonomic dysfunction may be disturbed at several levels. An increasing body of experimental information (64–70) and a limited amount of clinical data (12–15, 71–74) suggest that cardiac abnormalities predisposing to SCD (such as prior myocardial infarction) are accompanied by changes in autonomic function within the heart. Several patterns of regional changes in response to sympathetic stimulation have been reported in different myocardial infarction models (65, 66, 68). Regionally altered β-adrenoceptor numbers and changes in coupling proteins and in adenylate cyclase activity have been observed in hearts with healed myocardial infarction (70). Experimental and clinical imaging studies have also shown a disruption of myocardial sympathetic innervation after acute myocardial infarction, with apparent reinnervation after convalescence (65, 67, 68, 71). Clinically, isoproterenol dependency for induction of sustained VT among cardiac arrest survivors and its prevention by β-adrenoceptor blocking drugs (72) suggest a role for autonomic variations in the genesis of potentially fatal arrhythmias.

At a systemic level, neurophysiologic alterations, which may modulate cardiac activity, have been proposed to identify subgroups at increased risk for SCD. Changes in heart rate variability or baroreceptor sensitivity have been studied in selected subgroups. Among myocardial infarction survivors (12, 15) and survivors of out-of-hospital cardiac arrest (14), altered heart rate variability has been suggested as a marker for SCD risk. Power spectrum analysis of heart rate variability in the frequency domain has suggested specific patterns that identify high-risk subgroups (15). A blunted baroreceptor response to phenylephrine infusion has also been suggested as a marker to identify subgroups at risk for SCD and VT after myocardial infarction (13).

Effects of Toxic Substances on the Heart

The risk of VF during chloroform anesthesia was the first recognized relationship between a clinically used substance and potentially fatal arrhythmias (75, 76). Subsequently, the relationship between antiarrhythmic drugs and proarrhythmic responses, initially described in terms of the risk of torsade de pointes and VF during quinidine therapy, identified a specific clinical circumstance in the ambulatory setting. It is now recognized that classical proarrhythmic responses of this type may occur with any of the class IA antiarrhythmic drugs with many class III drugs. More subtle, but possibly quite important, is the emerging number of clinically used substances that are *not* used as antiarrhythmic drugs, but that are recognized to have similar *proarrhythmic* responses. These include such diverse categories of medication as terfenadine, erythromycin, pentamidine, and a number of the psychotropic drugs. In addition, limited clinical data suggest an effect on QT interval and the risk of torsade de pointes in the susceptible individual for such diverse other substances as organic phosphates, insecticides, cocaine (77), and probucol (78). To the extent that these various substances have been studied for effects that might explain such responses, and the data are limited at this time, the one common denominator that appears to be emerging is that each of the offending substances prolongs QT intervals by an effect on repolarizing currents, such as the delayed rectifier current (77). The combination of an inherent ability to prolong action potential duration and variable individual susceptibility to this effect could explain the sporadic occurrence of these responses. It follows that identification of the offending channel dysfunction, coupled with an ability to identify individual susceptibility, might provide a method to identify risk prospectively. Unfortunately, because such events are more common in patients with underlying heart disease, the distinction between a proarrhythmic response and a clinical arrhythmia caused by the underlying disease becomes a difficult circumstance for identifying the magnitude of the problem in nature. Currently, it appears to be quite low; but this may be due to a sampling error related to confusion between the consequences of underlying diseases and the effects of substances in the environment.

Response Variables and Risk in the Susceptible Individual

The concept of response risk is an attempt to introduce principles of epidemiology to the disciplines of cardiac electrophysiology and myocardial cell membrane function. It is developed to test hypotheses on the mechanisms by which a specific individual having a conditioning risk factor is susceptible to arrhythmogenesis when exposed to a transient functional risk influence. Based on the premises that conditioning factors create a persistent substrate for arrhythmic risk and the transient functional factors serve an initiating role, the ultimate epidemiologic question relates to identification of those subjects whose inherent physiologic characteristics make the initiation of electrophysiologic instability more likely when these conditions are met. It assumes genetically based (or acquired) individual differences in responses of membrane channels, receptors, exchangers, and pumps, which may be clinically identifiable. That such conditions exist in nature has been shown in the biological model of the *Drosophila* mutant, which develops leg shaking when exposed to ether or environmental changes (79). Specific membrane channel defects have been identified, one being an abnormal I_{kA} channel, which is genetically determined to function abnormally on exposure to the inciting factor (80), and which therefore identifies a population subgroup at risk for this abnormal response. Other variations have I_{Na} abnormalities (79). In parallel, but not yet worked out genetically, is the clinical model of proarrhythmic response to class IA antiarrhythmic drugs, in which an idiosyncrasy to the class IA membrane-active antiarrhythmic agents is expressed as excessive prolongation of repolarization and generation of torsade de pointes. Delayed activation of I_K likely creates individual susceptibility on exposure (81), whereas the arrhythmia itself appears to be electrophysiologically mediated by $I_{Ca,L}$ (82). The ability to identify abnormal response characteristics of specific channels or receptors, under a variety of pathophysiologic conditions, holds the promise of identifying specific individuals at risk for potentially fatal arrhythmias under conditions of various exposures. This extends beyond proarrhythmic effects of antiarrhythmic drugs to include factors such as the response of specific channels to ischemia and reperfusion (54, 81, 82), as well as the response of previously conditioned hearts to other stimuli in their environment which influence channel function (77).

In summary, therefore, this quest toward the ultimate epidemiological achievement—identification of specific individuals at risk of responding abnormally to a specific stimulus—will provide increasing power to epidemiological approaches and yield increasingly greater resolution of subgroups at risk.

Summary and Conclusions

Classical epidemiology has provided a great deal of useful information regarding SCD and its prevention. The emphasis on specific population characteristics, the relationship between absolute numbers and relative risk, and the temporal modulation of risk, add power to epidemiological information. However, continued insight into the problem of SCD, and its control, will require an interaction with other disciples, both clinical and fundamental, in order to achieve greater resolution of risk. To this end, the roles of clinical and experimental electrophysiology and membrane function, as they influence identification of individuals at risk, are paramount.

Acknowledgments

This study was supported in part by Grants HL-28130 and HL-21735 (R.J.M.) from the National Heart, Lung, and Blood Institute, and by Grant 91G1A/70 from the Florida Affiliate of the American Heart Association (Palm Beach Chapter).

We thank Thelma L. Gottlieb for her invaluable assistance in the preparation of this manuscript.

References

1. Epstein, F.H., and Pisa, Z. (1979). International comparisons in ischemic heart disease mortality. *Proc. Conf. on the Decline in Coronary Heart Disease Mortality.* DHEW, NIH Publication No. 79-1610 (U.S. Government Printing Office, Washington, DC), pp. 58–88.

2. Working Group on Arteriosclerosis of the NHLBI. (1981). *Report of the Working Group on Arteriosclerosis of the National Heart, Lung, and Blood Institute. Volume 2: Patient Oriented Research—Fundamental and Applied, Sudden Cardiac Death.* DHEW, NIH Publication No. 83-2035 (Government Printing Office, Washington, DC), pp. 114–122.

3. Gillum, R.F. (1989). Sudden coronary deaths in the United States, 1980–1985. *Circulation* **79:**756–765.

4. Myerburg, R.J., and Castellanos, A. (1992). Cardiac arrest and sudden cardiac death, in *Heart Disease: A Textbook of Cardiovascular Medicine,* E. Braunwald, Ed. (W.B. Saunders Publishing Co., New York), 4th ed., chap. 26, pp. 756–789.

5. Myerburg, R.J., Kessler, K.M., and Castellanos, A. (1992). Sudden cardiac death: Structure, function, and time-dependence of risk. *Circulation* **85**(Suppl. 1)**:**1-2–1-10.

6. Myerburg, R.J., Kessler, K.M., and Castellanos, A. (1993). Progress in the control of sudden cardiac death: Applied clinical epidemiology, transient risk factors, and evaluation of interventions. Manuscript submitted for publication.

7. Kannel, W.B., and Thomas, H.E. (1982). Sudden coronary death: The Framingham study. *Ann. N.Y. Acad. Sci.* **382:**3–21.

8. Doyle, J.T., Kannel, W.B., McNamara, R.M., Quikenton, R., and Gordon, T. (1976). Factors related to suddenness of death from coronary heart disease: Combined Albany–Framingham Studies. *Am. J. Cardiol.* **37:**1073–1078.

9. Chiang, B., Perlman, H.V., Fulton, M., Ostrander, I.D., and Epstein, R.H. (1970). Predisposing factor in sudden cardiac death in Tecumseh, Michigan; a prospective study. *Circulation* **41:**31–37.

10. Demirovic, J. (1985). Risk factors in the incidence of sudden cardiac death and possibilities for its prevention. *Doctoral Thesis,* University of Belgrade Press, Belgrade, Yugoslavia.

11. Myerburg, R.J., and Demirovic, J. (1993). Epidemiology of sudden coronary death: A review. *Prog. Cardiovasc. Dis.*, in press.

12. Kleiger, R.E., Miller, J.P., Bigger, J.T., Moss, A.J., and the Multicenter Post-Infarction Research Groups. (1987). Decreased heart rate variability and its association with increased mortality after acute myocardial infarction. *Am. J. Cardiol.* **59:**256–262.

13. Le Rovere, M.T., Specchia, G., Mortara, A., and Schwartz, P.J. (1988). Baroreflex sensitivity, clinical correlates and cardiovascular mortality among patients with first myocardial infarction: A prospective study. *Circulation* **78:**816–824.

14. Huikuri, H.V., Linnaluoto, M.K., Valkama, J.O., Kessler, K.M., Takkunen, J.T., and Myerburg, R.J. (1990). Heart rate variability and its circadian rhythm in survivors of cardiac arrest. *Circulation* **82**(Suppl. III):111–237.

15. Bigger, J.T., Fleiss, J.L., Steinman, R.C., Rolnitzky, L.M., Kleiger, R.E., and Rottman, J.N. (1992). Frequency domain measures of heart period variability and mortality after myocardial infarction. *Circulation* **85:**164–171.

16. Bigger, J.T., Fleiss, J.L., Kleiger, R., Miller, J.P., Rolnitzky, L.M., and the Multicenter Post-Infarction Research Group. (1984). The relationships among ventricular arrhythmias, left ventricular dysfunction, and mortality in the 2 years after myocardial infarction. *Circulation* **69:**250–258.

17. Bigger, J.T. (1984). Antiarrhythmic therapy: An overview after myocardial infarction. *Am. J. Cardiol.* **53:**8B–16B.

18. Furukawa, T., Rozanski, J.J., Nogami, A., Moroe, K., Gosselin, A.J., and Lister, J.W. (1989). Time-dependent risk of and predictors for cardiac arrest recurrence in survivors of out-of-hospital cardiac arrest with chronic coronary artery disease. *Circulation* **80:**599–608.

19. Schechtman, K.B., Bipone, R.J., Kleiger, R.E., Gibson, R.S., Schwartz, D.J., Roberts, R., Yeng, P.M., Boden, W.E., and the Diltiazem Reinfarction Study Research Group. (1989). Risk stratification of patients with non-Q wave myocardial infarction. *Circulation* **80:**1148–1158.

20. The Cardiac Arrhythmia Suppression Trial (CAST) Investigators. (1989). Preliminary report: Effect of encainide and flecainide on mortality in a randomized trial of arrhythmia suppression after myocardial infarction. *N. Engl. J. Med.* **331:**406–412.

21. Echt, D.S., Liebson, P.R., Mitchell, B., Peters, R.W., Obias-Manno, D., Barker, A.H., Arensberg, D., Baker, A., Friedman, L., Greene, H.L., Huther, M.L., Richardson, D.W., and the CAST Investigators. (1991). Mortality and morbidity in patients receiving encainide, flecainide, or placebo. The Cardiac Arrhythmias Suppression Trial. *N. Engl. J. Med.* **324:**781–788.

22. Pfeffer, M.A., Braunwald, E., Moye, L.A., Basta, L., Brown, E.J., Jr., Cuddy, T.E., Davis, B.R., Geltman, E.M., Goldman, S., Flaker, G.C., Klein, M., Lamas, G.A., Packer, M., Rouleau, J., Rouleau, J.L., Rutherford, J., Wertheimer, J.H., Hawkins, C.M., and the SAVE Investigators. (1993). The effect of captopril on mortality and morbidity in patients with left ventricular dysfunction after myocardial infarction: Results of the survival and ventricular enlargement trial. *N. Engl. J. Med.*, in press.

23. Kannel, W.B., Doyle, J.T., McNamara, P.M., Quickenton, P., and Gordon, T. (1979). Precursors of sudden coronary death: Factors related to the incidence of sudden death. *Circulation* **51:**606–613.

24. Kuller, L.H. (1980). Sudden death: Definition and epidemiologic considerations. *Prog. Cardiovasc. Dis.* **23**:1–12.

25. Kjekshus, J. (1990). Arrhythmias and mortality in congestive heart failure. *Am. J. Cardiol.* **65**:42-1–48-1.

26. Moss, A.J., Schnitzler, R., Green, R., and DeCamilla, J. (1977). Ventricular arrhythmias 3 weeks after acute myocardial infarction. *Ann. Intern. Med.* **75**:837–842.

27. Vismara, L.A., Amsterdam, B.A., and Mason, D.T. (1975). Relation of ventricular arrhythmias in the late-hospital phase of acute myocardial infarction to sudden death after hospital discharge. *Am. J. Med.* **59**:6–12.

28. Ruberman, W., Weinblatt, M., Goldberg, J.D., Frank, C.W., Chaudhary, B.S., and Shapiro, S. (1981). Ventricular premature complexes and sudden death after myocardial infarction. *Circulation* **64**:297–305.

29. Schulze, R.A., Strauss, H.W., and Pitt, B. (1977). Sudden death in the year following myocardial infarction: Relationship of ventricular premature contractions in the late hospital phase and left ventricular ejection fraction. *Am. J. Med.* **62**:192–199.

30. Nikolic, G., Bishop, R.L., and Singh, J.B. (1984). Sudden death recorded during Holter monitoring. *Circulation* **66**:218–225.

31. Myerburg, R.J., Kessler, K.M., Luceri, R.M., Zaman, L., Trohman, R.G., Estes, D., and Castellanos, A. (1984). Classification of ventricular arrhythmias based on parallel hierarchies of frequency and form. *Am. J. Cardiol.* **54**:1355–1358.

32. Leciercq, J.F., Coumel, P.H., Maisonblanche, P., Cauchemez, B., Zimmwerman, M., Choutz, F., and Slama, R. (1986). Mise en evidence des mecanismes determinants de la morte subite: Enquete cooperative portant sur 69 cas enregistres par la methode de Holter. *Archiv. Mal Coeur* **79**:1024–1036.

33. Myerburg, R.J., Kessler, K.M., Bassett, A.L., and Castellanos, A. (1989). A biological approach to sudden cardiac death: Structure, function and cause. *Am. J. Cardiol.* **63**:1512–1516.

34. Kannel, W.B., and Thomas, H.E. (1982). Sudden coronary death: The Framingham Study. *Ann. N.Y. Acad. Sci.* **38**:3–21.

35. Cupples, L.A., Gagnon, D.R., and Kannel, W.B. (1992). Long- and short-term risk of sudden coronary death. *Circulation* **85**(Suppl. I):1-11–1-18.

36. Anderson, K.P. (1984). Sudden death, hypertension, and hypertrophy. *J. Cardiovasc. Pharm.* **6**(Suppl. III):S498–S503.

37. Messerli, F.H., Ventura, H.O., Elizardi, D.J., Dunn, F.G., and Frohlich, E.D. (1984). Hypertension and sudden death: Increased ventricular ectopic activity in left ventricular hypertrophy. *Am. J. Med.* **77**:18–22.

38. Furukawa, T., Myerburg, R.J., Furukawa, N., Kimura, S., and Bassett, A.L. (1990). Ionic mechanism of increased susceptibility of hypertrophied feline myocytes to metabolic inhibition. *Circulation* **82**(Suppl. III):111–522 (Abstract).

39. Furukawa, T., Bassett, A.L., Kimura, S., Furukawa, N., and Myerburg, R.J. (1990). "Reperfusion" early afterdepolarizations (EAD) in hypertrophied feline myocytes: Role of membrane currents. *Circulation* **82**(Suppl. III):111.

40. Ginzton, L.E., Conant, R., Rodrigues, D.M., and Laks, M.M. (1989). Functional significance of hypertrophy of the non-infarcted myocardium after myocardial infarction in humans. *Circulation* **80**:816–822.

41. Cox, M.M., Berman, I., Myerburg, R.J., Smets, M.J.D., and Kozlovskis, P.L. (1991). Monophometric mapping of regional myocyte diameters after healing of myocardial infarction in cats. *J. Mol. Cell Cardiol.* **23**:127–135.

42. Rosen, M.R., Janse, M.J., and Myerburg, R.J. (1987). Arrhythmias induced by coronary artery occlusion: What are the electrophysiologic mechanisms?, in *Life-Threatening Arrhythmias During Ischemia and Infarction*, D. Hearse, A. Manning, and M. Janse, Eds. (Raven Press, New York), chap. 2, pp. 11–47.

43. Baum, R.S., Alvarez, H., and Cobb, L.A. (1974). Survival after resuscitation from out-of-hospital ventricular fibrillation. *Circulation* **50**:1231–1235.

44. Myerburg, R.J., Kessler, K.M., Zaman, L., Conde, C.A., and Castellanos, A. (1982). Survivors of prehospital cardiac arrest. *J.A.M.A.* **247**:1485–1490.

45. Gottlieb, S.O., Weisfeldt, M.I., Ouyang, P., Mellits, E.D., and Gerstenblith, G. (1986). Silent ischemia as a marker for early unfavorable outcomes in patients with unstable angina. *N. Engl. J. Med.* **314**:1214.

46. Weintraub, R.M., Aroesty, J.M., Paulin, S., Levine, R.H., Markis, J.E., LaRaia, P.J., Cohen, S.I., and Kurland, G.S. (1979). Medically refractory unstable angina pectoris. 1. Long-term follow-up of patients undergoing intra-aortic balloon counterpulsation and operation. *Am. J. Cardiol.* **43**:877.

47. Mulcahy, R., Awadhi, A.H.A., deBuitieor, M., Tobin, G., Johnson, H., and Contoy, R. (1985). Natural history and prognosis of unstable angina. *Am. Heart J.* **109**:753.

48. Nademanee, K., Intarachot, V., Josephson, M.A., Rieders, D., Mody, F.V., and Singh, B.N. (1987). Prognostic significance of silent myocardial ischemia in patients with unstable angina. *J. Am. Coll. Cardiol.* **1**:1–9.

49. Myerburg, R.J., Kessler, K.M., Mallon, S.M., Cox, M.M., deMarchena, E., Interian, A., Jr., and Castellanos, A. (1992). Potentially fatal arrhythmias in patients with silent myocardial ischemia due to coronary artery spasm. *N. Engl. J. Med.* **326**:1451–1455.

50. Furukawa, T., Kimura, S., Furukawa, N., Bassett, A.L., and Myerburg, R.J. (1991). Role of cardiac ATP-regulated potassium channels in differential responses of endocardial and epicardial cells to ischemia. *Circ. Res.* **68**:1693–1702.

51. Furukawa, T., Myerburg, R.J., Furukawa, N., Kimura, S., and Bassett, A.L. (1990). Ionic mechanism of increased susceptibility of hypertrophied feline myocytes to metabolic inhibition. *Circulation* **82**(Suppl. III):III–522 (Abstract).

52. Ideker, R.E., Klein, G.J., Harrison, L., Smith, W.M., Kasell, J., Reimer, K.A., Wallace, A.G., and Gallagher, J.J. (1981). The transition to ventricular fibrillation induced by reperfusion after ischemia in the dog: A period of organized epicardial activation. *Circulation* **63**:1371–1379.

53. Priori, S.G., Mantica, M., Napolitano, C., and Schwartz, P.J. (1990). Early afterdepolarization induced in vivo by reperfusion of ischemic myocardium. *Circulation* **81**:1911–1920.

54. Furukawa, T., Bassett, A.L., Kimura, S., Furukawa, N., and Myerburg, R.J. (1990). Reperfusion early afterdepolarizations (EAD) in hypertrophied feline myocytes: Role of membrane currents. *Circulation* **82**(Suppl. III):111.

55. Koyha, T., Kimura, S., Myerburg, R.J., and Bassett, A.L. (1988). Susceptibility of hypertrophied rat hearts to ventricular fibrillation during acute ischemia. *J. Mol. Cell Cardiol.* **20**:159–168.

56. Packer, M. (1985). Sudden unexpected death in patients with congestive heart failure: A second frontier. *Circulation* **72**:681–685.

57. Multiple Risk Factor Intervention Trial Research Group. (1982). Multiple-risk factor intervention trial: Risk factor changes in mortality results. *J.A.M.A.* **248**:1465–1477.

58. Gettes, L.S. (1992). Electrolyte abnormalities underlying lethal and ventricular arrhythmias. *Circulation* **85**(Suppl. I):I-70–I-76.

59. Kimura, S., Bassett, A.L., Xi, H., Tomita, F., and Myerburg, R.J., (1993). Characteristics of ATP-sensitive K$^+$ channels in hypertrophied cells: Effects of pH. *Circulation,* in press.

60. Jackman, W.M., Friday, K.J., Anderson, J.L., Aliot, E.M., Clark, M., and Lazzara, R. (1988). The long QT syndrome: A critical review, new clinical observations, and a unifying hypothesis. *Prog. Cardiovasc. Dis.* **32**:115–172.

61. Robinson, J.S., Sloman, G., Mathew, T.H., and Gobie, A.J. (1965). Survival after resuscitation from cardiac arrest in acute myocardial infarction. *Am. Heart J.* **69**:740–747.

62. Lab, M.J. (1982). Contraction-excitation feedback in myocardium: Physiologic basis and clinical relevance. *Circ. Res.* **50**:757–766.

63. Calkins, H., Maughan, W.L., Weissman, H.F., Sugiura, S., Sagawa, K., and Levine, J.H. (1989). Effect of acute volume load on refractoriness and arrhythmia development in isolated chronically infarcted canine hearts. *Circulation* **79**:687–697.

64. Schwartz, P.J., La Rovere, T., and Vanoli, E. (1992). Autonomic nervous system and sudden cardiac death: Experimental basis and clinical observations for post-myocardial infarction risk stratification. *Circulation* **85**(Suppl. I):1-77–1-91.

65. Barber, M.J., Mueller, T.M., Henry, D.F., Felton, S.J., and Zipes, D.P. (1982). Transmural myocardial infarction in the dog produces sympathectomy in non-infarcted myocardium. *Circulation* **67**:787–796.

66. Gaide, M.S., Myerburg, R.J., Kozlovskis, P.L., and Bassett, A.L. (1983). Elevated sympathetic response of epicardium proximal to healed myocardial infarction. *Am. J. Physiol.* **14**:646–652.

67. Schwartz, P.J., Billman, G.E., and Stone, H.L. (1984). Autonomic mechanisms in ventricular fibrillation induced by myocardial ischemia during exercise in dogs with a healed myocardial infarction: An experimental preparation for sudden cardiac death. *Circulation* **69**:780–790.

68. Kammerling, J.J., Green, F.J., Watanabe, A.M., Inoue, H., Barber, M.J., Henry, D.P., and Zipes, D.P. (1987). Denervation supersensitivity of refractoriness in non-infarcted areas apical to transmural myocardial infarction. *Circulation* **76**:383–393.

69. Schwartz, P.J., Vanoli, E., Stramba-Badiale, M., De Ferrari, G.M., Billman, G.E., and Foreman, R.D. (1988). Autonomic mechanisms and sudden death:

New insights from analysis of baroreceptor reflexes in conscious dogs with and without a myocardial infarction. *Circulation* **78**:969–979.

70. Kozlovskis, P.L., Smets, M.J.D., Duncan, R.C., Bailey, B.K., Bassett, A.L., and Myerburg, R.J. (1990). Regional beta-adrenergic receptors and adenylate cyclase activity after healing of myocardial infarction in cats. *J. Mol. Cell Cardiol.* **22**:311–322.

71. Tull, M., Minardo, J., Mock, B.H., Weiner, R.E., Siddiqul, A.R., Zipes, D.P., and Wellman, H.N. (1987). SPECT with high purity 1-123-MIBG after transmural myocardial infarction (TMI), demonstrating sympathetic denervation followed by reinnervation in a dog model. *J. Nucl. Med.* **28**:669.

72. Interian, A., Fernandez, P., Robinson, E., Zeno, J., Garcia, O., Castellanos, A., and Myerburg, R.J. (1990). Long-term effect of propranolol in ventricular tachycardia/fibrillation patients with isoproterenol-dependent inducibility. *Circulation* **82**(Suppl. III):435.

73. Huikuri, H.V., Cox, M., Interian, A., Jr., Kessler, K.M., Castellanos, A., and Myerburg, R.J. (1989). Efficacy of intravenous propranolol for suppression of inducibility of ventricular tachyarrhythmias with different electrophysiologic characteristics in coronary artery disease. *Am. J. Cardiol.* **64**:1305–1309.

74. Huikuri, H.V., Zaman, L., Castellanos, A., Kessler, K.M., Cox, M., Glicksman, F., and Myerburg, R.J. (1989). Changes in spontaneous sinus node rate as an estimate of cardiac autonomic tone during stable and unstable ventricular tachycardia. *J. Am. Coll. Cardiol.* **13**:646–652.

75. Hill, I.G.W. (1932). Human heart in anaesthesia: Electrocardiographic study. *Edinburgh Med. J.* **39**:533–553.

76. Hill, I.G.W. (1932). Cardiac irregularities during chloroform anaesthesia. *Lancet* **1**:1139–1142.

77. Kimura, S., Bassett, A.L., Xi, H., and Myerburg, R.J. (1992). Early afterdepolarizations and triggered activity induced by cocaine: A possible mechanism of cocaine arrhythmogenesis. *Circulation* **85**:2227–2235.

78. Gohn, D.C., and Simmons, T.W. (1992). Polymorphic ventricular tachycardia (torsades de pointes) associated with the use of probucol. *N. Engl. J. Med.* **326**:1435–1436.

79. Tanouye, M.A., Kamb, C.A., Iverson, L.E., and Salkoff, L. (1986). Genetic and molecular biology of ion channels in *Drosophila*. *Ann. Rev. Neurosci.* **9**:255–276.

80. Iverson, L.E., Tanouye, M.A., Lester, H.A., Davidson, N., and Rudy, B. (1988). A-type potassium channels expressed from Shaker Iocus cDNA. *Proc. Natl. Acad. Sci. U.S.A.* **85**:5723–5727.

81. Roden, D.M., Bennett, P.B., Snyders, D.J., Balser, J.R., and Hondeghem, L.M. (1988). Quinidine delays I_k activation in guinea pig ventricular myocytes. *Circ. Res.* **62**:1055–1058.

82. January, C.R., and Riddle, J.M. (1989). Early afterdepolarizations: Mechanisms of induction and block: a role for L-type Ca^{++} current. *Circ. Res.* **64**:977–990.

3

Autonomic Markers for Sudden Cardiac Death

Peter J. Schwartz

During the last two decades, compelling evidence has been provided for the existence of a tight relationship between the autonomic nervous system and sudden cardiac death (1–5). Interest in this relationship has focused primarily on the electrophysiologic mechanisms involved (1, 3, 6, 7) and on the evidence that ventricular fibrillation could be enhanced by sympathetic (5, 8, 9) and antagonized by vagal activity (10–12).

For a while, the clinical implications of these concepts were applied only to therapy; examples are the widespread use of β-blockers after myocardial infarction (13) and the more recent use of left cardiac sympathetic denervation for selected populations at high risk for sudden death (14, 15). Further, based on a growing body of experimental data, the time was ripe for examining the possibility that functional aspects of cardiac innervation could contribute to the identification of patients at high risk for sudden cardiac death.

Major progress occurred as a consequence of the first experimental (16) observations that suggested that analysis of autonomic tone and reflexes might have *prognostic* value in identifying individuals following myocardial infarction and who were at high risk for subsequent cardiac death. These initial observations have been followed by several larger studies that confirmed and reinforced this concept.

In this chapter, some of the most critical studies are reviewed supporting the concept that the analysis of vagal tone and reflexes carries important prognostic information that contributes, together with the traditional risk factors, to a more accurate identification of the high-risk patient. Also discussed are some recent experimental and clinical observations that have provided new perspectives for understanding neural pathophysiological mechanisms underlying the onset of lethal arrhythmias and the development of new approaches to risk stratification of patients with coronary artery disease. More extensive and detailed information is given in several recent reviews that constitute the data base for this study (17–21).

Heart Rate Variability

Heart rate variability (often referred to as "heart period variability") is usually regarded as an index of "tonic" vagal activity. It should be remembered that heart rate changes are the consequence of the interplay, at the sinus node level, between the acetylcholine released by vagal nerves and the norepinephrine released by sympathetic nerves.

Clinical Studies

In 1978, in Melbourne, Wolf et al. (22) first reported an association between heart period (RR) variability and mortality in 176 patients with acute myocardial infarction. Their study showed that heart period variance, measured over a period <30 sec, predicted mortality over the next 9 to 14 days. The study included only a small number of deaths, so that the strength of the association was not estimated precisely. Relevant herein is the fact that Wolf et al. mentioned vagal activity only in association with the faster heart rate of the patients with reduced sinus arrhythmia. They did not relate their finding to a potential causal relationship between reduced vagal activity and increased mortality.

The study by Kleiger et al. (23) called general attention to the importance of heart period variability, reporting a strong association between the standard deviation of the normal RR intervals (SDNN) and all-cause mortality after myocardial infarction. Of the 867 patients enrolled in a natural history study of myocardial infarction (The Multicenter Postmyocardial Infarction Program), 808 had Holter recordings suitable for calculation of heart period variability. SDNN < 50 msec was found in 15.5% of the patients, and this subgroup had a mortality rate of 34.4%, compared with a 12.3% mortality rate for patients with SDNN $ 50 msec; the relative risk was 2.8 (see Fig. 1). SDNN correlated weakly but significantly with age, heart rate, and measures of left ventricular function, but it did not correlate with ventricular arrhythmias. Of all the Holter variables, SDNN had the strongest association with all-cause mortality. For other risk predictors (age, New York Heart Association functional class, rales in coronary care unit, left ventricular ejection fraction, and ventricular arrhythmias), SDNN was still significantly associated with the deaths that occurred over the next 4 years. This result is definitive because of the large population and the 127 deaths that occurred during follow-up. SDNN measures both the slow and fast oscillations in the RR interval, and it does not, therefore, provide specific information on the vagal or sympathetic modulation of the RR interval. However, its independence from left ventricular function and ventricular arrhythmias does suggest that it provides information about a different lethal force, probably involving the autonomic nervous system.

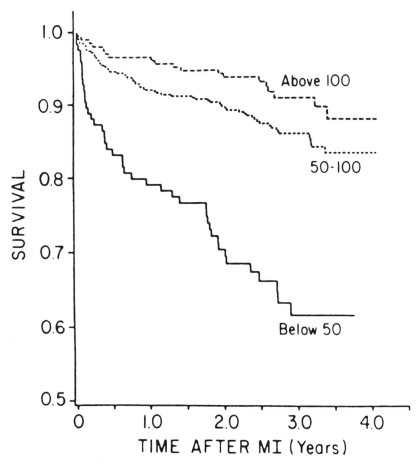

Figure 1. Survival after myocardial infarction (MI) for patients grouped according to the SDNN computed over a 24-hr period <50, 50–100, and >100. [From Kleiger et al. (23).]

A further and more detailed spectral analysis has recently been performed by Bigger et al. (24), who reanalyzed 24-hr ECG recordings from 715 patients participating in the Multicenter Postmyocardial Infarction Program. Estimates of mortality rates were precise, because there were 119 deaths in the 715 patient study group, 88 of which were classified as cardiac failure and 68 as arrhythmic. After adjustment for important covariates in a Cox regression model, ultra low–and low-frequency power were still strongly and significantly associated with death. Low- and high-frequency power were not strongly associated with death after adjusting for these covariates. Very low frequency power was more strongly associated with arrhythmic death than with all-cause mortality or cardiac failure death, before and after adjustment with covariates. Combining measures of heart period variability with left ventricular ejection fraction or ventricular arrhythmias identified small subgroups of postinfarction patients with a 2.5-year mortality rate > 50% (Fig. 2). This study suggested that slow cyclic variability was a stronger predictor than the high-frequency variability that reflects vagal tone. The physiologic mechanism for ultra low-frequency modulation of RR intervals is not yet known.

A contribution came also from Odemuyiwa et al. (25), who studied 385 survivors of myocardial infarction to compare the sensitivity and specificity of left ventricular ejection fraction and a heart rate variability index. The index used was a time domain measure derived from the frequency distribution of normal RR intervals in a 24-hr ECG recording, a measure dominated by ultra low-frequency information. This group concluded that,

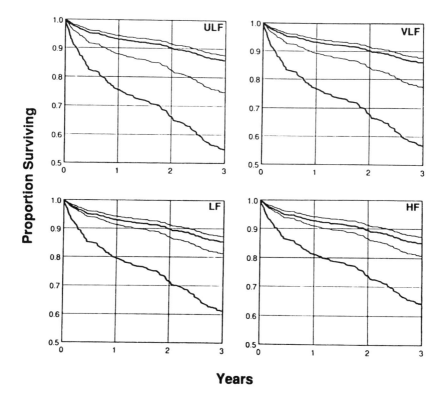

Years

Figure 2. Survival curves for 673 postinfarction patients in the high or low category for the four mutually exclusive frequency domain measures of heart rate variability [ultra low–frequency (ULF), very low-frequency (VLF), low-frequency (LF), and high-frequency (HF) power] using all-cause mortality as the endpoint. Thick lines represent unadjusted heart period variability data, and thin lines represent data adjusted for the five covariates: age, New York Heart Association functional class, rales in the coronary care unit, radionuclide ejection fraction, and the frequency of ventricular premature complexes. In each panel, the top two curves are for patients in the high category, and the lower two curves are for patients in the low category [From Bigger et al. (24).]

although left ventricular ejection fraction and heart rate variability index had similar sensitivities and specificity for all-cause mortality, the heart rate index was a better predictor of sudden death, or arrhythmic events. This suggests that heart period variability predicts arrhythmic events better than nonarrhythmic events.

In another study from the same group, Farrell et al. (26) examined 416 survivors of myocardial infarction to investigate the prognostic value of heart period variability in combination with ventricular arrhythmias found in a Holter recording of positive, signal-averaged ECGs. They hypothesized that the combination of abnormal autonomic tone and an arrhythmogenic substrate would be an excellent predictor of arrhythmic events (26). Their results apply to current practice, because their observations were made after postmyocardial infarction thrombolysis had become routine. During a mean follow-up of 612 days, there were 24 arrhythmic events, 47 cardiac deaths, and 40 nonfatal myocardial infarctions. The best univariate predictors of cardiac death were heart rate variability index [relative risk = 7 (95% confidence interval 4, 12)] and Killip class $ 2 [relative risk = 6 (95% confidence interval 3, 10)]. Left ventricular ejection fraction, positive exercise test, and ventricular arrhythmias in the Holter recording were all substantially weaker predictors of cardiac death. The best univariate predictor of arrhythmic events (arrhythmic deaths) was heart rate variability index (relative risk = 32), followed by signal-averaged ECG (relative risk = 7) and frequent or repetitive ventricular premature complexes in the Holter recording (relative risk = 5). Left ventricular ejection fraction and Killip class were weaker predictors of arrhythmic events. These results again suggest that heart rate variability has specificity for predicting arrhythmic events (i.e., it predicts arrhythmic events better than it predicts cardiac death or nonfatal reinfarction). Even though variability index is significantly associated with a positive, signal-averaged ECG, these two risk predictors each have substantial predictive power independent of each other. The prediction of arrhythmic events by a heart rate variability index also seems independent of left ventricular ejection fraction values or a positive exercise test.

Experimental Studies

At variance with the evolution of information on baroreflex sensitivity (BRS), as described herein, experimental studies on heart rate variability and risk for sudden death followed; they did not precede the critical clinical investigation.

Clinical extrapolation of experimental findings depends largely on the characteristics of the animal preparation in which the study is performed. This makes necessary a brief recapitulation of the animal model used for the studies that provided a breakthrough in our understanding of the complex relationship between the autonomic nervous system, acute myocardial ischemia, and life-threatening arrhythmias. The model therefore played a key role in demonstrating the prognostic value of BRS. Because it was also used to study heart rate variability, it seems appropriate to describe it herein.

Three elements involved often in the genesis of malignant arrhythmias in man are present in the experimental model reported in 1984 by Schwartz et al. (27): (a) healed myocardial infarction that acts as a substrate, (b) a transient episode of acute myocardial ischemia, and (c) physiologically elevated sympathetic activity that acts as a trigger. Briefly, 1 month after an anterior wall myocardial infarction, chronically instrumented dogs are exposed to a submaximal exercise stress test. Whenever heart rate reaches ~220 beats/min, a 2-min occlusion of the circumflex coronary artery is initiated by means of an occluder previously positioned around the vessel. After 1 min, exercise ends, but the occlusion is continued for one additional minute. This "exercise and ischemia test" produces ventricular fibrillation in >50% of the animals; whenever this occurs, the dogs are immediately defibrillated using steel paddles placed on the chest before the test. An important feature of the model is the very high reproducibility of the outcome and fibrillation in "susceptible" or survival in "resistant" animals in subsequent tests.

Using this preparation, Hull et al. (28) examined the prognostic value of heart rate variability, measured over a 30-min period. The model was used to predict the outcome (ventricular fibrillation or survival) during a brief ischemic episode in conscious dogs with a 1-month-old myocardial infarction. The study was performed on 50 dogs, 25 of which developed ventricular fibrillation (susceptible) and 25 of which survived (resistant). Heart rate variability, measured a few days before exposing the animals to the exercise and ischemia regime, was significantly lower among susceptible dogs than among the resistant ones (106 ± 9 vs. 209 ± 13 msec, $P <$ 0.001). As shown in Fig. 3, this difference was independent of the difference in heart rate; the results remained unchanged when they used the coefficient of variance, which corrects for heart rate.

These experimental data confirm in dogs what Kleiger et al. (23) had demonstrated in man. Agreement between the two studies underlines the clinical applicability of this canine model to the problem of sudden death, an important observation for studies that do not yet have a clinical counterpart. The study by Hull et al. (28) also provided a new and important piece of information. The novel observation comes from an internal control performed with 18 resistant and 15 susceptible dogs before and after myocardial infarction. It was found that before infarction, susceptible and resistant dogs had almost an identical heart rate variability (226 ± 30 vs. 233 ± 30 msec), but that myocardial infarction produced a significant reduction in susceptible, but not resistant dogs (Fig. 4).

Thus, although heart rate variability effectively distinguishes between individuals at high and at low risk *after* myocardial infarction, its analysis

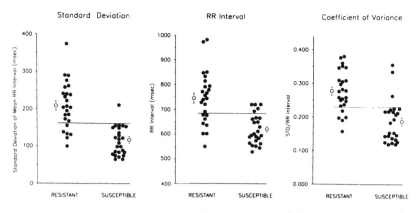

Figure 3. Scattergrams of the standard deviation (STD) of the mean, RR intervals (**left**), and RR interval (**center**) and coefficient of variance (**right**) in 25 dogs resistant (left aspect of the diagrams) and 25 dogs susceptible (right aspect of the diagrams) to sudden death 1 month after myocardial infarction. Group mean values (±SEM) (open circles) are displayed adjacent to the scatter data; discriminator placed at the midpoint of group mean values, $P < 0.05$. [From Hull et al. (28).]

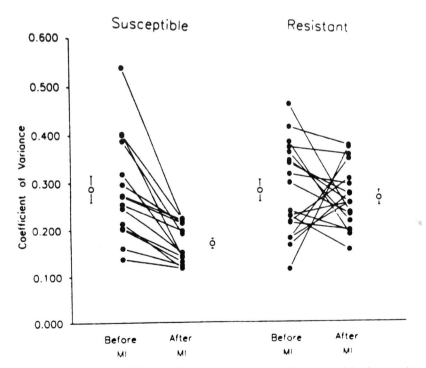

Figure 4. Scatter plots of the coefficient of variance in 15 susceptible dogs and in 18 resistant dogs before and 1 month after myocardial infarction. [From Hull et al. (28).]

41

before myocardial infarction could not predict the outcome during a subsequent ischemic episode. As a consequence, it is unlikely heart rate variability will have high predictive value in the absence of an earlier infarction. This represents a major difference with respect to our analysis of (BRS), as described in the next section.

BRS

BRS is usually regarded as a measure of "vagal reflex activity," because it quantifies the capability to increase cardiac vagal efferent activity in response to an increase in arterial blood pressure. As is the case with heart rate variability, the parameter measured is heart rate or, more precisely, duration of the R-R interval. BRS is expressed in milliseconds of increase in the R-R interval consequent to an increase of 1 mm Hg in arterial blood pressure. The method was initially described by Smyth et al. (29) for clinical hypertension studies, and the pressor agent most frequently used is the α-agonist, phenylephrine.

In 1982 Billman et al. (16) published the first study suggesting that depressed BRS was closely associated with increased risk for ventricular fibrillation in conscious dogs that had previously experienced myocardial infarction. The definitive demonstration was provided in 1988 by Schwartz et al. (3) in an unusually large ($N = 192$) experimental study involving the clinically relevant canine model for sudden death described earlier (27). Results from this work paved the way for the clinical studies that followed shortly and contributed significantly to the concept that depressed vagal activity may often be the harbinger of cardiac mortality.

Experimental Studies

After the initial serendipitous observation that survival in this preparation was often associated with vagally mediated reflex reductions in heart rate during myocardial ischemia, it became logical to evaluate vagal reflexes before exposing the dogs to the "exercise and ischemia" regime.

The most relevant finding on the issue of early identification of individuals at high risk for sudden death was that BRS was significantly lower in susceptible than in resistant dogs. After the first observation in a small study (27), more definitive results were published in 1988 (30) based on a large number of conscious and infarcted dogs ($N = 192$). As illustrated in Figs. 5 and 6, BRS was 17.7 ± 6.0 msec/mm Hg in resistant dogs and 9.1 ± 6.5 in the susceptible group ($P < 0.001$). This indicates that the capability of reflexly increasing vagal activity, as reflected in BRS, was significantly lower in those animals at higher risk of developing ventricular fibrillation. This study also allowed a calculation of the risk of developing ventricular fibrillation from a given value of BRS. For example, the risk of

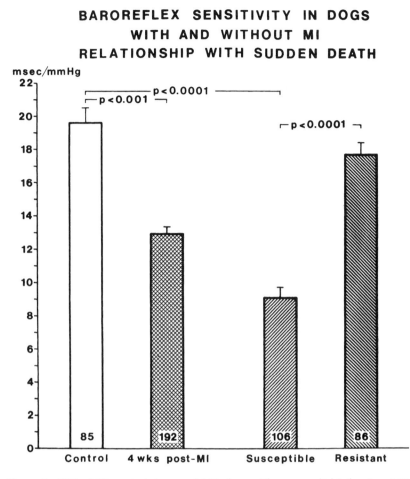

**BAROREFLEX SENSITIVITY IN DOGS
WITH AND WITHOUT MI
RELATIONSHIP WITH SUDDEN DEATH**

Figure 5. BRS of 85 control dogs and 192 dogs with myocardial infarction (MI). Former are without myocardial infarction, whereas the latter are tested 4 weeks after the production of an anterior myocardial infarction. Among the animals with myocardial infarction, 106 were susceptible and 86 were resistant to ventricular fibrillation during the exercise and ischemia test. BRSs are shown in the third and fourth columns. [From Schwartz et al. (30).]

sudden death during the exercise and ischemia test increased from 12% for a BRS > 20 msec/mm Hg to 91% for a BRS < 9 msec/mm Hg. Sensitivity was 58%, and both specificity and predictive value exceeded 90%.

A completely unexpected finding emerged from a further analysis on the group of dogs in which BRS was assessed before and after myocardial infarction. Contrary to expectation, reductions in BRS after myocardial infarction were not significantly different between resistant and susceptible dogs, and when analyzed further, we showed that the difference in BRS

BAROREFLEX SENSITIVITY AND SUDDEN DEATH

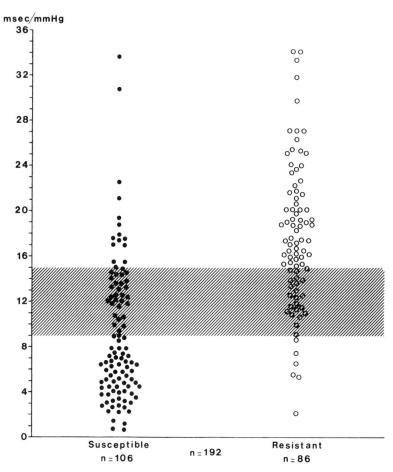

Figure 6. Plot of BRS in 192 dogs after infarction and its relation with susceptibility to sudden death. Dashed area is an arbitrary gray zone. Less than 9 msec/mm Hg, 91% of the dogs were susceptible to sudden death, whereas at >15 msec/mm Hg, 80% of the dogs survived during the exercise and ischemia test. Note the large number of animals with BRS <9 msec/mm Hg. [From Schwartz et al. (30).]

between the two groups was already present before infarction. Indeed, Fig. 7 shows that, of 68 dogs studied *before* myocardial infarction, those that would have died either during recovery from anterior myocardial infarction or during the exercise and ischemia test, already had a lower BRS compared with the dogs that would have survived.

Before this study, the possibility that analysis of autonomic reflexes in normal individuals might identify a subgroup at increased risk for sudden

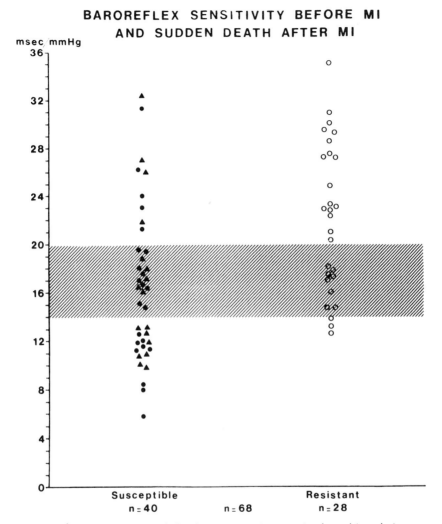

Figure 7. BRS before myocardial infarction (MI) in 68 animals and its relation with susceptibility to sudden death after myocardial infarction. In this case, the arbitrary gray zone extends from 14 to 20 msec/mm Hg. ●, dogs susceptible to sudden death during the exercise and ischemia test. ▲, dogs that died suddenly during the first 4 weeks after myocardial infarction. ○, dogs that survived during the exercise and ischemia test. Note how few animals have a BRS <9 msec/mm Hg. [From Schwartz et al. (30).]

death following myocardial infarction had not been considered. The intriguing new concept is that the individual autonomic make-up under normal conditions is characterized by such a wide range of reflex responses, exemplified by the large differences in BRS, as to allow prognostic inference about death following myocardial infarction. Myocardial infarction, besides creating an arrhythmogenic substrate, displaces the entire range of vagal responses (BRS) toward lower values, thus enhancing conditions associated with higher risk. Individual animals already at the lower end of the normal distribution of baroreflex responses find themselves, after a myocardial infarction, with very low BRS values and, thus, at very high risk for sudden death.

This finding that a depressed BRS accurately identifies a group of animals at very high risk for sudden death represents the first application of using autonomic neural parameters to obtain a more accurate prognosis of specific individuals.

Clinical Studies

The clinical implications of these experimental results immediately led to the design of the first study to test the applicability to man of the observations made with conscious dogs. The hypothesis tested was that BRS was correlated with cardiac mortality and sudden death in patients.

In the first study, La Rovere et al. (31) evaluated BRS in 78 patients with a 1-month-old myocardial infarction. This study was performed in a cardiac rehabilitation center, using entry criteria that favored enrollment of patients at relatively low risk. All patients had survived by 30 days their first myocardial infarction, were below age 65, and were able to perform a maximal exercise stress test following pharmacological washout (i.e., after all drugs had been withheld for at least 5 half-lives). These entry criteria were apparently correct, because 2-year mortality for the entire group was only 9%. During an average follow-up of 2 years, seven patients died; four of them suddenly. We found that their BRS was markedly lower (2.4 ± 1.5 vs. 8.2 ± 4.8 msec/mm Hg, P = .004) when we compared them with 71 survivors (Fig. 8). When mortality was correlated with the presence or absence of a markedly depressed BRS # 3.0 msec/mm Hg (i.e., 1 SD below the group mean), a striking difference became evident (Table 1): the risk of dying was 17 times greater for patients who 1 month after a myocardial infarction had a depressed BRS. This conclusion must be interpreted with caution, however, because of the small number of patients (N = 10) with depressed BRS. The difference in mortality, nevertheless, was sufficiently large to have meaningful implications.

The possibility that a reduced BRS represents nothing more than reduced left ventricular function is ruled out by the complete lack of correlation between BRS and left ventricular ejection fraction, assessed during left ventriculography (Fig. 9). Of special interest is the relationship between BRS, ejection fraction, and mortality (Fig. 10). It is evident that, within the group of patients with reduced left ventricular ejection fraction, risk of death was increased when there was the coexistence of a depressed BRS. This suggests that depressed pump function represents an important substrate on which unfavorable alterations in autonomic balance (i.e.,

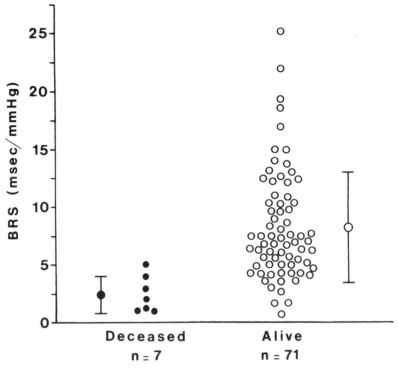

Figure 8. Plot of relation between BRS and cardiovascular mortality. Besides the clear difference in BRS ($P = 0.004$) between the deceased patients and the survivors, it is notable that, whereas all deceased patients had a reduced BRS, four of them were in the extreme lower end of the distribution of BRS for the entire population. [Updated and modified from La Rovere et al. (31).]

Table 1. BRS and Mortality

	N	Mortality %
Whole population	78	8.9
BRS > 3.0 msec/mm Hg	68	2.9
BRS # 3.0 msec/mm Hg	10	50.0

reduced vagal activity and increased sympathetic activity) can more easily act as a trigger for lethal arrhythmias. If so, these two parameters would act synergistically to seriously enhance risk. Should this hypothesis be confirmed, new perspectives for postmyocardial infarction risk stratification would be opened. This may also have practical consequences in choosing entry criteria in large mortality trials where the ability to identify not only a high-risk group, but also a group more likely to encounter death because of a specific mechanism (e.g., substrate versus autonomic trigger) becomes progressively more important.

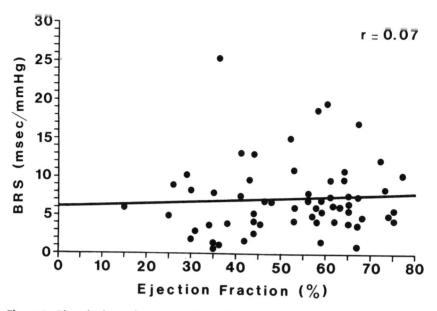

Figure 9. Plot of relation between BRS and left ventricular ejection fraction at rest. [From La Rovere et al. (31).]

Because of the small size of the population in this work, it is important to observe the results of similar studies by different groups. Our findings are supported by a recent study by Farrell et al. (32). Using the same methods we described (31), they measured BRS and heart rate variability in 68 patients who had experienced a myocardial infarction 7 to 10 days earlier. They also assessed the presence of late potentials and used programmed ventricular stimulation to evaluate the inducibility of sustained monomorphic ventricular tachycardia. An important methodological note is the striking similarity of the correlations between BRS and age ($r = -0.57$, $P < 0.001$ vs. $r = -0.53$, $P < 0.001$) and between BRS and left ventricular ejection fraction [$r = 0.07$ (NS) vs. $r = 0.035$ (NS)] in the two studies. BRS was found to be the most significant predictor of induction of sustained monomorphic ventricular tachycardia at programmed ventricular stimulation. During follow-up there were major arrhythmic events in five cases (clinical ventricular tachycardia with and without sudden death); they were all correctly identified by depressed BRS and by inducibility during electrical testing. There was an impressive difference in BRS when the patients with major arrhythmic events during follow-up were compared to those without events (0.9 ± 0.8 vs. 7.4 ± 4.6 msec/mm Hg, $P = 0.002$). Farrell et al. conclude that their study "confirms that depressed BRS identifies a subgroup at high risk for arrhythmic events following myocardial infarction" and, interestingly, add that "programmed electrical stimulation may be safely limited to this group without any loss of predictive accuracy."

RELATIONSHIP AMONG BRS, EF AND MORTALITY

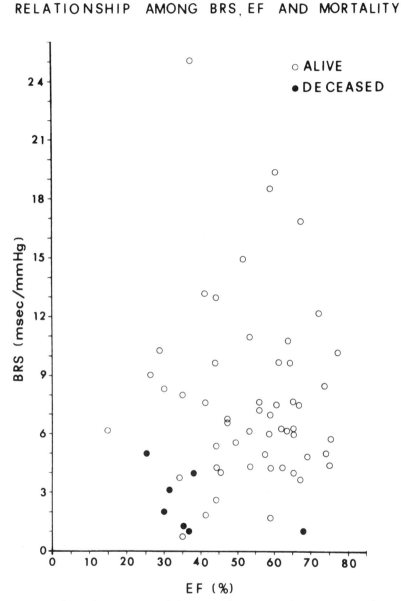

Figure 10. Relation between BRS, left ventricular ejection fraction (EF), and cardiovascular mortality. It is evident that, among patients with depressed left ventricular function, the prediction of mortality is enhanced by analysis of BRS. [Updated and modified from La Rovere et al. (31).]

49

The initial observations by Farrell et al. (33) have now been extended. During 1-year follow-up of 122 patients, there were 10 major arrhythmic events, including 5 with sudden death. The striking feature of this second study is that patients with a depressed BRS (<3 msec/mm Hg) had a relative risk of 23 for arrhythmic events during the follow-up, superior to any other variable, including the different measures of heart rate variability (relative risk of 10). Another important contribution of this study is the suggestion (Fig. 11) that a depressed BRS is particularly effective in identifying patients at risk for major arrhythmic events and for sudden death and that it is less effective when the risk is related to cardiac deaths in general.

The amount of progress achieved in predictive reliability accrued over such a brief time is very impressive. When one examines together the pioneering study by La Rovere et al. (31) and the two significant contributions by Farrell et al. (32, 33), it becomes highly likely that the clinical use of BRS should contribute substantially to postmyocardial infarction risk stratification.

Pathophysiological Considerations

The preceding studies have in turn raised several further issues. Two are addressed herein: the issue "markers" and that of implications for antifibrillatory interventions.

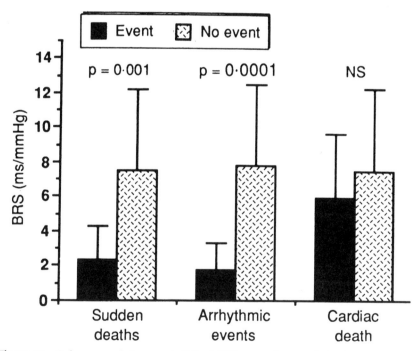

Figure 11. Column graph (mean ± SD) of BRS according to clinical events. Arrhythmic events include sudden deaths and ventricular fibrillation. [From Farrell et al. (33).]

Markers of Vagal Activity

BRS and heart rate variability are considered "markers" of reflex and of tonic vagal activity, respectively. The validity of many of the concepts generated by the analysis of these indirect events depends on how informative they are about levels of "true" cardiac vagal activity.

The only way to study vagal activity directly, as opposed to "markers," is to record the activity of single vagal fibers directed mostly to the sinus node (34, 35). Efferent vagal activity in these fibers in modulated by both vagal and sympathetic afferent activity (35) and receives a major input from the carotid sinus nerve, thus representing the efferent part of the baroreceptive reflex (Fig. 12). By means of this experimental paradigm, we have assessed directly the relationship between tonic and reflex vagal activity and susceptibility to sudden death (36).

In 17 anesthetized cats, cardiac vagal activity (single fiber) was recorded under control conditions, during blood pressure increases elicted by phenylephrine, and during a 60-min occlusion of the left anterior descending coronary artery. Ventricular fibrillation occurred within 3 min of occlusion in 9 cats defined as "susceptible," whereas the remaining 8 survived and were defined "resistant." Whereas resting vagal activity ("tonic") was similar in the two groups (1.48 ± 0.30 vs. 1.58 ± 0.35), the reflex increase following blood pressure elevation was markedly smaller in the susceptible animals (80 ± 14% vs. 246 ± 66%, $P < 0.05$) (Fig. 13). Also, vagal activity did not change in the susceptible animals (-18%) during the first 2 min of coronary occlusion; it markedly increased in the resistant animals (100%, $P < 0.05$).

These data from anesthetized animals agree with our observations on conscious dogs made using "markers" of vagal activity. This study shows that animals that survive coronary artery occlusion are capable of reflexly increasing vagal activity during acute myocardial ischemia and that outcome can be predicted by analysis of the reflex response to a baroreceptive stimulus, but not by analysis of tonic activity. "Tonic" vagal activity, as defined herein, is the resting activity seen in anesthetized animals; only with caution can this be extrapolated to the conscious state.

Antifibrillatory Effect of Vagal Activity

Based on experimental and clinical data regarding the relationship between reduced vagal activity and susceptibility to ventricular fibrillation, one would expect a protective effect to be associated with augmented vagal activity. We have explored this possibility using both electrical and pharmacologic means.

Interest in previous reports on the antifibrillatory potential of vagal stimulation (4, 8, 37) has been limited by the use of anesthesia in most

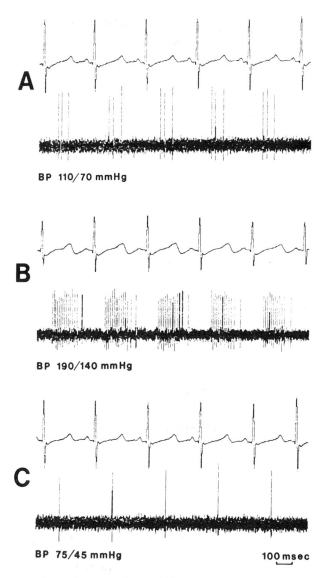

BP 110/70 mmHg

BP 190/140 mmHg

BP 75/45 mmHg 100 msec

Figure 12. Recordings showing effects of blood pressure increase (by aortic occlusion) and sympathetic afferent activation (by electrical stimulation) of the cut central end of the left inferior cardiac nerve, on the discharge of a single efferent vagal fiber in an intact, anesthetized cat. Broken line indicates stenosis of the aorta, and solid line indicates sympathetic stimulation. The two strips are continuous recordings. Tracings in each section from **top** to **bottom** are as follows: respiration, systemic arterial blood pressure, electrocardiogram, and neural activity. This vagal fiber begins to fire only in response to blood pressure elevation (baroreceptor reflex), and the concurrent afferent sympathetic stimulation is able to interfere with this response. [Modified from Schwartz et al. (35).]

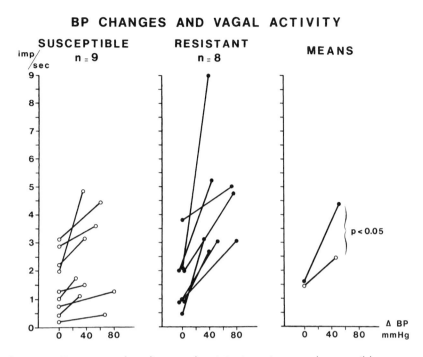

BP CHANGES AND VAGAL ACTIVITY

Figure 13. Responses of cardiac vagal activity in resistant and susceptible cats, during increases in mean blood pressure (BP) following phenylephrine injection. The **left** and **middle** panels show individual responses, whereas the **right** panel shows the mean response of each group. Values are expressed as imp/sec. Open circles, susceptible cats; filled circles, resistant cats. [From Cerati and Schwartz (36).]

experiments, the lack of an effective cardioselective muscarinic agonist, and the widely held view that electrical stimulation of the vagus in conscious animals was not feasible. We developed a chronically implantable device that is placed around the cervical right vagus that allows effective stimulation without discomfort (38). One month after myocardial infarction, 54 dogs were identified as "susceptible" using exercise and ischemia testing: they all developed ventricular fibrillation. They were then allocated to randomized groups in which the exercise and ischemia test was repeated under control conditions or following implantation of the vagal device (11). Vagal stimulation in the latter group was initiated shortly after onset of occlusion of the circumflex coronary artery, whereas the dogs were performing submaximal exercise stress. In the control group, 22 of 24 (92%) dogs again developed ventricular fibrillation during a second exercise and ischemia test. By contrast, during vagal stimulation, ventricular fibrillation occurred again in only 3 of 30 dogs (10%) and recurred in 26 (87%) during an additional exercise and ischemia test performed once more in the absence of vagal stimulation. The difference in the incidence of ventricular fibrillation was

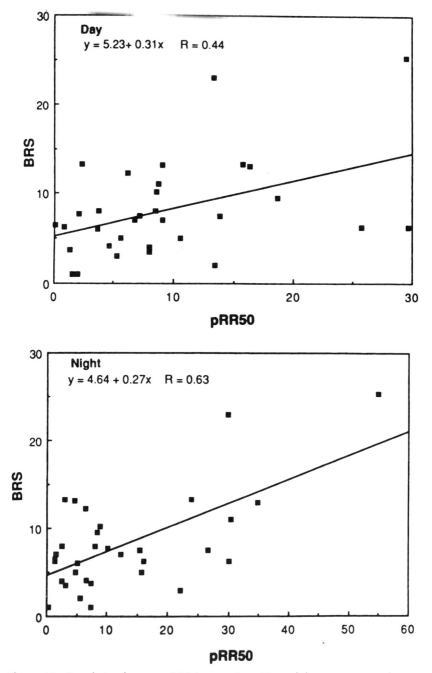

Figure 14. Correlation between BRS in msec/mm Hg and the percentage of successive normal RR intervals differing >50 msec (pRR50) plotted separately for day and night. [From Bigger et al. (42).]

between the two types of measurement, as preliminary data indicate, it would be logical to use only the noninvasive method. This could represent a major advance in the clinical use of BRS testing.

The entire community awaits the results of ATRAMI, as data are accumulated and analyzed over the coming years. This trial has considerable potential to advance understanding and treatment of the problems of sudden cardiac death and should help guide our use of these tools for some years to come. It illustrates extraordinarily well the potential resulting from applying experimental concepts to clinical realities.

References

1. Schwartz, P.J., Brown, A.M., Malliani, A., and Zanchetti, A., Eds. (1978). *Neural Mechanisms in Cardiac Arrhythmias* (Raven Press, New York), pp. 1–442.

2. Lown, B. (1979). Sudden cardiac death: The major challenge confronting contemporary cardiology. *Am. J. Cardiol.* **43:**313–320.

3. Corr, P.B., Yamada, K.A., and Witkowski, F.X. (1986). Mechanisms controlling cardiac autonomic function and their relation to arrhythmogenesis, in *The Heart and Cardiovascular System*, H.A. Fozzard, E. Haber, R.B. Jennings, A.M. Katz, and H.E. Morgan, Eds. (Raven Press, New York), pp. 1343–1403.

4. Schwartz, P.J., and Stramba-Badiale, M. (1988). Parasympathetic nervous system and cardiac arrhythmias, in *Neurocardiology*, H.E. Kulbertus and G. Frank, Eds. (Futura Publishing Co., Mount Kisco, NY), pp. 179–200.

5. Schwartz, P.J., and Priori, S.G. (1990). Sympathetic nervous system and cardiac arrhythmias, in *Cardiac Electrophysiology. From Cell to Bedside*, D.P. Zipes and J. Jalife, Eds. (W.B. Saunders Co., Philadelphia), pp. 330–343.

6. Lown, B., and Verrier, R.L. (1976). Neural activity and ventricular fibrillation. *N. Engl. J. Med.* **294:**1165–1170.

7. Schwartz, P.J., and Stone, H.L. (1982). The role of the autonomic nervous system in sudden coronary death. *Ann. N.Y. Acad. Sci.* **382:**162–181.

8. Verrier, R.L., and Lown, B. (1978). Sympathetic-parasympathetic interactions and ventricular electrical stability, in *Neural Mechanisms in Cardiac Arrhythmias*, P.J. Schwartz, A.M. Brown, A. Malliani, and A. Zanchetti, Eds. (Raven Press, New York), pp. 75–85.

9. Schwartz, P.J., and Vanoli, E. (1981). Cardiac arrhythmias elicited by interaction between acute myocardial ischemia and sympathetic hyperactivity: A new experimental model for the study of antiarrhythmic drugs. *J. Cardiovasc. Pharmacol.* **3:**1251–1259.

10. Kolman, B.S., Verrier, R.L., and Lown, B. (1975). The effect of vagus nerve stimulation upon vulnerability of the canine ventricle: Role of the sympathetic-parasympathetic interactions. *Circulation* **52:**578–585.

11. Vanoli, E, De Ferrari, G.M., Stramba-Badiale, M., Hull, S.S. Jr., Foreman, R.D., and Schwartz, P.J. (1991). Vagal stimulation and prevention of

sudden death in conscious dogs with a healed myocardial infarction. *Circ. Res.* **68**:1471–1481.

12. De Ferrari, G.M., Vanoli, E., Stramba-Badiale, M., Hull, S.S., Jr., Foreman, R.D., and Schwartz, P.J. (1991). Vagal reflexes and survival during acute myocardial ischemia in conscious dogs with healed myocardial infarction. *Am. J. Physiol.* **261**:H63–H69.

13. Yusuf, S., and Teo, K.K. (1991). Approaches to prevention of sudden death: Need for fundamental reevaluation. *J. Cardiovasc. Electrophysiol.* **2**(Suppl):S233–S239.

14. Schwartz, P.J., Locati, E.H., Moss, A.J., Crampton, R.S., Trazzi, R., and Ruberti, U. (1991). Left cardiac sympathetic denervation in the therapy of the congenital long QT syndrome. A worldwide report. *Circulation* **84**:503–511.

15. Schwartz, P.J., Motolese, M., Pollavini, G., Malliani, A., Ruberti, U., Trazzi, R., Bartorelli, C., Zanchetti, A., Lotto, A., and The Sudden Death Italian Prevention Group. (1992). Prevention of sudden cardiac death after a first myocardial infarction by pharmacological or surgical antiadrenergic interventions. *J. Cardiovasc. Electrophysiol.* **3**:2–16.

16. Billman, G.E., Schwartz, P.J., and Stone, H.L. (1982). Baroreceptor reflex control of heart rate: A predictor of sudden cardiac death. *Circulation* **66**:874–880.

17. Schwartz, P.J., La Rovere, M.T., and Vanoli, E. (1992). Autonomic nervous system and sudden cardiac death. *Circulation* **85**(Suppl. I):I77–I91.

18. Schwartz, P.J., La Rovere, M.T., Mortara, A., and Vanoli, E. (1992). Autonomic nervous system and sudden cardiac death. A rational basis for postmyocardial infarction risk stratification, in *Sudden Cardiac Death*, M. Akhtar, Ed. (Andover Medical Publishers, Inc., Wayne, PA), in press.

19. De Ferrari, G.M., Vanoli, E., and Schwartz, P.J. (1993). Vagal activity and ventricular fibrillation, in *Vagal Control of the Heart*, M.N. Levy and P.J. Schwartz, Eds. (Futura Publishing Co., Mount Kisco, NY), in press.

20. Vanoli, E., La Rovere, M.T., Mortara, A., and Schwartz, P.J. (1993). Methods for assessment of vagal reflexes, in *Vagal Control of the Heart*, M.N. Levy and P.J. Schwartz, Eds. (Futura Publishing Co., Mount Kisco, NY), in press.

21. Bigger, J.T., and Schwartz, P.J. (1993). Markers of vagal activity and the prediction of cardiac death after myocardial infarction, in *Vagal Control of the Heart*, M.N. Levy and P.J. Schwartz, Eds. (Futura Publishing Co., Mount Kisco, NY), in press.

22. Wolf, M., Varigos, G., Hunt, D., and Sloman, J. (1978). Sinus arrhythmia in acute myocardial infarction. *Med. J. Austral.* **2**:52–53.

23. Kleiger, R.E., Miller, J.P., Bigger, J.T., Jr., Moss, A.J., and the Multicenter Postinfarction Research Group. (1987). Decreased heart rate variability and its association with increased mortality after acute myocardial infarction. *Am. J. Cardiol.* **59**:256–262.

24. Bigger, J.T., Jr., Fleiss, J.L., Steinman, R.C., Rolnitzky, L.M., Kleiger, R.E., and Rottman, J.N. (1992). Frequency domain measures of heart period variability and mortality after myocardial infarction. *Circulation* **85**:164–171.

25. Odemuyiwa, O., Malik, M., Farrell, T., Bashir, Y., Poloniecki, J., and Camm, A.J. (1991). Comparison of the predictive characteristics of heart rate variability index and left ventricular ejection fraction for all-cause mortality, arrhythmic events and sudden death after acute myocardial infarction. *Am. J. Cardiol.* **68:** 434–439.

26. Farrell, T.G., Bashir, Y., Cripps, T., Malik, M., Poloniecki, J., Bennett, E.D., Ward, D.E., and Camm, A.J. (1991). Risk stratification for arrhythmic events in postinfarction patients based on heart rate variability, ambulatory electrocardiographic variables and the signal-averaged electrocardiogram. *J. Am. Coll. Cardiol.* **18:**687–697.

27. Schwartz, P.J., Billman, G.E., and Stone, HL. (1984). Autonomic mechanisms in ventricular fibrillation induced by myocardial ischemia during exercise in dogs with a healed myocardial infarction. An experimental preparation for sudden cardiac death. *Circulation* **69:**780–790.

28. Hull, S.S., Evans, A.R., Vanoli, E., Adamson, P.B., Stramba-Badiale, M., Albert, D.E., Foreman, R.D., and Schwartz, P.J. (1990). Heart rate variability before and after myocardial infarction in conscious dogs at high and low risk of sudden death. *J. Am. Coll. Cardiol.* **16:**978–985.

29. Smyth, H.S., Sleight, P., and Pickering, G.W. (1969). Reflex regulation of arterial pressure during sleep in man: A quantitative method of assessing baroreflex sensitivity. *Circ. Res.* **24:**109–121.

30. Schwartz, P.J., Vanoli, E., Stramba-Badiale, M., De Ferrari, G.M., Billman, G.E., and Foreman, R.D. (1988). Autonomic mechanisms and sudden death. New insight from the analysis of baroreceptor reflexes in conscious dogs with and without a myocardial infarction. *Circulation* **78:** 969–979.

31. La Rovere, M.T., Specchia, G., Mortara, A., and Schwartz, P.J. (1988). Baroreflex sensitivity, clinical correlates and cardiovascular mortality among patients with a first myocardial infarction: A prospective study. *Circulation* **78:**816–824.

32. Farrell, T.G., Paul, V., Cripps, T.R., Malik, M., Bennett, E.D., Ward, D., and Camm, A.J. (1991). Baroreflex sensitivity and electrophysiological correlates in patients after acute myocardial infarction. *Circulation* **83:**945–952.

33. Farrell, T.G., Odemuyiwa, O., Bashir, Y., Cripps, T.R., Malik, M., Ward, D.E., and Camm, A.J. (1992). Prognostic value of baroreflex sensitivity testing after acute myocardial infarction. *Br. Heart J.* **67:**129–137.

34. Kunze, D.L. (1972). Reflex discharge patterns of cardiac vagal efferent fibres. *J. Physiol.* **222:**1–15.

35. Schwartz, P.J., Pagani, M., Lombardi, F., Malliani, A., and Brown, A.M. (1973). A cardiocardiac sympatho-vagal reflex in the cat. *Circ. Res.* **32:**215–220.

36. Cerati, D., and Schwartz, P.J. (1991). Single cardiac vagal fiber activity, acute myocardial ischemia, and risk for sudden death. *Circ. Res.* **69:**1389–1401.

37. Verrier, R.L. (1986). Neurochemical approaches to the prevention of ventricular fibrillation. *Fed. Proc.* **45:** 2191–2196.

38. Stramba-Badiale, M., Vanoli, E., De Ferrari, G.M., Cerati, D., Foreman, R.D., and Schwartz, P.J. (1991). Sympathetic-parasympathetic interaction

and accentuated antagonism in conscious dogs. *Am. J. Physiol.* **260:**H335–H340.

39. Schwartz, P.J., Vanoli, E., Zaza, A., and Zuanetti, G. (1985). The effect of antiarrhythmic drugs on life-threatening arrhythmias induced by the interaction between acute myocardial ischemia and sympathetic hyperactivity. *Am. Heart J.* **109:**937–948.

40. De Ferrari, G.M., Vanoli, E., Curcuruto, P., Tommasini, G., and Schwartz, P.J. (1992). Prevention of life-threatening arrhythmias by pharmacologic stimulation of the muscarinic receptors with oxotremorine. *Am. Heart J.* **124:**883–890.

41. De Ferrari, G.M., Salvati, P., Grossoni, M., Ukmar, G., Vaga, L., Patrono, C., and Schwartz, P.J. (1993). Pharmacologic modulation of the autonomic nervous system in the prevention of sudden cardiac death. *J. Am. Coll. Cardiol.*, manuscript submitted for publication.

42. Bigger, J.T., Jr., La Rovere, M.T., Steinman, R.C., Fleiss, J.L., Rottman, J.N., Rolnitzky, L.M., and Schwartz, P.J. (1989). Comparison of baroreflex sensitivity and heart period variability after myocardial infarction. *J. Am. Coll. Cardiol.* **14:**1511–1518.

43. Pagani, M., Lombardi, F., Guzzetti, S., Rimoldi, O., Furlan, R., Pizzinelli, P., Sandrone, G., Malfatto, G., Dell'Orto, S., Piccaluga, E., Turiel, M., Baselli, G., Cerutti, S., and Malliani, A. (1986). Power spectral analysis of heart rate and arterial pressure variabilities as a marker of sympatho-vagal interaction in man and conscious dog. *Cir. Res.* **59:**178–193.

44. Pomeranz, M., Macaulay, R.J.B., Caudill, M.A., Kutz, I., Adam, D., Gordon, D., Kilborn, K.M., Barger, A.C., Shannon, D.C., Cohen, R.J., and Benson, M. (1985). Assessment of autonomic function in humans by heart rate spectral analysis. *Am. J. Physiol.* **248:**H151–H153.

4

Autonomic Mechanisms Underlying Arrhythmogenesis and Sudden Cardiac Death in Ischemic Heart Disease

Douglas P. Zipes

$\mathbf{T}$wo major sets of nerves link the heart to the central nervous system, carrying information *from* the heart over neural afferents and *to* the heart over neural efferents (1, 2). These nerves, the parasympathetic (vagus) and sympathetic nerves, are part of normal functional control pathways and also can affect the development of cardiac arrhythmias. The mechanisms by which this happens are incompletely understood. This chapter therefore deals with some of the fundamentals of these various interactions.

Autonomic Innervation of the Heart

Although significant overlap and complex patterns of innervation exist, in general, autonomic neural input to the heart exhibits some degree of "sidedness." The right sympathetic and vagus nerves affect the sinus node pacemaker region of the right atrium more than they modulate the atrioventricular (AV) node conducting portion of the heart, whereas the left sympathetic and vagus nerves affect the AV node more than the sinus node (3).

Recent functional studies of intracardiac neural pathways indicate that afferent vagal fibers cross the AV groove in the superficial subepicardium and then penetrate the myocardium, at which point they are probably located in the subendocardium. In contrast, afferent sympathetic fibers appear to be located in the superficial subepicardium throughout most of their course (Fig. 1). Similarly, sympathetic efferents are superficially placed, whereas most efferent vagal fibers in route to the ventricle cross the AV groove within 0.25 to 0.5 mm of the epicardial surface and dive intramurally, where they are located in the subendocardium (4). Vagal efferent fibers crossing the AV groove are probably postganglionic axons with the ganglion cells located in the atria (5).

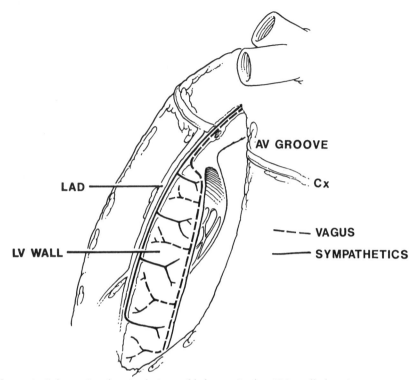

Figure 1. Schematic of sagittal view of left ventricular (LV) wall showing pathways of vagal and sympathetic afferent and efferent nerves. Postganglionic sympathetic axons are located superficially in periadventia of coronary arteries; postganglionic vagal axons cross the AV groove in subepicardium but are located in subendocardium. Cx, circumflex coronary artery; LAD, left ventricular descending coronary artery.

Pericardium

Because the vagal fibers for part of their course, and sympathetic fibers throughout most of their course, are located in the superficial subepicardium, it might be possible for substances in the pericardial fluid that bathes these fibers to modulate their function. Instilling hexamethonium (500 µM), a ganglionic blocker, into the pericardial sac results in block of efferent vagal responses but not efferent sympathetic responses, proving that only vagal ganglia are located on the epicardium (Fig. 2). Sympathetic ganglia are located in the paravertebral sympathetic chain and would not be expected to be affected by pericardial fluid. In contrast, tetrodotoxin (5 µM), a sodium channel blocker that interrupts axonal neurotransmission, when instilled in the pericardial space, suppresses changes in refractoriness induced by both efferent vagal and sympathetic stimulation (Fig. 2). Tetrodotoxin does not block postjunctional responses produced by intravenous methacholine or norepinephrine, indicating that the postjunc-

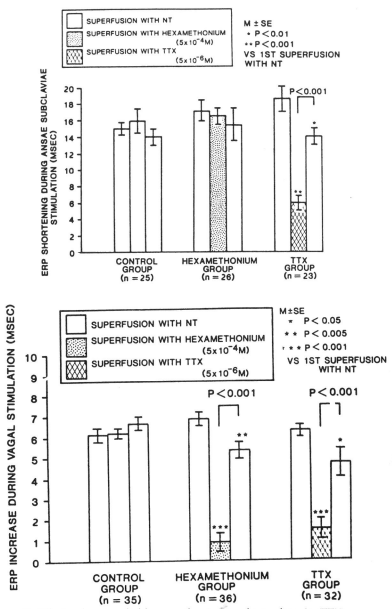

Figure 2. Effects of pericardial hexamethonium and tetrodotoxin (TTX).
Top: Effects of epicardial superfusion with hexamethonium and tetrodotoxin on ansae subclaviae-induced prolongation of ventricular refractoriness. **Bottom:** Effects of epicardial superfusion with hexamethonium and tetrodotoxin on changes in ventricular refractoriness induced by bilateral vagal stimulation. ERP, effective refractory period; NT, normal Tyrode's solution; n, number of test sites. [From Zipes (4).]

tional target tissue, (i.e., the myocardium) is not directly affected by this intervention (6) (Fig. 3). These neural responses to pericardial instillation of hexamethonium and tetrodotoxin prove that substances in the pericardial fluid can modulate neural activity to the heart.

Interestingly, the pericardium is capable of synthesizing prostaglandins as a response to several stimuli, including the introduction of arachidonic acid into the pericardial sac. Pericardial prostaglandins reduce sympathetic efferent action on the heart, thereby modulating sympathetic acceleration of sinus rate, AV nodal conduction, and refractory period shortening of the myocardium. Because these prostaglandin-induced changes do not blunt the response to intravenous infusion of norepinephrine, the actions of the pericardial prostaglandin are due to prejunctional modulation of cardiac sympathetic neurotransmission rather than to an alteration in postjunctional (myocardial) responsiveness. Thus, increased concentration of prostaglandins in the pericardial fluid in response to various stimuli could constitute a physiological negative feedback control mechanism that regulates efferent sympathetic stimulation of the heart (7).

Pericardial prostaglandins do not reduce cardiac responses to efferent vagal stimulation or afferent vagal or sympathetic reflexes produced from the heart. Such autonomic changes elicited by pericardial prostaglandins

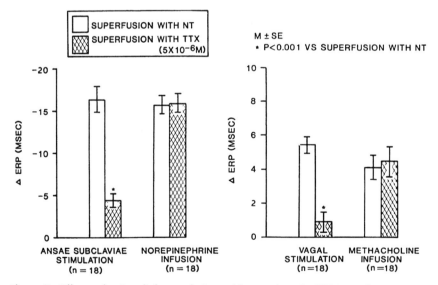

Figure 3. Effects of epicardial superfusion with tetrodotoxin (TTX) on changes in ventricular effective refractory period (ΔERP) induced by neural stimulation and by intravenous administration of norepinephrine (0.25 μg/kg/min) and methacholine (12.5 or 25 μg/kg/min). The effects of vagal stimulation and methacholine on the effective refractory period were determined during intravenous infusion of norepinephrine (0.125 μg/kg/min). NT, normal Tyrode's solution; n, number of test sites. [From Blomquist et al. (5).]

could be antiarrhythmic by preserving efferent vagal actions while reducing efferent sympathetic effects. In fact, pericardial prostaglandins can prevent ventricular fibrillation induced by reperfusion of an occluded coronary artery during sympathetic stimulation (8) (Fig. 4). Whether such pericardial modulation of sympathetic actions on the heart is important clinically is not known.

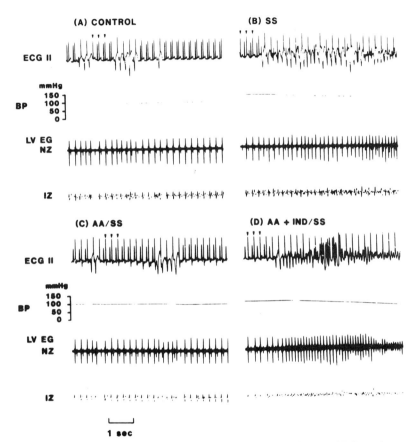

Figure 4. Tracings from a dog showing the effect of stimulation of bilateral ansae subclaviae (SS) on reperfusion-induced ventricular fibrillation and reversal by epicardial superfusion with arachidonic acid solution. Simultaneous recordings of lead II electrocardiogram (ECG II), mean arterial blood pressure (BP), and local bipolar electrograms (EG) of the left ventricular (LV), normal (NZ), and ischemic (IZ) zones immediately after reperfusion are shown. Arrows in the ECG II indicate the stimuli from right atrial pacing to maintain a constant heart rate. AA, epicardial superfusion with Tyrode's solution containing arachidonic acid (3μg/ml); AA plus IND, epicardial superfusion with arachidonic acid (3 μg/ml) plus indomethacin (3μg/ml). In (**A**) and (**C**), only nonsustained ventricular tachycardia developed. In (**B**) and (**D**), ventricular fibrillation resulted. [From Miyazaki et al. (7).]

Effects of Myocardial Ischemia and Infarction on Neurotransmission To and From the Heart

Afferent Reflexes

Myocardial ischemia or infarction and reperfusion can trigger afferent cardiac reflexes (9). However, ischemia or infraction, in addition to stimulating mechanosensitive and chemosensitive sensory nerve endings in the ischemic myocardium, can impair neurotransmission (10, 11). Axons can become ischemic, infarcted or dysfunctional, because they lie in an ischemic myocardial milieu that can adversely effect neural function. This can result in loss of normal neural responsiveness in the area of the ischemia or infarction. In addition, myocardium apical to the site of ischemia or infarction, but not otherwise involved in the process, can lose normal neural function because nerve fibers serving the apex, but traveling through ischemic segment located more basally, can develop impaired function. Thus, myocardial injury that was either functional and transient, or anatomical and permanent, can disrupt autonomic neural transmission to the infarction and sites distal to it, resulting in areas of regional denervation (12, 13). This interaction between ischemically damaged myocardium and altered neural innervation can cause cardiac arrhythmias (14–17).

Ample evidence in animals supports these possibilities. Myocardial ischemia or infarction has been shown to interrupt cardiac reflexes soon after the onset of coronary occlusion. Several minutes after creating transmural myocardial ischemia, the sympathetic reflex elicited from the epicardium of the ischemic area or apical to it becomes interrupted or attenuated when the myocardial blood flow in the epicardial test site decreases to ~ 40% or less of the control value (Fig. 5). In contrast, nontransmural ischemia does not attenuate the epicardial sympathetic reflex, but does attenuate the vagal vasodepressor response, as would be expected from the functional pathways described in Fig. 1. A 15-min coronary occlusion followed by reperfusion produces reversible attenuation of vagal and sympathetic epicardial reflexes. Loss of these reflex responses so quickly after the onset of ischemia and their return with reperfusion suggests initial functional neural impairment (10, 11).

Because myocardial ischemia and infarction have been shown to trigger cardiac reflexes, and because these considerations indicate that inhibition of reflexes can also result, it is likely that the resultant physiological response to ischemia or infarction is a balance between these inhibiting and activating conditions.

These observations from experimental animals may be relevant to real clinical situations. For example, the mechanism responsible for painless ischemia is unknown. Because afferent sympathetic fibers appear to mediate cardiac pain sensation, it is possible that some patients have a form of "autodenervation." Ischemia could interrupt afferent neurotransmission

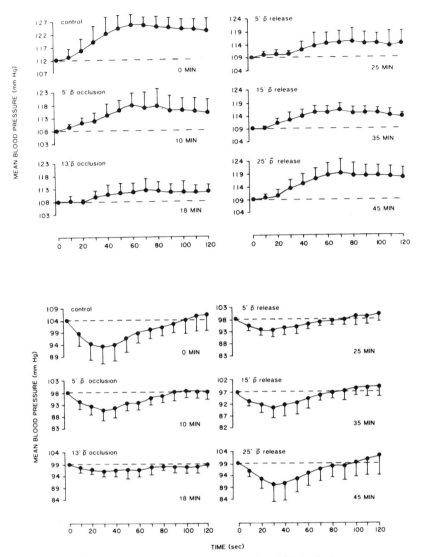

Figure 5. Top: Changes in vasopressor response to bradykinin during snare occlusion of multiple coronary arteries and after reperfusion. Mean arterial pressure is shown on ordinate. Dotted line is baseline value (i.e., average of mean arterial blood pressure when bradykinin was applied at 0 sec). Brackets indicate standard deviation for changes in mean arterial blood pressure from the baseline value. Small numbers to the **left** indicate time after occlusion or release. Large numbers to the **right** indicate number of minutes elapsed from determination of control value (0 min). **Bottom:** Changes in vasodepressor response to nicotine during snare occlusion of a diagonal branch and after reperfusion. [From Inoue et al. (11).]

with elimination of pain perception, Recovery of neurotransmission would occur with reperfusion, so that another episode of ischemia, perhaps localized differently and sparing the epicardium, might then produce anginal pain in the same subject.

Efferent Responses

Transmural myocardial ischemia or infarction also alters efferent sympathetic and vagal presynaptic function, in a fashion similar to that noted for afferent reflexes, and produces efferent sympathetic and vagal denervation at the infarct site, as well as at noninfarcted sites apical to that zone (12, 13). Subendocardial infarction that spares the epicardium interrupts vagal innervation, but not sympathetic transmission, consistent with the diagram noted in Fig. 1. The noninfarcted myocardial rim overlying a subendocardial infarction also has a transiently depressed response to sympathetic nerve stimulation, possibly due to local factors released by the adjacent infarct (18).

Heterogeneous loss of functional efferent sympathetic innervation in noninfarcted apical sites occurs as early as 5 to 20 min after transmural ischemia created by coronary occlusion, with more complete denervation progressing with time. Some sites may undergo partial denervation initially, which evolves as the occlusion is maintained (Fig. 6). Importantly, the activity of tyrosine hydroxylase, a neurochemical marker for sympathetic innervation, decreases significantly in the ischemic left ventricle only after ~ 5 hr of ligation of the left anterior descending coronary artery. Ischemia-produced efferent vagal denervation follows a time course similar to that for efferent sympathetic denervation. However, the activity of the enzyme critical for synthesis of acetylcholine, choline acetyltransferase, does not decrease significantly until many hours after coronary ligation (19).

The mechanisms responsible for loss of afferent and efferent neural responses is not known. However, accumulation of metabolites in the ischemic myocardium through which the nerves pass is sufficient to produce neural dysfunction in myocardium apical to the ischemic site. Support for this concept comes from studies replicating the denervation response by perfusing a coronary artery with a hypoxic Tyrode's solution containing 12 mM potassium and 10 μM, adenosine with a pH of 6.8. A similar result can be achieved by infusing this solution into the pericardial sac. Thus, ischemia of the nerves themselves is not necessary to produce neural dysfunction; accumulation of metabolites in the ischemic myocardium through which the nerves pass is sufficient to produce neural dysfunction in myocardium apical to the ischemia (20). These experiments may explain the functional derangement in neural activity occurring initially, with measurable decreases in transmitter concentration or enzyme activity lagging behind and following the onset of actual neural damage as the infarction develops and progresses over time.

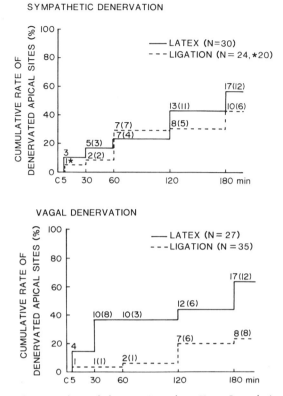

Figure 6. Sympathetic and vagal denervation plots. **Top:** Cumulative percentage of sympathetically denervated apical sites divided by number of total apical test sites (N) shown on ordinate as function of time. Solid line indicates data from dogs with latex coronary injection; dashed line indicates data from dogs with coronary ligation; numbers without parentheses indicate the cumulative number of denervated test sites (total number of sites that had shown shortening of effective refractory period #2 msec at least once by that moment of determination); numbers in parentheses indicate the number of test sites that showed shortening of effective refractory period #2 msec at that moment of determination. Presentation in this manner is necessary because some sites showed variation in response around cutoff value. For example, 120 to 180 min after latex injection, four new sites (17 − 13) became denervated, whereas only 12 of the 17 sites still exhibited shortening of effective refractory period #2 msec at 180 min. The remaining five sites that had shown shortening of effective refractory period #2 msec at least once by 120 min now exhibited refractory period shortening >2 msec at 180 min after infarction. Cumulative rate of denervated sites did not differ between dogs receiving latex injection and those receiving coronary artery ligation (*P* = 0.41). C, control before coronary occlusion. *Data from one dog that developed ventricular fibrillation were not included at 5 min after ligation. **Bottom:** Plot showing cumulative percentage of vagally denervated apical sites is shown as in top panel and was greater in dogs receiving latex injection than in dogs with ligation of coronary arteries (*P* < 0.002). [From Inoue and Zipes (13).]

Modulation of Extracellular Potassium Changes During Ischemia

Because these observations suggest that accumulation of extracellular potassium during ischemia, along with pH reduction and accumulation of such substances as adenosine, may be important in the development of subsequent sympathetic denervation, our laboratory determined the effects of various interventions on extracellular potassium accumulation during acute myocardial ischemia. We found that sympathetic neural stimulation increased the extracellular potassium concentration evoked by 5 minutes of left anterior descending coronary artery occlusions at most sites in the ischemic myocardium (Fig. 7). Interestingly, however, intravenously infused norepinephrine decreased extracellular potassium concentration during 5 min of left anterior descending occlusion (21). Because both sympathetic neural stimulation and norepinephrine infusion increased myocardial blood flow in ischemic and normal myocardium, it is unlikely that alterations in blood flow alone are responsible for the disparate effects of sympathetic stimulation and norepinephrine infusion on ischemia-induced increases in extracellular potassium concentration. It is possible that substances other than norepinephrine, (e.g., neuropeptide Y) that are released from sympathetic nerve terminals may modify cardiac function globally and at the cellular level to enhance extracellular potassium accumulation during acute myocardial ischemia.

In another series of studies (22), we investigated the role of ATP-sensitive potassium channels in modulating the efferent autonomic response during acute myocardial ischemia/infarction. We found that the ATP-sensitive potassium channel blocker, glibenclamide, increased the extent of cumulative denervation at test sites apical to the area of ischemia/

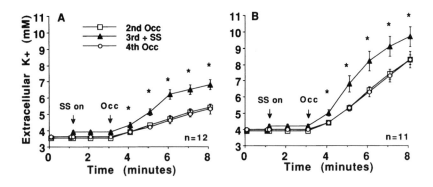

Figure 7. Effects of sympathetic stimulation (SS) at sites where the extracellular K^+ concentration increased to <7 mM (**A**) or >7mM (**B**) during the second and fourth occlusions (Occ). Sympathetic stimulation was begun 2 min before the third occlusion only. Data are from 23 K^+ electrodes in 11 dogs. Values are mean ± SEM (*$P < 0.03$). [From Warner et al. (21).]

infarction during a 3-hr period, whereas the ATP-sensitive potassium channel opener, pinacidil, reduced the extent of denervation. Infarct size was similar in both groups. These results suggest that the opening of ATP-sensitive potassium channels exerts a protective effect by reducing the extent of sympathetic denervation after acute myocardial ischemia/infarction. The mechanism by which this occurs is not known, but may relate to the marked shortening of cardiac action potential duration that could reduce calcium entry into the cells, which in turn could decease ATP consumption and delay ischemic cell death. Glibendamide, by blocking ATP-sensitive potassium channels, deceases action potential shortening during ischemia and could contribute to intracellular calcium overload, whereas ATP-sensitive potassium channel openers, such as pinacidil, encourage shortening of action potential duration, which could reduce intracellular calcium accumulation and preserve cellular function.

Preconditioning Ischemia

The extent of denervation can be reduced by myocardial preconditioning ischemia (23). Transient ischemia can condition the heart to resist the denervating effects subsequently of prolonged ischemia or infarction. For example, four 5-min episodes of coronary occlusion and reperfusion preserve the efferent sympathetic response during the first hour of the subsequent sustained ischemia and preserve the efferent vagal response for at least 3 hr (24). The mechanism responsible for preconditioning ischemia is not known, but does not appear to be related to reduced pH or adenosine. We tested this hypothesis by intracoronary perfusion of Tyrode's solution containing ischemic metabolites composed of 12 mM potassium, (pH 6.8) and 10 μM adenosine. In contrast to the results obtained by four 5-min periods of coronary artery occlusion and reperfusion, in dogs receiving the ischemic perfusion noted previously, effective refractory period shortening induced by sympathetic stimulation became significantly attenuated at apical sites after coronary artery occlusion (25). Thus, brief exposure of the left ventricular myocardium to ischemic metabolites before a subsequent permanent coronary artery occlusion did not trigger these mechanisms responsible for protection against efferent sympathetic denervation apical to an area of transmural myocardial infarction/ischemia.

Denervation Supersensitivity

Supersensitivity in denervated areas of the myocardium follows several days after the coronary artery occlusion and is manifest by an exaggerated shortening of refractoriness during both norepinephrine and isoproterenol infusions, with an upward and leftward shift in the dose-response curves in the apical denervated regions of the ventricle (26, 27). Such denervation supersensitivity elicits inhomogeneous autonomic and electrophysiological changes and makes the heart vulnerable to electrical induction of ventricular arrhythmias. Propranolol significantly attentuates this vulnerability (14). β-adrenoceptor blockade following myocardial infarction in humans may reduce the incidence of sudden cardiac death in part by attenuating the effects of denervation supersensitivity on dispersion of refractoriness, conduction changes, or other regional electrophysiologic properties.

Regional sympathetic denervation and supersensitivity can also modulate drug actions and cause the drugs to affect the myocardium heterogeneously. (28) Such changes can set the stage for proarrhythmic responses.

The mechanism responsible for this type of postganglionic sympathetic supersensitivity is not clear, because there is no difference in denervated apical myocardium, compared with normal vasomyocardium, in the density of β-adrenergic receptors, their dissociation constants, adenylate cyclase activity, or G-protein synthesis (29).

Effects of Sympathetic Scintigraphy

In an effort to explore a procedure by which sympathetic denervation could be detected noninvasively, we investigated whether ^{123}I-labeled meta-iodobenzylguanidine (MIBG), a guanethanine analog taken up by sympathetic nerve terminals, could provide a scintigraphic image that would detect apical sympathetic denervation and a possible reinnervation. To test this, we subjected dogs to MIBG imaging at various times after epicardial phenol application to interrupt sympathetic nerves or after transmural myocardial infarction. The results of MIBG scintigraphy were then correlated with electrophysiological responses obtained during ansae subclaviae stimulation and norepinephrine infusion to establish the presence of neural denervation, reinnervation, and supersensitivity. Thallium images were obtained concurrently to outline areas of normal blood flow and cell viability. When an MIBG/thallium mismatch occurred, (i.e., apical defects in the MIBG scan were associated with either a normal thallium scan or a thallium defect that was smaller than the MIBG defect), dogs were found to have apical sympathetic denervation. We established that the results of MIBG scintigraphy correlated accurately with the presence of denervation. Further, MIBG defects were noted to disappear in dogs ~8 to 17 weeks later, and electrophysiologic evaluation at that time established that reinnervation had occurred. Despite this evidence of reinnervation, denervation supersensitivity was still present (30).

Studies with MIBG scintigraphy in humans have also shown MIBG/thallium mismatch after myocardial infarction similar to those changes found in the animal studies (31, 32). For example, we found that 10 of 12 patients with spontaneous ventricular tachyarrhythmias after myocardial infarction exhibited regions of thallium-201 uptake, indicating that viable perfused myocardium was present with no MIBG uptake (31). Such a finding is consistent with sympathetic denervation. We have followed a group of patients with sympathetic denervation after myocardial infarction and have noted that reinnervation occurs, partially or completely, about 6 months later (33). Recent data indicate that regional cardiac sympathetic denervation can also occur in patients with ventricular tachycardia in the absence of coronary disease (34). How important these areas of regional sympathetic denervation are in patients after myocardial infarction and whether they can be a cause of sudden cardiac death (35) await further investigation.

Conclusions

The studies presented herein represent only a minor segment of the literature involving the autonomic nervous system and cardiac arrhythmias. More extensive reviews can be found elsewhere (1–4). However, the previous studies attempt to explain how ischemia can modify the autonomic nervous system and, in turn, how the autonomic nervous system can modify ischemia. Understanding these processes, with their resultant effects on cardiac excitable properties, will help provide a basis for understanding how vagal and sympathetic nerves promote, precipitate, or prevent the development of cardiac arrhythmias.

Acknowledgments

This study was supported in part by the Herman C. Crannert Fund; by Grants HL-42370 and HL-07182 from the National Heart, Lung, and Blood Institute of the National Institutes of Health; by the U.S. Public Health Service; and by the American Heart Association (Indiana Affiliate, Inc.).

References

1. Corr, P.B., Yamada, K.A., and Witkowski, F.X. (1986). Mechanisms controlling cardiac autonomic function and their relation to arrhythmogenesis, in H.A. Fozzard, E. Haber, R.B. Jennings, A.M. Katz, H.E. Morgan, Eds., *The Heart and Cardiovascular System* (Raven Press, New York).

2. Kulbertus, H.E., and Franck, G., Eds. (1988). *Neurocardiology* (Futura Publishing Co., Mt. Kisco, NY).

3. Randall, W.C., and Ardell, J.L. (1985). Selective parasympathectomy of automatic and conductile tissues of the canine heart. *Am. J. Physiol.* **248**(*Heart Circ. Physiol.* 17):H61–H68.

4. Zipes, D.P. (1990). Influence of myocardial ischemia and infarction on autonomic innervation of the heart. *Circulation.* **82**:1095–1105.

5. Blomquist, T.M., Priola, D.V., Romero, A.M. (1987). Source of intrinsic innervation of canine ventricles: A functional study. *Am. J. Physiol.* **252**(*Heart Circ. Physiol.*):H638–H644.

6. Miyazaki, T., Pride, H.P., and Zipes, D.P. (1989). Modulation of cardiac autonomic neurotransmission by epicardial superfusion. Effects of hexamethonium and tetrodotoxin. *Circ. Res.* **65:**1212–1219.

7. Miyazaki, T., Pride, H.P., and Zipes, D.P. (1990). Prostaglandins in the pericardial fluid modulate neural regulation of cardiac electrophysiologic properties. *Circ. Res.* **66:**163–175.

8. Miyazaki, T., and Zipes, D.P. (1990). Pericardial prostaglandin biosynthesis prevents the increased incidence of reperfusion-induced ventricular fibrillation produced by efferent sympathetic stimulation in dogs. *Circulation* **82:**1008–1019.

9. Thames, M.D., and Minisi, A.J. (1989). Reflex responses to myocardial ischemia and reperfusion: Role of prostaglandins. *Circulation* **80:**1878–1885.

10. Barber, M.J., Mueller, T.M., Davies, B.G., Gill, R.M., and Zipes, D.P. (1985). Interruption of sympathetic and vagal-mediated afferent responses by transmural myocardial infarction. *Circulation* **72:**623–631.

11. Inoue, H., Skale, B.T., and Zipes, D.P. (1988). Effects of myocardial ischemia and infarction on cardiac afferent sympathetic and vagal reflexes in the dog. *Am. J. Physiol.* **255**(*Heart Circ. Physiol.* 24):H26–H36.

12. Barber, M.J., Mueller, T.M., Henry, D.P., Felten, S.Y., and Zipes, D.P. (1983). Transmural myocardial infarction in the dog produces sympathectomy in noninfarcted myocardium. *Circulation* **67:**787–796.

13. Inoue, H., and Zipes, D.P. (1988). Time course of denervation of efferent sympathetic and vagal nerves after occlusion of the coronary artery in the canine heart. *Circ. Res.* **62:**1111–1120.

14. Inoue, H., and Zipes, D.P. (1987). Results of sympathetic denervation in the canine heart: Supersensitivity that may be arrhythmogenic. *Circulation* **75:**877–887.

15. Herre, J.M., Wetstein, L., Lin, Y.L., Mills, A.S., Dae, M., and Thames, M.D. (1988). Effect of transmural versus nontransmural myocardial infarction on inducibility of ventricular arrhythmais during sympathetic stimulation in dogs. *J. Am. Coll. Cardiol.* **11:**414–421.

16. Butrous, G.S., Gough, W.D., Restivo, M., et al. (1992). Adrenergic effects on reentrant ventricular rhythms in subacute myocardial infarction. *Circulation* **86:**247–254.

17. Cinca, J., Worner, F., Bardaji, A., et al. (1991). Induced ventricular arrhythmias in regionally denervated porcine heart with healed myocardial infarction. *Cardiovasc. Res.* **25:**568–593.

18. Martins, J.B., Lewis, R., Wenbt, B., Lund, D.D., and Schmid, P.G. (1989). Subendocardial infarction produces epicardial parasympathetic denervation in canine left ventricle. *Am. J. Physiol.* **256**(*Heart Circ. Physiol.* 25):H859–H866.

19. Schmid, P.G., Greif, B.J., Lund, D.D., and Roskoski, R., Jr. (1982). Tyrosine hydroxylase and choline acetyltransferase activities in ischemic canine heart. *Am. J. Physiol.* **243:**H788–H795.

20. Miyazaki, T., and Zipes, D.P. (1990). Presynaptic modulation of efferent sympathetic and vagal neurotransmission in the canine heart by hypoxia, high K^+, low pH and adenosine: Possible relevance to ischemia-induced denervation. *Circ. Res.* **66:**289–301.

21. Warner, M.R., Kroeker, T.S., and Zipes, D.P. (1982). Sympathetic stimulation and norepinephrine infusion modulate extracellular postassium concentration during acute myocardial ischemia. *Circ. Res.* **71**:1078–1087.

22. Ito, M., Pride, H.P., and Zipes, D.P. (1992). ATP-sensitive potassium channel opener protects against autonomic denervation early after acute coronary occlusion. *PACE* **15**:542.

23. Murray, C.E., Jennings, R.B., and Reimer, K.A. (1986). Preconditioning with ischemia: A delay of lethal cell injury in ischemic myocardium. *Circulation* **74**:1124–1136.

24. Miyazaki, T., and Zipes, D.P. (1989). Protection against autonomic denervation following acute myocardial infarction by preconditioning ischemia. *Circ. Res.* **64**:437–448.

25. Rubart, M., Pride, H.P., Warner, M.R., and Zipes, D.P. (1993). Simulated ischemia does not protect against efferent sympathetic denervation following acute myocardial infarction in canine hearts. *J. Cardiovasc. Electrophysiol.*, in press.

26. Kammerling, J.J., Green, F.J., Watanabe, A.M., Inoue, H., Barber, M.J., Henry, D.P., and Zipes, D.P. (1987). Denervation supersensitivity of refractoriness in noninfarcted areas apical to transmural myocardial infarction. *Circulation* **76**:383–393.

27. Martins, J.B. (1988). Time course of sympathetic denervation supersensitivity in canine ventricular recovery. *Am. J. Physiol.* **255**(*Heart Circ. Physiol.* 24):H577–H586.

28. Stanton, M.S., and Zipes, D.P. (1991). Modulation of drug effects by regional sympathetic denervation and supersensitivity. *Circulation* **84**:1709–1714.

29. Warner, M.R., Wisler, P.L., Hodges, T.D., Watanabe, A.M., and Zipes, D.P. (1993). Mechanisms of denervation supersensitivity in regionally denervated canine hearts. *Am. J. Physiol.*, in press.

30. Minardo, J.D., Tuli, M.M., Mock, B.H., Weiner, R.E., Pride, H.P., Wellman, H.N., and Zipes, D.P. (1988). Scintigraphic and electrophysiologic evidence of canine myocardial sympathetic denervation and reinnervation produced by myocardial infarction on phenol application. *Circulation* **78**:1008–1019.

31. Stanton, M.S., Tuli, M.M., Heger, J.J., Miles, W.M., Mock, B.H., Wellman, H.N., and Zipes, D.P. (1989). Regional sympathetic denervation after MI in humans detected noninvasively using I-123 metaiodobenzylguanidine (MIBG). *J. Am. Coll. Cardiol.* **14**:1519–1526.

32. McGhie, I., Corbett, J.R., Akers, M.S., Kahn, J.K., et al. (1989). Detection of regional depletion of myocardial catecholaine stores following acute myocardial infarction using I-123 metaiodobenzylguanidine. *J. Nucl. Med.* **30**:810.

33. Mitrani, R.M., Burt, R.W., Klein, L.S., Miles, W.M., Hackett, F.K., Witt, R.M., Schauwecker, D.S., Wellman, H.N., and Zipes, D.P. (1992). Regional cardiac sympathetic denervation and reinnervation following myocardial infarction in humans, *Circulation* **86**(Suppl. 1):982.

34. Mitrani, R., Klein, L.S., Miles, W.M., Burt, R.W., Wellman, H.N., and Zipes, D.P. (1992). Regional cardiac sympathetic denervation in patients with

ventricular tachycardia in the absence of coronary artery disease. *PACE*
15:538.

35. Zipes, D.P. Sympathetic stimulation and arrhythmias. *N. Engl. J. Med.*
325:656–657 (Editorial).

PART TWO

Ion Channels and Cardiovascular Function

The human heart derives its essential function of rhythmic contractility from the propagated action potential initiated by cells of the sino-atrial node. Normal function requires that automaticity be regular and propagation be orderly and coordinated. Sudden cardiac death, as defined and elaborated in the Part 1 chapter, is usually due to ventricular fibrillation (VF), an extreme example of electrical chaos.

The fundamental units of cardiac excitability are ion channels, complex glycoproteins embedded in the plasma membrane of cardiomyocytes. Ion channels conduct ions at rates sufficiently high that the flux through a single channel can be detected electrically using micropipettes in high resistance contact with the cell membrane (gigaseal patch clamp method). Because patch clamp technology is now widely available and isolation of single cardiomyocytes is now readily accomplished, functional studies have progressed rapidly. In contrast, structural studies have lagged far behind because rich tissue sources of ion channels required for protein purification are, with rare exceptions, unavailable. The usual methods of isolating proteins do not provide sufficient material to identify the many different types of ion channels studied by functional methods. This situation changed dramatically with the introduction of recombinant DNA methods in the past decade. During this period, numerous ion channels have been cloned from a wide variety of tissues including those of the cardiovascular system. The primary amino acid sequences have been determined for many K^+, Na^+, Ca^{2+}, Cl^- and gap junction channel proteins. More importantly, studies using mutational analysis have made an auspicious beginning in assigning functional properties such as ion conduction and channel gating to specific domains in the protein.

In Chapter 5, Dr. Fozzard describes the currents that contribute to the cardiac action potential and focuses particularly on the sodium channel. The inward flow of Na^+ ions depolarizes the membrane and produces the upstroke of the action potential. Propagation of the action potential is also mediated by this inward Na^+ current which flows between cardiac cells via gap junctions. Having cloned and expressed cardiac Na^+ channels, Dr. Fozzard discusses the use of mutational analysis to identify amino acid residues responsible for sensitivity to tetrodotoxin and divalent cations. Based on these results, a model for the ion conduction pathway or pore of the Na^+ channel protein is proposed.

In Chapter 6, Dr. Marban considers the other major source of inward current in the heart, flow of calcium ions through L-type Ca^{2+} channels. Ca^{2+} entry contributes to the plateau of the action potential and triggers contraction. As might be anticipated from the central role of Ca^{2+} in excitation-contraction coupling, Ca^{2+} channels are highly regulated. In this chapter, Dr. Marban reviews modulation of the Ca^{2+} channel by phosphorylation using Mg-ATP as a substrate. In addition, a novel phosphorylation-independent role for Mg-ATP is presented.

Dr. Sanguinetti deals with the major source of outward current in the heart, flow through K^+ channels, in Chapter 7. The outward potassium current is by convention positive and repolarizes the plasma membrane of cardiomyocytes. This current is referred to as the delayed rectifier K^+ current and is shown to consist of slow and fast components, I_{Ks} and I_{Kr}, respectively, which can be distinguished both functionally and pharmacologically. The importance of this distinction is that specific blockers of I_{Kr} have been developed for use as Class III antiarrhythmic agents. In addition, the presence of delayed rectifiers which activate even faster than I_{Kr} have been discovered and these are discussed again in Chapter 15.

In Chapter 8, Dr. Vandenberg introduces inwardly rectifying K^+ channels. These channels are open at the resting potential, and are turned off during the depolarized plateau of the cardiac action potential so that they conduct relatively little current at this time. This behavior is very different from the delayed rectifier K^+ channels discussed in Chapter 7 which are activated by membrane depolarization. Inward rectifiers are therefore important regulators of resting potential and late repolarization. Inward rectification arises mainly from virtually instantaneous blockade of the channel upon depolarization by intracellular Mg^{2+}. An intrinsic gating process independent of Mg^{2+} blockade also appears to be involved. Since the Chantilly meeting, the inward rectifier proteins have been cloned from rat macrophages and rat kidney cells. These proteins show some sequence homology to voltage-dependent, delayed rectifying K^+ channels in the pore region but elsewhere the amino acid sequence is quite different. On a structural basis, they are considered to be members of a superfamily of K^+ channels.

Dr. Hume introduces cardiac Cl^- currents in Chapter 9. During the action potential, chloride ions flow inward producing by convention an outward current. Like the outward K^+ current, this Cl^- current shortens the cardiac action potential. Interestingly, this Cl^- current is dependent on cAMP. Work from Dr. Hume's laboratory suggests that the cystic fibrosis transmembrane regulator protein which is known to be regulated by cAMP, may be the same Cl^- channel.

In Chapter 10, Dr. Spray describes gap junction channels. In heart these channels are formed by connexin 43 protein subunits, are major pathways for the flow of electrical currents between cardiac cells and are therefore important for uniform propagation of the action potential. Flow of current through gap junction protein is highly regulated by phosphorylation mechanisms. Dr. Spray argues that gap junctions in heart appear to be targets for one of the most prevalent forms of heart disease in Latin America, Chaga's disease.

Arthur M. Brown & Peter M. Spooner

5

Cardiac Electrogenesis and the Sodium Channel

Harry A. Fozzard

There are many different types of cardiac ion channels and ion pumps, which altogether orchestrate a complex process that results in the cardiac cell's action potential. Different ion channel and transporter distributions are found in specific cardiac cell types, and together they generate a coordinated response of the whole heart. This electrical system produces an ordered sequence of events from the sinoatrial node pacemaker to the final ventricular activation. Because reliable cardiac electrogenesis is absolutely essential to life, the cardiac action potentials have little margin for error. They must be fail-safe, because malfunction of the system can be promptly lethal. In addition to this need for reliability, the action potentials also must adjust for heart rate, atrioventricular delay, and synchronous activation of contraction by alteration of their electrical function.

Three questions can be asked that are critical to cardiac electrogenesis. (1) *How do heart cells achieve the electrical reliability necessary for support of the circulation?* A partial answer may be in redundancy of functions. (2) *How do the cells adjust their electrical properties to regulate the rate of firing, the synchrony of activation, and the strength of contraction?* This process can involve modulation of channels and pumps by hormones and cytoplasmic second messengers. (3) *How does the electrical system malfunction when it generates life-threatening arrhythmias, and how can we restore balance?* This question was the theme of the ''Ion Channel'' symposium and the central topic of these proceedings.

This chapter seeks to identify the array of ion channels and transporters that underlie cardiac electrical behavior—the instruments in the action potential orchestra. Then we will explore in greater detail the characteristics of the sodium channel, which is the source of current for excitability in most heart cells. Subsequent chapters characterize other important channels and their modulation. Some references by the author for additional reading on the action potential and the sodium channel are Fozzard and Arnsdorf (1), Fozzard and Hanck (2), and Task Force on Arrhythmias (3).

The sodium current is generated by sodium ions flowing through highly selective channels into the cell, where the Na^+ concentration is kept low by the Na/K pump (4). The channel has voltage dependent gates that allow it to open in response to small changes in the transmembrane potential, generating a large current necessary for depolarization and conduction of the action potential. The voltage-dependent gates also allow the channel to close at the depolarized potentials, shutting off the current in a timely way (5). Its single-channel behavior can be measured and correlated with the whole-cell current. The channel's primary amino acid structure has been determined, and correlation between its structure and function (6) is the subject of a section in this symposium. The sodium channel is the site of action of many of our most powerful antiarrhythmic drugs, and we are now beginning to characterize their molecular actions. The sodium channel is important in its own right and as a model for understanding the action of drugs on other channels.

Cardiac Action Potential

Time Course of Voltage Change

A typical cardiac action potential is that of the Purkinje cell (Fig. 1). The rapid depolarization is called phase 0. After reaching an inside positive value of $+20$ to $+40$ mV, repolarization begins. The first, often rather

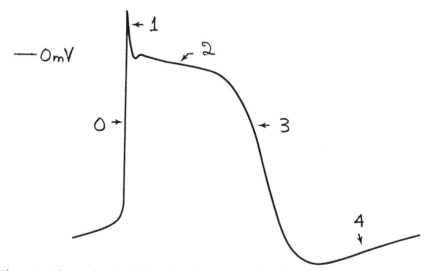

Figure 1. The cardiac Purkinje cell action potential can be used to identify the important segments of the action potential. Phase 0 is the depolarizing upstroke. Phase 1 is a rapid, partial repolarization immediately after the overshoot. Phase 2 is the plateau period that may last 200 to 400 msec. Phase 3 is final repolarization, and phase 4 is the resting or pacemaker period.

rapid, phase of repolarization is called phase 1. It is followed by a quasi–steady-state "plateau," phase 2, which may last for several hundred milliseconds. This phase is responsible for the long period of absolute refractoriness after excitation. The plateau is terminated by a rapid repolarization called phase 3. The resting potential of -90 to -60 mV is phase 4. It may be a steady potential, interrupted only by propagated action potentials. Alternatively, it may show a multicomponent depolarization to or toward the cell's excitatory threshold for another action potential, and this behavior is called the pacemaker potential. Under certain pathological conditions, abnormal depolarizations from the plateau or the resting potential can reach threshold (8).

There are at least six regions of the whole heart where cells possess different complements of ion channels, and consequently, they have differently shaped action potentials. The sinoatrial node (SAN) is specialized as the normal cardiac pacemaker, and it shows the fastest phase 4 pacemaker depolarization. The atrioventricular node (AVN) shows slow conduction, and the Purkinje system has the fastest conduction. Atrial and ventricular muscle have fairly rapid conduction of propagated action potentials and prolonged refractory periods. It has become apparent that ventricular muscle is not electrically homogeneous, with repolarization differing between endocardial and epicardial layers of cells.

Depolarizing Inward Currents

The primary depolarizing excitatory current in atrial, ventricular, and Purkinje cells is the sodium channel current I_{Na} (Fig. 2) (2). It activates quickly and generates a large current that supports a rapid conduction velocity. The principal excitatory current in the SAN and the AVN is calcium current through the L-type calcium channels. The I_{Ca} is smaller and it activates slower; consequently, I_{Ca} supports a slower conduction velocity (9). Sodium channels are present in the SAN, but they are mostly inactivated at the potentials normally present. There is also a second kind of calcium channel in heart cells, the T-type, but its role in excitation is not yet clear.

During the plateau period, the inward and outward currents are small and almost equal. The inward current component includes a slowly decaying calcium current and, in cells with sodium channels, a slowly decaying sodium current (10). The Na/Ca exchange system is rheogenic, because its stoichiometry is 3 Na^+ for 1 Ca^{2+} (11). The direction of the current depends on the electrochemical gradients for these two ions, which change during the plateau as a function of the voltage and the level of intracellular Ca^{2+}. During this period, Ca^{2+} release from the sarcoplasmic reticulum is high, and the exchanger favors efflux of Ca^{2+}, with a resulting inward current. This exchange current declines and disappears as the level of intracellular Ca^{2+} declines.

During phase 4 pacemaker depolarization, an inward current must flow. Two currents have been identified as important contributors. I_f is progressively activated by repolarization of the action potential (12). This channel is not very selective between Na^+ and K^+, but the current is mostly carried inward by Na^+, because of the large Na^+ electrochemical gradient at the pacemaker voltages. There is also a steady "background" inward current under some conditions, also carried by Na^+ (13). This background inward current can generate a pacemaker process when it is coupled with a decaying outward current. The relative contributions of these two inward currents for normal pacemaker behavior is not clear, but it may be an example of two systems to provide fail-safe operation of this critical pacemaker process.

There is evidence for a nonselective channel that is opened by elevated intracellular Ca^{2+}. It may be responsible for transient depolarizations from the resting potential after action potential repolarization under conditions of intracellular Ca^{2+} overload (14). The same conditions may activate the Na/Ca exchange system during the resting potential to produce Ca^{2+} efflux and a net phasic inward current (8).

Repolarizing Outward Currents

The outward currents are carried mainly, although not exclusively, by K^+. In the heart there is a large and growing number of potassium channel types, each with its own physiological role. The potassium channel that controls the resting potential is the "inward rectifier," and its current is called I_{IR} or I_{K1}. It is large in the voltage range near the resting potential but small during the plateau of the action potential because of its rectification. Its reopening during the latter part of the plateau may initiate phase 3 (15). This channel is not found in the SAN. The "delayed rectifier" current, called I_K, is carried by channels that activate slowly at depolarized potentials, and then play an important role in initiating repolarization in some cell types. There are probably several types of delayed rectifier channels (16). The early repolarization of phase 1 is produced by another group of potassium-channel types, called I_{to} or I_A, which activate transiently on depolarization. They may also influence the level of the plateau and, consequently, action potential duration (17). The SAN, AVN, and atrial muscle have special receptors for acetylcholine, the neurotransmitter of the vagus nerve. Acetylcholine binding to the receptor initiates a membrane process that results in the opening of a potassium channel with inward-rectifying properties (18). By this means, vagal nerve activity shortens the action potential and causes hyperpolarization of the resting potential. Acetylcholine can also slow the pacemaker process by acting on this channel or acting indirectly through modulation of the I_f channel (19). The Na/K pump is also rheogenic, and it generates a generally steady outward current that can influence the plateau duration and the resting and pacemaker potentials (20). This current is increased by cell loading with Na$^+$, which occurs with rapid pacing. It is decreased by low extracellular K$^+$ or by digitalis.

Two other outward currents need to be mentioned, one carried by K$^+$ ($I_{K(ATP)}$), and the other carried by Cl$^-$ (I_{Cl}). The $I_{K(ATP)}$ can be important under some metabolic conditions. This channel is kept shut by intracellular ATP, and it can be activated in ischemia, when ATP falls, ADP rises, and other metabolic changes favor channel opening. It is probably responsible for shortening of the action potential in severe ischemia (21). There is a chloride channel that is largely voltage-independent, but is activated by β-adrenergic stimulation (22). I_{Cl} can flow in either direction. The Cl$^-$ electrochemical gradient is about -50mV, so that the Cl$^-$ current would favor lowering the plateau and shortening the action potential, but it might also speed a pacemaker. These two channel types have not yet been reported in SAN cells. There are several other K$^+$ channel types that have been identified in heart cells, but it is premature to assign them a role as yet.

The dynamic electrical behavior of the cell is a complex of all these currents (Fig. 2). Reliability of excitation, repolarization, and pacemaker is perhaps related to a certain redundancy of current sources by the multiple channel and transporter types. Subtle modifications can be introduced by modulation of these different elements. This redundancy and the interactions between the currents make definitive identification of their separate functions during the plateau and the pacemaker phases very difficult. The commonly used methods of ion substitution, pharmacological blockade, and voltage clamp are insufficient. Careful characterization of the currents and study of interaction in mathematical models help, but they suffer from our incomplete understanding of their interdependencies. New methods will be required in order to complete our understanding of action potential behavior.

Sodium Channel

Na$^+$ Current

The sodium channel is the ingenious membrane molecular machine that endows cardiac cells with their property of excitability. It is shut at normal resting potentials of -80 to -90 mV. Upon modest depolarization (but not upon hyperpolarization) channels open, allowing flow of Na$^+$ from the extracellular solution into the cell under the driving force of the Na$^+$ electrical and chemical gradients. Entry of the positively charged ions makes the cytoplasm more positive, which opens more channels and makes the cell more positive in a positive feedback system. The current flows down the core of the long, narrow cells to depolarize adjacent membranes and

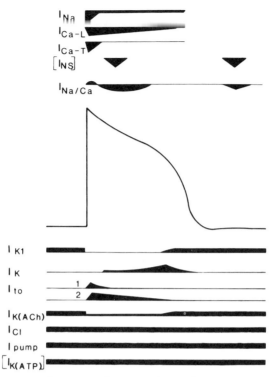

Figure 2. Time course of a ventricular or atrial muscle action potential with important inward (**top**) and outward (**bottom**) current sources. Inward current is defined as movement of positive charge from exterior to interior of the cell. The thickness of the line indicates the approximate timing of the current, but not the comparative magnitudes of each current. Currents identified in brackets are usually seen only under pathological conditions. I_{Na} is the inward excitatory current carried by Na^+ through a voltage-activated sodium channel. I_{Ca-L} is the calcium current that is activated regeneratively from a relatively depolarized threshold potential to produce depolarization and propagation in SAN and AVN cells. I_{Ca-T} is a calcium channel current activated at potentials between I_{NA} and I_{Ca-L} that contributes to depolarization in sinoatrial and His-Purkinje cells. [I_{NS}] is a nonselective cationic channel that produces an inward sodium current that may be activated by calcium overload. $I_{Na/Ca}$ represents Na-Ca exchange current of 1 Ca^{2+}/3 Na^+ countertransport; direction depends on membrane potential. I_{K1}, the "inward rectifier," is the K^+ channel current maintaining resting potential near K^+ equilibrium potential in atrial, AVN; His-Purkinje, ventricular, but not SAN cells. I_K, the "delayed rectifier," is the slowly activating, voltage-gated channel current primarily determining repolarization. I_{to} is a K^+ current that turns on rapidly, then inactivates. One component is activated by [Ca^{2+}]$_{in}$, the other is voltage-activated and modulated by neurotransmitters $I_{K(ACh)}$ is current carried by K^+, activated by acetylcholine, through a M_2 muscarinic G protein-sensitive channel [also called $I_{K(ADO)}$ because of its activation by adenosine]. I_{Cl} is a Cl current sensitive to β-adrenergic stimulation. I_{pump} represents current from electrogenic Na-K, and Ca, ATP-dependent pumps. [$I_{K(ATP)}$] is a K^+ current carried by an ATP-inhibited, metabolically regulated channel, which is activated during hypoxia. [From the Task Force on Arrhythmias (3).]

open their sodium channels. Because current can flow easily from cell to cell through gap junctions, the next cell is activated (23).

The peak intensity of the Na$^+$ current greatly exceeds any other normal cardiac membrane current, causing depolarization at the rate of 100 to 500 V/sec. Consequently, excitation and depolarization spread rapidly through the atria, the His-Purkinje system, and the ventricles at velocities of 0.5 to 3 M/sec (3). This rapid excitation is essential for the function of the cardiac muscular chamber, because the entire chamber must be activated and must contract conjointly in order to eject blood effectively.

The Na$^+$ current is normally very brief; inactivation occurs soon after the rapid voltage-dependent activation (Fig. 3). This is because the depolarization that causes the channels to open also initiates a process to close the channels to a new state from which they cannot be reopened until the membrane is repolarized for a time. Therefore, Na$^+$ current is intense but

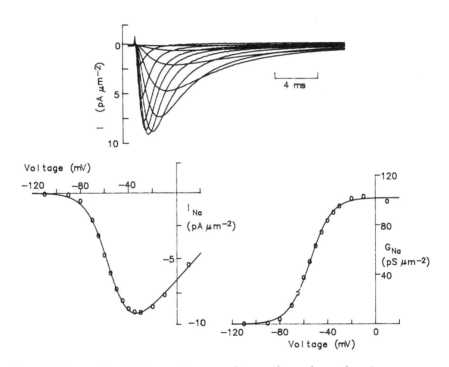

Figure 3. The cardiac Na$^+$ current measured in a voltage-clamped canine Purkinje cell. The **upper part** of the figure shows a family of Na$^+$ currents in response to voltage steps from -150 mV to various depolarized potentials above the current threshold. The current develops rapidly (Na$^+$ entry into the cell is reflected in a downward deflection of the current) and decays slowly back to a low level. The **lower left plot** shows the relationship of the peak Na$^+$ current versus the voltage step. The **lower right plot** is the current's voltage activation curve. Peak-activated conductance is calculated from the peak current and the Na$^+$ electrochemical driving force using Ohm's law. [From Fozzard (45).]

brief. After repolarization, a slow process of recovery occurs. This sequence of three channel states—closed but openable, open, and inactivated—is called the sodium channel cycle. Transitions between the states depend on voltage and time (Fig. 4).

The role of sodium channel activition in synchronizing the regular depolarization of atria and ventricles is critical. Premature activation finds the chamber incompletely relaxed and not yet refilled with blood. Disorganized activation produces an ineffective contraction. Under pathological conditions, slow conduction can result in reentry, an underlying degenerative process in ventricular tachycardia and ventricular fibrillation (24). This critical role for the sodium channel has made it the target for some of our most powerful antiarrhythmic drugs, such as lidocaine, which blocks the channel in a state-dependent way (25). This state dependence of drug affinity on channel state means that block is favored by opening of the channel, so that the drug is preferentially effective during rapid abnormal rhythms.

The Na^+ current in heart cells is similar to that in nerve cells, however with several important differences:

1. The cardiac Na^+ current is kinetically slower than that of nerve.

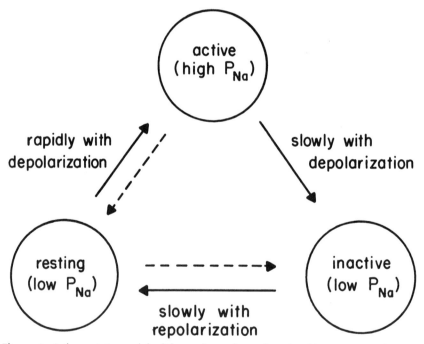

Figure 4. A three-state model of the sodium channel cycle. After recovery the channels are resting, but available for opening. Upon depolarization they become active (open), then they inactivate. Recovery requires repolarization.

2. It is resistant to blockade by the marine toxins saxitoxin and tetrodo-toxin.
3. It is sensitive to block by certain divalent ions, including cadmium (Cd) and zinc (Zn).
4. It appears to be more sensitive to local anesthetic drugs, such as lidocaine.

Single-Channel Properties

As we have seen, membrane currents are the integrated result of opening and closing of many individual channels. For many years we had to infer the properties of these individual channels, but the development of *patch clamp* techniques has made it possible to record the current from a single channel (26). This has revealed that many individual properties were correctly predicted on the basis of major recordings, but some were not. During the first recordings of single-channel openings, several characteristics were immediately obvious. The single-channel current at a chosen voltage was constant. The relationship between the current and the voltage was linear over a substantial range, so that we could say that open channel was *ohmic*, with a single-channel conductance of about 20 pS.

The second obvious property was that the same channel opened in different ways during sequential steps to the same voltage level. Sometimes it opened quickly after the depolarizing step, and sometimes it opened late. Sometimes it opened briefly, and sometimes it remained open for several mseconds. Sometimes it failed to open at all (Fig. 5). It must be expected that a single-channel molecule will behave *stochastically* (i.e., obeying the laws of probability). For the reaction

$$C \leftrightarrow O$$

the transition from C occurs when there is sufficient energy to convert to O. For the sodium channel at negative voltages, the probability is low, but it is increased by depolarization. In the same way, once the channel is open, it will have a certain probability of closing. If we measure a large population of single openings, we find that the open times show an exponential distribution, with characteristic time constants (means) for each voltage. In the same way, the latency to opening can be measured and shown to be a voltage function. A prediction of how this probabilistic behavior of single channels might result in whole cell currents can be made by taking the average behavior of single channel recordings during several hundred voltage steps. This average behavior, called the *ensemble*, for sodium channels results in a current that rises with time after depolarization and then gradually declines as openings become less frequent (Fig. 6). The ensemble follows the time course of the whole-cell current. In other words, the average behavior of one sodium channel sampled many times is the same as the behavior of many channels sampled once (27).

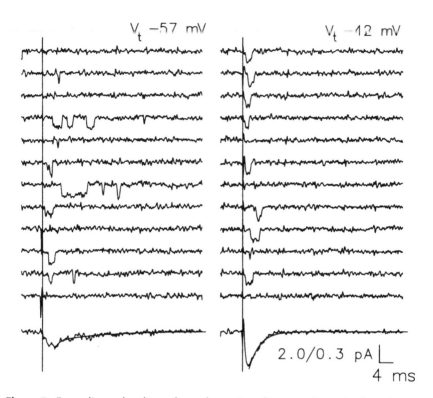

Figure 5. Recordings of sodium channel openings from a cell-attached patch containing only one sodium channel. A canine cardiac Purkinje cell was used, with 140 mM NaCl in the pipette. Each trace is the response to consecutive 45 msec depolarizing voltage steps to −57 mV **(left)** or −45 mV **(right)** at 1-sec intervals. The vertical line indicates the time of depolarization. The lowest traces in each set are average currents (ensembles) from recording of many single-channel openings. See text for more details. [From Scanley et al. (28).]

Our present concept of the kinetic behavior of the sodium channel can be illustrated using a Markov chain model of sequential configurational states. This model presumes that transitions between a number of conformations of the channel that are closed, open, or inactivated. The rate constants for the transitions are considered to be voltage-dependent (e.g., ref. 28) (Fig. 7).

Structure of the Sodium Channel

The brain sodium channel was one of the first to be cloned (29). It includes a 2,000 amino acid α-subunit and two smaller β-subunits. When the brain II α-subunit mRNA is expressed in *Xenopus* oocytes, voltage-dependent Na⁺ currents that are similar, but not identical, to those of the native sodium current are seen. Consequently, it is apparent that the

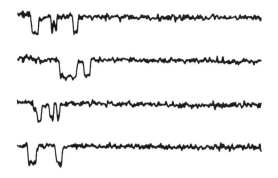

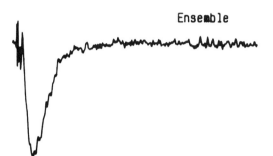

Ensemble

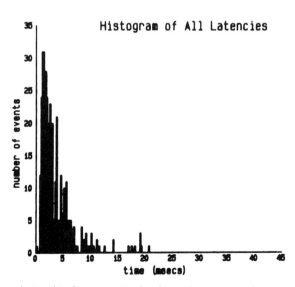

Figure 6. The relationship between single-channel openings, the ensemble current, and the time after depolarization until the channel opens (latency). It is apparent that the ensemble current decays with time, because fewer channels are opening. [From Fozzard et al. (46).]

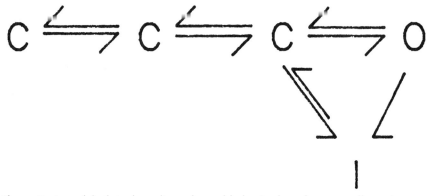

Figure 7. A model of single sodium channel behavior based on a small number of sequential configurational states of the channel protein. C is closed, O is open, and I is inactivated. The transitions between states are "memoryless" and voltage-dependent. This type of model is called a Markov chain.

α-subunit contains the ion transport part of the channel. Coexpression of the β_1-subunit corrects the rat brain II channel kinetics toward normal (30).

The cardiac sodium channel α-subunit has been cloned and is ~ 80% identical in structure (31). Its kinetic properties when expressed in the *Xenopus* oocyte (32) are close to those of native cardiac Na^+ currents. If a β-subunit is present in heart, then it does not appear to play an important kinetic role.

The channel's probable membrane topology is described by W. Catterall in a subsequent chapter. For comparison of channel structure with its function, we will focus on the parts of the channel that are thought to compose the outer vestibule and the pore. Modeling by Guy and others, in combination with mutation studies with the similar Shaker-type potassium channel (34), has identified the extracellular loop between S5 and S6 in each repeat region as the amino acids lining the outer opening vestibule or pore. These four loops are believed to fold back into the membrane in a hairpin fashion to form an eight-sided pore.

Much of the evidence from potassium channel studies for this structure is related to mutations that identify coordination sites for the extracellular blocking molecules TEA and charybdotoxin (35). An analogous approach to study the pore of the sodium channel is identification of the tetrodotoxin and saxitoxin binding sites. In addition to characterizing the pore, the toxin site is a good model for drug binding sites, such as those for clinically relevant local anesthetic antiarrhythmic drugs. Recently, Noda et al. (36) demonstrated involvement of a part of the S5–S6 loop in toxin binding by showing that neutralization of a glutamic acid (position 387 in the rat brain II channel) abolished toxin block. Neutralization of other negatively charged amino acids in nearby parts of the putative pore also alters toxin block (37).

A second set of clues about the properties of the pore has come from biophysical studies of Na^+ permeation and of divalent ion block. Both sorts of studies identify a "site" that is 20% to 30% into the membrane electrical field from the outside surface (38). In the context of Hille's 4-barrier, 3-well energetic model of the channel (39), divalent ions can enter the channel to the first energy well but cannot cross the high barrier into the cell. However, while at this site, they exclude Na^+, thereby blocking the channel. It seems likely that this blocking process explains why the normal concentrations of divalent ions in the intracellular solution have such a dramatic effect on excitability in heart and nerve. If the coordinating site for divalent ions could be located, it would identify that critical part of the pore. This site might also distinguish between the nerve and the cardiac isoforms of the channels, because the cardiac channel is much more sensitive to block by Cd and Zn than is nerve (40).

There is also reason to believe that the toxin site and the divalent ion site might overlap. Both monovalent and divalent ions displace toxin from the channel proteins. As expected, if the sites overlap, Cd and Zn are more effective in displacing the toxin from cardiac channels than from nerve channels (41). This inverse relationship between toxin sensitivity and divalent ion sensitivity could be explained if the same part of the channel structure is responsible.

Our laboratory was able to confirm that the characteristic low affinity for toxin and high affinity for Cd is a property of the cardiac α-subunit (42). This led us to examine the homology between the brain II, skeletal, and cardiac isoforms of the α-subunits. In the sequence identified by Terlau et al. (37) as important for toxin block, we found two amino acid differences (Fig. 8). All of the charged amino acids that they identified as important to toxin block are present in all three isoforms. Similar regions of repeats II–IV are identical in the isoforms, so they could not contribute to the functional differences. The presence of a positively charged arginine (RHI position 377) adjacent to a critical negative charge could be important. If the toxin interaction with the positively charged site was principally electrostatic, then this arginine should favor lower toxin affinity for the cardiac isoform. The second difference is a cysteine (RHI position 374) in place of a phenylalanine (brain II) or a tyrosine (skeletal). This cysteine was a good candidate for the Cd/Zn site.

We then made conservative mutations singly in each location, introducing the skeletal or brain II amino acid in place of the cardiac one. We found that the Cys–Tyr or the Cys–Phe changes simultaneously increased toxin affinity by almost 3 log units and decreased Cd sensitivity by almost 2 log units (43). The Arg–Asn mutation caused small changes in the opposite direction from a fit to the electrostatic model (Fig. 9). These results suggest that the divalent ions and the toxins have overlapping sites and that this part of the molecule is a critical part of the pore.

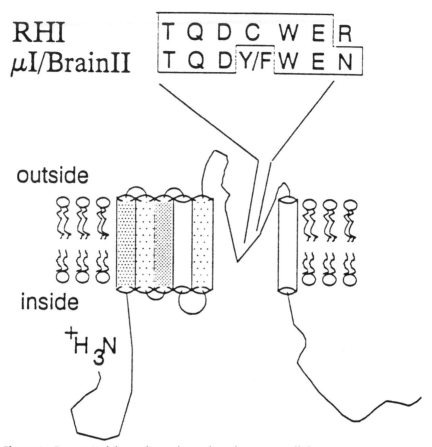

Figure 8. Repeat I of the sodium channel, with its intracellular amino terminus, six transmembrane helical segments, a part of the interconnecting loop to the next repeat, and an infolded segment between S5 and S6. Part of the infolded segment is believed to contribute to the lining of the pore. The seven amino-acid sequence comprising SS2 is shown, with the differences between the cardiac (RHI), skeletal (NI), and brain II isoforms. Abbreviations for the amino acids are C, Cys; D, Asp; E, Glu; F, Phe; N, Asn; Q, Gln; R, Arg; T, Thr; W, Trp; and Y, Tyr. [From Satin et al. (43).]

On the basis of our mutation studies and those of Terlau et al. (37), we can alter the potassium channel model of Durell and Guy (33) to suggest the amino acid sequences lining the sodium channel pore (Fig. 10). This alignment results in the formation of three rings of charges in the pore, similar to the three charged rings found in nicotinic acetylcholine channels (44). The outer and intermediate rings are good candidates for divalent ion binding sites. The inner ring may function as the channel's selectivity filter, determining the passage of K^+ or Ca^{2+}. High-affinity Cd^+ block is likely to be near the intermediate ring, where it can interact with the

A

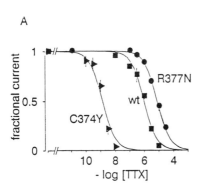

C

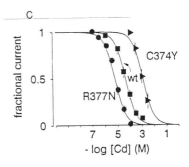

B

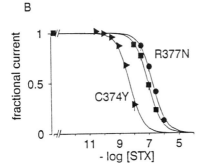

Figure 9. Log dose-response curves for the first pulse block of wild-type (wt) and SS2 mutant channels expressed in *Xenopus* oocytes for (**A**) tetrodotoxin (TTX); (**B**) saxitoxin (STX); and (**C**) Cd^{2+}. C374Y is the SS2 mutant with Cys at position 374 replaced by Tyr. R377N is with Arg at position 377 replaced by Asn. [From Satin et al. (43).]

A   B

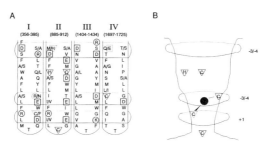

Figure 10. (**A**) A folding scheme for the sodium channel pore region. The amino acid single letter codes identify the primary sequences for portions of the S5–S6 loop from each of the four repeats. The numerical positions are from the RHI isoform. Residues in squares are negatively charged, and those in circles are positively charged. Histidines and cysteines are identified by triangles. Dashed lines indicate the amino acids in the cardiac isoform not conserved in the other isoforms and mutated in our studies. This alignment results in three possible charged rings from the juxtaposition of the four S5–S6 loops, indicated by the large boxes. (**B**) The putative channel region. Circles indicate the three charged rings, and the large dot is a possible location of the Cd^{2+} ion when bound in the channel at its high-affinity site. [From Doyle et al. (41).]

cysteine. Toxin is not tightly bound unless the channel has an aromatic amino acid at the equivalent of cardiac position 374. Although the proposed structure is largely speculative at this time, it offers a basis for further structure–function studies.

Summary

The cardiac action potential is the result of complex interactions of 10 or more ion channel or pump types. The primary cardiac excitatory current is through sodium channels. These channels have been studied extensively in recent years using whole-cell voltage and patch clamps. Several isoforms of this channel have been cloned and expressed. The cardiac sodium channel differs in its structure and function from the nerve sodium channel. Two differences—tetrodotoxin and saxitoxin affinities and divalent ion block by Cd and Zn—can be traced to specific amino acids, thereby identifying the channel's pore region. These studies lead to a suggested model for the lining of the sodium channel pore and selectivity filter, and they provide insight into the nature of sites to which drug binding to the channel can be targeted.

References

1. Fozzard, H.A., and Arnsdorf, M.F. (1992). Cardiac electrophysiology, in *The Heart and the Cardiovascular System*, H.A. Fozzard, E. Haber, R.B. Jennings, A.M. Katz, and H.E. Morgan, Eds. (Raven Press, New York), 2nd ed., chap. 3, pp. 63–110.

2. Fozzard, H.A., and Hanck, D.A. (1992). Sodium channels, in *The Heart and the Cardiovascular System*, H.A. Fozzard, E. Haber, R.B. Jennings, A.M. Katz, and H.E. Morgan, Eds. (Raven Press, New York), 2nd ed., chap. 41, pp. 1091–1119.

3. Task Force on Arrhythmias. (1992). The Sicilian gambit. *Circulation* **84:**1831–1851.

4. Hodgkin, L., and Huxley, A.F. (1952). A quantitative description of membrane current and its application to conduction and excitation in nerve. *J. Physiol.* **117:**500–544.

5 Armstrong, C.M. (1992). Voltage-dependent ion channels and their gating. *Physiol. Rev.* **72:**S5–S13.

6. Catterall, W.A. (1988). Structure and function of voltage sensitive ion channels. *Science* **242:**5060.

7. Baumgarten, C.M., and Fozzard, H.A. (1992). Cardiac resting and pacemaker potentials, in *The Heart and the Cardiovascular System*, H.A. Fozzard, E. Haber, R.B. Jennings, A.M. Katz, and H.E. Morgan, Eds. (Raven Press, New York), 2nd ed., chap. 38, pp. 963–1001.

8. January, C.T., and Fozzard, A. (1989). Delayed after depolarizations in heart muscle: Mechanisms and relevance. *Pharmacol. Rev.* **40:**219–227.

9. Pelzer, D., Pelzer, S., and McDonald, T.F. (1992). Calcium channels in Heart, in *The Heart and the Cardiovascular System,* H.A. Fozzard, E. Haber, R.B. Jennings, A.M. Katz, and H.E. Morgan, Eds. (Raven Press, New York), 2nd ed., chap. 40, pp. 1049–1090.

10. Carmeliet, E. (1987). Slow inactivation of the sodium current in rabbit cardiac Purkinje fibres. *Pflügers Arch.* **408:**18–26.

11. Sheu, S., and Blaustein, M.P. (1992). Sodium/calcium exchange, in *The Heart and Cardiovascular System,* H.A. Fozzard, E. Haber, R.B. Jennings, A.M. Katz, and H.E. Morgan, Eds. (Raven Press, New York), 2nd ed., chap. 36, pp. 903–944.

12. DiFrancesco, D., Ferroni, A., Mazzanti, M., and Tromba, C. (1986). Properties of the hyperpolarizing-activated current (if) in cells isolated from the rabbit sino-atrial node. *J. Physiol.* **377:**61–88.

13. Hagiqara, N., Irisawa, H., Kasanuki, H., and Hosoda, S. (1992). Background current in sino-atrial node cells of the rabbit heart. *J. Physiol.* **448:**53–72.

14. Ehara, T., Noma, A., and Ono, K. (1988). Calcium-activated non-selective cation channel in ventricular cells isolated from adult guinea-pig hearts. *J. Physiol.* **403:**117–133.

15. Shimoni, Y., Clark, R.B., and Giles, W.R. (1992). Role of an inwardly rectifying potassium current in rabbit ventricular action potential. *J. Physiol.* **448:**709–727.

16. Sanguinetti, M.C., and Jurkiewicz, N.K. (1990). Two components of cardiac delayed rectifier K^+ current. Differential sensitivity to block by class III antiarrhythmic agents. *J. Gen. Physiol.* **96:**195–215.

17. Giles, W.R., and Iwazumi, Y.(1988). Comparison of potassium currents in rabbit atrial and ventricular cells. *J. Physiol.* **405:**123–145.

18. Sakmann, B., Nonma, A., and Trautwein, W. (1983). Acetylcholine activation of single muscarinic K^+ channels in isolated pacemaker cells of the mammalian heart. *Nature* **303:**250–253.

19. DiFrancesco, D. (1985). The cardiac hyperpolarizing-activated current, if. Origins and developments. *Prog. Biophys. Molec. Biol.* **46:**163–183.

20. Gadsby, D.C. (1984). The Na/K pump of cardiac cells. *Ann. Rev. Biophys. Bioeng.* **13:**373–378.

21. Carmeliet, E., Storms, L., and Vereecke, J. (1990). The ATP-dependent K-channel and metabolic inhibition, in *Cardiac Electrophysiology: From Cell to Bedside,* D.P. Zipes and J. Jalife, Eds. (W.B. Saunders Co., Philadelphia) pp. 103–108.

22. Harvey, R.D., Clark, C.D., and Hume, J.R. (1990). Chloride current in mammalian cardiac myocytes. Novel mechanism for autonomic regulation of action potential duration and resting membrane potential. *J. Gen. Physiol.* **95:**1077–1102.

23. Fozzard, H.A. (1979). Conduction of the action potential, in *Handbook of Physiology, Vol. I, The Heart; Section 2: The Cardiovascular System* (American Physiological Society, Bethesda, MD), pp. 335–356.

24. Janse, M. (1992). Reentrant arrhythymias, in *The Heart and the Cardiovascular System,* H.A. Fozzard, E. Haber, R.B. Jennings, A.M. Katz, and H.E. Morgan, Eds. (Raven Press, New York), 2nd ed., chap 79, pp. 2055–2095.

25. Grant, A.O., Starmer, C.F., and Strauss, H.C. (1984). Antiarrhythmic drug action. Blockade of the inward sodium current. *Circ. Res.* **55**:427–439.

26. Hamill, O.F., Marty, A., Neher, E., Sakmann, B., and Sigworth, F.J. (1981). Improved patch-clamp techniques for high-resolution current recording from cells and cell-free membrane patches. *Pflügers Arch.* **391**:85–100.

27. Hille, B.(1992). *Ionic Channels of Excitable Membranes* (Sinauer Associates, Inc., Sunderland, MA) pp. 65–70.

28. Scanley, B.E., Hanck, D.A., Chay, T., and Fozzard, H.A. (1990). Kinetic analysis of single sodium channels from canine cardiac Purkinje cells. *J. Gen. Physiol.* **95**:411–437.

29. Catterall, W.A. (1992). Cellular and molecular biology of voltage-gated sodium channels. *Physiol. Rev.* **72**:S15–S48.

30. Isom, L.L., DeJongh, K.S., Reber, B.F.X., Offord, J., Charbonneau, H., Walsh, K., Goldin, A.L., and Catterall, W.A. (1992). Primary structure and functional expression of the beta-1 subunit of the rat brain sodium channel. *Science* **256**:839–842.

31. Rogart, R.B., Cribbs, L.L., Muglia, L.K., Kephart, D.D., and Kaiser, M.W. (1989). Molecular cloning of a putative tetrodotoxin-resistant rat heart Na^+ channel isoform. *Proc. Natl. Acad. Sci. U.S.A.* **86**:8170–8174.

32. Satin, J., Kyle, J.W., Chen, M., Rogart, R.B., and Fozzard, H.A.(1992). The cloned cardiac Na channel submit expressed in Xenopus oocytes show gating and blocking properties of native channels. *J. Membr. Biol.* **130**:11–22.

33. Durell, S.R., and Guy, R. (1992). Atomic scale structure and functional models of voltage-gated potassium channels. *Biophys. J.* **62**:238–250.

34. Joho, R.H. (1992). Toward a molecular understanding of voltage-gated potassium channels. *J. Cardiovasc. Electrophys.* **3**:589–601.

35. Pongs, O. (1992). Molecular biology of voltage-dependent potassium channels. *Physiol. Rev.* **62**:S69–S88.

36. Noda, M., Suzuki, H., Numa, S., and Stuhmer, W. (1989). A single point mutation confers tetrodotoxin and saxitoxin insensitivity on the sodium channel II. *FEBS Lett.* **259**:213–216.

37. Terlau, H., Heinemann, S.H., Stuhmen, W., Pusch, M., Conti, F., Imoto, K., and Numa, S. (1991). Mapping the site of block by tetrodotoxin and saxitoxin of sodium channel II. *FEBS Lett.* **293**:9–96.

38. Sheets, M.F., and Hanck, D.A. (1992). Mechanisms of extracellular divalent and trivalent cation block of the sodium current in canine cardiac Purkinje cells. *J. Physiol.* **454**:299–320.

39. Hille, B.J. (1975). Ionic selectivity, saturation, and block in sodium channels. A four-barrier model. *J. Gen. Physiol.* **66**:535–560.

40. Ravindran, A., Schild, L., and Moczydlowski, E. (1991). Divalent cation selectivity for external block of voltage-dependent NA^+ channels prolonged by batrachotoxin. Zn^{2+} induces discrete substates in cardiac Na^+ channels. *J. Gen. Physiol.* **97**:89–115.

41. Doyle, D.D., Guo, Y., Lusting, S.L., Satin, J., Rogart, R.B., and Fozzard, H.A. (1993). Divalent cation competition with {3H} saxitoxin binding to tetrodotoxin-resistant and -sensitive sodium channels. A two-site structural model of ion/toxin interaction. *J. Gen. Physiol.* **101**:153–182.

42. Cribbs, L., Satin, J., Fozzard, H.A., and Rogart, R.B. (1990). Functional expression of the rat heart I Na^+ channel isoform. Demonstration of properties characteristic of native cardiac Na^+ channels. *FEBS Lett.* **275:**195–200.

43. Satin, J., Kyle, J.W., Chen, M., Bell, P., Cribbs, L.L., Fozzard, H.A., and Rogart, R.B. (1992). A mutant of TTX-resistant cardiac sodium channels with TTX-sensitive properties. *Science* **256:**1202–1205.

44. Konno, T., Busch, C., Vonkitzing, E., Imoto, K., Wang, F., Nakai, J., Mishina, M., and Sakmann, B. (1991). Rings of anionic amino acids as structural determinants of ion selectivity in the acetylcholine receptor channel. *Proc. R. Soc. Lond. (Biol).* **244:**137–144.

45. Fozzard, H.A. (1992). Cardiac sodium channel kinetics, in *Cardiac Electrophysiology, Circulation and Transport,* S. Sideman, R. Beyer, and A.G. Kleber, Eds. (Kluwer Academic, Boston, MA), pp. 137–144.

46. Fozzard, H.A., Hanck, D.A., Makielski, J.C., Scanley, B.E., and Sheets, M.F. (1987). Sodium channels in cardiac Purkinje cells. *Experientia* **43:**1162–1168.

6

Calcium Channels as Biosensors of Cellular Energy Metabolism: Effects of Magnesium and MgATP

Brian O'Rourke, Peter H. Backx, Rafael Mejía-Alvarez,
Gordon Tomaselli, John H. Lawrence, H. Bradley Nuss,
and Eduardo Marban

Although often taken for granted, the importance of Mg in the control of cell physiology cannot be overemphasized. Whether the cell is utilizing energy substrates, elevating or dissipating ion gradients across a membrane, contracting, or synthesizing nucleic acids and proteins, Mg participates in the process. The vital requirement for Mg^{2+} and Mg nucleotide complexes in supporting enzyme activity has long been recognized. More recently, a growing body of work has elucidated a number of mechanisms whereby ion channels can sense and respond to Mg^{2+} and Mg nucleotides. This chapter summarizes some of our results, demonstrating that L-type Ca^{2+} channels are subject to regulation by Mg nucleotides via a direct, phosphorylation-independent pathway in addition to the well-described cAMP-dependent route.

Chemical Properties of Mg: Effects on Enzyme Reactions

The widespread influence of Mg can be attributed to chemical properties that are unique among cations. Mg^{2+} has a relatively large charge for its small ionic radius [0.65 Å] in comparison to Ca^{2+} [0.99 Å], Na^+ [0.95 Å], and K^+ [1.33 Å; Pauling radii (1)], allowing it to polarize surrounding ligands without being polarized itself. As a consequence, Mg^{2+} readily forms complexes with highly electronegative electron donors, including phosphate, carboxylate, and amine groups. Mg^{2+} can therefore serve as a bridge between many types of molecules within the cell. By bringing molecules together, Mg^{2+} enhances reaction rates by reducing the unfavorable entropy associated with forming an intermediate complex. Mg^{2+} can also lower the enthalpy of activation by acting as a generalized acid catalyst. Both of these effects reduce the free energy of activation of the reaction (2). There are a number of schemes by which these general properties of Mg^{2+} influence physiological functions. Mg^{2+} can act on large intracellular polymers such as DNA, RNA, and proteins, by directly binding to these molecules. Notable examples of this mode of action include the stabilizing effects of Mg^{2+} on both the DNA helix and ribosomal RNA, and the allosteric activation of hexokinase, enolase, or pyruvate kinase (3). In a complex with ATP, its most abundant intracellular buffer, Mg functions as an allosteric effector by acting on nucleotide binding sites of proteins such as the DNA helicase of *Escherichia coli* (4), the mitochondrial F_1 ATPase (5), or phosphofructokinase (6). MgATP is also the substrate for a very large class of enzymes involved in phosphoryl transfer reactions, including nucleic acid polymerases, protein kinases, ion-motive ATPases, and myosin ATPase.

The precise role of magnesium at catalytically active sites has been analyzed in detail for several enzymes and can be subdivided into three major mechanistic schemes. First, Mg can form a metal bridge between the substrate and enzyme (simple: S–Mg–E or cyclic: $E < S^{Mg}$). Second, the substrate can form a bridge between the enzyme and Mg (E–S–Mg). Third, Mg may bind to the enzyme without interacting with the substrate (M–E–S) (7). Often, Mg^{2+} and MgATP can affect protein function by more than one of these mechanisms simultaneously. Adenylate cyclase is one example of an enzyme that utilizes MgATP as a substrate, but is also activated by the occupation of a metal binding site distal to the active site (8). Multiple actions of Mg on protein function may also explain the bimodal dependence of enzyme activity on Mg concentration, a common feature of kinase reactions (9).

Mg Effects on Ion Channels

Ion channel activity is often described by models analogous to those used for enzyme systems, with translocation of ions across the membrane the end result of the reaction (1). It is therefore not surprising that mechanisms for regulating ion channels can be similarly depicted. Some multiple modes of action of Mg on channel activity can then be described as follows:

1. Mg^{2+} can indirectly affect ion channel function by binding to negatively charged sites on the membrane. Screening of the surface charge on the membrane causes a perturbation of the electric field environment of the voltage sensors (gates) controlling channel opening, resulting in a shift in voltage-dependent properties (activation and inactivation). Mg^{2+} has a smaller surface charge screening effect than Ca^{2+}, because it has a lower affinity for the membrane binding sites (10).
2. Mg^{2+} can directly affect ion channel function by entering the channel pore to block ion flux. Although it has a small atomic radius, for most channels, Mg^{2+} is impermeant, because the free energy cost of dehydrat-

ing the ion is the largest among physiologically important ions. This open channel blocking effect plays a major role in the rectification properties of several channel types, including inwardly rectifying K$^+$ channels (11), acetylcholine-gated K$^+$ channels (12), and *N*-methyl D-aspartate receptors (13). In many cases, the straightforward blocking action of Mg^{2+} is also accompanied by an alteration of channel gating, resulting in somewhat complicated kinetic effects.

3. Mg, as part of the Mg nucleotide complex, can influence channel activity through direct interaction with the channel [e.g., ATP-sensitive K$^+$ channels (14), savcoplasmic reticulum Ca^{2+} release channels (15), and cystic fibrosis transmembrane conductance regulator (CFTR) Cl$^-$ channels (16)]. Regulation of channels via nucleotide binding sites can involve more than one mode of action depending on the type of channel, as will become evident in the discussion to follow.

4. Mg nucleotides serve as substrates for effector proteins catalyzing reactions involved in the regulation of ion channels. This can occur by at least four different routes: enzymes involved in phosphorylating channels (adenylate or guanylate cyclases, protein kinases); direct influences of effector products on channels [e.g., cyclic nucleotide-gated channels (17)]; interactions between nucleotide-activated proteins and channels [e.g., direct G-protein effects (18)]; and, moving farther up the regulatory cascade, by binding to specific Mg nucleotide receptors on the cell surface [e.g., purinergic receptor effects (19)].

This myriad of ways in which Mg may modulate ion channel activity is therefore reminiscent of the ion's critical role in mediating other cellular functions.

Magnesium and the Ca^{2+}-L Channel

L-type Ca^{2+} channels are subject to several of the modulatory actions of Mg mentioned previously. Direct channel blocking effects of both extracellular and intracellular Mg^{2+} have been observed (20). Furthermore, the rate of inactivation of inward Ba^{2+} or Na$^+$ currents through L-type Ca^{2+} channels has been reported to increase and the amplitude of the currents to decrease when intracellular Mg^{2+} was raised from 0.3 to 3 mM in frog cardiomyocytes (21). When Ca^{2+} is the charge carrier, raising intracellular Mg^{2+} also reduces the amplitude of I_{Ca} in guinea pig cardiomyocytes (22). In the frog, this effect is accentuated by prior channel phosphorylation, perhaps by altering the affinity of the Mg^{2+} binding site (21).

Although the role of MgATP in the cAMP-mediated phosphorylation of Ca^{2+} channels has been recognized, relatively little attention has been paid to investigating the effects of MgATP on L-type Ca^{2+} channels. Previous studies have shown that the inclusion of MgATP in sufficient quantities in intracellular solutions can retard the rate of "rundown" of Ca^{2+} current

(23) In addition, a positive correlation between intracellular MgATP and the amplitude of cardiac L-type Ca^{2+} currents has been reported (24). Both of these effects have been assumed to be related to the importance of MgATP as a substrate for phosphorylation.

With the knowledge that the modulatory effects of MgATP are often conducted via more than one mechanism, we explored the effects of intracellular MgATP on L-type Ca^{2+} currents, whereas Mg^{2+} was maintained well below physiological levels. MgATP was varied over a concentration range that may limit reactions involved in the regulation of Ca^{2+} channels. The effects of MgATP on Ca^{2+} current were then compared with the predominant mechanism for regulating Ca^{2+} channels, β-adrenergic receptor activation and cAMP-dependent phosphorylation.

Flash Photolysis as a Tool to Probe Mg-Dependent Action

In recent years, a variety of photosensitive compounds have been synthesized, which enable one alter the concentration of an active molecule in a few milliseconds or less. There are two main classes of compounds capable of chelating ("caging") divalent cations and subsequently releasing the ion upon exposure to ultraviolet light. Nitr-5 and its related compounds (e.g., nitr-2, nitr-7) are photosensitive Ca^{2+} buffers that have proven useful for the study of Ca^{2+}-mediated processes, because of their high selectivity for Ca^{2+} over Mg^{2+}, like the parent compound, BAPTA (25). Illumination of Nitr-5 generates an electron-withdrawing group near the chelation center, resulting in an increase in the K_D for Ca^{2+} binding from 0.145 to 6.3 μM. The second compound used to cage divalent cations is DM-nitrophen, a photosensitive derivative of EDTA (26). Unlike Nitr-5, DM-nitrophen has a high affinity for both Ca^{2+} and Mg^{2+} ($K_{D,Ca}$ = 5 nM; $K_{D,Mg}$ = 2.5 μM), and photolysis causes cleavage of the binding site into two halves, with a concomitant increase in the K_D's to ~3 mM. Both forms of caged Ca^{2+} have been successfully used to study the effects of a rapid jump in intracellular Ca^{2+} on Ca^{2+} currents (27–29). In cardiac cells, Ca^{2+} release can result in either inactivation or augmentation of the L-type Ca^{2+} current, depending on the magnitude or the method of increasing intracellular Ca^{2+} (28, 29).

A drawback of using DM-nitrophen caged Ca^{2+} is that one usually needs to omit Mg from the solution to avoid interference from Mg^{2+} binding to the chelator. The high concentration of total Mg in the cell and the lack of a good Mg^{2+}-selective buffer makes interpretation of the results that much more difficult. Although problematic when Ca^{2+} is the ion of interest, the Mg^{2+} binding capability of DM-nitrophen can be turned into an advantage in the study of Mg^{2+}-dependent processes. The technical problem of Ca^{2+} binding to DM-nitrophen can be easily solved by the inclusion of a readily available highly Ca^{2+}-selective buffer like BAPTA. Caged Mg^{2+} has been used to study the activation of Na^+ pump proteins by MgATP in isolated canine kidney membranes (30), but until the present studies, it does not appear to have been used in intact cells. As in the Na$^+$ pump studies, the effects attributed to MgATP following the photolysis of caged Mg^{2+} can be confirmed by photolyzing caged ATP in the presence of Mg^{2+}.

Effects of Photolysis of Caged Mg^{2+} on L-Type Ca^{2+} Currents

Figure 1 depicts the striking effect of photolysis of the Mg–DM-nitrophen complex on cardiac L-type Ca^{2+} current (I$_{Ca}$) in guinea pig ventricular myocytes. In this experiment, Mg, ATP, and DM-nitrophen concentrations in the intracellular solution were selected so that the calculated intracellular Mg^{2+} would rise from 0.16 μM before a flash to 76 μM after complete photolysis. MgATP would correspondingly rise from 2.9 μM to 365 μM. A clear biphasic effect on I$_{Ca}$ amplitude ensued after a flash (marked by the arrow in Fig. 1A), consisting of an immediate inhibition of the current followed by a slower sustained upregulatory response. A similar effect, albeit of a lesser magnitude, was observed after a second flash as a result of destruction of the remaining unphotolyzed DM-nitrophen. The lack of an increase in subsequent flashes confirmed the completeness of the photolysis. The increase in current amplitude was not accompanied by alterations in the kinetics of activation of the current (see raw current records shown at the top of Fig. 1A) and no statistically significant effects on the inactivation rate of the current were observed when longer test pulses were used (not shown).

As a confirmation that Ca^{2+} flux through the pore was not required for the upregulatory response, Ca^{2+} was replaced with Ba^{2+} in the extracellular solution. Very similar results were obtained under these conditions (Fig. 1B), confirming that the response could not be attributed to Ca^{2+} acting as an intracellular second messenger (which was highly unlikely in any case, given the presence of excess BAPTA in the pipet solution). This experiment also ruled out interactions between Ca^{2+} and sites in and around the pore potentially responsible for Ca^{2+}-dependent inactivation (27, 31) or facilitation (32).

Because the change in Mg^{2+} after photolysis was relatively small in the experiments previously discussed, screening of negative surface charges on the cytosolic face of the sarcolemma should have been negligible. This was confirmed by examining the effect of Mg^{2+} release on I$_{Ca}$ over a wide range of test potentials. As shown in Fig. 2A, I$_{Ca}$ was enhanced over the entire range of the current-voltage curve, with only a slightly greater effect evident at negative potentials. In addition, the specific nature of the effect of Mg^{2+} release on Ca^{2+} channels as compared with the effect on Na$^+$ channels (Fig. 2B) argues against a significant contribution of surface charge screening. Furthermore, it is unlikely that I$_{Ca}$ enhancement was the result of a direct effect of Mg^{2+} on the channel; the change in intracellular

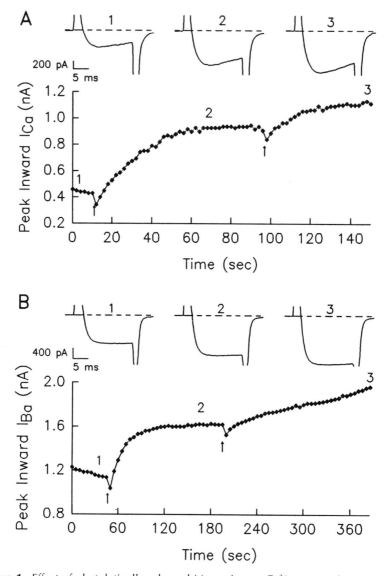

Figure 1. Effect of photolytically released Mg on L-type Ca^{2+} currents in guinea pig ventricular myocytes. (**A**) Flash photolysis of intracellular caged Mg^{2+} (indicated by arrows) in the presence of BAPTA evokes a biphasic effect on I_{Ca} (2 mM external Ca^{2+}). After a transient inhibition of the current, sustained upregulation of I_{Ca} was observed. The effect was maximal after two flashes. Each value in the time course represents the peak inward current for brief depolarizations from -40 mV to 0 mV. Raw current records [**top** of (**A**)] for the indicated times demonstrate that there is little effect of the Mg^{2+} release on the kinetics of I_{Ca}. (**B**) The analogous experiment conducted with 2 mM Ba^{2+} instead of Ca^{2+} in the external solution.

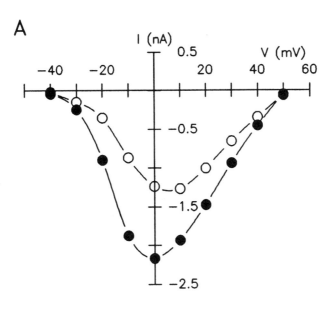

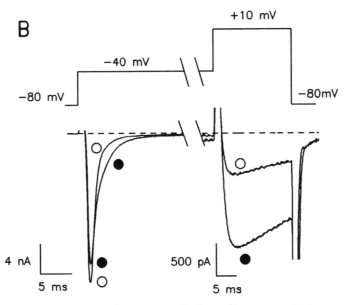

Figure 2. Response to Mg²⁺ release is specific for Ca²⁺ current. (**A**) Current-voltage relationship for I_{Ca} before and after photolysis (○, before flash; ●, after flash) of caged Mg. I_{Ca} increased over the entire range of test potentials with a minimal hyperpolarizing shift of the current activation curve. (**B**) I_{Ca} in the test pulse to 10 mV substantially increases in response to Mg²⁺ release (○, before flash; ●, after flash) without an increase in I_{Na} in the inactivating prepulse to −40 mV. The reduction in I_{Na} occurred slowly during the experiment and was not correlated with the timing of the flashes.

Mg^{2+} was small (well below the millimolar range), and the effect was directionally opposite to that expected for an increase in intracellular Mg^{2+}.

Role of ATP and Phosphorylation in the Response to Mg^{2+} Release

The next likely candidate as a mediator of the observed effect was MgATP. Two different strategies were used to confirm that MgATP was required. First, Mg^{2+} release was initiated after cytosolic ATP was depleted by omitting ATP from the intracellular solution and inducing ATP degradation by including the mitochondrial uncoupler dinitrophenol. As shown in Fig. 3A, Mg^{2+} release after this intervention did not support the upregulatory response. The second strategy was to keep Mg^{2+} in the physiological range and to increase rapidly cytosolic MgATP by photolysis of caged ATP. This resulted in enhancement of I_{Ca} amplitude with a time course and magnitude reminiscent of that observed after Mg^{2+} release (Fig. 3B), supporting the idea that a direct relationship exists between MgATP levels and I_{Ca} amplitude.

With the wealth of information linking cAMP-dependent phosphorylation pathway with L-type Ca^{2+} channel activity in the heart (33, 34), it was of interest to determine if phosphorylation plays a role in the MgATP-induced upregulatory phenomenon. Two different methods were used to block phosphorylation of the Ca^{2+} channels. First, myocytes were equilibrated with intracellular solutions containing high concentrations of non-hydrolyzable ATP analogs. By competing with ATP at the active site of regulatory kinases (35), these analogs can effectively prevent channel phosphorylation, provided that care is taken to reduce endogenous ATP production (34). In an initial set of experiments, this precaution was met by uncoupling mitochondrial function with dinitrophenol in the absence of any exogenous fuel substrate. Under these nonphosphorylating conditions, intracellular release of Mg in the presence of either adenylylmethylenediphosphate (AMP-PCP) or adenylylimidodiphosphate (AMP-PNP) still resulted in marked enhancement of I_{Ca} amplitude (Fig. 4A). In other experiments, an even more stringent blockade of endogenous ATP generation was used. In addition to inhibiting mitochondrial function, glycolytic flux was blocked by adding 2-deoxyglucose to the extracellular medium, and an inhibitor of myokinase was added to the intracellular solution. These interventions resulted in gradual contracture of the myocytes, presumably as a consequence of degradation of residual ATP to levels inducing rigor cross-bridge formation (36). The upregulation of calcium current following Mg^{2+} release was not significantly diminished by the prior development of rigor (Fig. 4A), suggesting that the Mg nucleotide itself may have a direct, phosphorylation-independent effect on Ca^{2+} channel activity.

The second strategy to support the conclusion that Ca^{2+} channels could be modulated by MgATP via a phosphorylation-independent pathway

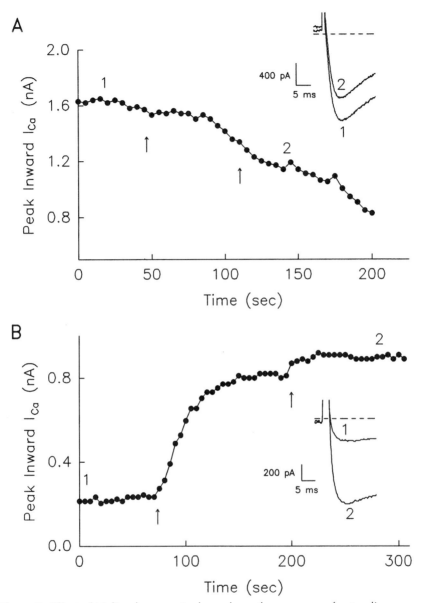

Figure 3. Effect of Mg²⁺ release on I_{Ca} depends on the presence of cytosolic nucleotides. (**A**) In cells dialyzed without ATP in the internal solution and subjected to metabolic inhibition (200 μM dinitrophenol), the upregulatory response was not observed after Mg²⁺ release from caged Mg. (**B**) In the presence of 0.8 mM internal Mg²⁺, photolysis of 1 mM caged ATP induced an upregulatory response similar to the effect of caged Mg. In (A) and (B), insets depict superimposed current records for the indicated points on the time course before [1] and after [2] flashes.

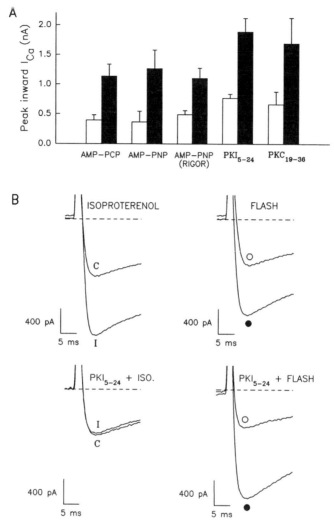

Figure 4. Upregulation of I_{Ca} by Mg^{2+} release does not depend on phosphorylation. (**A**) Replacement of ATP with nonhydrolyzable ATP analogs (the three groups on the **left-hand side** of the figure) or inclusion of peptide inhibitors of protein kinase A or C (the two groups to the right) does not attenuate the response to Mg^{2+} release. Values indicate the mean ± SEM for an N of 4 or more in each group (□, before flashes; ■, after flashes). (**B**) Exposure to 100 nM isoproterenol increases the peak inward Ca^{2+} current in a cell equilibrated with caged Mg^{2+} and ATP (**upper left:** C, before isoproterenol; I, during isoproterenol). After washout of the isoproterenol, an increase of similar magnitude was observed in response to photolysis of caged Mg^{2+} (**upper right:** O, before flash; ●, after flash) . In a different cell, PKI_{5-24}) was added to the internal solution, resulting in inhibition of the isoproterenol response (**lower left**), but not the response to Mg^{2+} release (**lower right**).

was to use specific peptide blockers of the kinases normally associated with channel regulation. The inclusion of an active 20 amino acid peptide fragment of the protein kinase A inhibitor protein (PKI$_{5-24}$) (37) completely suppressed the effect of 100 nM isoproterenol on I_{Ca}, but did not alter the response to photolysis of caged Mg^{2+} (Fig. 4B). Additionally, in the absence of PKI$_{5-24}$, the observation that the cell could still respond robustly to isoproterenol in the low Mg condition (before the flash) suggests that the Mg^{2+} and MgATP requirements for the cAMP-dependent pathway are likely to be lower than those of the phosphorylation-independent pathway. Previous reports have suggested that intracellular ATP enhances I_{Ca} with a K$_D$ in the millimolar range (24). The effects of ATP on channel phosphorylation were proposed to account for these earlier findings. That conclusion may be subject to reinterpretation in light of present results.

The large amount of Ca^{2+} buffer present in our experiments, as well as the observation that the response occurred in the presence of Ba^{2+}, made it highly unlikely that calmodulin-dependent kinases or protein kinase C were involved in the response to Mg^{2+} release. Nevertheless, protein kinase C has been reported to increase the activity of L-type Ca^{2+} channels in single channel patches (38), so a specific peptide inhibitor was used to rule out this possibility as well. Intracellular equilibration with 10 µM PKC$_{19-36}$ (39), containing the pseudosubstrate inhibitor portion of the kinase, did not alter the effect of caged Mg photolysis on I_{Ca} (Fig. 4, A and B). We also observed no effect of phorbol myristate acetate, a protein kinase C activator, on Ca^{2+} current, regardless of whether or not the peptide inhibitor was present.

Effects of Mg Nucleotides on Single Ca^{2+} Channels

An increase in whole-cell Ca^{2+} current can occur by several different means when one examines underlying single channel events. Macroscopic current (I) is the product of the number of channels in the membrane available for opening (N), the probability that a channel will open (P$_0$), and the single channel conductance of the channel (i), or $I = N \cdot P_0 \cdot i$. For example, activation of the cAMP-dependent phosphorylation pathway results in an increase in channel availability (seen as an increase in the number of openings during a depolarizing pulse) and an increase in probability of opening. The latter is manifested both as an increase in the frequency of openings during a depolarizing pulse (33) and an increase in the number of long openings (40). An example of the effect of β-adrenergic receptor stimulation on single L-type Ca^{2+} channel activity is depicted in Fig. 5. Under control conditions, single-channel openings (Fig. 5; left panel) are quite brief and often do not occur at all during depolarizations to the various test potentials shown to the left of the records. In contrast, exposure to 1 µM isoproterenol increases channel availability (as evidenced by a reduction in the number of blank sweeps; middle and

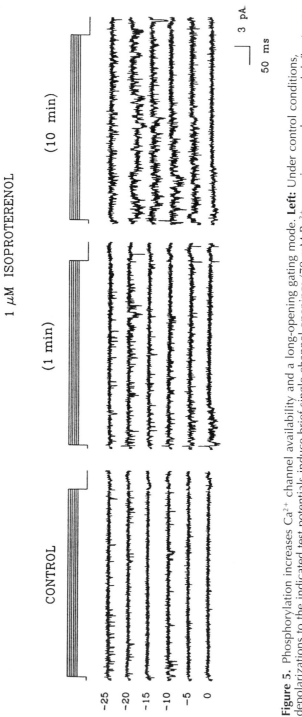

Figure 5. Phosphorylation increases Ca²⁺ channel availability and a long-opening gating mode. **Left:** Under control conditions, depolarizations to the indicated test potentials induce brief single-channel openings (70 mM Ba²⁺; openings are downward deflections). Pulses without an opening are often observed. **Middle:** Soon after exposure to isoproterenol, the percentage of pulses showing channel activity increases and the frequency of channel reopening during a pulse are greater. **Right:** Prolonged exposure reveals an increase in the occurrence of openings of a longer duration.

right panels) and increases the occurrence of a long-opening mode of the channel (right panel of Fig. 5). At present, experiments are under way to delineate which effect on single-channel activity underlies the phosphorylation-independent effect of Mg nucleotides on the whole-cell Ca^{2+} current. Properly conducting the necessary experiments requires recording single Ca^{2+} channel currents, while simultaneously dialyzing the intracellular space with caged Mg^{2+} and AMP-PNP. Our preliminary results indicate that rapidly increasing MgAMP-PNP concentration results in an increase in the number of active sweeps and in the frequency of reopening during a depolarization, similar to the some of the effects of isoproterenol. No changes in the amplitude of the single-channel currents or in the occurrence of the long-opening mode of the channel were observed (unpublished data).

Ion channels as MgATP Sensors

Elucidation of the phosphorylation-independent pathway does not diminish the importance of cAMP-dependent phosphorylation as the primary mechanism for increasing Ca^{2+} channel activity in the heart. However, it does stimulate speculation as to the supplementary role of MgATP in linking metabolism to Ca^{2+} influx. As pointed out by Goldhaber et al. (41), cytosolic Ca^{2+} transients are reduced in ventricular myocytes during metabolic inhibition as a result of both a reduction in I_{Ca} and impaired coupling between the Ca^{2+} current and SR Ca^{2+} release, even though the caffeine-releasable pool of Ca^{2+} is actually greater than the control condition. Similarly, Taniguchi et al. (42) reported that I_{Ca} depression induced by metabolic inhibition could be reversed by injection of ATP. During times of metabolic stress, the ability of the Ca^{2+} channels to sense MgATP levels may serve as a protective mechanism to reduce the metabolic demand associated with Ca^{2+} removal by cutting back on the trigger for Ca^{2+} release. This type of stop-gap regulation would be conducted at no energy cost to the cell and would function even when the phosphorylation pathway is in high gear. One situation where this may occur is during ischemia, where cytosolic Mg^{2+} rises, MgATP falls (43) and the sympathetic nerves are in overdrive. The overall picture of ion channel activity at this time may include inhibition of the sarcoplasmic reticulum Ca^{2+} release channels (15), activation of ATP-sensitive K^+ channels (44), and perhaps a reduction in Ca^{2+} current as a result of both the drop in MgATP and the rise in Mg^{2+}.

Close coupling between energy metabolism and Ca^{2+} channel activity has also been reported in mouse pancreatic β-cells. In these insulin-producing cells, secretion is triggered by a rise in extracellular glucose concentration. Glucose metabolism leads to depolarization of the cell membrane by closing ATP-sensitive K^+ channels and also results in direct enhancement

Table 1. Comparison of intracellular Mg_i^{2+} nucleotides or Mg nucleotide complexes on several ion channel types.*

Channel	Mg_i^{2+}	(Mg) ATP		(Mg) AMPPxP		Phosphorylation
K_{ATP}	↓	No	↓	No	↓	↑
SR Ca^{2+} release	↓	No	↑	No	↑	Yes
Cl^- (CFTR)	?	Yes	↑	No	No	↑
Gap junction	↓	Yes	↑	Yes	↑	Yes
L-type Ca^{2+}	↓	Yes	↑	Yes	↑	↑

*Arrows indicate positive or negative effects on channel activity. Yes or no indicates whether a given effect requires the Mg nucleotide complex (in the case of the second and third columns) or is phosphorylated without a clear functional effect (fourth column).

of Ca^{2+} channel activity (45). Phosphorylation-independent modulation of the Ca^{2+} channels by MgATP may play a role in this response.

Because direct, phosphorylation-independent effects of MgATP on Ca^{2+} channels is a novel idea, it is useful to compare the working hypothesis with the regulatory schemes of other known ATP-sensitive channels. First, the ATP-sensitive K^+ channel is regulated in a complex manner by Mg^{2+} and nucleotides. ATP or AMP-PNP inhibit channel opening without a requirement for magnesium, whereas MgADP may act to open the channel after it has become dephosphorylated (46). Mg^{2+} also inhibits channel opening. A second example is the Ca^{2+} release channel of the sarcoplasmic reticulum. ATP or AMP-PNP facilitate channel opening without requiring magnesium, whereas Mg^{2+} inhibits opening (15). A third regulatory design is found for CFTR. Cl^- currents through this channel are activated by MgATP directly through a nucleotide binding domain, but only when the channel has been previously phosphorylated. MgAMP-PNP does not support the activation of the CFTR currents (16). The comparisons among nucleotide-regulated channels are summarized in Table 1. The effect of Mg nucleotides on Ca^{2+} channels may represent a fourth modulatory mechanism in that it requires the Mg nucleotide complex but does not require a nucleotide with a transferable γ-phosphate. Criteria analogous to these are common among enzymes modulated by allosteric effectors (4, 6, 47). Although it has been reported that L-type Ca^{2+} channel preparations from cardiac and skeletal muscle are photoaffinity-labeled by 8-azido-ATP (48), it is not known whether MgATP binding sites exist on the Ca^{2+} channel itself. Alternative hypotheses include Mg nucleotide action on proteins associated with the channel (49) or on sites distant from the channel, but capable of producing a second messenger.

Summary

Mg undoubtedly fulfills a unique role in the coordination of cellular activities. The balance between Mg^{2+} and MgATP profoundly alters enzyme

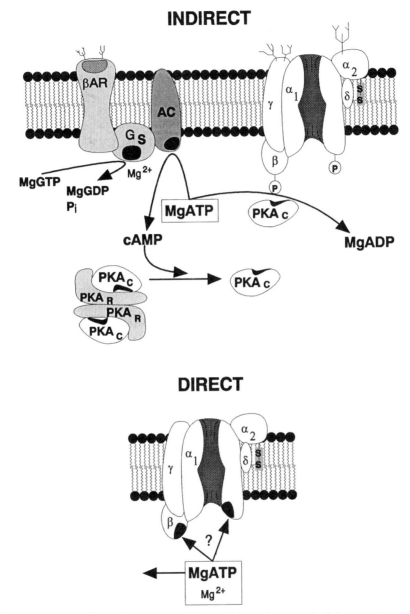

Figure 6. Top: Mg^{2+} and Mg nucleotides participate in several of the reaction steps involved in the indirect regulatory pathway leading from β-adrenergic receptor occupation (βAR) to phosphorylation of the Ca^{2+} channel. MgGTP is required for G-protein (G_S) activation, whereas MgATP serves as the substrate for both adenylate cyclase (AC) and the catalytic subunit of protein kinase A (PKA_C). Mg^{2+} serves as an activator of both the G-protein and adenylate cyclase. **Bottom:** Mg^{2+} and MgATP may also act directly on the Ca^{2+} channel or on associated proteins with the two species mediating opposite effects on channel activity.

function, including pathways responsible for the regulation of ion channels. Cardiac L-type Ca^{2+} channels are particularly sensitive to the stimulation of receptors that initiate a cascade involving the generation of cAMP, and ultimately, phosphorylation of the channel protein. Each step of this indirect mechanism, including receptor activation, G-protein activation, cAMP generation by adenylate cyclase, and the protein kinase A phosphorylation step, requires either Mg^{2+}, an Mg nucleotide, or both (Fig. 6, upper panel). Another effect of MgATP may be to activate the Ca^{2+} channels by a more direct, phosphorylation-independent route (Fig. 6, lower panel). Presumably, this mechanism could enable the Ca^{2+} channel to sense local MgATP concentration during times of metabolic stress, thus serving as a brake on further Ca^{2+} entry, regardless of the phosphorylation state of the channels. When energy production is slowed, a decrease in MgATP and the corresponding increase in intracellular Mg^{2+} are likely to participate in negative feedback control of cardiac L-type Ca^{2+} channel activity.

References

1. Hille, B. (1992). *Ionic Channels of Excitable Membranes* (Sinauer Associates, Inc., Sunderland, MA).

2. Ingraham, L.L., and Green, D.E. (1958). Role of magnesium in enzyme-catalyzed syntheses involving adenosine triphosphate. *Science* **128:**310–312.

3. Vernon, W.B., and Wacker, W.E.C. (1978). Magnesium metabolism, in *Recent Advances in Clinical Biochemistry*, K.G. M.M. Alberti, Ed. (Churchill Livingstone, Edinburgh), pp. 39–71.

4. Wong, I., and Lohman, T.M. (1992). Allosteric effects of nucleotide cofactors on *Escherichia coli* rep helicase-DNA binding. *Science* **256:**350–355.

5. Ulrich., F. (1964). Kinetic studies of the activation of mitochondrial adenosine triphosphate by Mg^{2+}. *J. Biol. Chem.* **239:**3532–3536.

6. Roberts, D., and Kellett, G.L. (1980). The kinetics of effector binding to phosphofructokinase. *Biochem. J.* **189:**561–567.

7. Mildvan, A.S. (1970). Metals in enzyme catalysis, in *The Enzymes*, P.D. Boyer, Ed. (Academic Press, New York), pp. 445–536.

8. Cech, S.Y., Broaddus, W.C., and Maguire, M.E. (1980). Adenylate cyclase: The role of magnesium and other divalent cations. *Mol. Cell. Biochem.* **33:**67–92.

9. Garner, P.S. and Rosett, T. (1973). The influence of Mg^{2+}/adenine nucleotide ratios and absolute concentration of Mg^{2+}/adenine nucleotide on the observed velocity of some kinase reactions. *FEBS Lett.* **34:**243–246.

10. Kass, R.S., and Krafte, D.S. (1987). Negative surface charge density near heart calcium channels. Relevance to block by dihydropyridines. *J. Gen. Physiol.* **89:**629–644.

11. Vandenberg, C.A. (1987). Inward rectification of a potassium channel in cardiac ventricular cells depends on internal magnesium ions. *Proc. Natl. Acad. Sci. U.S.A.* **84:**2560–2564.

12. Horie, M., and Irisawa, H. (1989). Dual effects of intracellular magnesium on muscarinic potassium channel current in single guinea-pig atrial cells. *J. Physiol.* **408**:313–332.

13. Mayer, M.L., and Westbrook, G.L. (1987). Permeation and block of N-methyl-D-aspartic acid receptor channels by divalent cations in mouse cultured central neurones. *J. Physiol.* **394**:501–527.

14. Findlay, I. (1987). The effects of magnesium upon adenosine triphosphate-sensitive potassium channels in a rat insulin-secreting cell line. *J. Physiol.* **391**:611–629.

15. Meissner, G., and Henderson, J.S. (1987). Rapid calcium release from cardiac sarcoplasmic reticulum vesicles is dependent on Ca^{2+} and is modulated by Mg^{2+}, adenine nucleotide, and calmodulin. *J. Biol. Chem.* **262**:3065–3073.

16. Anderson, M.P., Berger, H.A., Rich, D.P., Gregory, R.J., Smith, A.E., and Welsh, M.J. (1991). Nucleoside triphosphates are required to open the CFTR chloride channel. *Cell* **67**:775–784.

17. Goulding, E.H., Ngai, J., Kramer, R.H., Colicos, S., Axel, R., Siegelbaum, S.A., and Chess, A. (1992). Molecular cloning and single channel properties of the cyclic nucleotide-gated channel from catfish olfactory neurons. *Neuron* **8**:45–58.

18. Brown, A.M., and Birnbaumer, L. (1988). Direct G protein gating of ion channels. *Am. J. Physiol.* **254**:H401–H410.

19. Burnstock, G. (1981). *Purinergic Receptors* (Chapman and Hill, London).

20. Lansman, J.B., Hess, P., and Tsien, R.W. (1986). Blockade of current through single calcium channels by Cd^{2+}, Mg^{2+}, and Ca^{2+}. Voltage and concentration dependence of calcium entry into the pore. *J. Gen. Physiol* **88**:321–347.

21. Hartzell, H.C., and White, R.E. (1989). Effects of magnesium on inactivation of the voltage-gated calcium current in cardiac myocytes. *J. Physiol.* **94**:745–767.

22. Agus, Z.S., Kelepouris, E., Dukes, I., and Morad, M. (1989). Cytosolic magnesium modulates calcium channel activity in mammalian ventricular cells. *Am. J. Physiol.* **256**:C452–C455.

23. Belles, B., Malécot, C.O., Hescheler, J., and Trautwein, W. (1988). "Rundown" of the Ca current during long whole-cell recordings in guinea pig heart cells: role of phosphorylation and intracellular calcium. *Pflügers Arch.* **411**:353–360.

24. Irisawa, H., and Kokubun, S. (1983). Modulation by intracellular ATP and cyclic AMP of the slow inward current in isolated single ventricular cells of the guinea-pig. *J. Physiol.* **338**:321–337.

25. Adams, S.R., Kao, J.P.Y., Grynkiewicz, G., Minta, A., and Tsien, R.Y. (1988). Biologically useful chelators that release Ca^{2+} upon illumination. *J. Am. Chem. Soc.* **110**:3212–3220.

26. Kaplan, J.H., and Ellis-Davies, G.C.R. (1988). Photolabile chelators for the rapid photorelease of divalent cations. *Proc. Natl. Acad. Sci. U.S.A.* **85**:6571–6575.

27. Morad, M., Davies, N.W., Kaplan, J.H., and Luy, H.D. (1988). Inactivation and block of calcium channels by photo-released Ca^{2+} in dorsal root ganglion neurons. *Science* **241:**842–844.

28. Hadley, R.W., and Lederer, W.J. (1991). Ca^{2+} and voltage inactivate Ca^{2+} channels in guinea-pig ventricular myocytes through independent mechanisms. *J. Physiol.* **444:**257–268.

29. Gurney, A.M., Charnet, P., Pye, J.M., and Nargeot, J. (1989). Augmentation of cardiac calcium current by flash photolysis of intracellular caged-Ca^{2+} molecules. *Nature* **341:**65–68.

30. Klodos, I., and Forbush, B., III. (1988). Rapid conformational changes of the Na/K pump revealed by a fluorescent dye. *J. Gen. Physiol.* **92:**46a (Abstract).

31. Yue, D.T., Backx, P.H., and Imredy, J.P. (1990). Calcium-sensitive inactivation in the gating of single calcium channels. *Science* **250:**1735–1738.

32. Zygmunt, A.C., and Maylie, J. (1990). Stimulation-dependent facilitation of the high threshold calcium current in guinea-pig ventricular myocytes. *J. Physiol.* **428:**653–671.

33. Tsien, R.W., Bean, B.P., Hess, P., Lansman, J.B., Nilius, B., and Nowycky, M.C. (1986). Mechanisms of calcium channel modulation by β-adrenergic agents and dihydropyridine calcium agonists. *J. Mol. Cell. Cardiol.* **18:**691–710.

34. Kameyama, M., Hofmann, F., and Trautwein, W. (1985). On the mechanism of β-adrenergic regulation of the Ca channel in the guinea-pig heart. *Pflügers Arch.* **405:**285–293.

35. Yount, R.G., Babcock, D., Ballantyne, W., and Ojala, D. (1971). Adenylyl imidodiphosphate, an adenosine triphosphate analog containing a P-N-P linkage. *Biochemistry* **10:**2484–2489.

36. Fabiato, A., and Fabiato, F. (1975). Effects of magnesium on contractile activation of skinned cardiac cells. *J. Physiol.* **249:**497–517.

37. Cheng, H.-C., Van Patten, S.M., Smith, A.J., and Walsh, D.A. (1985). An active twenty-amino-acid-residue peptide derived from the inhibitor protein of the cyclic AMP-dependent protein kinase. *Biochem. J.* **231:**655–661.

38. Lacerda, A.E., Rampe, D., and Brown, A.M. (1988). Effects of protein kinase C activators on cardiac Ca^{2+} channels. *Nature* **335:**249–251.

39. House, C., and Kemp, B.E. (1987). Protein kinase C contains a pseudosubstrate prototope in its regulatory domain. *Science* **238:**1726–1728.

40. Yue, D.T., Herzig, S., and Marban, E. (1990). β-Adrenergic stimulation of calcium channels occurs by potentiation of high-activity gating modes. *Proc. Natl. Acad. Sci. U.S.A.* **87:**753–757.

41. Goldhaber, J.I., Parker, J.M., and Weiss, J.N. (1991). Mechanisms of excitation-contraction coupling failure during metabolic inhibition in guinea-pig ventricular myocytes. *J. Physiol.* **443:**371–386.

42. Taniguchi, J., Noma, A., and Irisawa, H. (1983). Modification of the cardiac action potential by intracellular injection of adenosine triphosphate and related substances in guinea pig single ventricular cells. *Circ. Res.* **53:**131–139.

43. Borchgrevink, P.C., Bergan, A.S., Bakoy, O.E., and Jynge, P. (1989). Magnesium and reperfusion of ischemic rat heart assessed by ^{31}P-NMR. *Am. J. Physiol.* **256:**H195–H204.

44. Venkatesh, N., Lamp, S.T., and Weiss, J.N. (1991). Sulfonylureas, ATP-sensitive K$^+$ channels, and cellular K$^+$ loss during hypoxia, ischemia, and metabolic inhibition in mammalian ventricle. *Circ. Res.* **69:**623–637.

45. Smith, P.A., Rorsman, P., and Ashcroft, F.M. (1989). Modulation of dihydropyridine-sensitive Ca^{2+} channels by glucose metabolism in mouse pancreatic β-cells. *Nature* **342:**550–553.

46. Tung, R.T., and Kurachi, Y. (1991). On the mechanism of nucleotide diphosphate activation of the ATP-sensitive [K+] channel in ventricular cell of guinea-pig. *J. Physiol.* **437:**239–256.

47. Hammes, G.G., and Wu, C.-W. (1974). Kinetics of allosteric enzymes. *Ann. Rev. Biophys. Bioeng.* **3:**1–33.

48. Murphy, B.J., and Tuana, B.S. (1989). Phosphorylation and the identification of a protein kinase activity associated with the dihydrophyridine receptor isolated from rabbit heart and skeletal muscle. *Ann. N.Y. Acad. Sci.* **560:**391–394.

49. Kim, K.C., Caswell, A.H., Talvenheimo, J.A., and Brandt, N.R. (1990). Isolation of a terminal cisterna protein which may link the dihydropyridine receptor to the junctional foot protein in skeletal muscle. *Biochemistry* **29:**9281–9289.

7

Delayed Rectifier Potassium Channels of Cardiac Muscle

M. C. Sanguinetti and N. K. Jurkiewicz

The action potentials of cardiac myocytes are characterized by a prolonged depolarized state and a plateau phase (phase 2) that can last up to a few hundred milliseconds in some cell types. This is in contrast to the action potential of nerve cells that lasts only a few tens of milliseconds. This results from the simultaneous rapid inactivation of depolarizing inward currents (I_{Na} and I_{Ca}) and the relatively rapid activation of one or both of two distinct types of repolarizing outward K^+ channels: transient outward (I_{to}) and delayed outward rectifier (I_K) K^+ channels. I_{to} channels open (activate) almost immediately upon a shift in membrane potential to more positive levels and close (inactivate) within several milliseconds after opening. I_K channels also activate in response to a positive shift in membrane potential, but only after a distinct, albeit sometimes brief, delay. In addition, I_K channels do not inactivate appreciably and exhibit a property referred to as "rectification," meaning that the slope conductance either increases or decreases as the membrane is depolarized, in contrast to an ohmic (i.e., linear) current–voltage (I–V) relationship. Cardiac cells also have rapidly inactivating Na^+ and Ca^{2+} inward currents, and most have both I_{to} and I_K channels. The cellular basis for the long plateau phase of cardiac myocytes is complex (1), but results primarily from inward ("anomalous") rectification and/or very slow activation of multiple types of K^+ channels. The conductance of inward rectifier K^+ current (I_{K1}) in atrial and ventricular cells is high at negative membrane potentials and, as such, "clamps" the resting potential near E_K, the equilibrium potential for K^+ (about -85 mV). Upon depolarization, I_{K1} channels close almost instantly. I_{K1} channels remain closed throughout the plateau phase and do not contribute to the repolarization process until later in the action potential cycle. Thus, it is the activation of other outward K^+ channels during the plateau phase that initiates repolarization and the return of the membrane potential to a level (about -20 mV) where I_{K1} channels can again open and contribute to terminal (phase 3) repolarization.

Pacemaker sinoatrial node cells, like myocardial cells, also have a multitude of different currents that determine action potential configuration, including a delayed rectifier I_K current, which initiates a gradual repolarization from the plateau phase (Fig. 1). Overall, I_K channels thus represent a diverse group that have only recently been clearly distinguished from one another. To date, three distinct types of I_K channels have been identified in isolated cardiac cells based on differences in rate of activation, rectification properties, and pharmacology using whole-cell voltage clamp techniques. These types are (1) slowly activating, outwardly rectifying I_K (I_{Ks}, I_{x2}); (2) rapidly activating, inwardly rectifying I_K (I_{Kr}, I_{x1}); and (3) rapidly activating, outwardly rectifying I_K (I_{RAK}, HK2). This classification does not imply the existence of only three classes of I_K channel proteins. For example, I_{RAK} and HK2 are strikingly different in primary amino acid sequence, despite somewhat similar electrophysiological properties. It is important to note that the height and duration of the plateau phase differ markedly between different regions of the heart and between species. For example, in most vertebrate species that have been investigated, cardiac Purkinje cells have a much longer plateau phase than ventricular cells, which in turn is longer than atrial cells. The types of I_K and their relative magnitude in a given cell is in part responsible for the observed tissue- and species-dependent differences in action potential duration. A description of each delayed rectifier K^+ channel type and their pharmacological modulation by antiarrhythmic agents is the focus of this chapter.

I_K of Multicellular Preparations

The first detailed description of cardiac delayed rectifier current was made in 1969 by Noble and Tsien (2), who concluded that in Purkinje fibers this current had two distinct components, which they termed i_{x1} and i_{x2}. The reversal potentials of both current components were significantly different from E_K, such that the channels were believed to be only poorly K^+ selective. For this reason, the currents were termed i_x and not i_K. Both current components were characterized by a slow onset of activation, but whereas the fully activated I–V relationship of i_{x2} was linear, i_{x1} was an inward rectifier. Two components of I_K were also described in a sucrose-gap clamp study of cat ventricular trabeculae by McDonald and Trautwein (3). Subsequent studies showed that these initial experiments were complicated by inadequate space clamp and the effects of K^+ accumulation between cells of this multicellular tissue during long lasting voltage clamp pulses (4–6). These investigators concluded that at least the slower component (i_{x2}) was probably an experimental artifact, and that only a single delayed outward current existed in cardiac Purkinje fibers. More recently it was suggested that the multiexponential nature of delayed rectifier activation could easily be accounted for by assuming a multistate scheme for the activation of a single population of I_K channels (7, 8).

RABBIT SA NODAL CELL

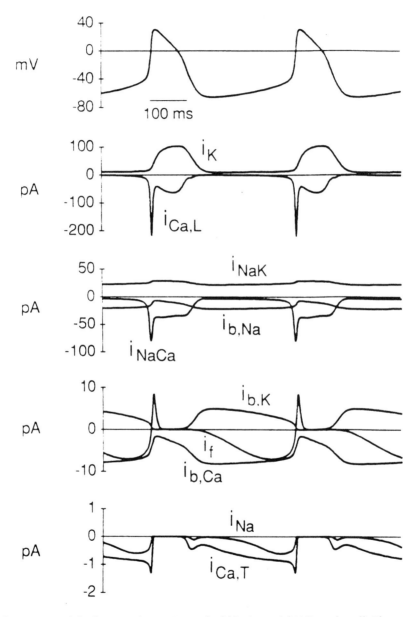

Figure 1. Model of pacemaker activity of rabbit sinoatrial (SA) node cell. The most prominent outward current during the plateau and phase 3 repolarization is I_K. Note that the pA scale is different for each panel. [From Wilders et al. (70).]

123

I_K: Single-Cell Studies

The most detailed studies of I_K in the last decade have used single myocytes isolated from the hearts of frogs (9, 10), chicks (11, 12), guinea pigs (8, 13), and rabbits (14, 15). In the frog and guinea pig, I_K activates very slowly, requiring many seconds to reach a pseudo–steady-state and has a nearly ohmic I–V relationship (8–10, 13). In contrast, I_K of single rabbit nodal and Purkinje cells activates more rapidly and exhibits strong inward rectification (14, 15). The I_K of cell aggregates of chick heart has both an ohmic and a rectifying component. When the same preparation was disaggregated into single cells, only the nonrectifying component was observed using similar voltage clamp protocols (12). It is obvious from the heterogeneity in properties of delayed rectifier current recorded from different species that multiple types of K^+ channels contribute to the whole-cell current commonly referred to as I_K.

I_{Ks} and I_{Kr}

The existence of multiple types of I_K in a single cell was recently proposed based on specific block of one type by a group of structurally related class III antiarrhythmic drugs. Class III antiarrhythmic agents are characterized by their ability to prolong action potential duration, most often a result of blocking one or more repolarizing K^+ currents. Sotalol, a β-adrenergic receptor blocker and class III agent, was shown to be a relatively specific blocker of I_K (IC_{50} = 10 μM) in rabbit Purkinje fibers (16). The block of I_K in these fibers correlated well with the concentrations required to prolong action potential duration. In our initial attempt to duplicate this finding, we discovered that d-sotalol had little or no effect on I_K recorded from isolated guinea pig ventricular cells. A similar lack of effect was demonstrated for E-4031 (17), a more potent analog of sotalol. Both agents are methanesulfonanilides, but E-4031 is 750 times more potent in prolonging effective refractory period and action potential duration (18). In these initial experiments, I_K was quantified by measuring the magni-tude of slowly activating current during long pulses to test potentials >40 mV. The only effect of these agents using this pulse protocol was a slight decrease in the amplitude of the tail current measured on repolarization to the holding potential. This result could be interpreted to mean that either E-4031 blocked I_K in a voltage-dependent manner (assuming a single-channel type) or that the drug blocked a small K^+ current other than the dominant I_K. One way to detect if an outward K^+ current represents the net conductance of multiple types of K^+ channels is to determine if the amplitude of tail current increases in proportion to the outward current during test pulses of progressively increasing duration. This protocol is commonly referred to as an envelope of tails test (2). The ratio of tail current relative to that measured during a test depolarization would be constant if I_K was a single current. In the example shown in Fig. 2, I_K was recorded during steps to 40 mV (V_{test}) followed by return to a holding potential of -40 mV (V_{tail}). Assuming a K$^+$ selective channel and $E_K = -90$ mV: predicted ratio = $(V_{tail} - E_K)/(V_{test} - E_K) = 0.38$. Using this pulse protocol the ratio of tail current/outward current ($\Delta I_{Ktail}/\Delta I_K$) is not constant under control conditions, being larger at short versus long test

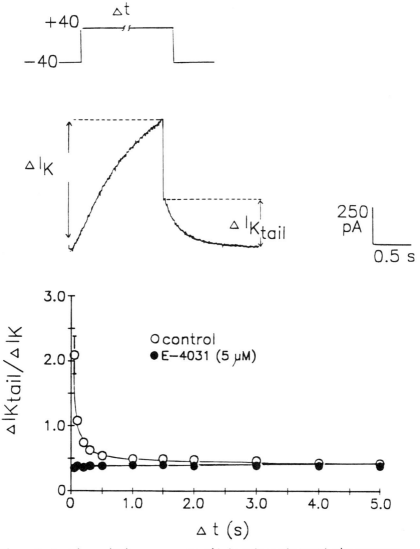

Figure 2. Test for multiple components of I_K in guinea pig ventricular myocyte (envelope of tails test). Ratio of tail current to outward current during pulse ($\Delta I_{Ktail}/\Delta I_K$) decreases as pulse duration is increased in control. After exposure to E-4031 the ratio is constant and equal to 0.38 (17).

depolarizations. In the presence of E-4031 the envelope of tails test is satisfied (Fig. 2), meaning that the ratio is constant regardless of pulse duration and that this ratio (0.38) is equal to the predicted value. This finding was the same as that reported previously, where La^{3+} was shown to effect the envelope of tails test similar to E-4031 (19). As expected, treatment of cells with La^{3+} prevents block of the rectifying component of I_K normally observed with E-4031 (Fig. 3) (20). The component of I_K that was sensitive to block by sotalol, E-4031, and La^{3+} was characterized further and shown to strikingly resemble the properties of I_K as described in rabbit single sinoatrial and atrioventricular node cells by Shibasaki (14). I_K of rabbit isolated nodal cells activates more rapidly than net I_K of guinea pig myocytes and displays inward rectification (Fig. 4). The intense inward rectification of I_{Kr} explains the envelope of tails test. At 40 mV, I_{Kr} rectifies strongly and, therefore, carries very little current. However, upon repolarization to -40 mV, I_{Kr} deactivates slowly, thereby contributing more than I_{Ks} to the net tail current following short test depolarizations. The current blocked by E-4031 and La^{3+} was named I_{Kr} to indicate its strong *rectifying* properties and *rapid* rate of activation (17). We refer to the much larger drug-insensitive current as I_{Ks} to denote its *slow* onset of activation. More than 20 years after it was first suggested, then later discounted, that cardiac I_K was resolved into two distinct components (2–6), development of specific blockers of one of these components has thus revived the concept that multiple types of I_K exist in mammalian myocytes.

I_{Kr} of guinea pig myocytes is also similar to I_K of rabbit nodal cells with respect to its midpoint of activation, slope factor of the activation curve, and sensitivity to β-adrenergic agonists and methanesulfonanilides. These properties of I_{Ks}, I_{Kr}, and rabbit I_K are summarized in Table 1. Another distinctive property of guinea pig I_{Kr} and rabbit I_K is the effect of extracellular K^+ on current magnitude. Exposure of cells to K^+-free saline increases I_{Ks}, as predicted by the increase in the driving force for K^+ (21). In contrast, I_{Kr} is greatly reduced by this change in extracellular $[K^+]$. This is similar to the effect of extracellular $[K^+]$ on I_K recorded from cells isolated from rabbit Purkinje fibers (15). The mechanism of this modulation by extracellular K^+ is unknown, but may involve competition with Na^+ for an external blocking site (15). Evidence for multiple components of I_K in guinea pig atrial cells was also obtained by single channel analysis (22). In the presence of 150 mM extracellular K^+, two distinct channels were discerned (3 and 10 pS), with kinetics of deactivation consistent with one representing I_{Ks} (3 pS) and the other representing I_{Kr} (10 pS). The single channel conductance of rabbit nodal I_K [11 pS (14)] is almost identical to the large conductance I_K channel in guinea pig atrial cells. The conductance of I_{Ks} channels in guinea pig ventricular cells is below the level of detection, but was estimated to be ≤ 1 pS (23).

The activation of I_K by isoproterenol and other β-adrenergic receptor agonists has been well studied in frog and guinea pig cardiac myocytes.

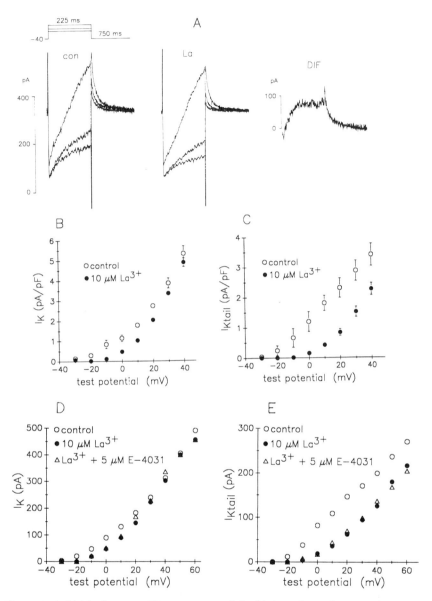

Figure 3. La^{3+} blocks a specific component (I$_{Kr}$) of I$_K$ in guinea pig myocytes.
(A) Currents recorded during pulses to 0, 10, and 30 mV in control (con) and
after addition of 10 μM La^{3+}. La^{3+}-sensitive current (DIF) for pulse to 10 mV is
shown at **right. (B, C)** Time-dependent currents (B) and tail currents (C) for five
cells using pulse protocol shown in (A). **(D, E)** E-4031 has no effect on currents
after treatment of cell with 10 μM La^{3+}. [Adapted from Sanguinetti and Jurkiewicz
(20).]

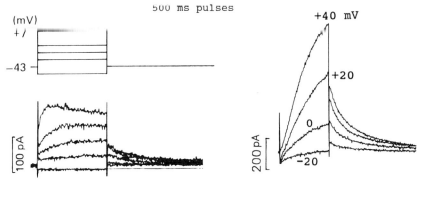

Figure 4. Delayed rectifiier K⁺ currents recorded during 500 msec pulses of isolated rabbit nodal and guinea pig ventricular cells. [Adapted from Shibasaki (14).]

Table 1. Comparison of delayed rectifier K^+ currents of guinea pig and rabbit cardiac myocytes

	GUINEA PIG		RABBIT
	I_{Ks}	I_{Kr}	I_K
τ activation (@ 0 mV)	400, 2400 msec	50 msec	50 msec
τ deactivation (@ −40 mV)	400 msec	170 msec	210 msec
Midpoint of activation	20 mV	−22 mV	−25 mV
Slope factor of activation	12.7 mV	7.5 mV	7.4 mV
Rectification	Slight	Marked (inward)	Marked (inward)
Single-channel conductance (150 mM K^+_0)	<1–3 pS	10 pS	11 pS
Effect of K^+_0 removal on current magnitude	Increase	Decrease	Decrease
Activation by β-agonists (1 μM isoproterenol)	Yes (250%–280%)	No	Partial (0%–36%)
Block by dofetilide	No (@ 100 μM)	Yes (IC_{50} = 32 nM)	Yes (IC_{50} = 4 nM)
Block by 10 μM La^{3+}	No	Yes	?
References	13,17,20–23,28	17,20–22,28,60	14,15,27,66

The maximal increase in I_K by these agents has been reported to be from 250% to 280% in guinea pig cells (24, 25) and from 50% to 100% in frog atria (26), but only minor increases occur in rabbit nodal cells (27). This is consistent with the interpretation that β-adrenergic receptor stimulation enhances I_{Ks}, but not I_{Kr} (28), and that rabbit nodal cells have only a minor I_{Ks} component. In guinea pig nodal cells the only measurable I_K had properties described for I_{Ks}, but not I_{Kr} (29), once again illustrating the species-dependent expression of the two channel types.

Fully activated I_{Ks} is about 11-fold greater than I_{Kr} in guinea pig myocytes (Fig. 5). From this comparison it might seem that I_{Ks} is the primary current responsible for repolarization in these cells. However, full activation of I_{Ks} requires many seconds, whereas I_{Kr} activates with a $\tau < 50$ msec at 0 mV. During the time course of a normal action potential, the two currents activate to equivalent magnitudes (17), and thus may contribute almost equally to repolarization. However, the relative role of each current in determining the rate of repolarization depends on stimulation rate.

I_{sK}: Comparison with I_{Ks}

A channel with many properties consistent with its identity as I_{Ks} was recently expression cloned from rat kidney (30) and subsequently cloned by PCR techniques from mammalian heart (31). This channel protein, dubbed I_{sK} (30) or minK (32, 33), is only 130 (rat), or 129 (mouse, human) amino acids in length and has a single putative transmembrane spanning region (30–32). I_{sK} has no obvious homology with other known channel proteins. When RNA encoding this protein is expressed in *Xenopus* oocytes, an extremely slow activating, K^+ selective, voltage-dependent outward current is induced. Skepticism existed regarding the claim that I_{sK} mRNA encoded a channel, because conceivably similar results could be obtained if it coded for some modulatory protein that greatly increased the open probability or expression of some endogenous channel. The most compelling evidence that the I_{sK} gene does indeed code for a channel is the finding that point mutations in the putative transmembrane region alter cation selectivity and block by tetraethylammonium (TEA) and Ba^{2+} (33). Changing the phenylalanine at position 55 to a threonine increased the permeability of the expressed channels to NH_4^+ and Cs^+ (e.g., P_K/P_{Cs} decreased from 16.4 in wild type channels to 4.6 in the point mutant). The initial report that such a small protein could form a functional and selective channel was surprising. Even more astounding, however, was the report that injection of mRNA encoding a double deletion mutant (positions 10–39 and 94–130 deleted) still resulted in expression of I_{sK} current (34). This mutant is only 63 amino acids in length and includes the entire putative transmembrane region. It represents the ultimate "minK" channel.

Both I_{Ks} and I_{sK} are activated by an increase in intracellular $[Ca^{2+}]$ (35, 36). Activators of protein kinase C, such as phorbol esters and diacylglycerol

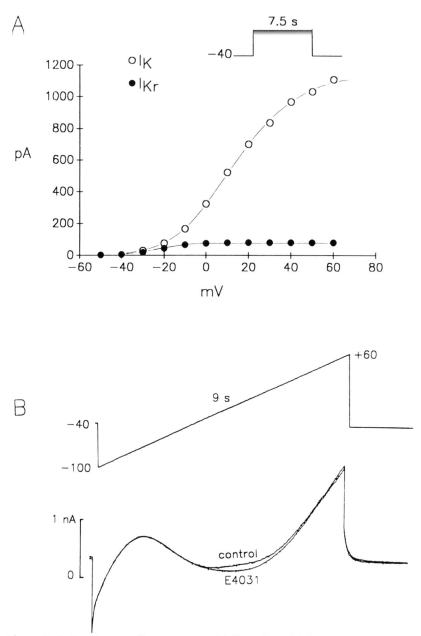

Figure 5. I_{Kr} is only a small component of fully activated I_K in guinea pig ventricular myocytes. **(A)** Voltage-dependence of activation of I_K and I_{Kr}. Plot shows tail current amplitude of I_K following 7.5-sec pulses to the indicated test potential. I_{Kr} represents the component of net I_K sensitive to block by 5 μM E-4031. Drug-insensitive current represents I_{Ks}. **(B)** Net currents activated during 9-sec voltage ramp from −100 mV to 60 mV. Note that E-4031 only blocks a small component of total current.

analogs, inhibit I_{sK}, an action that is prevented by the protein kinase C inhibitor staurosporine (37, 38). The inhibition of I_{sK} by protein kinase C activation is not observed when the channel is mutated within the consensus site for protein kinase C phosphorylation by substitution of alanine for the wild-type serine at position 103 (37). Receptor activation of phospholipase C, which stimulates production of both inositol triphosphate (IP_3) and diacylglycerol (DAG), enhances I_{sK} (39). For example, the net effect of hormones such as serotonin and endothelin is to increase I_{sK}. This implies that the effect of IP_3 (presumedly release of intracellular Ca^{2+}) overcomes the decrease in current that would otherwise occur via simultaneous activation of protein kinase C by DAG (39). In contrast to I_{sK} expressed in *Xenopus* oocytes, stimulation of protein kinase C by DAG or phorbol esters enhances I_{Ks} in isolated cardiac myocytes (40–42). Stimulation of protein kinase A by cAMP, 8-bromo-cAMP, forskolin, or the catalytic subunit of protein kinase A rapidly increases the magnitude of I_{Ks} several-fold in myocytes (24, 25, 40, 42). Both 8-bromo-cAMP and forskolin slowly increase rat I_{sK} expressed in *Xenopus* oocytes (43). These agents still increase I_{sK} in oocytes injected with site-directed mutants of the protein kinase A consensus site, suggesting that modulation occurs by some mechanism other than direct channel phosphorylation (43). In contrast, neither 8-bromo-cAMP nor forskolin have any effect on mouse I_{sK} expresed in oocytes (38).

I_{sK} is blocked by Ba^{2+} (31, 38), La^{3+} (31), and clofilium (31, 38) at concentrations similar to those required to block I_{Ks} in isolated cardiac myocytes (20, 44). In common with I_{Ks}, sotalol at a concentration of 300 µM has no effect on I_{sK} (38). However, in contrast to I_{Ks} of myocytes (45, 46), I_{sK} is not blocked by 4-aminopyridine (3 mM), amiodarone, bretylium, or tedisamil (38). This apparent discrepancy in sensitivity to modulators of I_{sK} and I_{Ks} may be caused by the difference in preparations (oocytes versus myocytes) more than any real differences between the channel proteins. A more quantitative comparison of the pharmacology of I_{Ks} and I_{sK} must await the successful transfection of mammalian cells with I_{sK}.

Embryonic Chick Heart I_K

Embryonic chick heart also has two distinct I_K channels with properties analogous to I_{Kr} and I_{Ks}, but the single-channel conductance of these channels is much greater than that observed in guinea pig myocytes. A very slowly activating K^+ current was recorded from 7- to 12-day-old ventricle ($\tau = 6$ sec at -20 mV) (47) and atria ($\tau = 2$ sec at -20 mV) (12). This current is also like I_{Ks} in that it has a half-point for activation of 15 mV with a slope factor of 10.3 mV, and it does not inactivate (47). The chick equivalent of I_{Ks} has a single-channel conductance of 15 pS and is blocked by both 4-aminopyridine and Ba^{2+} ($IC_{50} = 1$ mM) (46). Another I_K that is activated at more negative potentials (half-point = -40 mV) and exhibits inward rectification has been described in chick ventricle (47, 48) and in aggregates of chick atrial cells (11). This I_{Kr}-like current has a single-channel conductance of 63 pS. Oddly, the I_{Ks} equivalent (called I_{x2}), but not the I_{Kr}-like current (called I_{x1}), was observed during whole-cell voltage clamp of isolated chick atria (12). It is unclear why I_{x1} was observed in cell aggregates but not in isolated cells.

Rapidly Activating, Outwardly Rectifying I_{Ks}

I_{RAK}

The action potentials of rat myocytes are somewhat unusual in that they lack a plateau phase, because repolarization is very rapid, requiring only 4 msec in atrial cells and 27 msec in ventricular cells (49). The lack of a plateau phase in rat cardiac action potentials is caused by the presence of a very large transient outward K^+ current and a rapidly activating, ohmic I_K. The rat atrial I_K (I_{RAK}) is an outward rectifier with very rapid kinetics of activation and very slow inactivation (Fig. 6). I_{RAK} activates with a time constant of ~2 msec at 40 mV (assuming n^4 activation) and has a half-point for activation of -1.5 mV with a slope factor of 13.7 mV. The half-point for steady-state, slow inactivation is -41 mV (slope factor $= 9.4$ mV) (49). This property distinguishes I_{RAK} from all other cardiac I_K's, which either do not inactivate or do so only at much more positive membrane potentials. I_{RAK} is blocked by 4-aminopyridine ($IC_{50} = 0.6$mM), Ba^{2+} (IC_{50}

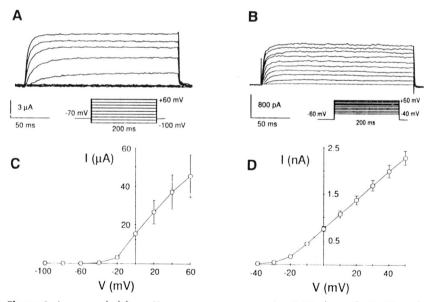

Figure 6. I_{RAK} recorded from *Xenopus* oocyte expressing RAK channels (**A, C**) and from single adult rat atrial cells (**B, D**). [From Paulmichl et al. (50).]

= 10 mM), and TEA ($IC_{50} > 50$ mM) (50). A similar current has been described in rat ventricular cells based on its relative (compared to a much larger I_{to}) sensitivity to block by TEA and insensitivity to block by 4-AP (51). The rat ventricular I_K is 50% inactivated at -70 mV.

A channel has been cloned and expressed from rat atria, which, when expressed in *Xenopus* oocytes, has a voltage-dependence and kinetics very similar to I_{RAK} (Fig. 6) (50). The primary sequence of this protein (RAK = rat heart Kv1.2) has been deduced and is very similar to the cloned rat brain K current, BK2. RAK is 499 amino acids in length and has a relative molecular weight of 56,766 with six potential transmembrane-spanning domains. Based on Northern blot analysis, the channel is much more abundant in rat atria than in ventricle (50), consistent with the relative magnitude of the current in cells isolated from the two tissues.

HK2

A current similar to I_{RAK} has been recorded in cells transfected with human cDNA encoding the HK2 channel (52). HK2 (human cardiac Kv1.5) is 605 amino acids in length and has a relative molecular weight of 66,640 (53). Similar to RAK, HK2 has six putative transmembrane regions as determined by hydropathy analysis and is more abundant in human atria than in ventricle. HK2 is 86% identical to its rat Kv1.5 homolog and shares 96% identity within the putative transmembrane domains (53). When expressed in mouse Ltk⁻ cells, HK2 activates with a time constant of ~2 msec at 50 mV and has a half-point for activation of -10 mV (52). Also similar to I_{RAK}, HK2 is an outward rectifier that exhibits only very slow inactivation. HK2 is blocked by the antiarrhythmic agent quinidine with an IC_{50} of 9 μM when assayed at a test potential of 0 mV. The current is also blocked by the class III antiarrhythmic agent clofilium at concentrations <1 μM (52).

I_{Kp}

A very rapidly activating outward K^+ current has been described in guinea pig ventricular myocytes by Yue and Marban (54). This current was named I_{Kp} because it activates during step depolarizations to *plateau* potentials. I_{Kp} rapidly activates ($\tau < 10$ msec) but does not inactivate during pulses as long as 600 msec. I_{Kp} has a single-channel conductance of 14 pS when recorded in the presence of 1 mM external K^+ (54). Open probability is independent of intracellular $[Ca^{2+}]$ over a range of 0.1 nM to 5 μM. Like I_{RAK}, I_{Kp} is blocked by Ba^{2+} (complete block at 1 mM) but is insensitive to TEA (no block at 135 mM). However, unlike I_{RAK}, I_{Kp} does not exhibit steady-state inactivation. I_{Kp} would not be considered to be an I_K subtype in the strictest sense, because it activates upon depolarization without a measurable delay.

A rapidly activating (τ = 10 to 40 msec), slowly inactivating, outwardly rectifying K$^+$ current has also been described in 3-day-old chick ventricle (48). The single-channel conductance of this channel is 21 pS in 5.4 mM external K$^+$ and has a half-point for activation of -5 mV.

Table 2 summarizes the classification and major properties of cardiac I$_K$ channels.

Block of Delayed Rectifier K$^+$ Channels as an Antiarrhythmic Mechanism

Reentrant-based malignant ventricular arrhythmias are believed to be the leading cause of sudden cardiac death (55). In animal models of sudden cardiac death, drugs that act by specifically prolonging action potential duration (class III) have demonstrated potential therapeutic utility (56, 57). The most recently developed agents of this class are analogs of sotalol that are dramatically more potent and mechanistically specific. For example, as previously discussed, E-4031 blocks I$_{Kr}$, but not I$_{Ks}$, in guinea pig cardiac myocytes and is far more potent than sotalol. Several other methane-sulfonanilide class III antiarrhythmic agents (e.g. dofetilide, L-691,121) more potent than E-4031 are being developed (Fig. 7). [^{3}H]Dofetilide binds with high affinity to guinea pig ventricular membranes with a K_d of 23 nM (58) or 70 nM (59), a concentration similar to its IC$_{50}$ (32 nM) for block of I$_{Kr}$ (60). Structurally related agents competitively displace [^{3}H]dofetilide from specific binding sites on guinea pig ventricular myocytes with K_i's and a rank order of affinity consistent with their in vitro class III activity (58, 59). These data further support the notion that specific block of I$_{Kr}$ is the mechanism of action of these recently developed class III agents.

Rate-Dependent Effects of Class III Agents

Most if not all class III antiarrhythmic agents prolong action potential duration; this effect is more pronounced at slow heart rates. This rate-dependent effect has been termed "reverse use dependence" (61) and is observed not only in isolated tissue preparations (18, 62), but also in patients instrumented with electrodes to record monophasic action potentials (63). Several potential mechanisms could account for the reverse use dependence of I$_{Kr}$ blockers. These agents could either preferentially block I$_{Kr}$ channels in their closed state (during diastole), or unblock from the open state (during systole). Alternatively, reverse use dependence could result from a nearly constant block of I$_{Kr}$ if other repolarizing currents increase in magnitude and thus lessen the impact of I$_{Kr}$ block at fast heart rates. The mechanism of rate-dependent prolongation of action potential duration by dofetilide has been investigated in guinea pig myocytes (60). Dofetilide (1 μM) lengthened action potential duration more when cells were paced

Table 2. Classification of cardiac-delayed rectifier K⁺ channels

Channel	Activation	Rectification	Cloned?#	No. of Amino Acids	M_r	References
I_{Ks} (I_{sk}) (Kvs1.1) (I_{x2})	Very slow (τ = 1–30 sec)	Outward	Yes	130 (rat) 129 (human)	14,699	30,31,38
I_{Kr} (I_{x1})	Rapid/slow (τ = 10–200 msec)	Inward	No			17
I_{RAK} (Kv1.2)	Very rapid (τ = 1–10 msec)	Outward	Yes	499 (rat)	56,766	50
HK2	Very rapid	Outward	Yes	605 (human)	66,640	52,53
I_{Kp}	Very rapid	Outward	No			54

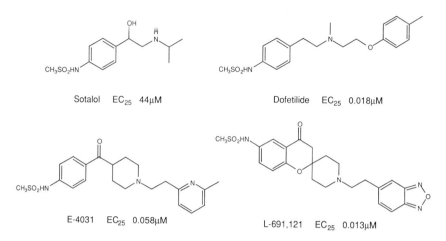

Figure 7. Structures of class III antiarrhythmic agents. EC_{25} is the concentration required to lengthen effective refractory period by 25% in ferret-isolated papillary muscles (18).

at 30/min (44 msec increase) than when paced at 240/min (21 msec increase). Yet block of I_{Kr} by 1 μM dofetilde was the same in cells paced at either 30 pulses/min or 240 pulses/min (Fig. 8). Although the magnitude of I_{K1} was the same at both pacing rates, I_{Ks} deactivation was incomplete during rapid pacing (Fig. 9), resulting in accumulation of I_{Ks} channels in the open state. Thus, the increase in I_{Ks} at fast pulsing rates offset the rate-independent block of I_{Kr}, resulting in the observed reverse use dependence of the drug. A rate-dependent increase in I_{K1} would also be expected to hasten repolarization in the intact heart. Inmulticellular tissue, accumulation of K^+ in intercellular spaces would enhance outward I_{K1} because the magnitude of this current is dependent on extracellular $[K^+]$ (conductance proportional to square root of $[K^+]_0$) (64).

Proarrhythmic Risk Associated with I_K Block

E-4031 nearly completely blocks I_K in isolated cat and rabbit ventricular myocytes (65, 66), implying that in these cells, I_{Ks} is either very small or absent. I_K of these cells activates much slower than I_{Kr} of guinea pig and rabbit nodal cells but shares the property of intense inward rectification. Complete block of the current primarily responsible for normal action potential repolarization should produce early afterdepolarizations (EADs) and lethal arrhythmias. The in vivo effects of class III agents in rabbits confirms this obvious prediction. When rabbits were administered class III agents such as clofilium, sematilide, or dofetilide, a strong correlation was observed between the dose required to prolong QT interval and that which resulted in ventricular tachyarrhythmia (67). Administration of large doses

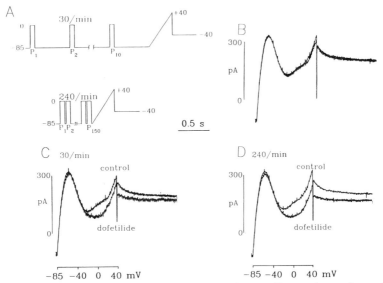

Figure 8. Dofetilide block of I_{Kr} is not rate-dependent. Cell was clamped at -85 mV, and conditioning pulses (200 msec to 0 mV) were applied at a rate of either 30/min (10 pulses) or 240/min (150 pulses). Following the conditioning train of pulses, a 1-sec voltage ramp was applied from -85 mV to 40 mV. **(A)** Pulse protocols. **(B)** Currents recorded during ramps following both conditioning pulse trains in the absence of drug. Outward I_{K1} peaks at -60 mV and declines to near 0 at -20 mV, followed by progressive activation of I_K throughout the remainder of the voltage ramp. **(C, D)** Dofetilide (1 μM) blocks a component of I_K (I_{Kr}) equally at both stimulation rates. Currents were bathed in a nominally Ca^{2+}-free saline (to reduce magnitude of I_{Ks} during ramp) containing nisoldipine (to block Ca^{2+} current). [From Jurkiewicz and Sanguinetti (60).]

of dofetilide to dogs has not been associated with proarrhythmic activity (68). The relative risk of drug-induced ventricular tachycardia or torsades de pointes may reflect the species-dependent magnitude of I_{Kr} compared with other repolarizing K^+ currents activated during the plateau phase of cardiac action potentials. If I_{Kr} is the only or dominant repolarizing current activated during the plateau, then excessive block would increase the likelihood of spontaneous EADs, especially in the setting of bradycardia or hypokalemia (69). The potential proarrhythmic risk of new class III agents could be better predicted if there was more complete knowledge of the K^+ currents responsible for repolarization of human ventricular action potentials in normal and diseased cells.

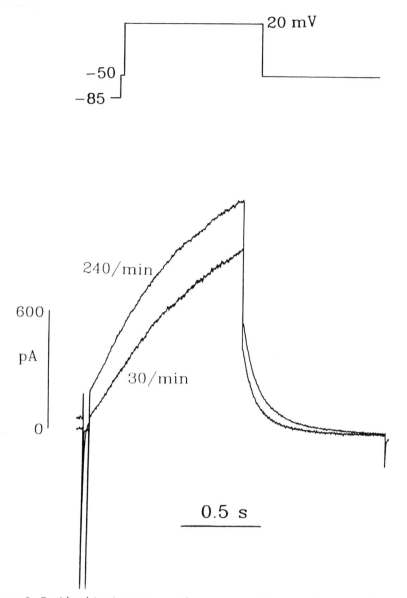

Figure 9. Rapid pulsing increases I_{Ks}. The same conditioning pulse protocols shown in Fig. 8A were followed by 1-sec test pulses to 20 mV. Cell was bathed in a K⁺-free saline plus nisoldipine to eliminate I_{K1} and block of Ca^{2+} current. Deactivation of I_{Ks} was incomplete following the 240/min train of pulses that resulted in a 25% increase in current relative to that measured following the 30/min train of pulses. This increase in I_{Ks} is in part responsible for rate-dependent decreases of action potential duration. [Adapted from Jurkiewicz and Sanguinetti (60).]

Acknowledgment

We thank Maureen Bechtel for typing the manuscript.

References

1. Gintant, G.A., Cohen, I.S., Datyner, N.B., and Cline, R.P. (1992). Time dependent outward currents in the heart, in *The Heart and Cardiovascular System* (Raven Press, New York), p. 1121.

2. Noble, D., and Tsien, R.W. (1969). Outward membrane currents activated in the plateau range of potentials in cardiac Purkinje fibers. *J. Physiol. (Lond.)* **200:**205.

3. McDonald, T.F., and Trautwein, W. (1978). The potassium current underlying delayed rectification in cat ventricular muscle. *J. Physiol. (Lond.)* **274:**217.

4. Attwell, D.E., and Cohen, I. (1977). Progress biophysics. *Mol. Biol.* **31:**201.

5. Johnson, E.A., and Lieberman, M. (1971). Heart: Excitation and contraction. *Ann. Rev. Physiol.* **33:**479.

6. Cohen, L., and Kline, R. (1982). K fluctuations in the extracellular spaces of cardiac muscle. Evidence from the voltage clamp and extracellular K-sensitive electrodes. *Circ. Res.* **50:**1.

7. Bennett, P.B., McKinney, L.C., Kass, R.S., and Begenisich, T. (1985). Delayed rectification in the calf cardiac Purkinje fiber. Evidence for multiple state kinetics. *Biophys. J.* **48:**553.

8. Balser, J.R., Bennett, P.B., and Roden, D.M. (1990). Time-dependent outward current in guinea pig ventricular myocytes. Gating kinetics of the delayed rectifier. *J. Gen. Physiol.* **96:**835.

9. Hume, J.R., Giles, W., Robinson, K., Shibata, E.F., Nathan, R.D., Kanai, K., and Rasmusson, R. (1986). A time-dependent K current in single cardiac cells from bullfrog atrium. *J. Gen. Physiol.* **88:**777.

10. Simmons, M.A., Creazzo, T., and Hartzell, H.C. (1986). A time-dependent and voltage-sensitive K^+ current in single cells from frog atrium. *J. Gen. Physiol.* **88:**739.

11. Shrier, A., and Clay, J.R. (1986). Repolarization currents in embryonic chick atrial heart cell aggregates. *Biophys. J.* **50:**861.

12. Clay, J.R., Hill, C.E., Roitman, D., and Shrier, A. (1988). Repolarization current in embryonic chick atrial heart cells. *J. Physiol. (Lond.)* **403:**525.

13. Matsuura, H., Ehara, T., and Imoto, Y. (1987). An analysis of the delayed outward current in single ventricular cells of the guinea pig. *Pflügers Arch.* **410:**596.

14. Shibasaki, T. (1987). Conductance and kinetics of delayed rectifier potassium channels in nodal cells of the rabbit heart. *J. Physiol. (Lond.)* **387:**227.

15. Scamps, F., and Carmeliet, E. (1989). Delayed K^+ current and delayed K^+ current and external K^+ in single cardiac Purkinje cells. *Am. J. Physiol.* **257:**C1086.

16. Carmeliet, E. (1985). Electrophysiologic and voltage clamp analysis of the effects of sotalol on isolated cardiac muscle and Purkinje fibers. *J. Pharmacol. Exp. Ther.* **232:**817.

17. Sanguinetti, M.C., and Jurkiewicz, N.K. (1990). Two components of cardiac delayed rectifier K+ current. Differential sensitivity to block by class III antiarrhythmic agents. *J. Gen. Physiol.* **96**:195.

18. Baskin, E.P., Serik, C.M., Wallace, A.A., Brookes, L.M., Selnick, H.G., Claremond, D.A., and Lynch, J.J. (1991). Effects of new and potent methanesulfonanilide class III antiarrhythmic agents on myocardial refractoriness and contractility in isolated cardiac muscle. *J. Cardiovasc. Pharmacol.* **18**:406.

19. Balser, J., and Roden, D. (1988). Lanthum-sensitive current contaminates Ik in guinea pig ventricular myocytes. *Biophys. J.* **53**:642a (Abstract).

20. Sanguinetti, M.C., and Jurkiewicz, N.K. (1992). Lanthanum blocks a specific component of IK and screens membrane change in cardiac cells. *Am. J. Physiol.* **259**:H1881.

21. Sanguinetti, M.C., and Jurkiewicz, N.K. (1992). Role of external Ca^{2+} and K^+ in gating of cardiac delayed rectifier K^+ currents. *Pflügers Arch.* **420**:180.

22. Horie, M., Hayashi, S., and Kawai, C. (1990). Two types of delayed rectifying K^+ channels in atrial cells of guinea pig heart. *Jap. J. Physiol.* **40**:479.

23. Walsh, K.B., Arena, J.P., Kwok, W.-M., Freeman, L., and Kass, R.S. (1991). Delayed-rectifier potassium channel activity in isolated membrane patches of guinea pig ventricular myocytes. *Am. J. Physiol.* **260**:H1390.

24. Walsh, K.B., Begenisich, T.B., and Kass, R.B. (1989). Beta-adrenergic modulation of cardiac ion channels. Differential temperature sensitivity of potassium and calcium currents. *J. Gen. Physiol.* **93**:841.

25. Yazawa, K., and Kameyama, M. (1990). Mechanism of receptor-mediated modulation of the delayed outward potassium current in guinea-pig ventricular myocytes. *J. Physiol. (Lond.)* **421**:135.

26. Duchatelle-Gourdon, L., Hartzell, H.C., and Lagrutta, A.A. (1989). Modulation of the delayed rectifier potassium current in frog cardiomyocytes by beta-adrenergic agonists and magnesium. *J. Physiol. (Lond.)* **415**:251.

27. Noma, A., Kotake, H., and Irisawa, H. (1980). Slow inward current and its role mediating the choronotropic effect of epinephrine in the rabbit sinoatrial node. *Pflügers Arch.* **38**:1.

28. Sanguinetti, M.C., Jurkiewicz, N.K., Scott, A., and Siegl, P.K.S. (1991). Isoproterenol antagonizes prolongation of refractory period by the class III antiarrhythmic agent E-4031 in guinea pig myocytes. Mechanism of action. *Circ. Res.* **68**:77.

29. Anumonwo, J.M.B., Freeman, L.C., Kwok, W.M., and Kass, R.S. (1992). Delayed rectification in single cells isolated from guinea pig sinoatrial node. *Am. J. Physiol.* **262**:H921.

30. Takumi, T., Ohkubo, H., and Nakanishi, S. (1988). Cloning of a membrane protein that induces a slow voltage-gated potassium current. *Science* **242**:1042.

31. Folander, K., Smith, J.S., Antanavage, J., Bennett, C., Stein, R.B., and Swanson, R. (1990). Cloning and expression of the delayed-rectifier IsK channel from neonatal rat heart and diethylstilbestrol-primed rat uterus. *Proc. Natl. Acad. Sci. U.S.A.* **87**:2975.

32. Hausdorff, S.F., Goldstein, S.A.N., Rushin, E.E., and Miller, C. (1991). Functional characterization of a minimal K+ channel expressed from a synthetic gene. *Biochemistry* **30**:3341.

33. Goldstein, S.A.N., and Miller, C. (1991). Site-specific mutations in a minimal voltage-dependent K$^+$ channel alter ion selectivity and open-channel block. *Neuron* **7**:403.

34. Takumi, T., Moriyoshi, K., Aramori, L., Ishii, T., Oiki, S., Okada, Y., Ohkubo, H., and Nakanishi, S. (1991). Alteration of channel activities and gating by mutations of slow ISK potassium channel. *J. Biol. Chem.* **266**:22192.

35. Tohse, N. (1990). Calcium-sensitive delayed rectifier potassium current in guinea pig ventricular cells. *Am. J. Physiol.* **258**:H1200.

36. Busch, A.E., Kavanaugh, M.P., Varnum, M.D., Adelman, J.P., and North, R.A. (1992). Regulation by second messengers of the slowly activating, voltage-dependent potassium current expressed in *Xenopus* oocytes. *J. Physiol. (Lond.)* **450**:491.

37. Busch, A.E., Varnum, M.D., North, R.A., and Adelman, J.P. (1992). An amino acid mutation in a potassium channel that prevents inhibition by protein kinase C. *Science* **255**:1705.

38. Honore, E., Attali, B., Romey, G., Heurteaux, C., Ricard, P., Lesage, F., Lazdunski, M., and Barhanin, J. (1991). Cloning, expression, pharmacology and regulation of a delayed rectifier K$^+$ channel in mouse heart. *EMBO J.* **10**:2805.

39. Honore, E., Attali, B., Lesage, F., Barhanin, J., and Lazdunski, M. (1992). Receptor-mediated regulation of IsK, a very slowly activating, voltage-dependent K+ channel in *Xenopus* oocytes. *Biochem. Biophys. Res. Commun.* **184**:1135.

40. Walsh, K.B., and Kass, R.S. (1988). Regulation of a heart potassium channel by protein kinase A and C. *Science* **242**:67.

41. Tohse, N., Kameyama, M., Sekiguchi, K., Shearman, M.S., and Kanno, M. (1990). Protein kinase C activation enhances the delayed rectifier potassium current in guinea-pig heart cells. *J. Mol. Cell. Cardiol.* **22**:725.

42. Walsh, K.B., and Kass, R.S. (1991). Distinct voltage-dependent regulation of a heart-delayed IK by protein kinases A and C. *Am. J. Physiol.* **261**:C1081.

43. Blumenthal, E.M., and Kaczmarek, L.K. (1992). Modulation by cAMP of a slowly activating potassium channel expressed in *Xenopus* oocytes. *Neuroscience* **12**:290.

44. Arena, J.P., and Kass, R.S. (1988). Lock of heart potassium channels by clofilium and its tertiary. Analogs: Relationship between drug structure and type of channel blocker. *Mol. Pharmacol.* **34**:60.

45. Balser, J.R., Bennett, P.B. Hondeghem, L.M., and Roden, D.M. (1991). Suppression of time-dependent outward current in guinea pig ventricular myocytes. Actions of a quinidine and amiodarone. *Circ. Res.* **69**:519.

46. Dukes, L.A., Cleeman, L., and Morad, M. (1990). Tedisamil blocks the transient and delayed rectifier K$^+$ currents in mammalian cardiac and glial cells. *J. Pharmacol. Exp. Ther.* **254**:560.

47. Clapham, D.E., and Logothetis, D.E. (1988). Delayed rectifier K$^+$ current in embryonic chick heart ventricle. *Am. J. Physiol.* **254**:H192.

48. Josephson, L.R., and Sperelakis, N. (1989). Two types of outward K$^+$ channel currents in early embryonic chick ventricular myocytes. *J. Dev. Physiol.* **12**:201.

49. Boyle, W.A., and Nerbonne, J.M. (1991). A novel type of depolarization-activated K$^+$ current in isolated adult rat atrial myocytes. *Am. J. Physiol.* **260**:H1246.

8

Cardiac Inward Rectifier Potassium Channel

Carol A. Vandenberg

$\mathbf{I}$nwardly rectifying potassium channels are characterized by asymmetry in their potassium conductance. They carry large inward currents at potentials negative to the potassium equilibrium potential (E_K) and relatively small currents at potentials positive to E_K. This class of potassium currents was first discovered by Katz (1) in skeletal muscle, and the property was termed "anomalous rectification." The anomaly was that the K^+ conductance increased with hyperpolarization and decreased with depolarization, opposite to the conductance expected from the potassium gradient and opposite to the effect of voltage on the delayed rectifier potassium currents.

The phenomenon of inward rectification is a prominent feature of many cardiac potassium currents. These include: (i) K_1, the inward rectifier potassium channel that shows strong rectification (2–7), (ii) K_{ACh}, the G-protein–coupled channel modulated by neurotransmitters with moderate rectification (8), (iii) K_{ATP}, the ATP-regulated channel with modest rectification (9), and (iv) K_{Na}, the Na-activated potassium channel also with modest rectification (10). The focus of this review is on the inward rectifier potassium channel K_1.

Physiological Role of the Inward Rectifier K_1

Inwardly rectifying potassium currents are found in cardiac and skeletal muscle, glial cells, many neurons, macrophages, and invertebrate oocytes. Proposed roles include maintenance of long duration action potentials, determination of cell resting potential, involvement in action potential repolarization, modulation of membrane excitability, and transport of potassium by glial cells (11–13).

In the heart, the inward rectifier K_1 is present in high abundance in cardiac atrial, ventricular, and Purkinje cells (14–16) but is absent in pacemaker cells in the sinoatrial and atrioventricular nodes (14, 17). The more positive resting potential of nodal cells has been attributed to the lack of I_{K1}. Inward rectifier current I_{K1} is much larger in ventricle than in atrium, based on both whole-cell measurements (15, 16) and single-channel densities (15). In ventricular cells, K_1 channels provide the major potassium conductance, whereas in atrial cells other potassium channels also contribute significantly to the potassium conductance. The less strongly rectifying properties of the atrial K^+ conductance, caused by the presence of transient K^+ channels, delayed rectifier K^+ channels, K_{ACh} and K_{Ca} in addition to K_1, account for its shorter duration action potential (15, 16).

Measurement of I_{K1} during cardiac ventricular action potentials shows that I_{K1} is the current that generates the resting potential and modulates the final phase of repolarization of the action potential (13, 18, 19). Selective blockage of I_{K1} causes an increase in action potential duration together with a decreased rate of repolarization and a more positive cell resting potential (16). Significant I_{K1} current has been measured also at subthreshold levels of depolarization, suggesting the involvement of I_{K1} in the modulation of cell excitability (19, 20).

The large spike of outward current due to I_{K1} during ventricular action potential repolarization is illustrated in Fig. 1A from Shimoni, et al. (13). Rabbit ventricular myocytes were voltage-clamped using action potentials as the command voltage. Current through the inward rectifier was prominent during the late phase of repolarization and was present at the resting potential. The current-voltage relationship (Fig. 1B) shows that the current rectified strongly and displayed a negative slope conductance for potentials more positive than -65 mV, confirming its identity as I_{K1}. The inward

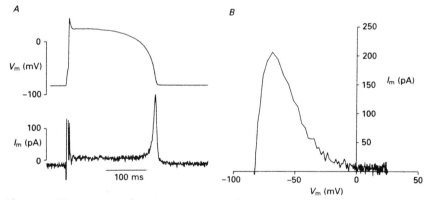

Figure 1. Time course of I_{K1} during a ventricular action potential. In action potential voltage-clamp experiments, single rabbit ventricular myocytes were voltage-clamped using action potentials as the command signal. I_{K1} was measured as the difference between currents recorded in normal 5.4 mM K^+-containing Tyrode solution and currents in K^+-free bathing solution. **(A)** Time course of the action potential (upper record) and the corresponding I_{K1} (lower record). **(B)** Current-voltage relationship during the plateau and repolarization phases of the action potential. [From Shimoni et al. (13).]

rectifier I_{K1} carries little outward current during the action potential plateau, which permits long duration ventricular action potentials and minimizes both cell potassium loss and extracellular potassium accumulation. As the cell begins to repolarize, the negative slope conductance of the inward rectifier acts as a threshold to promote rapid repolarization. In the region of negative-slope conductance, the increasing conductance of I_{K1} during repolarization increases the rate of repolarization, causing further increases in the conductance of I_{K1}. The resulting large outward I_{K1} current of 100–250 pA over a narrow voltage range is responsible for the rapid rate of late repolarization in ventricular myocytes (13). In atrial cells, these functions are shared by K_1 and other ion channels (15, 16).

Properties of the Inward Rectifier Current

The whole-cell characteristics of the cardiac inward rectifier show many similarities to inwardly rectifying currents that were first described in detail in skeletal muscle and in invertebrate oocytes (21–23; reviewed in refs. 11 and 24). Distinguishing features of the inwardly rectifying potassium current are: (i) selectivity to potassium, (ii) block by external Ba^{2+} and Cs^+, (iii) inward rectification, (iv) dependence of rectification on external potassium concentration, (v) square-root dependence of conductance on external potassium concentration, and (vi) "inactivation" that is dependent on external Na^+.

Selectivity

The current I_{K1} is potassium-selective. The reversal potential showed a nearly Nernstian dependence on extracellular potassium concentration when K^+ was substituted with Na^+ in whole-cell experiments or extrapolated from single-channel measurements (7, 25, 26). Estimates of the selectivity to K^+ compared with Na^+ were 1:0.007 from reversal potential measurements (26). Permeability ratios calculated from peak inward currents showed highest permeability to K^+ compared with other monovalent ions. The relative monovalent permeabilities were $K^+:Rb^+:NH_4^+:Cs^+$ of 1.0:0.5:0.3:0.15 (27). Permeability ratios measured in the steady state were considerably lower, which was attributed to steady-state block of the currents by external Ca^{2+} or Mg^{2+}. The relative steady-state permeabilities were $K^+:Rb^+:NH_4^+:Cs^+:Na^+:Li^+$ of $1.0:0.21:0.06:0.01:<0.005:<0.001$ (27).

External Block

A variety of cations are effective blockers of I_{K1} when applied externally (5, 25, 27–31). Ba^{2+} or Cs^+ are commonly used to identify I_{K1} by measuring difference currents before and after the addition of blocker. Channel block is time- and voltage-dependent. Block is faster and more complete with increasing hyperpolarization (25). The voltage dependence of these blockers and their ability to shorten channel open time and cause flickery interruption of single-channel currents are consistent with the suggestion that they act as open channel blockers (6, 25, 32).

Inward Rectification

Currents through the inward rectifier exhibit distinct inward rectification (2–7). The amplitude of inward current elicited by hyperpolarization is large, and the amplitude of outward current measured for a depolarizing voltage step is small. The typical characteristics of I_{K1} in response to voltage steps are illustrated in Fig. 2 from Ishihara et al. (33). Inward rectifier currents were recorded from single guinea pig ventricular myocytes with the oil gap voltage clamp method. With an approximately 11-fold K^+ gradient of 160 mM $[K^+]_i$ and 14 mM $[K^+]_o$, the current was evident as a large, inward current at potentials below E_K and as a smaller, outward current positive to E_K (Fig. 2A, left). Rectification upon depolarization was instantaneous. Upon hyperpolarization, a component of time-dependent activation of the current was observed at the beginning of the hyperpolarization, followed by slower inactivation. The extent of inactivation was low in this Na^+-free external solution. As expected from a K^+-selective channel, the amplitude of I_{K1} was suppressed when currents were recorded in the absence of external K^+ (Fig. 2A, right). The isochronal I–V relationship (Fig. 2B) showed that I_{K1}, recorded as the difference between currents in 14 mM $[K^+]_o$ (filled

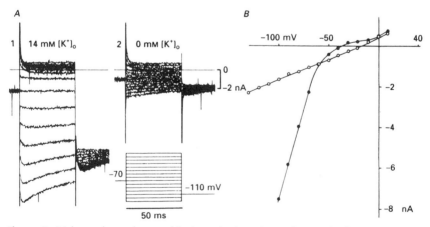

Figure 2. Voltage-dependence of I_{K1} in a single guinea-pig ventricular myocyte. **(A)** Currents elicited by voltage steps using the oil-gap clamp were recorded in solutions containing 14 mM $[K^+]_o$ **(left)** and 0 mM $[K^+]_o$ **(right)**. **(B)** The I–V relationship was measured near the end of the test pulse in 14 mM $[K^+]_o$ (filled circles) and in 0 mM $[K^+]_o$ (open circles). [From Ishihara et al. (33).]

circles) and 0 mM $[K^+]_o$ (open circles), reversed sign at the potassium equilibrium potential. Outward current was recorded positive to E_K, which exhibited a negative slope-conductance region characteristic of I_{K1}. The amplitude of this outward current is small relative to the inward current, but is of significant magnitude to promote action potential repolarization (Fig. 1).

Single-channel currents have been recorded with properties that identify them as the K_1 channel (6, 7, 32, 34–41). The K_1 channel has a single channel conductance of 25–30 pS in isotonic KCl. The channel displays slow gating kinetics at potentials negative to E_K with long open times on the order of tens to hundreds of milliseconds (34, 35). Single K_1 currents show abrupt inward rectification at a potential near E_K when measured in the steady state or in response to voltage ramps. The single-channel current-voltage relationship from a cell-attached patch is shown in Fig. 3A from

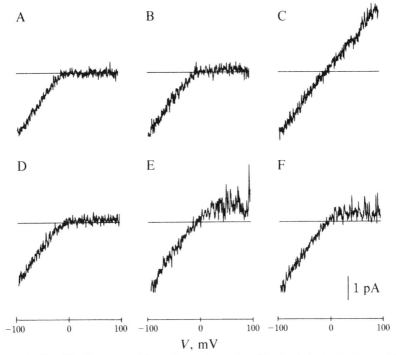

Figure 3. Rectification caused by voltage-dependent block of single K_1 channel by Mg^{2+}. The single-channel current-voltage relationship of the K_1 channel in a guinea-pig ventricular myocyte was measured by applying a voltage ramp. The patch pipet and bathing solution contained isotonic K^+. **(A)** Cell-attached record. **(B)** The patch was excised in an inside-out configuration into isotonic K^+ bathing solution containing 1.2 mM $[Mg^{2+}]_i$. **(C–F)** The bathing solution was exchanged to internal solutions containing **(C)** ~0.2 μM $[Mg^{2+}]_i$ that eliminated rectification, **(D)** 1.2 mM $[Mg^{2+}]_i$ that restored rectification, and **(E and F)** 17 μM $[Mg^{2+}]_i$ that gave an intermediate degree of rectification. [From Vandenberg (36).]

Vandenberg (36). The single-channel current was measured in response to a linear voltage ramp from -100 to 100 mV in 100 msec. Inward single-channel currents were readily observed, but outward currents from mammalian K_I have not been reported in cell-attached patches under normal intracellular ionic conditions (7, 34–37; see, however, ref. 42 for chick myocytes). Based on the relative amplitudes of inward and outward currents from whole-cell measurements, the outward single-channel current is expected to be small. The calculated maximal outward current is ~0.05 pA (7), an amplitude that would be difficult to resolve. The absence of detectable, outward, single-channel current might also be attributed to the ionic conditions used in single-channel experiments. High $[K^+]_o$ in the cell-attached patch pipettes generally has been used to increase the channel conductance for inward current. As a consequence, E_K and channel rectification were shifted toward more positive potentials, placing them in a voltage range where internal divalent block could decrease the magnitude of outward single-channel current (36, 40, 43).

Dependence of Rectification on $[K^+]_o$

A characteristic feature of the inward rectifier is that external K^+ influences rectification of the current. Unlike the voltage-dependent properties of many ion channels that depend primarily on the potential, the conductance change during rectification was found to depend on both the membrane potential and the external K^+ concentration (2, 3, 7, 15, 25, 26, 36, 40, 44, 45). For low concentrations of external K^+, the conductance shifted along the voltage axis approximately in parallel with the change in E_K (7, 15, 26, 36, 40, 44, 45), whereas for high external K^+ concentrations, the conductance shifted in the direction of the change in E_K; however, the magnitude of the shift was less than the change in E_K (36, 40). In contrast, changes in the concentration of internal K^+ were not found to alter greatly the voltage at which the conductance rectified (36, 40, 44, 45; see, however, ref. 46), but instead slowed the activation and deactivation kinetics (44, 45). These properties are in agreement with the inward rectifiers of skeletal muscle and starfish egg, in which the conductance depended also on membrane potential and $[K^+]_o$, but not on $[K^+]_i$ (22, 23).

A consequence of the shift of rectification with the concentration of external K^+ is that the current-voltage relationship exhibits crossover of the outward currents (7, 15, 25, 26). That is, outward current is larger at a given potential for higher $[K^+]_o$, because the negative-slope conductance region of the I–V is shifted along the voltage axis.

Dependence of Conductance on $[K^+]_o$

The conductance of the inward rectifier depends approximately on the square root of the external K^+ concentration (6, 7, 47). This property has been interpreted as reflecting the multi-ion nature of the pore (43).

Inactivation

Upon hyperpolarization of myocytes bathed in physiological saline, the inward current activates rapidly and then slowly declines. This "inactivation" of the current was found to be largely due to voltage-dependent block of the channel by external Na^+ (29–31) as found also in tunicate egg (48) and skeletal muscle (49). Substitution of external Na^+ with choline, Tris, or sucrose reduced, but did not completely eliminate inactivation. External Ca^{2+} and Mg^{2+} may also block I_{K1} under some circumstances. When current was carried by K^+, these divalent cations did not cause channel inactivation, but in the absence of K^+, when Cs^+ was the current carrier, Mg^{2+} and Ca^{2+} were able to block inward Cs^+ current (27). Single-channel currents from cell-attached patches have also been reported to undergo a time-dependent decline in open probability upon hyperpolarization (6, 32, 34, 35), although Na^+ was absent from the pipet solutions. It has been suggested that inactivation of single-channel current in the absence of Na^+ in some cases may be due to the composition of the recording pipets, because its occurrence was related to the types of pipets used (50).

Mechanisms of Rectification

Several mechanisms have been proposed to explain channel rectification, including an intrinsic channel gate (34, 51) with binding sites for K^+ that control the opening and closing of the gate (45, 52, 53), an asymmetric pathway for potassium permeation through the open channel (23, 54), or blockage of the channel by an intracellular blocking particle or ion (36–40, 43, 55, 56). It appears now that more than one processes is involved in rectification. Block of the open channel by intracellular magnesium causes rectification of the channel on a fast time scale, and a second process that may be channel gating contributes to rectification on a slower time scale.

Channel Block by Intracellular Magnesium

A blocking model for channel rectification was proposed by Armstrong (55) based on studies of quaternary ammonium block of delayed rectifier K^+ channels in squid axon. Voltage-dependent, open-channel block by intracellular cations would be expected to produce inward rectification as charged blocking particles are driven into the open channel at positive potentials. Hille and Schwarz (43) showed that a blocking model also can account for the dependence of rectification on external potassium concentration. They showed theoretically that, as external $[K^+]$ is increased, block by an internal monovalent would cause a shift in the I–V relationship in parallel with the change in the potassium equilibrium potential. For a divalent blocker, the rectification voltage also would shift in the direction of the change in E_K, but the magnitude of the shift would be less because of the higher valence, and thus greater voltage dependence for entry of a divalent blocker than the monovalent permeant ion.

In cell-attached patches, inward rectification can be observed in single-channel currents. The single-channel current records consist of well-defined, long openings at potentials negative to the potassium equilibrium potential. However, at potentials positive to E_K, no outward current could be recorded (7, 34–37). Voltage jumps to positive potentials indicated that the kinetics of rectification are fast. At 1.5 msec after a voltage jump to 45 mV, there was no difference between records that had one or no channels open at negative potentials immediately before the pulse (7). This suggested that rectification occurred with a time constant <1 msec.

The blocker model of rectification was examined by Vandenberg (36) and Matsuda et al. (37) at the single-channel level by exchanging the internal solution to remove possible blocking particles. This was accomplished using both excised inside-out patches (36) and "open" cell-attached patches (36, 37), in which the distal end of the myocyte was permeabilized to permit exchange of the intracellular solution. Figure 2, from Vandenberg (36), shows the strongly rectifying current-voltage relationship from a single channel in a cell-attached patch (Fig. 2A). The I–V relationship was measured from a single channel in response to a linear voltage ramp. Rectification was maintained when the patch was excised into a solution containing 1.2 mM Mg^{2+} (Fig. 2B). Single-channel rectification was removed upon exchange to an internal solution containing no divalent cations (Fig. 2C). The appearance of a linear, single-channel I–V relationship eliminated the hypothesis that rectification is due to an asymmetric permeation pathway for potassium. Instantaneous rectification was also removed in whole-cell experiments when cells were perfused with low divalent-containing solutions (33, 37, 46, 57).

Internal magnesium ions were identified as the blocking particles responsible for inward rectification (36–38; reviewed in ref. 58). Rectification was restored by the addition of magnesium to the internal solution. As shown in Fig. 2D, the addition of 1.2 mM Mg^{2+} restored the normal extent of rectification, whereas 17 μM Mg^{2+} gave partial rectification (Fig. 2, E and F). Increased noise of the outward currents in the single-channel records during the voltage ramp resulted from rapid block and unblock of the channel, causing flickery interruptions in the single-channel current (Fig. 2, E and F). The steady-state block of the channel was increased both by positive potential and by increased Mg^{2+} concentration. The voltage and Mg^{2+} dependence of the block was fitted by a single-site blocking model (59) with a K_d (0 mV) of 37 μM and a blocking site for Mg^{2+} located 0.57 of the electrical distance from the intracellular side of the membrane (38).

Magnesium is not the only intracellular ion capable of blocking the channel to produce rectification, but it is likely to be of major importance physiologically because of its high concentration in the cell. There is general agreement that the concentration of cytosolic free magnesium in vertebrate myocardium is between 0.5 and 1.0 mM (60). Thus, physiological concentrations of magnesium are sufficient to cause the rectification observed in a cell-attached patch.

Calcium and barium also block the inward rectifier (36, 61). Micromolar concentrations of internal Ca^{2+} were reported to block the outward K^+ current in excised patches and to favor the appearance of channel substates of lower conductance (61). Estimates of the ability of Ca^{2+} to block outward current indicate that its blocking affinity is similar to that of Mg^{2+} (Vandenberg, unpublished observations). Block or channel modulation by Ca^{2+} may play a role in rectification, particularly during the transient increases in intracellular Ca^{2+} associated with cell contraction. However, even peak Ca^{2+} concentrations are much lower than the steady-state concentration of Mg^{2+}, suggesting that the ability of Ca^{2+} to modulate channel function may be more important than its blocking ability.

The effects of external and internal K^+ on Mg^{2+} block of the inward rectifier were examined by Matsuda (40). Rectification of single-channel conductance due to Mg^{2+} block was shifted on the voltage axis for changes in external, but not internal K^+ concentration. External K^+ increased the unblocking rate and decreased the blocking rate, suggesting that permeant ions from the opposite side of the membrane could speed the exit of blocker from the channel and also compete with the blocker for binding to the blocking site. In agreement with the predictions of Hille and Schwarz (43) for divalent ion block, rectification of the conductance shifted along the voltage axis less than the change in E_K when external K^+ was changed (40).

Among cardiac potassium channels, open-channel block by intracellular Mg^{2+} is a common mechanism of rectification. The G-protein coupled K channel regulated by muscarinic agonists K_{ACh} (62, 63), the ATP-regulated K channel K_{ATP} (64, 65), and the Na-activated K channel K_{Na} (66) all show voltage-dependent block by intracellular Mg^{2+} with K_d's of ~0.3 mM (62, 63), 2–6 mM (64, 65), and 5–10 mM (66), respectively at 40 mV in isotonic K^+. The rectification of these channels is less pronounced than for the inward rectifier K_1. They show larger outward currents, because their Mg^{2+} dissociation constants are more than an order of magnitude greater than the K_d for block of K_1. Block of K_{ATP} and K_{Na} channels by intracellular Na^+ also contributes to their rectification (64–66).

Subconductance States

An interesting feature of the inward rectifier channels was revealed by blocking ions. Matsuda (38) discovered that substates in single-channel conductance were produced during block of the channel by internal Mg^{2+}. The single-channel current level fluctuated between the full open state, the full closed state, and two substates of intermediate amplitude. The conductances of the substates were ⅓ and ⅔ the conductance of the full open state. The occurrence of equally spaced conductance amplitudes suggested that the channel was composed of three identical conducting units that each could be blocked by Mg^{2+}. Increasing the Mg^{2+} concentration or raising the membrane potential caused the lower-conductance states and closed state to be populated for greater proportions of time. A quantitative comparison of the state dwell times revealed that the state occupancies followed approximately the binomial distribution, consistent with the behavior of three independent identical conducting units (38). Block of the channel by external Cs^+ or Rb^+ supported this model (39). Figure 4A from Matsuda (39) shows the transitions among sublevels for a single channel blocked by external Cs^+. Three sublevels of equal conductance were present with external block (Fig. 4B), and hyperpolarization promoted occupancy of the lower conductance states. As with internal block, the state distribution for external block conformed approximately to the expected binomial relationship. Unexpectedly, however, only a small fraction of the channels displayed sublevels when blocked by external ions, whereas most of the channels exhibited transitions only from the fully open and fully closed states (39). Apparently the inward rectifier is a "triple-barreled" channel with three equally conducting units that function nearly independently when blocked by internal ions. With respect to external block, they are sometimes independent but usually function nonindependently.

The concentration and voltage dependences of the blocking rates indicated that Mg^{2+}, Cs^+, and Rb^+ act as open channel blockers, blocking the passage of permeant ions by binding to a site in the channel located in the membrane field (38, 39). The rates of block and unblock were calculated for block by external and internal ions. The blocking rate at a given membrane potential increased with the concentration of blocking ion concentration, and for Cs^+ or Rb^+ block was shown to be linearly related to the concentration of blocker. The effect of voltage was to alter the rate of block consistent with the blocking site being located in the membrane field. The blocking rate increased with depolarization for block by the internal blocker Mg^{2+}, and the rate increased with hyperpolarization for the external blockers Cs^+ and Rb^+. The unblocking rates were nearly independent of the concentration of blocking ions, and were less dependent on the membrane voltage.

Substates have also been reported in amplitudes other than those predicted by the triple-barrel model. The occurrence of substates in channel conductance was reported first as spontaneous sublevels in the inward single-channel current in cell-attached patches (6, 7). These spontaneous sublevels of inward current were at 65%–85% of main current amplitude (6) and at four approximately equally spaced levels (7). Substates of four current levels have also been reported for outward currents blocked by internal Ca^{2+} (61).

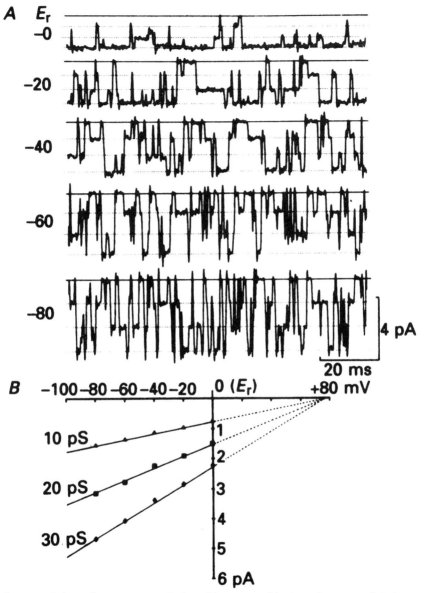

Figure 4. Subconductance states induced by current blockage by external Cs⁺. Single-channel currents were recorded in a cell-attached patch on a guinea-pig ventricular myocyte. The patch pipet contained isotonic K⁺ solution with 20 μM Cs⁺. The cell was bathed in 5.4 mM K⁺ Tyrode solution. **(A)** Currents were recorded at various holding potentials, as indicated at **left,** expressed relative to the cell resting potential (E_r). The zero current level is shown with the solid lines, and levels at one-third, two-thirds, and the full-open state are shown with dashed lines. **(B)** Current-voltage relationship of the channel substates and full-open level. [From Matsuda et al. (39).]

Channel Gating

The cardiac inward rectifier was at one time thought of as a time-independent, "background" potassium current. However, like the inward rectifiers of invertebrate egg (11) and vertebrate skeletal muscle (24), the cardiac current I_{K1} shows distinct time dependence (33, 34, 53, 67–69). Upon hyperpolarization, the inward rectifier current shows two components: an instantaneous current jump that is followed by a rapid, time-dependent increase in current. The time-dependent component has been attributed to an intrinsic gating process that activates upon hyperpolarization and deactivates upon depolarization (33, 34, 53, 69). To identify the contributions of intracellular divalent block and channel gating to the rectification process, Ishihara et al. (33) measured the currents through guinea-pig ventricular myocytes during perfusion of the cell with intracellular solutions of various free magnesium concentrations. In the presence of 500 μM Mg^{2+}, the outward current on depolarization was instantaneously rectified. When internal Mg^{2+} was buffered at 2 μM, the current was instantaneously ohmic (33), as reported previously in single-channel measurements with submicromolar internal Mg^{2+} (36–38) and in whole-cell measurements with 15 μM Mg^{2+} (37, 46). The initial jump in outward current was followed by an exponential decrease in current, attributed to intrinsic gating of the channel.

The relative amounts of current that were blocked by Mg^{2+} and that were closed by a gating process could be separated based on their time-dependences (33). Currents blocked by Mg^{2+} rectified instantaneously upon depolarization at 500 μM $[Mg^{2+}]_i$ and activated instantaneously upon repolarization. Currents closed by a gating process declined more slowly upon depolarization and gave rise to the time-dependent activation upon repolarization. Figure 5 shows that both voltage and internal Mg^{2+} are important in determining the amplitude of the time-dependent component (33). The current was allowed to rectify during a 40-msec prepulse to voltages in the range of -25 to 65 mV relative to E_K, and the relative amounts of time-dependent and instantaneously activatable current were then measured upon repolarization. With a low concentration of internal Mg^{2+} (2 μM), the amplitude of the time-dependent component increased with increasing depolarization of the prepulse (Fig. 5, left). This was interpreted as time-dependent gating during the 40-msec prepulse, which caused more complete deactivation as the potential became more depolarized. At a physiological concentration of internal Mg^{2+} (500 μM), the amount of time-dependent component was similar for prepulses to voltages near E_K, but the instantaneous component dominated for depolarized potentials (Fig. 5, right).

It was concluded that instantaneous inward rectification on depolarization is due to Mg^{2+} block at physiological concentrations of Mg^{2+} (33). During maintained depolarization, channels that were instantaneously

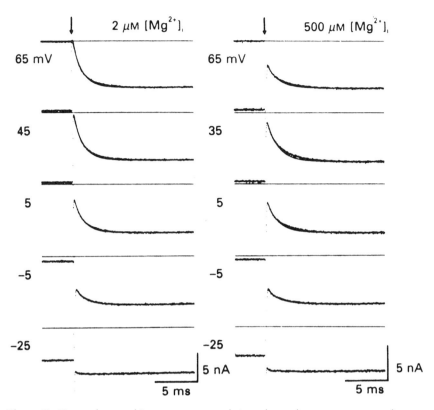

Figure 5. Dependence of instantaneous and time-dependent components of currents activated by hyperpolarization on the amplitude of the preceding depolarization and the $[Mg^{2+}]_i$. The membrane was depolarized for 40 msec to the indicated prepulse voltages (relative to the reversal potential) and then jumped back to the holding potential of V_0-35 mV at the arrow. Potentials are expressed relative to the reversal potential V_0 of approximately -50 to -60 mV. The same cell was perfused with 2 μM $[Mg^{2+}]_i$ **(left)** and 500 μM $[Mg^{2+}]_i$ **(right)**. Currents were recorded in 14 mM $[K^+]_o$, with subtraction of background currents in K^+-free external solution. [From Ishihara et al. (33).]

blocked by Mg^{2+} could later reopen and slowly move to the closed state. Inward rectification caused both the Mg^{2+} block and a gating process. The gating process is most important for rectification at potentials near E_K or for very long depolarizations.

In the presence of channel gating, the effect of open channel block has interesting consequences on the steady-state current magnitude. Matsuda (38) showed that, with low $[Mg^{2+}]_i$, the steady-state outward current was larger than in its absence. These results were explained by a model in which all three of the conducting units are required to be unblocked before the channel can gate to the closed state (33, 38, 53). Partial block of the channels, at a potential when they would otherwise close, has the somewhat unexpected consequence of increased outward current (33, 38, 53).

The nature of the gating process has not yet been clarified. Channel gating has been assumed to be an intrinsic property of the channel, unrelated to channel block, because it was present when intracellular Mg^{2+} was buffered to micromolar levels (33, 37). However, gating was largely, but not completely, removed when intracellular solutions were buffered to submicromolar divalent ion concentrations. Gating was nearly eliminated in excised inside-out patches (36), and in whole-cell recordings in which the cell was buffered to submicromolar Mg^{2+} concentrations (57). In "open" cell-attached patches, exchange of internal solution more slowly removed rectification (36, 38). After instantaneous rectification was removed, the channels still closed in a time- and voltage-dependent manner. However, the closing rate became slower with time after opening the cell to the bath solution, suggesting that a soluble substance associated with the gating process could be washed away during solution exchange. This soluble factor might be a modulatory enzyme or cofactor able to alter the rate of an intrinsic gating mechanism, or perhaps another blocking particle.

Mitra and Morad (27) suggested that the time-dependent activation of I_{K1} may not represent intrinsic gating, but rather that it could reflect the exit rate of blocking divalent cations. They showed that removal of extracellular and most of the intracellular divalent cations eliminated time-dependent activation and inactivation of inward currents when the current carrier was Cs^+.

A model of channel rectification must account for the dependence of channel rectification on external potassium ion concentration. For blocking models, this relationship is explained by voltage-dependent entry of permeant and blocking ions into the open channel (43). For intrinsic gating models, the strong dependence of rectification on $[K^+]_o$ has been modeled assuming binding of K^+ ions to regulatory sites that control the gating of the channel (44, 45, 52). Pennefather et al. (45) proposed that binding of external K^+ to closed channels is required before channels open. Upon channel opening, it was suggested that additional K^+ may bind to the channel with higher affinity and decrease the channel closing rate.

Modulation of Inward Rectifier Channel

Several lines of evidence indicate that I_{K1} is modulated, and that its activity can be influenced by adrenergic stimulation, ATP, and Ca^{2+}.

Adrenergic agonists have been reported to regulate the activity of I_{K1}. In canine Purkinje cells, Tromba and Cohen (70) showed that isoproterenol increased the rate of inactivation of I_{K1}, causing a shift of the isochronal I–V relationship to the right. The effect was mimicked by membrane permeable cAMP analogs but was not blocked by classical blockers of α_1-, α_2-, or β-adrenergic receptors. It was suggested that the action of isoproterenol may be mediated through a novel class of adrenergic receptors.

Modulation of I_{K1} by α_1-adrenergic receptors was demonstrated by Fedida et al. (71) in rabbit ventricular myocytes. Adrenergic stimulation caused a dose-dependent reduction in inward and outward I_{K1} that was blocked by the α_1-antagonist prazosin. It was not affected by preincubation with pertussis toxin, suggesting that the modulation does not occur via a pertussis toxin-sensitive G protein.

Involvement of ATP in regulating the K_1 channel was suggested by its ability to maintain channel activity. In inside-out patches and "open" cell-attached patches, the activity of the inward rectifier declined when ATP was removed from the internal solution (72, 73). The decline in open-state probability could be reversed by reapplying ATP (73). The hydrolysis-resistant analog AMPPNP was ineffective in promoting recovery of the channel activity, consistent with the hypothesis that ion channel activity is maintained by phosphorylation (73).

The effect of internal Ca^{2+} as a channel modulator was examined in inside-out patches. Internal Ca^{2+} increased channel rectification by decreasing the outward current (61). Ca^{2+} also promoted a rapid decline in single-channel activity in excised patches (36).

Because changes in the concentration of intracellular Ca^{2+} occur during the action potential, it is possible that Ca^{2+} transients may have a physiological role in regulating I_{K1}. In beating embryonic chick cardiac cells, outward current from single inward rectifier channels was decreased by external Ca^{2+} in the patch pipet (42). Mazzanti and DeFelice (42) speculated that Ca^{2+} entering the cell during the action potential caused increased inward rectification. Delmar et al. (74) also suggested that dynamic changes in I_{K1} may occur with stimulation of the myocyte. They showed that repetitive activity decreased Cs^+-sensitive current, believed to be caused in part to I_{K1}. Ca^{2+} channel blockers, such as Co^{2+} or ryanodine, blocked this change, suggesting that increases in cytosolic Ca^{2+} during repetitive stimulation may regulate outward current through I_{K1}.

Expression of Inward Rectifier Current in *Xenopus* Oocytes

Until recently, there was no molecular or biochemical information on the composition of the inward rectifier channel protein. Biochemical studies have been hindered by the lack of a specific high-affinity ligand for the channel and the low abundance of channels in the cell membrane (typically $0.5-1/\mu m^2$; refs. 6 and 7). Isolation of channel cDNAs by homology to known delayed rectifier potassium channels has yielded numerous cDNAs encoding delayed rectifier K^+ channels, but none that encode channels of the inward rectifier type.

An alternative strategy to isolate the cDNA for the inward rectifier is to use a functional expression system. Two approaches that have been successful in the isolation of cDNAs coding for potassium channels (75–78) are cloning by functional expression in *Xenopus* oocytes (79) and cloning by complementation in yeast (75, 76). Both methods rely on the identification of a source of mRNA that is rich in transcript coding for the channel of interest. This mRNA is then used in the construction of a cDNA library that is subsequently screened for functional expression.

Inwardly rectifying K^+ current has been expressed in *Xenopus* oocytes using mRNA isolated from carp olfactory epithelium (80), rat basophilic leukemia cells RBL-2H3 (81), canine hippocampus (82), and murine macrophage J774.1 cells (83). The currents expressed in oocytes retained the properties of the native inward rectifier currents. Expressed inward rectifier currents were K^+ selective, were blockable by external Ba^{2+} or Cs^+, showed distinct inward rectification, and the voltage at which the conductance rectified depended on the concentration of external K^+ (80–83). The conductance also showed the expected square-root dependence on external $[K^+]$ (83). The dependence of conductance and rectification of the currents expressed from J774.1 mRNA are shown in Fig. 6 from Perier et al. (83). The currents were of large magnitude, and the shift in the voltage-dependence of rectification with external $[K^+]$ was retained in the expressed currents (Fig. 6). The currents from the olfactory epithelium, RBL cells, and J774.1 cells all showed rapid activation upon hyperpolarization (80, 81, 84), characteristic of the cardiac current I_{K1}, whereas the hippocampal current activated more slowly (83), like inward rectifiers in invertebrate oocytes. Expression of inward rectifier current was found to be specific for an mRNA size-class of 4–5 kb for RBL and J774.1 cells (81, 83) and ~4 kb for canine hippocampus. The single-channel conductance of the inward rectifier channel in the native membranes of the RBL-2H3 cells (84) and J774.1 cells (85) was identical to the cardiac K_1 channel. In J774.1 cells, the ability of internal Mg^{2+} to cause rectification of the single-channel current (86), and the ability of Na^+ to promote channel inactivation at negative potentials (85), suggest that the macrophage inward rectifier is similar to the cardiac inward rectifier.

Conclusions

The cardiac inward rectifier channel K_1 is involved in maintenance of long duration cardiac action potentials, action potential repolarization, and generation of the resting potential. The strong inwardly rectifying character of I_{K1} is an important factor in these functions. Inward rectification is caused by open-channel block by intracellular Mg^{2+} and a process that resembles channel gating. Channel blocking properties indicate that the inward rectifier may be a triple-barreled channel composed of three pores. Modulation of the channel by neurotransmitters and intracellular second messengers also may play an important role in channel function. Isolation of a cDNA encoding an inwardly rectifying channel will pave the way for

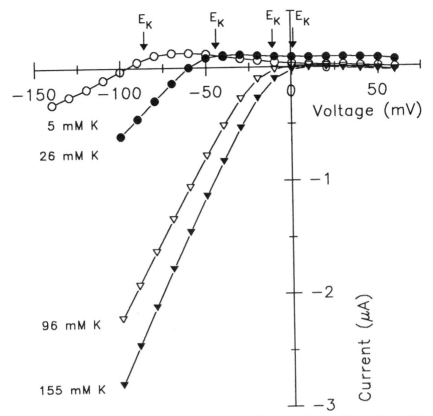

Figure 6. Dependence of conductance and rectification of inwardly rectifying K^+ currents expressed in *Xenopus* oocytes on $[K^+]_o$. Current versus voltage relationship of Ba^{2+}-sensitive currents expressed following injection of size-fractionated mRNA (4 ± 1 kb) from the murine macrophage cell line J774.1. Currents were recorded in external solutions of various K^+ concentrations, as indicated. [From Perier et al. (83).]

a molecular understanding of the structure and function of the inward rectifier.

Note Added in Proof

Using *Xenopus* oocyte expression cloning, Kubo et al. (87) recently have succeeded in isolating a cDNA encoding an inward rectifier channel from J774 cells. The deduced amino acid sequence predicts a protein of 428 amino acids with two hydrophobic putative transmembrane domains. Between the hydrophobic domains, the protein has a region of homology with the H5 pore-forming domain of the *Shaker* potassium channels. Oocytes injected with transcripts produced from this clone expressed inwardly rectifying currents that were sensitive to block by external Ba^{2+}, Cs^+, and Na^+.

These studies now make possible a molecular characterization of the structure and function of the inward rectifier channels.

Acknowledgments

This work was supported by the National Institutes of Health Grant HL41656 and by the American Heart Association (California Affiliate). I thank K. Coulter and F. Perier for their comments and suggestions.

References

1. Katz, B. (1949). Les constantes electriques de la membrane du muscle. *Arch. Sci. Physiol.* **3**:285–300.

2. Noble, D. (1965). Electrical properties of cardiac muscle attributable to inward going (anomalous) rectification. *J. Cell Comp. Physiol.* **66**:127–136.

3. McAllister, R.E., and Noble, D. (1966). The time and voltage dependence of the slow outward current in cardiac Purkinje fibres. *J. Physiol.* **186**:632–662.

4. Noble, D., and Tsien, R.W. (1968). The kinetics and rectifier properties of the slow potassium current in cardiac Purkinje fibers. *J. Physiol.* **195**:185–214.

5. Isenberg, G. (1976). Cardiac Purkinje fibers: Cesium as a tool to block inward rectifying potassium currents. *Pflügers Arch.* **391**:85–100.

6. Kameyama, M., Kiyosue, T., and Soejima, M. (1983). Single-channel analysis of the inward rectifier K current in the rabbit ventricular cells. *Japan. J. Physiol.* **33**:1039–1056.

7. Sakmann, B., and Trube, G. (1984). Conductance properties of single inwardly rectifying potassium channels in ventricular cells from guinea-pig heart. *J. Physiol.* **347**:641–657.

8. Noma, A. (1987). Chemical-receptor-dependent potassium channels in cardiac muscles, in *Electrophysiology of Single Cardiac Cells*, D. Noble and T. Powell, Eds. (Academic Press, London), pp. 223–246.

9. Ashcroft, F. M. (1988). Adenosine 5-triphosphate-sensitive potassium channels. *Annu. Rev. Neurosci.* **11**:97–118.

10. Kameyama, M., Kakei, M., Sato, R., Shibasaki, H., and Irisawa, H. (1984). Intracellular Na$^+$ activates a K$^+$ channel in mammalian cardiac cells. *Nature* **309**:354–356.

11. Hagiwara, S. (1983). *Membrane Potential-Dependent Ion Channels in Cell Membrane. Phylogenetic and Developmental Approaches.* (Raven Press, New York).

12. Brew, H., Gray, P.T.A., Mobbs, P., and Attwell, D. (1986). Endfeet of retinal glial cells have higher densities of ion channels that mediate K$^+$ buffering. *Nature* **324**:466–468.

13. Shimoni, Y., Clark, R.B., and Giles, W. R. (1992). Role of an inwardly rectifying potassium current in rabbit ventricular action potential. *J. Physiol.* **448**:709–727.

14. Noma, A., Nakayama, T., Kurachi, Y., and Irisawa, H. (1984). Resting K conductances in pacemaker and non-pacemaker heart cells of the rabbit. *Japan. J. Physiol.* **34**:245–254.

15. Hume, J.R., and Uehara, A. (1985). Ionic basis of the different action potential configurations of single guinea-pig atrial and ventricular myocytes. *J. Physiol.* **268:**525–544.

16. Giles, W.R., and Imaizumi, Y. (1988). Comparison of potassium currents in rabbit atrial and ventricular cells. *J. Physiol.* **405:**123–145.

17. Irisawa, H., Nakayama, T., and Noma, A. (1987). Membrane currents of single pacemaker cells from rabbit S-A and A-V nodes, in *Electrophysiology of Single Cardiac Cells,* D. Noble and T. Powell, Eds. (Academic Press, London), pp. 167–186.

18. Mazzanti, M., and DeFelice, L.J. (1988). K channel kinetics during the spontaneous heart beat in embryonic chick ventricle cells. *Biophys. J.* **54:**1139–1148.

19. Ibarra, J., Morley, G.E., and Delmar, M. (1991). Dynamics of the inward rectifier K$^+$ current during the action potential of guinea pig ventricular myocytes. *Biophys. J.* **60:**1534–1539.

20. Tourneur, Y. (1986). Action potential–like responses due to the inward rectifying potassium channel. *J. Membr. Biol.* **90:**115–122.

21. Hagiwara, S., and Takahashi, K. (1974). The anomalous rectification and cation selectivity of the membrane of a starfish egg cell. *J. Membr. Biol.* **18:**61–80.

22. Hagiwara, S., and Yoshii, M. (1979). Effects of internal potassium and sodium on the anomalous rectification of the starfish egg as examined by internal perfusion. *J. Physiol.* **292:**251–265.

23. Leech, C.A., and Stanfield, P.R. (1981). Inward rectification in frog skeletal muscle fibres and its dependence on membrane potential and external potassium. *J. Physiol.* **319:**295–309.

24. Stanfield, P.R., Standen, N.B., Leech, C.A., and Ashcroft, F.M. (1981). Inward rectification in skeletal muscle fibres. *Adv. Physiol. Sci.* **5:**247–262.

25. DiFrancesco, D., Ferroni, A., and Viscentin, S. (1984). Barium-induced blockade of the inward rectifier in calf Purkinje fibers. *Pflügers Arch.* **402:**446–453.

26. Shah, A.K., Cohen, I.S., and Datyner, N.B. (1987). Background K$^+$ current in isolated canine cardiac Purkinje myocytes. *Biophys. J.* **52:**519–525.

27. Mitra, R.L., and Morad, M. (1991). Permeance of Cs$^+$ and Rb$^+$ through the inwardly rectifying K$^+$ channel in guinea pig ventricular myocytes. *J. Membr. Biol.* **122:**33–42.

28. Cleeman, L., and Morad, M. (1976). Extracellular potassium accumulation and inward-going potassium rectification in voltage-clamped ventricular muscle. *Science* **191:**90–92.

29. Biermans, G., Vereecke, J., and Carmeliet, E. (1987). The mechanism of the inactivation of the inward-rectifying K current during hyperpolarizing steps in guinea-pig ventricular myocytes. *Pflügers Arch.* **410:**604–613.

30. Biermans, G., Vereecke, J., and Carmeliet, E. (1989). Effect of external K on the block of the inward rectifier during hyperpolarization in guinea-pig ventricular myocytes by external Na. *Biomed. Biochim. Acta* **48:**S358-S363.

31. Harvey, R.D., and Ten Eick, R.E. (1989). Voltage-dependent block of cardiac inward-rectifying potassium current by monovalent cations. *J. Gen. Physiol.* **94:**349–361.

32. Sakmann, B., and Trube, G. (1984). Voltage-dependent inactivation of inwardly rectifying single-channel currents in the guinea-pig heart cell membrane. *J. Physiol.* **347:**659–683.

33. Ishihara, K., Mitsuiye, T., Noma, A., and Takano, M. (1989). The Mg^{2+} block and intrinsic gating underlying inward rectification of the K^+ current in guinea-pig cardiac myocytes. *J. Physiol.* **419:**297–320.

34. Kurachi, Y. (1985). Voltage-dependent activation of the inward-rectifier potassium channel in the ventricular cell membrane of guinea-pig heart. *J. Physiol.* **366:**365–385.

35. Payet, M.D., Rousseau, E., and Sauve, R. (1985). Single-channel analysis of a potassium inward rectifier in myocytes of newborn rat heart. *J. Membr. Biol.* **53:**143–156.

36. Vandenberg, C.A. (1987). Inward rectification of a potassium channel in cardiac ventricular cells depends on internal magnesium ions. *Proc. Natl. Acad. Sci. U.S.A.* **84:**2560–2564.

37. Matsuda, H., Saigusa, A., and Irisawa, H. (1987). Ohmic conductance through the inwardly rectifying K channel and blocking by internal Mg^{2+}. *Nature* **325:**156–159.

38. Matsuda, H. (1988). Open-state substructure of inwardly rectifying potassium channels revealed by magnesium block in guinea-pig heart cells. *J. Physiol.* **397:**237–258.

39. Matsuda, H., Matsuura, H., and Noma, A. (1989). Triple-barrel structure of inwardly rectifying K^+ channels revealed by Cs^+ and Rb^+ block in guinea-pig heart cells. *J. Physiol.* **413:**139–157.

40. Matsuda, H. (1991). Effects of external and internal K^+ ions on magnesium block of inwardly rectifying K^+ channels in guinea-pig heart cells. *J. Physiol.* **435:**83–99.

41. Josephson, I.R., and Brown, A.M. (1986). Inwardly rectifying single-channel and whole cell K^+ currents in rat ventricular myocytes. *J. Membr. Biol.* **94:**19–35.

42. Mazzanti, M., and DeFelice, L.J. (1990). Ca modulates outward current through I_{K1} channels. *J. Membr. Biol.* **116:**41–45.

43. Hille, B., and Schwarz, W. (1978). Potassium channels as multi-ion single-file pores. *J. Gen. Physiol.* **72:**409–442.

44. Cohen, I.S., DiFrancesco, D., Pennefather, P., and Mulrine, N.K. (1989). Internal and external K help gate the inward rectifier. *Biophys. J.* **55:**197–202.

45. Pennefather, P., Oliva, C., and Mulrine, N. (1992). Origin of the potassium and voltage dependence of the cardiac inwardly rectifying K-current (I_{K1}). *Biophys. J.* **61:**448–462.

46. Saigusa, A., and Matsuda, H. (1988). Outward currents through the inwardly rectifying potassium channel of guinea-pig ventricular cells. *Japan. J. Physiol.* **38:**77–91.

47. Daut, J. (1982). The passive electrical properties of guinea-pig ventricular muscle as examined with a voltage-clamp technique. *J. Physiol.* **330:**221–242.

48. Ohmori, H. (1978). Inactivation kinetics and steady-state current noise in the anomalous rectifier of tunicate egg cell membranes. *J. Physiol.* **281:**77–99.

49. Standen, N.B., and Stanfield, P.R. (1979). Potassium depletion and sodium block of potassium currents under hyperpolarization in frog sartorius muscle. *J. Physiol.* **294:**497–520.

50. Trube, G. (1986). Inactivation of inwardly rectifying potassium channels in the heart. *Neurosci. Lett. (Suppl.)* **26:**S8.

51. Gunning, R. (1983). Kinetics of inward rectifier gating in the eggs of the marine polychaete, *Neanthes arenaceodentata. J. Physiol.* **342:**437–451.

52. Ciani, S., Krasne, S., Miyazaki, S., and Hagiwara, S. (1978). A model for anomalous rectification: Electrochemical-potential-dependent gating of membrane channels. *J. Membr. Biol.* **44:**103–134.

53. Oliva, C., Cohen, I.S., and Pennefather, P. (1990). The mechanism of rectification of I_{K1} in canine Purkinje myocytes. *J. Gen. Physiol.* **96:**299–318.

54. Woodbury, J.W. (1971). Eyring rate theory model of the current-voltage relationships of ion channels in excitable membranes, in *Chemical Dynamics: Papers in Honor of Henry Eyring,* J.O. Hirschfelder, Ed. (Wiley, New York), pp. 601–617.

55. Armstrong, C.M. (1969). Inactivation of the potassium conductance and related phenomena caused by quaternary ammonium ion injection in squid axons. *J. Gen. Physiol.* **54:**553–575.

56. Standen, N. B., and Stanfield, P.R. (1978). Inward rectification in skeletal muscle: A blocking particle model. *Pflügers Arch.* **378:**173–176.

57. O'Rourke, B., Backx, P.H., and Marban, E. (1992). Phosphorylation-independent modulation of L-type calcium channels by magnesium-nucleotide complexes. *Science* **257:**245–248.

58. Matsuda, H. (1991). Magnesium gating of the inwardly rectifying K^+ channel. *Annu. Rev. Physiol.* **53:**289–298.

59. Woodhull, A.M. (1973). Ionic blockage of sodium channels in nerve. *J. Gen. Physiol.* **61:**687–708.

60. Murphy, E., Freudenrich, C.C., and Lieberman, M. (1991). Cellular magnesium and Na/Mg exchange in heart cells. *Annu. Rev. Physiol.* **53:**273–287.

61. Mazzanti, M., and DiFrancesco, D. (1989). Intracellular Ca modulates K-inward rectification in cardiac myocytes. *Pflügers Arch.* **413:**322–324.

62. Horie, M., and Irisawa, H. (1987). Rectification of muscarinic K^+ current by magnesium ion in guinea-pig atrial cells. *Am. J. Physiol.* **253:**H210–214.

63. Horie, M., and Irisawa, H. (1989). Dual effects of intracellular magnesium on muscarinic potassium channel current in single guinea-pig atrial cells. *J. Physiol.* **408:**313–332.

64. Findlay, I. (1987). ATP-sensitive K^+ channels in rat ventricular myocytes are blocked and inactivated by internal divalent cations. *Pflügers Arch.* **410:**313–320.

65. Horie, M., Irisawa, H., and Noma, A. (1987). Voltage-dependent magnesium block of adenosine-triphosphate-sensitive potassium channel in guinea-pig ventricular cells. *J. Physiol.* **287:**251–272.

66. Wang, Z., Kimitsuki, T., and Noma, A. (1991). Conductance properties of the Na^+-activated K^+ channel in guinea-pig ventricular cells. *J. Physiol.* **433:**241–257.

67. Horowicz, P., Gage, P.W., and Eisenberg, R.S. (1968). The role of the electrochemical gradient in determining potassium fluxes in frog striated muscle. *J. Gen. Physiol.* **51**:1935–2035.

68. Carmeliet, E. (1982). Induction and removal of inward-going rectification in sheep Purkinje fibers. *J. Physiol.* **327**:285–308.

69. Tourneur, Y., Mitra, R., Morad, M., and Rougier, O. (1987). Activation properties of the inward-rectifying potassium channel on mammalian heart cells. *J. Membr. Biol.* **97**:127–135.

70. Tromba, C., and Cohen, I.S. (1990). A novel action of isoproterenol to inactivate a cardiac K^+ current is not blocked by beta and alpha adrenergic blockers. *Biophys. J.* **58**:791–795.

71. Fedida, D., Braun, A.P., and Giles, W.R. (1991). Alpha₁-adrenoceptors reduce background K^+ current in rabbit ventricular myocytes. *J. Physiol.* **441**:673–684.

72. Kakei, M., Noma, A., and Shibasaki, T. (1985). Properties of adenosine-triphosphate–regulated potassium channels in guinea-pig ventricular cells. *J. Physiol.* **363**:441–462.

73. Takano, M., Qin, D., and Noma, A. (1990). ATP-dependent decay and recovery of K^+ channels in guinea pig cardiac myocytes. *Am. J. Physiol.* **258**:H45-H50.

74. Delmar, M., Ibarra, J., Davidenko, J., Lorente, P., and Jalife, J. (1991). Dynamics of the background outward current of single guinea-pig ventricular myocytes. *Circul. Res.* **69**:1316–1326.

75. Anderson, J.A., Huprikar, S.S., Kochian, L.V., Lucas, W.J., and Gaber, R.F. (1992). Functional expression of a probable *Arabidopsis thaliana* potassium channel in *Saccharomyces cerevisiae*. *Proc. Natl. Acad. Sci. U.S.A.* **89**:3736–3740.

76. Sentenac, H., Bonnaud, N., Minet, M., Lacroute, F., Salmon, J.-M., Gaymard, F., and Grignon, C. (1992). Cloning and expression in yeast of a plant potassium ion transport system. *Science* **256**:663–665.

77. Takumi, T., Ohkubo, H., and Nakanishi, S. (1988). Cloning of a membrane protein that induces a slow voltage-gated potassium current. *Science* **242**:1042–1045.

78. Frech, G.C., VanDongen, A.M., Schuster, G., Brown, A.M., and Joho, R.H. (1989). A novel potassium channel with delayed rectifier properties isolated from rat brain by expression cloning. *Nature* **340**:642–645.

79. Frech, G.C., and Joho, R.H. (1992). Isolation of ion channel genes by expression cloning in *Xenopus* oocytes. *Meth. Enzymol.* **207**:592–604.

80. Yoshii, K., and Kurihara, K. (1989). Inward rectifier produced by *Xenopus* oocytes injected with mRNA extracted from carp olfactory epithelium. *Synapse* **3**:234–238.

81. Lewis, D.L., Ikeda, S.R., Aryee, D., and Joho, R.H. (1991). Expression of an inwardly rectifying K^+ channel from rat basophilic leukemia cell mRNA in *Xenopus* oocytes. *FEBS Lett.* **290**:17–21.

82. Cui, J., Mandel, G., DiFrancesco, D., Kline, R.P., Pennefather, P., Datyner, N.B., Haspel, H.C., and Cohen, I.S. (1992). Expression and characterization of a canine hippocampal inwardly rectifying K^+ current in *Xenopus* oocytes. *J. Physiol.* **457**:229–246.

83. Perier, F., Coulter, K.L., Radeke, C.M., and Vandenberg, C.A. (1992). Expression of an inwardly rectifying potassium channel in *Xenopus* oocytes. *J. Neurochem.* **59:**1971–1974.

84. Lindau, M., and Fernandez, J.M. (1986). A patch-clamp study of histamine-secreting cells. *J. Gen. Physiol.* **88:**349–368.

85. McKinney, L.C., and Gallin, E.K. (1988). Inwardly rectifying whole-cell and single-channel K currents in the murine macrophage cell line J774.1. *J. Membr. Biol.* **116:**47–56.

86. Coulter, K.L., and Vandenberg, C.A. (1993). Rectification of inwardly rectifying potassium channels in the murine macrophage cell line J774.1: Dependence on internal magnesium and channel gating. *Biophys. J.* **64:**A201.

87. Kubo, Y., Baldwin, T.J., Jan, Y.N., and Jan, L.Y. (1993). Primary structure and functional expression of a mouse inwardly rectifying potassium channel. *Nature,* in press.

9

Molecular Physiology of cAMP-Dependent Chloride Channels in Heart

Joseph R. Hume, Paul C. Levesque, Pádraig J. Hart,
Stephen S. Tsung, Todd Chapman, and
Burton Horowitz

β-Adrenergic modulation of the cardiac action potential is generally believed to involve stimulation of protein kinase A (PKA), resulting in phosphorylation of a number of sarcolemmal ion channels. Abundant evidence is available that shows that sarcolemmal Ca^{2+} channels (1–3), delayed rectifier K^+ channels (4, 5), Na^+ channels (6, 7), and pacemaker (I_f) channels (8) are modulated. These effects in some cases are mediated by a direct G-protein pathway (9), an indirect cAMP-dependent PKA pathway (2, 10–12), or a direct effect of cAMP on the channel protein (13). The recent discovery of cAMP-dependent Cl^- channels in heart (14, 15) suggests another important mechanism for β-adrenergic modulation of the cardiac action potential. Anion substitution experiments suggest that activation of Cl^- channels (in cells with a physiological Cl^- gradient) can produce significant outward membrane current during the action potential plateau and thereby contribute to shortening of the action potential plateau and duration (16). Thus cAMP-dependent Cl^- channels may represent a new potentially important target site for the development of class III antiarrhythmic agents. An arrhythmogenic role of Cl^- channel activation in ischemia and reperfusion-induced ventricular fibrillation has been confirmed in a recent study (17).

Despite recent advances in our understanding of the mechanism of modulation of specific sarcolemmal ion channels by β-adrenergic stimulation in the heart, the effects of β-adrenergic stimulation on the shape and duration of the cardiac action potential are variable and unpredictable. Depending on experimental conditions, isoproterenol can either prolong or shorten the action potential in the same species, that is believed to be due primarily to the modulation of both Ca^{2+} and K^+ currents that have opposing effects on repolarization and the action potential plateau (18,

10). Presumably activation of cAMP-dependent Cl⁻ current [$I_{Cl(cAMP)}$] is another important factor that can also play a major role in the repolarization phase of the action potential.

Although there appear to be differences in the properties of Cl⁻ channels in different preparations, the cAMP-activated Cl⁻ conductance in cardiac muscle (20) has many properties in common with the Cl⁻ conductance observed in epithelial cells (21, 22) or *Xenopus* oocytes (23, 24) expressing the cystic fibrosis transmembrane regulator (CFTR) gene product. Both the CFTR-mediated (21, 23) and cardiac Cl⁻ currents (20) are time-independent and exhibit similar rectification properties. The cAMP-activated Cl⁻ channels from heart (25) have the same anion selectivity (bromide > Cl⁻ > iodide > fluoride) as the CFTR-generated channel (22, 26), and both channels are regulated through the cAMP-dependent PKA pathway (14, 15, 27). A novel dependence on nucleoside triphosphates has recently been demonstrated for Cl⁻ channel activation in both epithelial cells (28) and heart (29). Finally, cardiac and CFTR Cl⁻ channels exhibit a similar sensitivity to Cl⁻ channel blockers (15, 16, 30, 31) and have similar single-channel conductances: 8–13 pS (22, 23, 29, 32). These similarities raise the issue of whether or not CFTR Cl⁻ channels and cardiac cAMP-dependent Cl⁻ channels are structurally similar proteins.

This chapter reviews recent data on the physiological role of cAMP-dependent Cl⁻ channel activation during the cardiac action potential, as well as recent new molecular data on the structure of the cAMP-dependent Cl⁻ channel protein in heart and its relationship to the known structure of the CFTR gene product. Detailed reviews describing the physiological (20) and molecular properties (33) of cardiac Cl⁻ channels have been published previously.

Results

Physiological Role of cAMP-Dependent Cl⁻ Channels

Estimates of Cl⁻ activity, a^i_{Cl}, in cardiac muscle place the equilibrium potential, E_{Cl}, in the range of -65 to -45 mV under normal physiological conditions (34). Because this value represents a membrane potential range that can be both negative and positive to the actual membrane potential during the normal cardiac cycle, membrane Cl⁻ channels may contribute both inward and outward current during the cardiac action potential. At membrane potentials negative to E_{Cl}, activation of $I_{Cl(cAMP)}$ would be expected to produce an inward current that would depolarize the resting membrane potential, whereas during the action potential plateau, activation of $I_{Cl(cAMP)}$ would be expected to produce an outward current and accelerate repolarization. The degree to which activation of $I_{Cl(cAMP)}$ depolarizes the resting potential or accelerates action potential repolarization depends on the actual value of E_{Cl} and the magnitude of the Cl⁻ conductance relative to the total membrane conductance.

Two general approaches have been used to determine the effects of cAMP-dependent Cl⁻ channel activation on the resting membrane potential and action potential in ventricular myocytes. The first examined β-adrenergic stimulation effects on the action potential under conditions where the Cl⁻ gradient across the membrane was varied and activation of other membrane channels, in particular, delayed rectifier K⁺ channels, was prevented (16). β-Adrenergic modulation of I_K was minimized by conducting experiments at 20°C, because low temperatures are known to attenuate this response (35). The major effects of β-adrenergic stimulation on the action potential at 20°C might therefore be expected to reflect primarily β-adrenergic modulation of Ca^{2+} and Cl⁻ currents. To distinguish between these, the effects of isoproterenol were examined using two different Cl⁻ gradients. As shown in Fig. 1A, with $E_{Cl} = -49$ mV, isoproterenol produced a very small depolarization of the resting membrane potential but a significant shortening of the action potential duration. Under this condition, activation of $I_{Cl(cAMP)}$ opposes the effects of β-adrenergic stimulation of I_{Ca}, which would tend to lengthen the action potential duration. With $E_{Cl} = 0$ mV, isoproterenol produces a pronounced depolarization of the resting potential, often resulting in induction of spontaneous activity (Fig. 1B). Under this condition, with a reduced driving force for Cl⁻ at the plateau range of potentials, β-adrenergic stimulation of I_{Ca} predominates, causing a prolongation of the action potential duration.

The second approach to investigate the effects of Cl⁻ channel activation on cardiac resting and action potentials utilized the Cl⁻ channel blocker, 9-anthracene carboxylic acid (9-AC), an agent that inhibits cAMP-dependent Cl⁻ currents in guinea-pig ventricular myocytes (36). Experiments were conducted using an asymmetrical Cl⁻ gradient (estimated $E_{Cl} = -50$ mV), believed to mimic physiological conditions. Ca^{2+} channel modulation was prevented by continuous exposure of cells to 1 μM nisoldipine, and K⁺ channel modulation was prevented by conducting experiments at 20°C. Exposure of cells to isoproterenol under these conditions reduced the height of the plateau and caused a marked shortening of action potential duration (Fig. 2A). These effects of isoproterenol on the action potential are similar to those expected from activation of outward Cl⁻ current during the action potential plateau. In some cells there was a slight depolarization of the membrane potential. That these changes in the action potential can be attributed primarily to activation of Cl⁻ channels is supported by the observation that these effects of isoproterenol on action potential plateau and duration were nearly completely reversed by simultaneous exposure to the Cl⁻ channel antagonist, 9-AC (Fig. 2A). Similar results were observed in four other cells.

To test whether this concentration of 9-AC might be relatively selective for Cl⁻ channels, the effects of 9-AC on the ventricular action potential in

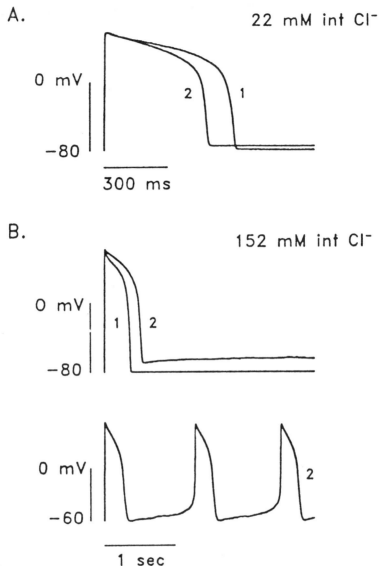

Figure 1. Effect of altering the Cl⁻ gradient on isoproterenol-induced changes of the guinea-pig ventricular action potential. **(A)** $E_{Cl} = -49$ mV ($Cl_i^- = 22$ mM, Cl_o^- $= 151.4$ mM). Action potentials were elicited by intracellular (int) current injection at a frequency of 0.25 Hz. An example of an action potential recorded in the control (trace 1) and following exposure to isoproterenol (1 μM; trace 2) are superimposed. **(B, top)** $E_{Cl} = 0$ mV ($Cl_i^- = 152$ mM, $Cl_o^- = 151.4$ mM) in a different cell. With this symmetrical Cl⁻ gradient, isoproterenol caused a prolongation of the action potential plateau and duration (trace 2) compared with the control (trace 1), and a significant depolarization of the resting membrane potential that eventually resulted in the initiation of spontaneous action potentials **(B, bottom).** Experiments were conducted at 20°C. [From Harvey et al. (16).]

A.

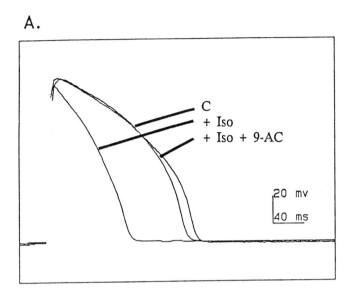

B.

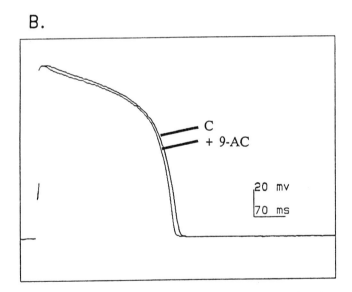

Figure 2. Effect of 9-AC on guinea-pig ventricular action potential in the presence (**A**) and absence of β-adrenergic stimulation (**B**). In (A), cell was continuously exposed to nisoldipine (1 μM) to block Ca^{2+} currents, and the bath temperature was maintained at 20°C to prevent β-adrenergic modulation of K^+ currents. In (B), nisoldipine was not present; bath temperature was maintained at 20°C. Stimulation frequency for action potentials was 0.05 Hz. [Adapted from Levesque et al. (36).]

the absence of β-adrenergic stimulation were examined. Because there is little basal $I_{Cl(cAMP)}$ present in the absence of β-stimulation (27), any significant effects of this agent on the action potential under these unstimulated conditions would strongly suggest additional nonselective effects of 9-AC on other ion channels, such as Ca^{2+} and K^+ channels. As shown in Fig. 2B, 200 μM 9-AC, in the absence of β-adrenergic stimulation, produced little or no change in the action potential. Similar results were observed in a total of five cells, suggesting that this dose of 9-AC may be rather selective for cAMP-dependent Cl^- channels. Consistent with this conclusion is the finding that, in voltage-clamp experiments utilizing the perforated patch technique to study L-type Ca^{2+} currents directly, 200 μM 9-AC failed to produce any significant effect (36).

These data suggest that under normal conditions (with E_{Cl} in the range of -65 to -45 mV) the major physiological role of activating $I_{Cl(cAMP)}$ is to minimize (oppose) the significant action potential prolongation associated with β-adrenergic stimulation of I_{Ca}. Thus, β-adrenergic stimulation can augment Ca^{2+} entry into cardiac cells with small or minimal changes in action potential duration. Also under these conditions, only small changes in the resting membrane potential would occur in response to activation of $I_{Cl(cAMP)}$, because the Cl^- conductance at the resting membrane potential is small relative to the large background K^+ conductance found in ventricular myocytes. This conclusion has been confirmed in recent experiments on intact guinea-pig papillary muscles (37). These effects of $I_{Cl(cAMP)}$ on resting membrane potential and action potential, though, are critically dependent on the actual value of E_{Cl}, which will vary in different areas of the heart under normal conditions, as well as the magnitude of the Cl^- conductance relative to the total membrane conductance. The relative distribution of cAMP-dependent Cl^- channels in different areas of the heart or in different species may vary. A recent study conducted in cells isolated from different regions of the rabbit heart suggests that cAMP-dependent Cl^- channels are much more abundantly expressed in ventricle compared with atria and sinoatrial node (38). Another very interesting finding of this study was a higher density of cAMP-dependent channels in the epicardial region of the ventricle compared with the endocardial region, suggesting that this may be an important determinant of the shorter action potential duration of epicardial tissue.

Molecular Biology of Cardiac cAMP-Dependent Cl⁻ Channels

As previously described, there are numerous similarities in the electrophysiological properties of cardiac cAMP-dependent Cl^- channels and CFTR Cl^- channels. These similarities raise the question of whether a similar CFTR channel protein is responsible for the cAMP-dependent Cl^- conductance in heart. To investigate this question, the polymerase chain reaction (PCR) technique was used to clone a portion of cDNA homologous to CFTR expressed in heart, and attempts were made to express functionally cAMP-dependent Cl⁻ channels in *Xenopus* oocytes injected with poly A$^+$ mRNA extracted from rabbit and guinea-pig ventricular tissue (39).

Poly A$^+$ mRNA was isolated from freshly dissected rabbit ventricle and converted to single-stranded cDNA using oligo(dT) primers. The cDNA was used as a template for enzymatic amplification primed by oligonucleotides designed to hybridize to both ends of the first nucleotide-binding domain (NBD1) of CFTR (Fig. 3A). NBD1 is critical for normal functioning of CFTR, because ATP hydrolysis by NBD1 is necessary for channel opening (26), and the majority of missense mutations that cause cystic fibrosis are found in this ATP-binding domain (40). The amplification products were

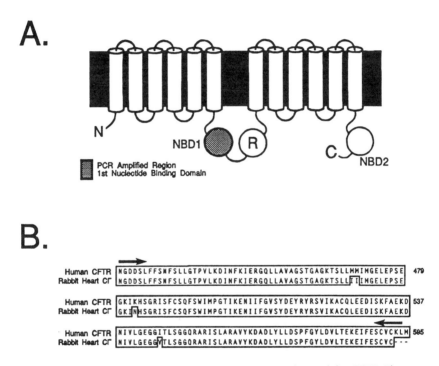

Figure 3. **(A)** Diagram representing the membrane topology of the CFTR Cl⁻ channel. The regulatory (R) and NBD1, NBD2 domains are cytoplasmically oriented. Shaded region (NBD1) represents the domain amplified by PCR. mRNA was isolated from samples of rabbit ventricle and a complementary strand of DNA synthesized. The mRNA was degraded and PCR primers allowed to anneal to the first-strand cDNA. PCR was then performed and products of expected size cloned. **(B)** Amino acid sequence of heart Cl⁻ channel: comparison of amino acid sequence of NBD1 of human CFTR with rabbit heart Cl⁻ channel PCR product. Arrows indicate the position and direction of PCR primer sequences. [From Levesque et al. (39).]

analyzed on 3% agarose by electrophoresis. A prominent band was present with a molecular weight of ~550 base pairs (bp). This size closely corresponds to the expected distance between the primer hybridization sequences (21). The band was excised from the gel, and DNA fragments were purified. These fragments were subcloned, and the DNA sequences were determined. The PCR product, termed rabCF6, and human CFTR gene share ~93% sequence homology over the 550 bp cDNA fragment (41). The deduced amino acid sequence displays only four different residues when compared with human CFTR, corresponding to 98% identity (Fig. 3B). This degree of identity far exceeds homologies between the nucleotide binding domains of other nucleotide binding proteins.

RabCF6, which has a high degree of homology to NBD1, was used as a probe in Northern blot analysis to test for expression in pancreas and in cardiac muscle from several species. Pancreas was used in the analysis, because CFTR is expressed quite strongly in this tissue (41), and we wanted to compare hybridization bands resulting from our heart probe to the CFTR signal. Poly A$^+$ mRNA was prepared from freshly dissected dog pancreas, human atrium, and guinea-pig and rabbit ventricles. Autoradiograms resulting from the hybridizations are shown in Fig. 4. The PCR product hybridized to a transcript of ~6.5 kb in dog pancreas, rabbit, guinea-pig, and human heart. A CFTR-specific probe used in a previous

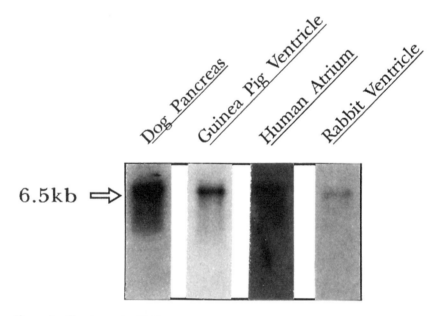

Figure 4. Cl$^-$ channel mRNA expression in heart and pancreas. Autoradiograms of Northern blots containing mRNA from dog pancreas, guinea-pig ventricle, human atrium, and rabbit ventricle. Blots were probed with the PCR amplification product from rabbit heart. [From Levesque et al. (39).]

study (41) hybridized to transcripts of 6.5 kb in several different tissues affected in cystic fibrosis, including airway epithelia and pancreas. The results of our Northern analysis suggest that the heart and CFTR cAMP-activated Cl⁻ channel transcripts are the same size, because our heart probe hybridized to 6.5 kb transcripts expressed in heart and pancreas. Although expression of CFTR mRNA was detectable by Northern analysis from the tissues listed using rabCF6 as a labeled probe, it was undetectable in mRNA prepared from dog atrium and ventricle, rabbit atrium, and guinea-pig atrium when probed with rabCF6 on the same blots. Similar samples of mRNA, when PCR amplified using NBD1 specific primers, did not yield CFTR specific amplification products. Either CFTR is not expressed in these tissues, the expression level is too low to be detected, or NBD1 primer annealing is not efficient on these RNA samples. It is interesting to note that electrophysiological studies failed to elicit cAMP-dependent Cl⁻ currents in dog ventricle (37) and rabbit atrium (38).

In recent experiments, PCR was also used employing primers homologous to regions other than NBD1. Primers were synthesized homologous to regions immediately proximal to transmembrane segment 7 and distal to transmembrane segment 12. These primers should amplify a fragment of 944 bp, which encompasses the regions encoding the carboxy terminal transmembrane segments 7 through 12 (Fig. 5). When rabbit ventricle, guinea-pig ventricle, or dog pancreas mRNA (cDNA) was used as a template, a fragment of the appropriate size (944 bp) was generated. These tissues have been shown to exhibit a cAMP-dependent Cl⁻ conductance. In contrast, using rabbit atrium or guinea-pig atrium mRNA as the template, the 944 bp fragment could not be detected. It is noteworthy that rabbit (38) and guinea-pig atrial cells (Levesque and Hume, unpublished observations) do not exhibit a significant cAMP-dependent Cl⁻ conductance. The 944 bp amplification product generated from rabbit ventricle mRNA (cDNA) was subcloned and the DNA sequence determined. As in the NBD1 region, the nucleotide sequence of the 6 carboxy terminal transmembrane segments are remarkably similar to CFTR (Fig. 5). The few differences observed could be attributed to species diversity, given that the CFTR is reported from human (41), and we have used rabbit for these studies.

Expression of cAMP-Dependent Cl⁻ Channels in Xenopus Oocytes

Xenopus oocytes were used to express the cAMP-regulated Cl⁻ conductance from mammalian heart and pancreas functionally (39). Oocytes were injected with 46 nl of poly A⁺ mRNA (1 mg/1 ml) extracted from rabbit and guinea-pig ventricle or dog pancreas. A two-microelectrode voltage-clamp technique was used to assay oocytes for expression of an exogenous cAMP-activated Cl⁻ conductance. Native oocyte membranes contain a transient Cl⁻ conductance that is activated by Ca²⁺ influx through voltage-

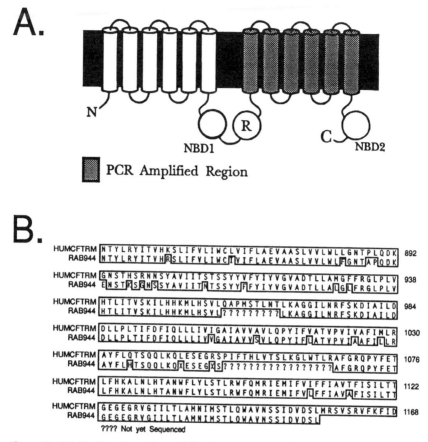

Figure 5. (A) Predicted topology of the CFTR gene product. Shaded area was amplified from rabbit ventricle cDNA by the PCR reaction, cloned, and its DNA sequence determined **(B)**. HUMCFTRM, cDNA cloned by Riordan et al. (41) from epithelial cells; RAB944, rabbit ventricle PCR amplification product.

dependent channels (42). Thus, all current recordings were made in Ca^{2+}-free external solutions to prevent activation of Ca^{2+}-activated Cl^- channels, which might otherwise interfere with efforts to detect expression of exogenous Cl^- currents. Figure 6 shows results obtained from an oocyte that was injected with rabbit ventricle mRNA 3 days before voltage-clamping. Currents elicited under control conditions (100 mM Cl^-_{out}; zero-Ca^{2+}_{out}) during 500 msec steps from -120 mV to 60 mV in 30 mV increments from a holding potential of -60 mV are shown in Fig. 6A. The endogenous Ca^{2+}-activated Cl^- conductance was nearly undetectable in the absence of external Ca^{2+}. The same voltage protocol elicited time-independent currents following addition of 100 μM 8-Br-cAMP to the bath (Fig. 6B). This conductance was never observed in noninjected control oocytes ($N = 12$). The prolonged time course of activation of the conductance by bath

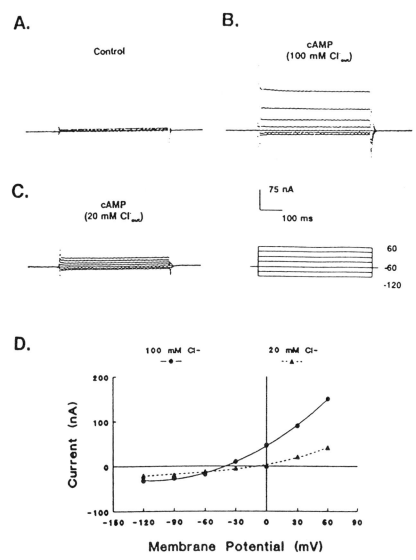

Figure 6. Effects of cAMP and external Cl⁻ on membrane currents in oocytes injected with mRNA from rabbit ventricle. Currents were recorded 96 hr after injecting oocytes with 46 nl of poly A⁺ mRNA (1 mg/1 ml) extracted from rabbit ventricle. **(A)** Endogenous Ca^{2+}-activated Cl⁻ currents were negligible during 500 msec voltage-clamp steps from −120 mV to 60 mV (30 mV increments) from a holding potential of −60 mV in the absence of external Ca^{2+}. **(B)** The same voltage protocol elicited time-independent currents after incubating the oocyte in 8-bromo-cAMP (100 μM) for 35 min. The cAMP-activated conductance was not observed in noninjected control oocytes. **(C)** Partially substituting external Cl⁻ with aspartate attenuated cAMP-activated currents. **(D)** Reducing external Cl⁻ shifted the current-voltage relationship of the cAMP-induced currents. [From Levesque et al. (39).]

application of 8-Br-cAMP (35 min) is expected, due to the slow permeation of this compound across the oocyte membrane. Replacing 80% of bath Cl^- with aspartate markedly attenuated the cAMP-activated currents (Fig. 6C), suggesting that the conductance is anion selective. The current-voltage curve of the cAMP-induced currents (Fig. 6D) was outwardly rectifying, and the reversal potential was near -36 mV, which is close to the predicted value for Cl^- assuming an intraoocyte $[Cl^-]$ of 30 mM (42). A similar cAMP-activated Cl^- conductance was also observed in oocytes injected with mRNA from guinea-pig ventricle and dog pancreas (not shown).

Summary

The ability of β-adrenergic stimulation to simultaneously activate L-type Ca^{2+} channels, delayed rectifier K^+ channels and Cl^- channels means that β-stimulation has the potential to prolong, shorten, or produce minimal changes in the action potential duration of ventricular myocardium. Activation of cAMP-dependent Cl^- channels may act normally to minimize the rather significant action potential prolongation associated with β-adrenergic stimulation of Ca^{2+} channels, thus allowing β-stimulation to produce large increases in Ca^{2+} entry into cardiac cells with minimal changes in action potential duration. Agents that selectively antagonize delayed rectifier K^+ channels have class III antiarrhythmic activity (43), and cAMP-dependent Cl^- channels may represent a new target site for the development of class III agents (20). In our studies, 9-AC appears to be an effective antagonist of cAMP-dependent Cl^- channels in heart. This compound, therefore, may represent a prototype for the development of new class III antiarrhythmic agents.

Molecular studies investigating the structure of the cAMP-dependent Cl^- channel in heart have begun only recently, but the available data provide convincing evidence that there are marked similarities in the structure of this protein and the known structure of the CFTR Cl^- channel in pancreas and various epithelia. Although future work is required to obtain a complete clone of the heart Cl^- channel, it is safe to conclude at this time that CFTR is in fact expressed in the heart of several species and is the molecular equivalent of the cAMP-dependent Cl^- channel. Future studies will reveal whether the heart CFTR channel is identical to the epithelial CFTR Cl^- channel and whether in patients with cystic fibrosis a similar mutated form of CFTR is expressed in heart, as has been documented in various epithelia (40).

Acknowledgments

This study was supported by the National Institutes of Health (NIH) Grant HL-30143 (J.R.H.). P.C.L. was supported by an NIH postdoctoral fellowship, and S.S.T. was supported by a Medical Student Research Fellowship (NIDDK Grant DK-07478-11).

10

Cardiovascular gap junctions: Gating properties, function, and dysfunction

D. C. Spray, M. B. Rook, A. P. Moreno, J. C. Sáez,
G. J. Christ, A. C. Campos de Carvalho, and G. I. Fishman

Gap junction channels span the membranes of adjacent cells to provide a private pathway for intercelluar diffusion that is not accessible to extracellular space (for recent general reviews, see refs. 1–3). Through these channels pass anions, cations, and neutral molecules with molecular weights below $\sim$1,000 Da; there is thus little charge selectivity. In the heart, the role that gap junctions play is primarily in coordination and conduction of electrical activity, and the most relevant permeant ion is probably K^+, because of its high cytosolic abundance and mobility. In smooth muscle (and perhaps also between endothelium and smooth muscle), the most relevant ion may be Ca^{2+} or other second messengers to which the channel is also freely permeable. Thus, depending on the cells involved, gap junctions may perform the functions of intercellular K^+, Ca^{2+}, or second messenger channels.

Communication Compartments of the Heart

From the standpoint of intercellular communication, and also with regard to function, the heart can be considered as an aggregate of communication compartments (schematized in Fig. 1). Pacemaking cells in the sinoatrial (SA) node are weakly coupled to other cells in this compartment because of the infrequent and small gap junctions between these cells (4, 5). It is very likely that the weakness of the coupling ensures that the pacemaking function is not weighed down by extensive electrotonic spread to other cells; the coupling *per se* permits coordinated and rhythmic activity among the SA nodal cells. The SA nodal compartment is weakly coupled to the working atrial muscle, in which the cells are rather well coupled through large gap junctions, giving rise to waves of contractions rapidly spreading throughout the atrial muscle mass (6).

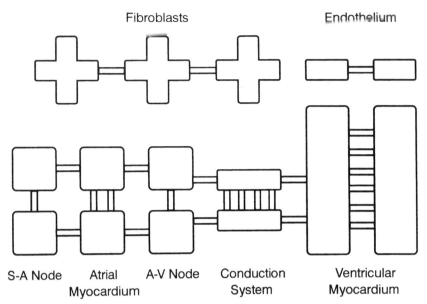

Figure 1. Intercellular communication compartments in the heart. Cells comprising cardiac tissue include fibroblasts and endothelium, as well as the cardiac cells specialized for pacemaking (SA and AV nodes), contraction (atrial and ventricular myocardium), and conduction (Purkinje system and His bundle). Strength of coupling within and between cardiac cell compartments (indicated diagrammatically by the parallel lines connecting blocks within compartments) varies from rather weak (nodal tissue) to very strong (conduction system, working myocardium). Coupling at the interfaces between compartments (horizontal lines connecting cell types in lower portion of figure) is generally weak, resulting in localized changes in conduction velocity in these regions (see text). Impulse generation and conduction occurs from left to right in the lower set of compartments. This model of connections within the heart was inspired by plasmodesmatograms developed by Dr. Aart von Bel to depict cellular interconnections in higher plants (104).

As previously mentioned, the differences in gap junctional area between pacemaker cells in the SA node and cells in the working atrial myocardium probably have an important functional correlate. Model studies in which a small number of pacemaker cells are required to drive a large number of surrounding atrial cells indicate that this can only be achieved if a gradient of electrical coupling exists between the weakly coupled pacemaking region and the well-coupled atrium (7). The model predicts that when the sinus nodal region is closely coupled to the atrium, the atrial cells will "clamp" the pacemaker cells to the resting potential typical for working myocardium, thus abolishing the spontaneous diastolic depolarization in the pacemaker cells. When the SA nodal-atrial electrotonic spread is too weak, the nodal cells will be pacing but not driving the atrium. In the model, a relatively narrow range of coupling gradients, lying between these two extremes, allows the pacemaker cells to pace *and* drive the mass of atrial cells. Whether such a gradient exists, and whether it is brought about by gradually incrementing gap junctional area from the SA node to the atrium, is still under investigation.

The electrically well-coupled myocytes in atria and ventricles are in complete electrical isolation from each other by the collagenous framework comprising the cardiac skeleton. These working regions can be considered as two virtually separate communication compartments. The only conduction pathway between these two compartments is the atrioventricular (AV) node and the ventricular conduction system (Fig. 1).

As in the SA node, cells within the AV node (especially in the central region) are weakly coupled to each other and to the ventricular conduction system by relatively sparse and small gap junctions, thus forming a separate communication compartment. The weak electrotonic coupling within the AV node and the increasing strength of coupling in the His-bundle and Purkinje system probably have functional meaning similar to that proposed for the SA node. Under normal conditions this configuration is responsible for the delay between atrial and ventricular activation (see, e.g., refs. 8 and 9). In the case of AV block, the gradient of coupling between AV node and ventricular myocardium ensures that the former can function as an accessory pacemaker for the latter. Under conditions of severe conduction failure, Purkinje cells can act as ventricular pacemaker cells; these cells, in contrast to nodal cells, are very well coupled through large gap junctions to each other as well as to the ventricular cell mass. This illustrates that, although differences in electrotonic coupling between pacemaker regions and working myocardium are very important in rhythm generation, there may be other mechanisms that support a small number of pacemaker cells in driving the large mass of working myocardium. For example, in Purkinje cells pacemaking and driving depend largely on their large inward (depolarizing) current, I_f, which is activated at potentials negative to about -60 mV and which can be found in most of the (potentially) pacemaking regions of the heart (10, 11).

Although by volume the myocytes in working myocardium comprise 70% to 80% of the tissue, estimates of their contribution to the actual number of cells forming the entire population range from 12% to 35% (12). The nonmyocyte cells include those comprising the cardiac blood vessels (endothelial cells in Fig. 1) and the ubiquitous fibroblastic cells interspersed between the cardiomyocytes. These data are taken from myocyte-rich regions of the heart; in other regions the contribution of fibroblasts to the total volume may exceed that of the myocytes (12). In particular, the SA and AV nodes contain a remarkable amount of connective tissue and fibroblasts (see, e.g., ref. 13). Moreover, injury to the heart (e.g., infarction) triggers invasion of fibroblasts in the affected region (14; De Maziere et al., manuscript in preparation). Fibroblasts in normal heart and in infarcted tissue are interconnected to one another by sparse and small but detectable gap junctions (15). Although, under culture conditions, cardiac fibroblasts readily intercalate with myocytes and are capable of passive impulse conduction through heterologous myocyte-fibroblast gap junctions (16, 17), no such interactions seem to be present in either normal (15) or infarcted hearts (De Maziere, personal communication). These observations suggest that cardiac fibroblasts may form a communication compartment that is completely separate from the myocardial compartments (see Fig. 1).

Although the cells in atrial and ventricular myocardium are electrically so well coupled that they might be regarded as an electrical syncytium, the spatial distribution of gap junction size in the intercalated disk is not uniform. This results in an anisotropy in axial resistance throughout the working myocardium, which favors conduction parallel to the fiber axis above conduction perpendicular to the fiber axis (18).

One of the factors involved in the emergence of arrhythmias during or after myocardial ischemia and infarction is a regional decrease in conduction velocity of the cardiac action potential (19). Apart from action potential amplitude and upstroke velocity (which are governed by the nonjunctional membranes), conduction velocity depends largely on the intercellular resistance, which is determined by how many gap junctions are present and how many of these junctional channels are open. As will be discussed later, gap junctional conductance is decreased under conditions of reduced intracellular pH, pCa, and ATP levels and altered fatty acid/lipid ratios in the cell membrane (19–21) such as those that occur during ischemia in the acute phase of infarction (19, 20, 22, 23). This regulation is a rapid process requiring only minutes or seconds.

It has been demonstrated that because of the naturally present anisotropy in conductance, a region of surviving myocardium surrounding a region of complete block is susceptible to reentrant ventricular tachycardias (24). In border zones of healing infarcts, these conditions can be further aggravated by a redistribution and a reduction of gap junction number and size, severely disturbing the normal conduction pattern in otherwise recovered tissue (25, 26). Moreover, comparison of conduction failure following potassium depolarization (which reduces nonjunctional excitability) with conduction failure following treatment with heptanol (which blocks gap junctions, see below) indicates that the anisotropic nature of gap junction distribution leads to exaggerated distances along conduction pathways when junctional conductance is reduced (27). The resulting tortuous pathway is hypothesized to lead to radical increases in susceptibility to arrhythmogenesis.

Composition and Structure of Gap Junctions and Their Genes

Gap junction channels are arrayed as plaques of hexagonally packed elements; this two-dimensional symmetry has facilitated structural studies.

Early evidence from x-ray diffraction of negatively stained material and more recently from low-angle electron scatter indicates hexagonal symmetry of the pore (28–30). Protein isolation from junctional membranes identified subunits now termed connexins (31), and perhaps the strongest dogma in the junctional field is that the channel is formed of six identical connexin subunits contributed by each cell that dock with high affinity but noncovalent interactions to form the pore (Fig. 2A).

cDNAs for ~12 mammalian connexins have now been cloned and sequenced, the most important of which in the cardiovascular system is connexin43, although there have been recent claims of minor expression of additional transcripts (32, 33). Figure 2B illustrates the membrane topology of connexin43 as deduced by controlled proteolysis and site-specific antibody binding to isolated junctional membranes (30, 34). Note that the general connexin motif spans the membrane four times, with both carboxyl and amino acid termini on the cytoplasmic portion of the molecule. The regions of the molecule with the highest homology among various members of the connexin family are the membrane spanning and extracellular domains. The least homology is on the cytoplasmic loop connecting the second and third transmembrane segments and on the cytoplasmic tail, and peptides corresponding to stretches of amino acids in these regions have been used to generate connexin-specific antibodies. Because these regions are the least homologous, it is within these regions that differences in sensitivity to gating stimuli of gap junctions in various cell types are thought to arise.

Members of the connexin multigene family all appear to share a characteristic chromosomal organization (35, 36), as shown in Fig. 2C. Each gene typically includes two exons, a short first exon containing only 5′-untranslated sequences and a longer second exon that encompasses the coding region and 3′-untranslated regions. The initiating methionine is located close to the beginning of the second exon. At present, there is no evidence for alternative splicing of any of the connexin genes. In fact, gap junction genes are distributed throughout the human genome, with connexin43 localized to chromosome 6 (and a connexin43 pseudogene to chromosome 5:329,30). The fact that the coding region is not interrupted by any introns limits the possibility for alternate splicing and has facilitated the molecular cloning of connexin isoforms using the polymerase chain reaction. Because of the absence of variably sized intronic sequence, amplification of genomic DNA using primers derived from highly conserved regions of connexin coding regions yields products of predictable length.

The regulation of connexin expression may be an important element in the control of junctional coupling. Transfection analysis of chimeric promoter-reporter genes into various cell types has been used to determine those sequences within the connexin43 gene, which determines both the strength and specificity of its transcriptional activity (37).

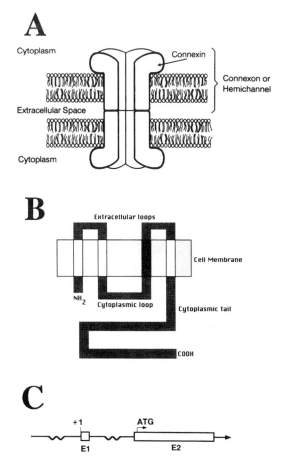

Figure 2. Composition of the cardiac gap junction channel and its gene. **(A)** Schematic diagram of longitudinal section of a gap junction channel. Each gap junction channel is formed by the union of two connexons or hemichannels, one contributed by each cell, across extracellular space. Each connexin is formed of six protein molecules termed connexins (lightly shaded); in cardiac tissue the predominant gap junction protein is connexin43, named for the length of its polypeptide (43 kDa) encoded by its cDNA sequence. **(B)** Membrane topology of connexin43 as deduced from hydrophobicity analysis, antibody binding to isolated gap junction membranes, and controlled proteolysis studies (see text for citations). Four transmembrane domains (the 1st, 2nd, and 4th are white in this drawing and the 3rd, which is most amphiphilic and most likely to line the pore, is black) are connected via two extracellular loops (which presumably dock with adjacent subunits to form high-affinity interactions across extracellular space) and a cytoplasmic loop or hinge. Both amino [NH_2 and carboxyl (COOH)] termini are on the cytoplasmic portion of the molecule. **(C)** Chromosomal organization of the connexins. Members of the connexin multigene family typically include a short first exon (E1) containing 5'-untranslated sequence and a longer second exon (E2) that encompasses the entire coding region and 3'-untranslated sequence. The start codon (ATG) is found close to the beginning of E2.

Portions of the human connexin43 5'-flanking sequence, the region of the gene most likely to regulate transcription, have been fused to luciferase reporter plasmids, introduced by calcium-phosphate coprecipitation into fetal rat cardiac myocytes and nonmyocytes, and subsequently analyzed for luciferase activity (37). These studies demonstrate that 100 base pairs of immediate 5'-flanking sequence are sufficient to drive expression of the luciferase reporter gene in both cell populations, although the activity is approximately 3-fold higher in the myocytes. Thus, this region appears to contain the connexin43 core promoter. Inclusion of an additional 75 base pair flanking sequence results in significantly higher levels of luciferase activity, suggesting the presence of a *cis*-acting positive element in this region.

Reporter gene activity has also been assessed by directly injecting plasmid DNA into adult rat hearts in vivo. High levels of luciferase activity are also observed in this system; however, the maximum expression is obtained with longer constructs containing 2.4 kb of 5'-flanking sequence. Further mapping of *cis*- and *trans*-acting elements will be useful in characterizing the molecular genetic mechanisms that determine steady-state levels of connexin43 in the normal and pathologic heart. This information undoubtedly will be helpful in understanding the contribution of altered connexin gene expression to cardiac conduction disturbances, including arrhythmogenesis.

Size of the Cardiac Gap Junction Channel

The size of a channel can be expressed in terms of its permeability to molecules of different radii or in terms of its electrical conductance where current is carried by cytoplasmic ions.

Gap junction channels are permable to molecules approaching 1 nm in radius, which includes the most abundant cytoplasmic ions, as well as second messengers such as cAMP, ATP, Ca^{2+}, and inositol triphosphate (IP_3). Calcium has been shown to permeate from one cell to another through gap junction channels in hepatocytes (where connexin32 is the major gap junction protein; e.g., ref. 38), as well as in astrocytes and smooth muscle (where connexin43 is abundant; e.g., refs. 39 and 40) and in ciliated epithelium (where the connexin type is unknown; ref. 41). The movement of Ca^{2+} between smooth muscle cells is illustrated in Fig. 3A, where Ca^{2+} concentrations in injected and adjacent human *corpus cavernosum* cells are measured using ratiometric methods with the fluorescent Ca^{2+} indicator, Fura2. Junctional flux is unaffected by changing extracellular Ca^{2+} (not shown) but is blocked by the uncoupling agent, heptanol, as is shown in Fig. 3B; thus, the pathway for this diffusion is gap junctional. The second messenger and Ca^{2+}-mobilizing molecule, IP_3, also traverses gap junction channels between cells (38), as does cAMP (42). Although the IP_3-elicited Ca^{2+} response in contiguous cells displays temporal and spatial patterns

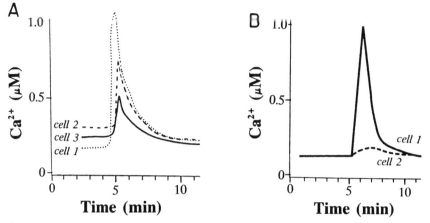

Figure 3. Gap junction permeability to calcium. Clusters of cultured human *corpus cavernosum* smooth muscle cells were loaded with the membrane permeant acetoxymethyl ester of the calcium-indicator dye, Fura2, and intracellular calcium was determined ratiometrically from video images in response to 350 and 380 nM excitation wavelengths. Each line in the graphs represents the Ca^{2+} level averaged over a selected area of a single cell. Corresponding to ~4 to 5 min on the abscissa of each graph, Ca^{2+} was injected into a single smooth muscle cell under conditions where Ca^{2+} was absent from the extracellular medium. **(A)** In response to Ca^{2+} injection into cell 1, Ca^{2+} levels in that cell and those adjacent to it (cells 2 and 3) rose transiently from baseline values of ~200 to 300 nM to peak levels of 0.5 to 1.1 μM and then returned to baseline levels. **(B)** In cells treated with 0.2 mM heptanol to reduce intercellular coupling, baseline Ca^{2+} levels were relatively unaffected. In response to Ca^{2+} injection, the Ca^{2+} level in that cell (cell 1) transiently increased to ~1 μM, but little Ca^{2+} elevation was detected in adjacent cells [cell 2 in this example modified from Christ et al. (39)].

that are different from those accompanying direct injection of Ca^{2+}, their occurrence indicates junctional permeability to this important second messenger molecule.

Channel conductances are more easily quantified than permeabilities. Study of the conductance of gap junction channels requires cell pairs such as neonatal cardiac myocytes (Fig. 4A), each of which is voltage clamped to a common holding potential, and junctional conductance (g_j) is calculated as the current recorded in one cell's clamp (I_j) in response to a command potential applied to the other cell (V_j, Fig. 4B). Under conditions where few channels are open, currents through individual gap junction channels are detected as equal-sized events of opposite polarity (Fig. 4C). Unitary junctional conductances (γ_j) are calculated by dividing the elemental currents (i_j) by the transjunctional driving force (V_j).

Typically, each individual cardiac gap junction channel has a conductance of 50 to 60 pS (equivalent to a resistance of ~17 to 20 × 10^9 Ohm) when measured with KCl- or CsCl-filled patch pipettes in pairs of isolated

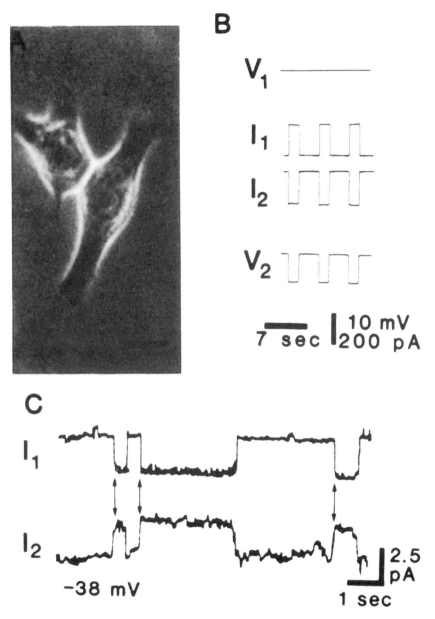

Figure 4. Measurement of junctional conductance and single-channel currents in pairs of neonatal rat cardiac myocytes. **(A)** Photograph of neonatal cardiac myocytes cultured for 24 hr. **(B)** Recording of junctional (I_1) and nonjunctional currents ($I_2 + I_1$) in response to a command voltage applied to cell 2 (V_2) in a pair of voltage clamped cells. **(C)** Recordings of single-channel currents between a pair of myocytes. Note that fluctuations (indicated by arrows) occur simultaneously, but with opposite polarities in the two cells' current records. Driving force in this record is -38 mV. [From Burt and Spray (43).]

cardiomyocytes (with lower values obtained when the pipettes contain larger and less mobile organic anions). There is now ample experimental evidence that this conductance corresponds to connexin43 gap junction channels (43, 44). Between neonatal rat heart cells an additional channel conductance of 20 to 30 pS (33 to 50 $\times$ 10^9 Ohm) has been reported (45), which could represent a subconductance state of the 60 pS channel (46) or a different gap junction channel type altogether [possibly connexins40 (33, 47), or 42 or 45 (32)]. Interestingly, cardiac fibroblasts are connected by gap junction channels of 20 to 30 pS (17, 48). The conductance of individual cardiac gap junction channels is thus on the order of, or even less than, that of ligand-gated ion channels and is much less than that of some voltage-sensitive but highly ion-selective channels, such as the maxi-K channel. This value for unitary conductance seems surprisingly low when the high permeability of gap junction channels is considered; however, very similar conductance values are predicted from calculations for a right cylindrical pore filled with cytoplasm extending through two membranes and extracellular space with morphological dimensions of gap junction channels (19). Because so many of these channels are usually present in parallel in a gap junctional plaque, total gap junctional conductance is sufficiently large to allow unimpeded action potential conduction under normal conditions (49).

Gating of Cardiac Gap Junction Channels

Unlike other membrane channels, macroscopic and single-channel gap junctional conductance in cardiac cells are independent of the membrane potential (i.e., the potential gradient from inside to outside the cell). Although initial studies concluded that gap junctions in mammalian heart were also insensitive to transjunctional (transcellular) voltage (43, 50–52), recent studies show that over larger voltage ranges and under favorable experimental conditions, a modest but conspicuous voltage dependence is present (4, 45, 48, 53, 54). It has been demonstrated, using the double whole-cell patch clamp technique, that in weakly to moderately coupled cardiac myocyte pairs ($g_j < 12$ nS) isolated from neonatal rat or hamster, gap junction channels tend to close during sustained transjunctional voltages ($>$0.5-sec duration) exceeding 40 to 50 mV (4, 45, 55). This decrease in junctional conductance is only partial, because a virtually voltage-insensitive residual component (termed g_{min}, or minimal junctional conductance; 49) always remains, which is 30% to 50% of the initial conductance (Fig. 5). Although residual conductances are characteristic for most types of gap junctions, the percentage of total junctional conductance that is voltage-insensitive (g_{min}/g_{max}) is much higher in tissues where connexin43 predominates (heart, smooth muscle, astrocytes, and various cell lines) than in cells connected by other connexin types (e.g., hepatocytes and Schwann cells) (56).

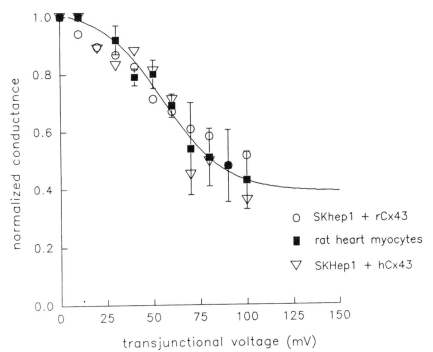

Figure 5. Voltage dependence of junctional conductance in rat cardiac myocytes (solid squares) and communication-deficient cells transfected with human (open triangles) and rat (open circles) connexin43. The smooth curve describes a Boltzmann relation, which fits best the rat myocyte data where V_0 = 55.2 mV, n = 1.5 gating charges, and g_{min} = 0.39 (see text for discussion).

Decline in junctional current during a long and large transjunctional voltage is primarily fit by a single exponential at each voltage. The junctional conductance/transjunctional voltage (G_j/V_j) relationship is well described by the Boltzmann equation, which predicts the change in proportion of channels in two states (open and closed) as a function of the energy difference between the states:

$$G_j = open/(open + closed) = \exp\left[-A(V_j - V_0)\right] - G_{min},$$

where A is a constant describing the degree of voltage sensitivity for which the number of equivalent gating charges (in the case of connexin43, ~2) can be obtained, and V_0 is the voltage at which half the voltage-sensitive channels are closed (~50 to 60 mV for connexin43).

Single-gap junction channel conductance is not dependent on transjunctional voltage and the time- and voltage-dependent reductions of g_j during a transjunctional voltage step are caused by a decrease in channel open probability (due to an increase of the mean closed time, together with a reduction of the mean open time).

Part of the observed differences originally obtained in various connex-in43-containing cell types with regard to voltage sensitivity is explained by the voltage ranges examined and the experimental conditions. In the double whole-cell voltage-clamp technique with patch electrodes that has been used to study the biophysics of gap junctional channels, electrode resistances to the cell interiors may cause considerable errors in voltage clamping the junctional membrane when junctional conductance is high (57). In addition, based on mathematical modeling, it has been proposed that cytosolic access resistance to the tightly packed channels in the gap junctional plaques also play an important role (58). With increasing junctional conductance, increasingly larger junctional currents must funnel into the gap junctional plaques leading to localized high current density in the cytosol near the channel mouths. This gives rise to an appreciable voltage drop in the cytosol, and, as a result, the channels sense less transjunctional voltage with increasing gap junctional size and higher conductance. Thus, in the working myocardium, where intercalated disks contain massive junctional plaques, the modest voltage dependence exhibited by small cardiac gap junctions is further reduced.

Although voltage sensitivity of the cardiac gap junction channel clearly is a biophysical property that distinguishes it from other junctional types, it is still not clear whether it has a functional meaning in either the normal or pathologic heart. It could be that it is a redundant or vestigial feature inherited from more voltage-dependent gap junctional ancestors or that this low degree of voltage dependence was selected for during evolution. On the other hand, it remains possible that even this weak voltage sensitivity can be involved in protecting still functional myocytes in an infarcted region from inexcitability and severe depolarization caused by the presence of adjacent severely damaged (and therefore depolarized) cells.

Cardiac gap junctions are more profoundly affected by other agents, including several whose concentrations have been shown to change during ischemia (e.g., ref. 17; Fig. 6). Under ischemic conditions, the intracellular concentrations of H^+ and divalent cations are rising, whereas, at the same time, the concentrations of cAMP and ATP are falling. This results in closure of the gap junctions and thus uncoupling of the affected region from the remaining tissue (see Fig. 6A for effect of intracellular acidification). Such regulatory mechanisms contribute to the "healing-over" phenomenon that protects intact tissue from permanent depolarization and inexcitability that might otherwise spread from an adjacent region seriously affected by ischemia. Both Ca^{2+} and H^{2+} ions affect junctional conductance (for review, see ref. 59), and in cardiac cells, calcium and hydrogen ions appear to act synergistically (60, 61), with increases in both $[Ca^{2+}]_i$ and $[H^+]_i$ being required for an effect. At low $[Ca]_i$ (60 to 240 nM), the junctions are barely pH-sensitive, but with increasing $[Ca]_i$ they become increasingly sensitive to $[H^+]_i$. Conversely, at high pH values, the junctions show hardly any sensitivity to a rise in $[Ca]_i$ (up to >1,000 nM, which is sufficient

196

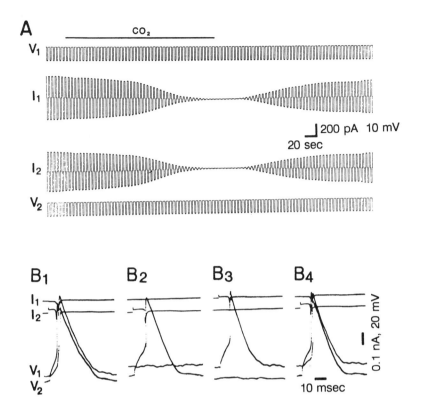

Figure 6. Gating of junctional conductance in pairs of cardiac myocytes by reduced intracellular pH (**A**) and halothane (**B**). Dual whole-cell voltage clamp recordings of a pair of myocytes during exposure to saline equilibrated with 100% CO_2 (applied during the bar atop figure). Upward-going currents in I_1 and I_2 are junctional and are reversibly reduced to very low values during CO_2 exposure. **B_1–B_4.** Current clamp experiment illustrating the blockade of action potential propagation between myocytes after exposure to 1.5 mM halothane. B_1: control, where excitation of cell 2 leads to depolarization and firing of cell 1. B_2 and B_3: after halothane treatment, when activation of either cell does not spread to the other. B_4, after recovery, when excitation once more spreads from cell 1 to cell 2. [(A) From Spray and Burt (19). (B) From Burt and Spray (67).]

to cause severe hypercontraction), but with increasing acidification the sensitivity to calcium increases dramatically. At a pH_i of ~6, cells will rapidly and completely uncouple when Ca_i levels approach 450 nM (data taken from ref. 61).

Gap junctional conductance is also reversibly reduced by a variety of lipophilic agents, including fatty acids that increase under ischemic conditions (22, 23), volatile anesthetics such as halothane (62), and short-chain alcohols such as heptanol and octanol (see ref. 20; Fig. 6B). The mechanism of action of these agents is still not completely understood, but it has been proposed on the basis of experiments with doxyl stearic acids of various lengths and side-chain positions that lipophilic compounds may interact at the interface of the membrane lipid with the channel protein (23). By doing so, the tertiary conformation of the channel is presumably perturbed enough to close completely. Alternatively or in addition, changes in membrane fluidity could contribute to altered gating behavior of the channels (63), or a lipophilic portion of the molecule could be affected directly.

Studies on the effects of Ca_i, pH, and lipophilic agents on the single-channel level have revealed that the single-channel conductance is not affected by any of these agents (44, 63, 64). Thus, as is the case with V_j, their effects must be caused by a decrease in open-channel probability. The precise way in which the gating parameters are changed by these agents is still under investigation, although recent experiments with halothane indicate that the mechanism for uncoupling is increased closed time (63).

Intracellular ATP has been reported to exert direct effects on cardiac gap junctions (64). However, cholinergic and β-adrenergic stimulation, which mediate the inotropic state of the heart (among other mechanisms) by raising the intracellular levels of cAMP and cGMP respectively, also regulate gap junctional conductance (65–69). In isolated heart cell pairs, treatment with agents that elevate cAMP (e.g., isoproternol or the membrane-permeant derivative 8-bromo-cAMP) may cause a ~50% increase of g_j, whereas agents that increase cGMP levels (e.g., carbachol or 8-bromo-cGMP) reduce g_j by ~25%. As will be discussed later in this chapter, connexin43 has a number of putative phosphorylation sites, and cyclic nucleotides are involved in a differential phosporylation of the gap junction channel. For the intact heart, an increase in junctional conductance, and thus conduction velocity, could contribute to the other inotropic effects of B-adrenergic stimulation. In addition, the increase in strength of coupling can be important in areas of the heart where the safety factor for impulse propagation is low, such as the Purkinje-ventricular junctions. The role of a g_j decrease resulting from cholinergic stimulation is not clear as yet, but it might participate in protective cell uncoupling during anoxia or ischemia. In this respect, it should be mentioned that, under conditions of calcium overload, g_j is reduced when cAMP levels are elevated (67, 68).

As will be discussed in more detail later, recent studies on the effects of gap junction channel phosphorylation have detected changes in amplitudes of single-channel currents. This suggests that the effects of cyclic nucleotides on gap junction channel gating through phosphorylation differ from other mediators such as pH, pCa, lipophilic agents, and voltage, in that they change unitary channel conductance instead of, or in addition to, affecting channel open probability.

Phosphorylation of Connexin43 in Neonatal Rat Cardiocytes

In primary cell cultures of rat neonatal cardiocytes, connexin43 shows a turnover of ~3 hr (70), and in Western blot analysis connexin43 is detected predominantly as two phosphorylated forms (connexin43-P_1 and connexin43-P_2) of slower electrophoretic mobility than the dephosphorylated form, Cx43-NP (70–72) (Fig. 7). The two phosphorylated forms are differentially phosphorylated, as demonstrated by two-dimensional phosphopeptide mapping (Sáez and Nairn, unpublished observations) and phosphorylation occurs almost exclusively in seryl residues (72). The turnover rate of phosphate groups on connexin43 is the same as the half-life of the protein, suggesting that phosphorylation is an early posttranslational event and that, once the protein is phosphorylated, it is not dephosphorylated during its life span (70). Nevertheless, treatment for only 30 min with okadaic acid (an inhibitor of phosphoprotein phosphatases), or with staurosporin (a protein kinase C and cyclic nucleotide-dependent protein kinase inhibitor) dramatically increases or decreases the phosphorylation state of Cx43-P_2 evaluated by $^{32}P_i$-incorporation (73). In these latter studies, it was also shown that, after inhibition with staurosporin, the state of phosphorylation of Cx43-P_2 was stimulated by treatment with a tumor-promoting phorbol ester known to activate protein kinase C. In addition, a synthetic peptide with sequence corresponding to residues 260–275 located in the carboxyl terminal of connexin43 was phosphorylated by protein kinase C in seryl residues 268 and 272. The synthetic peptide 260–275 was not phosphorylated by cAMP- or cGMP-dependent protein kinase. The functional effects observed after activation of those protein kinases might be related to differential phosphorylation of connexin43 occurring on other amino acid residues. It was also found that treatments that reduced or stimulated the state of phosphorylation of Cx-P_2 affected junctional conductance in the same direction (74). Therefore, these studies support the notion that changes in the state of phosphorylation of connexin43 gap junction subunits affect the functional state of the intercellular channels.

Gap Junctions During Heart Development

During the ontogeny of the heart, gap junctions between cardiac myocytes appear to be present in the precontactile stage. Although in rats the first evidence of synchronous electrical activity between cardiac myocytes is detected at the 3-somite stage (74), in chicks cardiac activity can be detected between the 7- and 9-somite stage (75). As early as the fourth day of chick development, gap junctions between cardiac myocytes are sensitive to transjunctional voltage, a feature that is gradually lost with increasing age (76), suggesting that the developmental expression of different connexins gives rise to gap junctions with different regulatory mechanisms. This notion has been supported by the detection of different connexins during chick heart organogenesis (77). Similar studies have not been reported for cardiac myocytes in mammals. The existence of connexins in addition to connexin43 in mammalian heart (connexin37 and connexin40 in rat; refs. 33 and 78) and connexin45 and connexin42 in dog (33) leaves

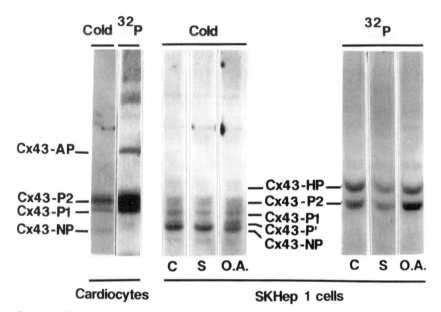

Figure 7. Phosphorylation of connexin43 in heart and in SKHep1 cells stably transfected with human connexin43. Connexin43 is a phosphoprotein in neonatal cardiac myocytes and in stably transfected SKHep1 cells, and its state of phosphorylation depends on the activity of protein kinases and protein phosphatases. Neonatal rat myocytes or SKHep1 cells transfected with the cDNA encoding the human connexin43 were incubated in $^{32}P_i$-(0.25 mCi/2 ml media/60 mm culture plate) for 2 hr or incubated in phosphate-free medium or phosphate-containing unlabeled ("cold") medium for the same period of time. Transfected cells were then treated with either staurosporin (300 nM) or okadaic acid (300 nM) for 20 min. Connexin43 was then immunoprecipitated, resolved in 8% sodium dodecyl sulfate-polyacrylamide gel electrophoresis and transferred to nitrocellulose. Lanes containing samples from cold cultures were incubated with anti-connexin43 antibody, developed with ^{125}I-protein A, autoradiographed (lane labeled Cold), and lanes containing samples from radiolabeled cells were autoradiographed (lane labeled ^{32}P). Immunoblots of neonatal rat cardiocytes showed that two major bands incorporated ^{32}P(Cx43-P1 and Cx43-P2), indicating that they are phosphorylated forms, and a minor band (Cx43-NP) that did not incorporate ^{32}P and which therefore corresponds to the dephosphorylated form. A protein aggregate of connexin43 (Cx43–AP) was variably detected. Immunoblots (Cold) of transfected SKHep1 cells showed at least five distinct bands: Cx43-NP corresponded to the dephosphorylated form and Cx43-P', Cx43-P1, Cx43-P2, and Cx43-P3 corresponded to phosphorylated forms of connexin43. The HP (higher electrophoretic mobility) form might correspond to that band recently described in other cell types that express connexin43 (113, 114). The lanes of radiolabeled cells showed two bands that comigrated with Cx43-P2 and Cx43-P3. Whereas treatment with staurosporin (S; cold) did not affect the immunoblot pattern of connexin43, treatment with okadaic acid (O.A.; cold) caused a slight reduction in Cx43-NP, with a concomitant increase in Cx43-P' form compared with control cultures (C; cold). The ^{32}P-incorporation into connexin43 was reduced by staurosporin (ST ^{32}P) and increased by okadaic acid (O.A.; ^{32}P).

open the possibility that mammalian cardiocytes also differentially express more than one connexin during organogenesis.

Morphological studies in mouse ventricles have shown short linear arrays of particles as early as the 10th embryonic day (79). Nonetheless, connexin43 is readily detected only by the 14th embryonic day (80). In rabbit, the highest gap junctional area is reached by the 1st postnatal week and is considerably reduced in adulthood (79, 81). At the molecular level, it has been shown that in whole rat heart (82) or in mouse ventricules (80) accumulation of connexin43 transcript precedes the increase in levels of its translation product detected by the 1st postnatal week. Later on, levels of connexin43 in the rat heart decline with increasing age, whereas levels of its transcript decrease to about half of the maximal levels and stay relatively contant during adulthood (82). Levels of connexin43 in mouse follow the variation in levels of its transcripts (80). The lag observed in both species between the increase in transcripts and levels of connexin43 detected 1 week postpartum suggests that the regulation of heart connexin43 during development is more likely to be determined by changes in the rate of transcription or stability of its mRNA than by changes in its turnover. The increase in connexin43 levels might be of functional relevance, because its abundance and distribution correlate well with the reported developmental increase in conduction velocity (83). Although connexin43 is predominantly in the phosphorylated format at all embryonic and postnatal ages studied (82) and is localized predominantly to the plasma membrane, it is likely that functional changes of gap junctions detected during development reflect changes in the number of available junctional channels.

Gating Properties of Connexin43—Use of Exogenous Expression

By comparing sequences of the connexins expressed in various tissues, specific regions of the channel molecules were hypothesized to be involved in the gating processes (19). In order to test these hypotheses using mutagenesis and also to determine the extent to which gating behavior was connexin-specific, one strategy has been to transfect communication-deficient cells stably with wild type and mutant connexins (44, 84). A vector containing cDNA encoding the wild type or mutant connexin (primarily human connexin43, the cloning and sequencing of which was described 2 years ago; ref. 44) was incorporated along with a selectable marker gene into a cell line in which endogenous gap junction expression was quite low (SKHep1, isolated by Dr. Fogh of Sloan Kettering from a highly metastatic human hepatoma). Colonies surviving selection for expression of the marker gene were subsequently injected with the dye Lucifer Yellow, a highly fluorescent dye molecule whose intercellular diffusion is commonly used to evidence gap junction presence. Northern blots of dye-coupled colonies indicated appropriate length transcript, and Southern blots have indicated stable incorporation of 5 to 10 connexin43 copies into the genome.

Voltage dependence of human connexin43 channels was analyzed by applying long transjunctional voltages (V_j's). Figure 5 shows that the parameters used to fit the Boltzmann relation to steady-state conductance for the transfectants are similar to those of rat heart cells. The parameters of the Boltzmann curve (85) are similar to those that have now been found in human *corpus cavernosum* (86), tracheal smooth muscle (87), and adult and neonatal mammalian atrial and ventricular tissue (4, 17, 48, 53), although the voltage sensitivity seems to be slightly higher in rat than in human tissues and for rat connexin43 expressed using the same transfection system as human connexin43 (54). Voltage dependence of rat connexin43 has not been detected in the *Xenopus* oocyte expression system, a difference among expression systems (88, 89) that remains mysterious but could arise from cytoplasmic access resistance or from differences in lipid environment or posttranslational processing in the oocyte system. For the voltage dependence of human connexin43, note that there is a minimal junctional conductance that persists, even at the highest V_j values (see 55, 56). The fraction of the conductance that is voltage-insensitive is a characteristic for each connexin type and is a constant fraction of the total junctional conductance, regardless of whether only a few or hundreds of channels are present. This suggests that either the rate constant of closing was saturating, so that channels of the same size continued to open and close but with a finite open probability, or that channel size was reduced at the highest V_js.

One way to examine the amplitude of the voltage-insensitive channels has involved the use of cell pairs where only a few channels were expressed by first applying a large V_j and then reducing g_j to low values by exposure to halothane. Under these conditions, unitary conductances were ~30 pS, which were smaller than those found at lower V_js, indicating that large transjunctional voltages drive the channel into a less voltage-dependent and smaller conductance state. This apparently voltage insensitive substate presumably accounts for the residual voltage-insensitive conductance, g_{min}, observed in cardiac myocytes (46).

Single channel measurements using driving forces of 40 to 50 mV, where open-channel probability is high, revealed multiple channel sizes. In addition to the occasional presence of the small 20 to 30 pS channels, two channel sizes (60 and 90 pS) are commonly detected in these transfected cells, examples of which are shown in Fig. 8. Histograms of hundreds of events recorded between individual cells show that both peaks are commonly present, and normalization of thousands of events measured in 14 cell pairs yields a histogram that is fit by the sum of three Gaussian distributions, the major ones having peaks at about 60 and 90 pS, and a smaller peak at 30 pS (90; see Fig. 8, top).

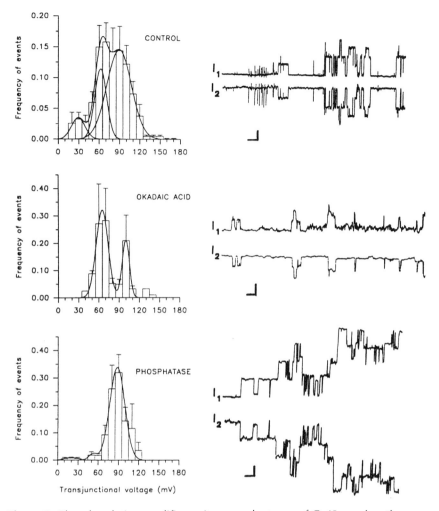

Figure 8. Phosphorylation modifies unitary conductance of Cx43 gap junction channels expressed in SKHep1 cells. Histograms on the **left** show the distribution of conductances present after halothane (2 mM) application to the bath. On the right are original traces of corresponding experiments; calibration bars are for 50 pS amplitude and 2 sec. **(Top)** Control experiments showing three unitary conductance sizes: 30, 60, and 90 pS. **(Middle)** 1 hr after okadaic acid (200 nM) was added to the bath, the most conspicuous events are of 60 pS. **(Bottom)** After alkaline phosphatase (*Escherichia coli*, 14 μg/ml) was dialyzed into one cell through the patch pipette; the most prominent peak in the histogram corresponds to channels of the large conductance size (90 pS).

This finding raised the question of how transfection with cDNA encoding a single gap junction protein resulted in channels of at least two sizes. The answer appears to lie in posttranslational processing of connexin43, which in heart (53, 70, 73) and other tissues (for review, see ref. 91) exhibits multiple electrophoretic mobilities. As shown in Fig. 7, Western blots of transfected cell homogenates detect multiple bands at 41 to 45 kDa, which collapse into a single 41 kDa band after treatment of the sample with alkaline phosphatase; phosphate label is incorporated into the upper bands but not into the bands treated with phosphatase.

To test the hypothesis that phosphorylation of human connexin43 affected unitary conductance, we recorded from cells treated with agents expected to increase phosphorylation (including phorbol esters to activate protein kinase C and okadaic acid to inhibit protein phosphatases) and found shifts in distribution to lower γ_j values. Treatment with a protein kinase inhibitor, staurosporine, and the placement of alkaline phosphatase into the pipette led to an increase in proportion of events of larger size (90; Fig. 8, middle and bottom). In order to determine whether these effects were directly correlated with phosphorylation of the human connexin43 molecule, cells were pretreated with radiolabeled inorganic phosphate for 1 hr and then exposed for 10 min to either staurosporine or okadaic acid. The Western blots of immunoprecipitated material indicate that these treatments led to only minor changes in total protein or relative distribution of the bands of different mobilities, but autoradiograms showed that incorporation of phosphate into the highest M_r forms was increased by okadaic acid and was decreased by staurosporine (Fig. 7). Tryptic digest of these bands showed that both were of the same protein with more or less incorporation of phosphate into the different peptides.

Phosphorylation also affects voltage sensitivity of the human connexin43 channel (90). Extent of phosphorylation does not appreciably affect steady-state voltage dependence, but dephosphorylation accelerates the time course of channel closure. Because steady-state voltage dependence is not affected, whereas the time course is, the forward and backward rate constants for this two-state system must be proportionately affected.

Other groups have hypothesized that phosphorylation of the gap junction channel might play a role in trafficking or assembly of the cardiac gap junction protein (70, 72, 92). To test this hypothesis, we first truncated the channel protein to various levels by inserting a stop codon in the cDNA sequence with which cells are transfected (84), and, more recently, we have been studying mutants where the phosphorylated serines are replaced by alanines. The truncation mutants were well expressed, and single channel sizes were increased by the elimination of a small portion of the carboxyl tail and decreased by larger deletion. These studies suggest that this portion of the molecule may be relevant for the channel's size but that the phosphorylation sites are unnecessary for appropriate assembly and functional activity (see also ref. 93).

Among the nine amino acid differences between human and rat connexin43 is a substitution of a SER in the rat sequence for an ALA in the human that has been suggested as a cGMP substrate (19, 44). Increasing the intracellular levels of cGMP in neonatal rat heart cells partially shifted unitary conductance from 60 pS to 30 pS (69), indicating that connexin43 probably has multiple conductance states that are regulated by different second messenger stimuli.

Gap Junction Disappearance in Cardiac Disease

Conductance of gap junction channels is decreased by many of the factors that have been found to change in the failing or ischemic heart (22), where pH is decreased, calcium is elevated, fatty acids and free radicals are generated, ATP and second messenger enzymes are reduced, and cells may be individually depolarized (generating transjunctional voltage). In addition to these acute effects mediated through channel gating, which can have profound effects on both conduction velocity and pathway anisotropy, long-term changes in gap junction expression can also result in conduction changes (for general consideration of long-term modulation of gap junctions, see ref. 94). Resculpting of ventricular bundles during aging is one example, where collagen deposition splits the aging heart into a maze of meandering conduction pathways (95). Similar resculpting may occur postinfarction (19, 25, 26), again favoring longitudinal over transverse conduction.

Chagas' disease, one of the most prevalent causes of heart disease in Latin America, is one example of a disease state in which studies on cultured cells have detected changes in gap junction distribution (96). In Central and South America, 10 to 20 million people are infected with the causative organism, *Trypanosoma cruzi*, a hemoflagellate protozoan parasite, and 50,000 deaths/year can be directly linked to the disease. Spread of excitation through the heart may be affected in both acute and chronic Chagas' disease, leading to arryhythmias and other conduction disturbances.

Infection of rat neonatal cardiac myocytes with *T. cruzi* is accompanied by marked disturbances in intercellular communication, which may underlie aberrant conduction patterns (96). Dye coupling and g_j are decreased between infected cells, and synchrony and rhythmicity of contractions in infected myocyte cultures are decreased compared with controls (Fig. 9, left). These functional alterations are associated with the disappearance of connexin43 from the appositional regions of the cell membranes of infected cells (Fig. 9, right). These findings would predict that infection of the heart with this parasite should result in a slowing of cardiac conduction and alter patterns of propagation as a consequence of decreased strength of electrotonic coupling.

Chronic Chagas' disease generally results in severe cardiomyopathy in which the integrity of both the myocardium and the conduction system

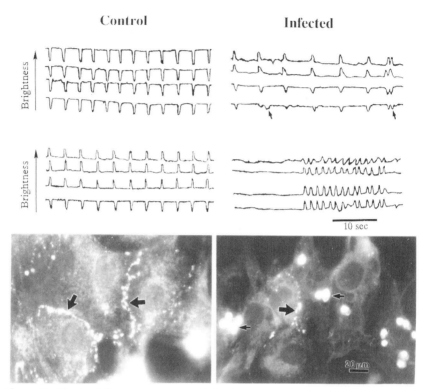

Figure 9. Effects of *Trypanosoma cruzi* infection on synchronous beating and gap junction distribution in cardiac myocytes in culture. **(Left)** Results of two experiments in which beat rates were recorded in matched control **(left)** and *T. cruzi*–infected **(right)** cardiac myocytes. Beat rates were recorded in multiple areas of a microscope field (40× magnification) using the brightness versus time utility program on an Image 1AT software package (Universal Imaging, Media, PA). Note that intervals between beats in control dishes are very constant, whereas in infected cultures beats are more irregular (even involving regional contractions, at arrows) and may be separated by long periods of quiescence **(bottom right). (Right)** Redistribution of connexin43 immunoreactivity in *T. cruzi*–infected myocardial cells. Control cells shown to the **left** illustrate the typical appositional staining with connexin43 antibody (large arrows). Infected cells are shown to the **right,** illustrating loss of the interfacial staining pattern between infected cells (small arrows indicate parasites). [From Campos de Carvalho et al. (96).]

is progressively compromised. In the chronic disease state, the presentation of conduction disturbances could result from decreased safety factor for intercellular communication as focal tissue damage exaggerates the effects of other factors that tend to fragment the conduction pathways within the aging heart.

Gap Junctions and Vascular Smooth Muscle

Although the physiological role for gap junctions in impulse propagation and contraction synchrony in heart are clear, the importance of gap junctions in the modulation of vasomotor tone is still considered controversial. This enigma results in large part from the disparity that has emerged between the numerous investigations that document the presence of gap junctions between vascular wall cells throughout the vascular tree (47, 97–100) and the relative paucity of studies demonstrating their physiological contribution to the modulation of tissue tone (101, 102). However, as outlined, recent evidence from a variety of laboratories suggests that gap junctions may indeed play a critical role in vascular physiology and dysfunction (103). In this regard, we will consider three types of cell-to-cell interactions that may modulate vasomotor tone: (1) smooth muscle cell–smooth muscle cell interactions; (2) endothelial cell–endothelial cell interactions; and (3) endothelial cell–smooth muscle cell interactions.

Intercellular Communication Among Vascular Smooth Muscle Cells

Recent experimental studies suggest that gap junctions may play a significant role in coordinating tone in vasculature subserving diverse functions. For example, functional gap junctions have been demonstrated between smooth muscle cells in large conduit vessels such as bovine, porcine, and rat aorta, in smaller conduit vessels such as pig coronary artery, and also in resistance vasculature such as rat mesentery. Moreover, gap junctions serve a prominent role in vascular tissue derived from the human *corpus cavernosum*, which is a specialized vascular resistence bed in the human penis. Although the role of gap junctions between smooth muscle cells in arterioles is less certain (104), the weight of experimental evidence emphasizes the potential diversity of functions that gap junctions may play in coordinating vasomotor activity between smooth muscle cells throughout the vasculature.

Most information concerning the function of gap junctions in vascular smooth muscle has been derived from studies performed on aorta, where there is ample evidence suggesting a physiological role for gap junctions in this tissue. For example, the presence of connexin43 mRNA as well as electrical coupling has been demonstrated in A7r5 cells, an aortic smooth muscle cell line (105). In addition, physiologically relevant second messengers were found to alter the gating properties of connexin43 in these cells. Fluorescent dye techniques have also demonstrated metabolic coupling among cultured aortic smooth muscle cells from diverse species following both enzymatic dissociation and explant cell culture (97, 98). Moreover, immunocytochemical studies have revealed an abundant distribution of gap junctions (connexin43) between smooth muscle cells throughout the intact Fischer 344 rat aorta (Christ et al., unpublished observations). Because intracellular recordings in both intact aorta (106) and cultured cells (98) reveal no spontaneous activity, the coordination of contractility and relaxation may be mediated largely by intercellular exchange of second messengers through gap junctions. Gap junctions have also been demonstrated between smooth muscle cells in smaller conduit arteries and resistance vasculature. In porcine coronary artery, for example, there is evidence for intercellular coupling among smooth muscle cells in the absence of morphological evidence for the presence of gap junctions (101). Such observations highlight the concept that small gap junction channels between adjacent smooth muscle cells are sufficient to provide physiologically relevant coupling, even when gap junctions are difficult to detect using transmission electron microscopy. Further evidence that gap junctions provide an important mechanism for coordinated contractile activity in vascular smooth muscle is derived from recent studies demonstrating that selective disruption of intercellular communication with heptanol abolishes fluorescent dye transfer among cultured vascular smooth muscle cells from rat mesenteric artery.

However, perhaps the most convincing evidence for the presence and physiological significance of gap junctions in vascular tissue derives from recent studies using intact tissues and cultured cells derived from human *corpus cavernosum*. These studies have demonstrated the following: (1) relatively small gap junctions formed of connexin43 ($\leq$0.25 μM) are found between corporal smooth muscle cells both in vitro and in situ (99); (2) electrophysiological studies have demonstrated that cultured corporal smooth muscle cells are well coupled electrically, exhibiting the three channel sizes characteristic of connexin43—that is, 30, 60, and 90 pS channels, respectively (86) (moreover, the distribution of channel sizes, and thus junctional conductance, is regulated by α_1-adrenergic receptor activation, as well as several physiologically relevant second messenger systems) (86); (3) calcium imaging studies using the calcium sensitive dye Fura2 have demonstrated that both calcium ions and IP_3 are freely diffusible through gap junctions between adjacent coporal smooth muscle cells in culture (39); (4) electrophysiological recordings of single corporal smooth muscle cells reveal the absence of action potentials, despite the presence of small inward calcium currents (107); and (5) consistent with the aforementioned observations, pharmacological studies on isolated corporal tissue strips have indicated that gap junctions contribute significantly to pharmacomechanical coupling and syncytial tissue contraction during activation of the α_1-adrenergic receptor (102). These findings have led to the model presented in Fig. 10, in which second messenger diffusion is hypothesized to underlie in large part the spread of contraction and relaxation among the cells.

Intercellular Communication Between Endothelial Cells

Endothelial cells form a continuous monolayer covering the vascular smooth muscle of the entire circulatory system. As such, intercellular communication among endothelial cells might provide an important mechanism for coordinating the extensive metabolic activity characteristic of these cells; especially in the microvasculature. In fact, gap junction messenger RNA (connexin43) and fluorescent dye transfer have been found among cultured endothelial cells from large conduit arteries such as bovine and

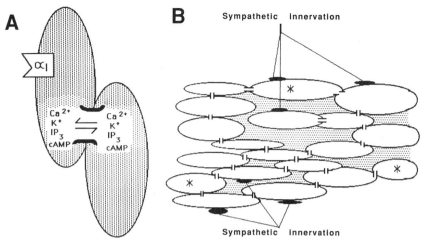

Figure 10. Schematic diagrams depicting the proposed role of gap junctions in coordinating α_1-adrenergic contraction in the smooth muscle. **(A)** Illustration of how second messengers known to be important modulators of smooth muscle contractility might be shared by diffusion through gap junctions between coupled cells. Stippled area emphasizes the potential continuity of the intracellular environments in the two respective cells. **(B)** Depicted is a group of smooth muscle cells connected by a network of small gap junctions that are a hallmark of this tissue; asterisks emphasize how smooth muscle cells in distant areas might be coupled with respect to both second messenger exchange and response generation, even if they were not directly activated by sympathetic stimulation. Stippled area outlines the extracellular space. For clarity and simplicity, endothelial cells are not shown.

porcine aorta, as well as in resistance vasculature from bovine brain and human *corpus cavernosum* (97, 108). Moreover, functional coupling has been demonstrated among endothelial cells in conduit arteries (109) and resistance arterioles (94) in situ. Additionally, intercellular communication among endothelial cells has been proposed to mediate the conduction of electrical and metabolic signals and to coordinate vasomotor activity among segments of the arteriolar network (104).

Intercellular Communication Between Endothelial Cells and Smooth Muscle Cells

Undoubtedly, heterocellular communication between endothelial and smooth muscle cells is the most controversial of the potential intercellular interactions among vascular wall cells. This is due in no small part to the fact that morphological evidence for such heterocellular gap junctions at points of myoendothelial contact is largely lacking. However, despite the sparsity of morphological data, several studies have demonstrated junctional transfer between endothelial and smooth muscle cells in vitro, as well as in both small and large vessels in vivo (108, 110, 111). In addition, another recent report has demonstrated the presence of myoendothelial junctions in vasculature and has postulated a significant role for heterocellular communication in mediating endothelium-dependent vasodilation (112). Such intercellular communication would seem to be an especially attractive mechanism for the transmission of endothelial vasoactive substances that are relatively labile (e.g., nitric oxide).

Taken together, the aforementioned information suggests that gap junctions are likely to play a physiologically important role in integrating and coordinating the tone of diverse vascular tissues. Such modulation may occur either homologous or heterologous gap junction-mediated intercellular communication. As such, it is not difficult to imagine that gap junctions could play a role in a diverse number of vascular disease states in which primary alterations to either the smooth muscle or endothelial cells are thought to be a significant factor. In fact, a partial list of vasculopathies that might be associated with altered intercellular communication could include such distinct diseases as coronary and cerebral vasospasm, Raynaud's syndrome, essential hypertension, the cardiovascular complications of diabetes mellitus, and perhaps erectile dysfunction as well.

Acknowledgments

The work from the laboratory cited herein was primarily supported by a grant from the National Institute of Health (HL-38449) to D.C.S. Additional support was provided by the New York Chapter of the American Heart Association (Grants-in-Aid to D.C.S., G.I.F., and A.P.M.; M.B.R. was supported by a Participating Laboratory Award). G.I.F. is the recipient of a Physician Scientist Award from the National Institutes of Health.

We thank F. Andrade for superb editorial and secretarial assistance. We acknowledge that the citations within the text are incomplete and apologize to the many authors whose uncited works have contributed enormously to the study of the role of gap junctions in aberrant conduction in heart.

References

1. Hertzberg, E.L., and, Johnson, R.G. (1988). *Gap Junctions* (Alan R. Liss, Inc., New York), pp. 1–548.

2. Hall, J.E., Zampighi, G., and Davis, R.M. (1993). *Gap Junctions: Progress in Cell Research* (Elsevier, New York), vol. 3.

3. Bennett, M.V., Barrio, L.C., Bargiello, T.A., Spray, D.C., Hertzberg, E., and Sáez, J.C. (1991). Gap junctions: New tools, new answers, new questions. *Neuron* **6**:305–320.

4. Anumonwo, J.M., Wang, H.Z., Trabka Janik, E., Dunham, B., Veenstra, R.D., Delmar, M., and Jalife, J. (1992). Gap junctional channels in adult mammalian sinus nodal cells. Immunolocalization and electrophysiology. *Circ. Res.* **71**:229–239.

5. Masson-Pévet, M., Bleeker, W.K., and Gros, D. (1979). The plasma membrane of leading pacemaker cells in the rabbit sinus node. *Circ. Res.* **45**:621.

6. Anderson, R.H., Ho, S.Y., Smith, A., and Becker, A.E. (1981). The intermodal atrial myocardium. *Anat. Rec.* **201**:75.

7. Joyner, R.W., and Van Capelle, F.J.L. (1986). Propagation through electrically coupled cells. How a small SA node drives a large atrium. *Biophys. J.* **50**:1157.

8. Sommer, J.R. (1983). Implications of structure and geometry on cardiac electrical activity. *Ann. Biomed. Engin.* **11**:149.

9. Rawling, D.A., Joyner, R.W., and Overhold, E.D. (1985). Variations in the functional electrical coupling between the subendocardial Purkinje and ventricular layers of the canine left ventricle. *Circ. Res.* **57**:252.

10. Di Francesco. (1985). The cardiac hyperpolarizing-activated current; origins and development. *Progr. Biophys. Mol. Biol.* **6**:163.

11. Bouman, L.N., and Jongsma, H.J. (1986). Structure and function of the sinoatrial node: A review. *Eur. Heart J.* **7**:94.

12. Severs, N.J. (1989). Constituent cells of the heart and isolated cell models in cardiovascular research, in *Isolated Adult Cardiomyocytes* (CRC Press, Boca Raton, FL), p. 3.

13. Opthof, T. (1988). The mammalian sino-atrial node. *Cardiovascular Drugs and Therapy* **1**:573.

14. Fishbein, M.C., Maclean, D., and Maroko, P.R. (1978). The histopathological evolution of myocardial infarction. *Chest* **73**:843.

15. De Maziere, A.M., van Ginneken, A.C., Wilders, R., Jongsma, H.J., and Bouman, L.N. (1992). Spatial and functional relationship between myocytes and fibroblasts in the rabbit sinoatrial node. *J. Mol. Cell. Cardiol.* **24**:567.

16. Burt, J.M., Frank, J.S., and Berns, M.W. (1982). Permeability and structural studies of heart cell gap junctions under normal and altered ionic conditions. *J. Membr. Biol.* **60**:227.

17. Rook, M.B., Jongsma, H.J., and de Jonge, B. (1988). Single channel currents of homo- and heterologous gap junctions between cardiac fibroblasts and myocytes. *Pflügers Arch.* **414**:95.

18. Spach, M.S., Dolber, P.C., and Heidlage, J.F. (1989). Interaction of inhomogeneities of repolarization with anisotropic propagation in dog atria. A mechanism for both preventing and initiating reentry. *Circ. Res.* **65**:1612.

19. Spray, D.C., and Burt, J.M. (1990). Structure-activity relations of the cardiac gap junction channel. *Am J. Physiol.* **258**:C195.

20. Page, E. (1992). Cardiac gap junctions, in *The Heart and Cardiovascular System*, H. Fozzard, et al., Eds. (Raven Press, New York), 2nd ed., p. 1003.

21. Janse, M.J., and Wit, A.L. (1989). Electrophysiological mechanisms of ventricular arrhythmias resulting from myocardial ischemia and infarction. *Physiol. Rev.* **69**:1049.

22. Gettes, L.S., and Cascio, W.E. (1992). Effect of acute ischemia on cardiac electrophysiology, in *The Heart and Cardiovascular System*, H. Fozzard, et al., Eds. (Raven Press, New York), 2nd ed., p. 2021.

23. Burt, J.M. (1991). Modulation of cardiac gap junction channel activity by the membrane lipid environment, in *Biophysics of Gap Junction Channels*, C. Peracchia, Ed. (CRC Press, Boca Raton, FL), p. 75.

24. Brugada, J., Boersma, L., Kirchhof, Ch.J.H., Heynen, V.V.T., and Allessie, M.A. (1991). Reentrant excitation around a fixed obstacle in uniform anisotropic ventricular myocardium. *Circ. Res.* **84:**1296.

25. Luke, R.A., and Saffitz, J.E. (1991). Remodeling of ventricular conduction pathways in healed canine infarct border zones. *J. Clin. Invest.* **87:**1594.

26. Smith, J.H., Green, C.R., Peters, N.S., Rothery, S., and Severs, N.J. (1991). Altered patterns of gap junction distribution in ischemic heart disease. An immunohistochemical study of human myocardium using laser scanning confocal microscopy. *Am. J. Path.* **139:**801.

27. Brugada, J., Mont, L., Boersma, L., Kirchhof, C., and Allessie, M.A. (1991). Differential effects of heptanol, potassium, and tetrodotocin on reentrant ventricular tachycardia around a fixed obstacle in anisotropic myocardium. *Circ. Res.* **84:**1307.

28. Makowski, L. (1988). X-ray diffraction studies of gap junction structure. *Adv. Cell. Biol.* **2:**119.

29. Unwin, N. (1989). The structure of ion channels in membranes of excitable cells. *Neuron* **3:**665.

30. Yeager, M., and Gilula, N.B. (1992). Membrane topology and quaternary structure of cardiac gap junction ion channels. *J. Mol. Biol.* **223:**929.

31. Beyer, E.C., Paul, D.L., and Goodenough, D.A. (1987). Connexin43: A protein from rat heart homologous to a gap junction protein from liver. *J. Cell. Biol.* **105:**2621.

32. Kanter, H.L., Saffitz, J.E., and Beyer, E.C. (1992). Cardiac myocytes express multiple gap junction proteins. *Circ. Res.* **70:**438.

33. Haefliger, J.A., Bruzzone, R., Jenkins, N.A., Gilbert, D.J., Copeland, N.G., and Paul, D.L. (1992). Four novel members of the connexin family of gap junction proteins. Molecular cloning, expression, and chromosome mapping. *J. Biol. Chem.* **267:**2057.

34. Yancey, S.B., John, S.A., Lal, R., Austin, B.J., and Revel, J.P. (1989). The 43-kD polypeptide of heart gap junctions: Immunolocalization, topology, and functional domains. *J. Cell. Biol.* **108:**2241.

35. Fishman, G.I., Eddy, R.L., Shows, T.B., Rosenthal, L., and Leinwand, L.A. (1991). The human connexin gene family of gap junction proteins: Distinct chromosomal locations but similar structures. *Genomics* **10:**250.

36. Willecke, K., Jungbluth, S., Dahl, E., Hennemann, H., Heynkes, R., and Grzeschik, K.H. (1990). Six genes of the human connexin gene family coding for gap junctional proteins are assigned to four different human chromosomes. *Eur. J. Cell. Biol.* **53:**275.

37. DeLeon, J.R., and Fishman, G.I. (1992). Connexin43 expression in cardiac myocytes and non-myocytes. *Circulation* **86:**1–624.

38. Sáez, J.C., Connor, J.A., Spray, D.C., and Bennett, M.V. (1989). Hepatocyte gap junctions are permeable to the second messenger, inositol 1,4,5-trisphosphate, and to calcium ions. *Proc. Natl. Acad. Sci. U.S.A.* **86:**2708.

39. Christ, G.J., Moreno, A.P., Melman, A., and Spray, D.C. (1992). Gap junction-mediated intercellular diffusion of Ca^{2+} in cultured human corporal smooth muscle cells. *Am. J. Physiol.* **263:**C1.

40. Finkbeiner, S. (1992). Calcium waves in astrocytes—filling in the gaps. *Neuron* **8:**1101.

41. Sanderson, M.J., Charles, A.C., and Dirksen, E.R. (1990). Mechanical stimulation and intercellular communication increases intracellular Ca^{2+} in epithelial cells. *Cell Regul.* **1**:585.

42. Tsien, R., and Weingart, R. (1976). Inotropic effect of cyclic AMP in calf ventricular muscle studied by a cut-end method. *J. Physiol.* **260**:117.

43. Burt, J.M., and Spray, D.C. (1988). Single-channel events and gating behavior of the cardiac gap junction channel. *Proc. Natl. Acad. Sci. U.S.A.* **85**:3431.

44. Fishman, G.I., Spray, D.C., and Leinwand, L.A. (1990). Molecular characterization and functional expression of the human cardiac gap junction channel. *J. Cell. Biol.* **111**:589.

45. Rook, M.B., Jongsma, H.J., and van Ginneken, A.C. (1988). Properties of single gap junctional channels between isolated neonatal rat heart cells. *Am. J. Physiol.* **255**:H770.

46. Moreno, A.P., Rook, M.B., and Spray, D.C. (1993). The multiple conductance states of mammalian connexin43. *Biophys. J.* **64**:A236.

47. Beyer, E.C., Reed, K.E., Westphale, E.M., Kanter, H.L., and Larson, D.M. (1992). Molecular cloning and expression of rat connexin40, a gap junction protein expressed in vascular smooth muscle. *J. Membr. Biol.* **127**:69.

48. Rook, M.B., Van Ginneken, A.C.G., de Jonge, B., El Aoumari, A., Gros, D., and Jongsma, H.J. (1992). Differences in gap junction channels between cardiac myocytes, fibroblasts, and heterologous pairs. *Am. J. Physiol.* **263**:C959–C977.

49. Maurer, P., and Weingart, R. (1988). Action potential transfer in cell pairs isolated from adult rat and guinea pig ventricles. *Circ. Res.* **63**:72.

50. White, N., Spray, D.C., Campos de Carvalho, A.C., Wittenberg, B.A., and Bennett, M.V.L. (1985). Some physiological and pharmacological properties of cardiac myocytes dissociated from adult rat. *Am. J. Physiol.* **249**:C447.

51. Kameyama, M. (1983). Electrical coupling between ventricular paired cells isolated from guinea pig heart. *J. Physiol.* **336**:345.

52. Weingart, R. (1986). Electrical properties of the nexal membrane studied in rat ventricular cell pairs. *J. Physiol.* **370**:267.

53. Lal, R., and Arnsdorf, M.F. (1992). Voltage-dependent gating and single-channel conductance of adult mammalian atrial gap junctions. *Circ. Res.* **71**:737.

54. Rook, M.P., Moreno, A.P., Fishman, G.I., and Spray, D.C. (1992). Rat and human connexin43 (Cx43) gap junction channels in stably transfected cells: comparison of unitary conductance and voltage sensitivity. *Biophys. J.* **61**:A505.

55. Spray, D.C., Harris, A.L., and Bennett, M.V. (1981). Equilibrium properties of a voltage-dependent junctional conductance. *J. Gen. Physiol.* **77**:75–94.

56. Spray, D.C., Bennett, M.V.L., Campos de Carvalho, A.C., Eghbali, B., Moreno, A., and Verselis, V. (1991). Voltage dependence of junctional conductance. *Biophysics of Gap Junction Channels* **97**.

57. Moreno, A.P., Eghbali, B., and Spray, D.C. (1991). Connexin32 gap junction channels in stably transfected cells: Unitary conductance. *Biophys. J.* **60**:1267.

58. Wilders, R., and Jongsma, H.J. (1992). Limitations of the dual voltage clamp method in assaying conductance and kinetics of gap junction channels. *Biophys. J.* **63**:942.

59. Spray, D.C., and Bennett, M.V. (1985). Physiology and pharmacology of gap junctions. *Ann. Rev. Physiol.* **47**:281.

60. Burt, J.M. (1987). Block of intercellular communication: interaction of intracellular H^+ and Ca^{2+}. *Am. J. Physiol.* **253**:C607.

61. White, R.L., Doeller, J.E., Verselis, V.K., and Wittenberg, B.A. (1990). Gap junctional conductance between pairs of ventricular myocytes is modulated synergistically by H^+ and Ca^{++}. *J. Gen. Physiol.* **95**:1061.

62. Burt, J.M., and Spray, D.C. (1989). Volatile anesthetics block intercellular communication between neonatal rat myocardial cells. *Circ. Res.* **65**:829.

63. Takens-Kwak, B.R., Jongsma, H.J., Rook, M.B., and van Ginneken, A.C. (1992). Mechanism of heptanol-induced uncoupling of cardiac gap junctions: A perforated patch-clamp study. *Am. J. Physiol.* **262**:C1531.

64. Sugiura, H., Toyama, J., Tsuboi, N., Kamiya, K., and Kodama, I. (1990). ATP directly affects junctional conductance between paired ventricular myocytes from guinea pig heart. *Circ. Res.* **66**:1095–1102.

65. De Mello, W.C., and van Loon, P. (1987). Influence of cyclic nucleotides on junctional permeability in atrial muscle. *J. Mol. Cell. Cardiol.* **19**:83.

66. De Mello, W.C. (1989). Increase in junctional conductance caused by isoproterenol in heart cell pairs is suppressed by cAMP dependent protein kinase inhibitors. *Biochem. Biophys. Res. Comm.* **154**:509.

67. Burt, J.M., and Spray, D.C. (1988). Inotropic agents modulate gap junctional conductance between cardiac myocytes. *Am. J. Physiol.* **254**:H1206.

68. Wojtczak, J. (1982). Influence of cyclic nucleotides on the internal longitudinal resistance of cow ventricular muscle induced by hypoxia. *Mol. Cell. Cardiol.* **14**:259.

69. Takens-Kwak, B.R., and Jongsma, H.J. Cardiac gap junctions: three distinct single channel conductances and their modulation by phosphorylating treatments. *Phlügers Arch.*, in press.

70. Laird, D.W., Puranam, K.L., and Revel, J.P. (1991). Turnover and phosphorylation dynamics of connexin43 gap junction protein in cultured cardiac myocytes. *Biochem. J.* **273**:67.

71. Laird, D.W., and Revel, J.P. (1990). Biochemical and immunochemical analysis of the arrangement of connexin43 in rat heart gap junction membranes. *J. Cell. Sci.* **97**:109.

72. Lau, A.F., Hatch Pigott, V., and Crow, D.S. (1991). Evidence that heart connexin43 is a phosphoprotein. *J. Mol. Cell. Cardiol.* **23**:659.

73. Sáez, J.C., Nairn, A.C., Czernik, D.C., Spray, D.C., and Hertzberg, E.L. (1988). Rat connexin43: Regulation by phosphorylation in heart, in *Gap Junctions. Progress in Cell Research*, J.E. Hall, G.A. Zampighi, and R.M. Davis, Eds. (Elsevier Science Publishers, Amsterdam), vol. 3.

74. Hirota, A., Kamino, K., Komuro, H., Sakai, T., and Yada, T. (1981). Early events in development of electrical activity and contraction in embryonic rat heart assessed by optical recording. *J. Physiol.* **369**:209.

75. Fuji, S., Hirota, A., and Kamino, K. (1981). Optical indications of pacemaker potential and rhythm generation in early embryonic chick heart. *J. Physiol.* **312**:253.

76. Veenstra, R.D. (1991). Developmental changes in regulation of embryonic chick heart gap junctions. *Membr. Biol.* **119**:253.

77. Beyer, E.C. (1990). Molecular cloning and developmental expression of two chick embryo gap junction proteins. *J. Biol. Chem.* **265**:14439.

78. Hennemann, H., Suchyna, T., Lichtenberg Frate, H., Jungbluth, S., Dahl, E., Schwarz, J., Nicholson, B.J., and Willecke, K. (1992). Molecular cloning and functional expression of mouse connexin40, a second gap junction gene preferentially expressed in lung. *J. Cell Biol.* **117**:1299.

79. Gros, D., Mocquard, J.P., Challice, C.E., and Schrevel, J. (1978). Formation and growth of gap junctions in mouse myocardium during ontogenesis: A freeze-cleave study. *J. Cell Sci.* **30**:45.

80. Fromaget, C., el Aoumari, A., Dupont, E., Briand, J.P. and Gros, D. (1990). Changes in the expression of connexin43, a cardiac gap junctional protein, during mouse heart development. *J. Mol. Cell. Cardiol.* **22**:1245.

81. Shibata, Y., Nakata, K., and Page, E. (1980). Ultrastructural changes during development of gap junctions in rabbit left ventricular myocardial cells. *J. Ultrastruct. Res.* **71**:258.

82. Fishman, G.I., Hertzberg, E.L., Spray, D.C., and Leinwand, L.A. (1991). Expression of connexin43 in the developing rat heart. *Circ. Res.* **68**:782.

83. van Kempen, M.J., Fromaget, C., Gros, D., Moorman, A.F., and Lamers, W.H. (1991). Spatial distribution of connexin43, the major cardiac gap junction protein, in the developing and adult rat heart. *Circ. Res.* **68**:1638.

84. Fishman, G.I., Moreno, A.P., Spray, D.C., and Leinwand, L.A. (1991). Functional analysis of human cardiac gap junction channel mutants. *Proc. Natl. Acad. Sci. U.S.A.* **88**:3525.

85. Spray, D.C., Moreno, A.P., Eghbali, B., Chanson, M., and Fishman, G.I. (1992). Gating of gap junction channels as revealed in cells stably transfected with wild type and mutant connexin cDNAs. *Biophys. J.* **62**:48.

86. Moreno, A.P., Campos de Carvalho, A.C., Christ, G., and Spray, D.C. (1993). Gap junctions between human *corpus cavernosum* smooth muscle cells: Gating properties and unitary conductance. *Am. J. Physiol.* **33**:C80.

87. DePalo, L.R., Spray, D.C., Hertzberg, E.L., Castaldi, M.C., Kotlikoff, M.I., and Kessler, J.A. (1992). Connexin43 expression and functional gap junction formation in cultured human airway smooth muscle cells. Manuscript submitted for publication.

88. Werner, R., Levine, E., Rabadan Diehl, C., and Dahl, G. (1989). Formation of hybrid cell-cell channels. *Proc. Natl. Acad. Sci. U.S.A.* **86**:5380.

89. Swenson, K.I., Jordan, J.R., Beyer, E.C., and Paul, D.L. (1989). Formation of gap junctions by expression of connexins in *Xenopus* oocyte pairs. *Cell* **57**:145.

90. Moreno, A.P., Fishman, G.I., and Spray, D.C. (1992). Phosphorylation shifts unitary conductance and modifies voltage dependent kinetics of human connexin43 gap junction channels. *Biophys. J.* **62**:51.

91. Sáez, J.C., Berthoud, V.M., Moreno, A.P., and Spray, D.C. (1992). Gap junctions: Multiplicity of controls in differentiated and undifferentiated cells and possible functional implications, in *Phosphoprotein Research,* S. Shenolikar and A.C. Narin, Eds. (Raven Press, New York), vol. 27, p. 163.

92. Musil, L.S., and Goodenough, D.A. (1991). Biochemical analysis of connexin43 intracellular transport, phosphorylation, and assembly into gap junctional plaques. *J. Cell. Biol.* **115**:1357.

93. Dunham, B., Liu, S., Taffet, S., Trabka Janik, E., Delmar, M., Petryshyn, R., Zheng, S., Perzova, R., and Vallano, M.L. (1992). Immunolocalization and expression of functional and nonfunctional cell-to-cell channels from wild-type and mutant rat heart connexin43 cDNA. *Circ. Res.* **70**:1233.

94. Spray D.C., Sáez, J.C., Burt, J.M., Watanabe, T., Reid, L.M., Hertzberg, E.L., and Bennett, M.V.L. (1988). Gap junctional conductance: Multiple sites of regulation, in *Gap Junctions,* E.L. Hertzberg and R.G. Johnson, Eds. (Alan R. Liss, Inc., New York), pp. 227–244.

95. Spach, M.S., and Dolber, P.C. (1986). Relating extracellular potentials and their derivatives to anisotropic propagation at a microscopic level in human cardiac muscle: Evidence for electrical uncoupling of side-to-side fiber connections with increasing age. *Circ. Res.* **58**:356.

96. Campos de Carvalho, A.C., Tanowitz, H.B., Wittner, M., Dermietzel, R., Roy, C., Hertzberg, E.L., and Spray, D.C. (1992). Gap junction distribution is altered between cardiac myocytes infected with *Trypanosoma cruzi. Circ. Res.* **70**:733.

97. Larson, D.M., Haudenschild, C.C., and Beyer, E.C. (1990). Gap junction messenger RNA expression by vascular wall cells. *Circ. Res.* **66**:1074.

98. Blennerhassett, M.G., Kannan, M.S., and Garfield, R.E. (1987). Functional characterization of cell-to-cell coupling in cultured rat aortic smooth muscle. *Cell Physiol.* **21**:C555.

99. Campos de Carvalho, A.C., Roy, C., Christ, G.J., Moreno, A.P., and Spray, D.C. (1992). Gap junctions formed of connexin43 are found between smooth muscle cells of human *corpus cavernosum. J. Urol.*, in press.

100. Mei-Ling, T., Loch-Caruso, R., and Webb, R.C. (1992). Characteristics of intracellular communication in mesenteric vascular smooth muscle cells from rats. *FASEB J.* **A970.**

101. Beny, J.L., and Connat, J.L. (1992). An electron-microscopic study of smooth muscle cell dye coupling in the pig coronary arteries. Role of gap junctions. *Circ. Res. Dev.* **70**:49–55.

102. Christ, G.J., Moreno, A.P., Parker, M.E., Gondre, C.M., Valcic, M., Melman, A., and Spray, D.C. (1991). Intercellular communication through gap junctions: A potential role in pharmacomechanical coupling and syncytial tissue contraction in vascular smooth muscle isolated from the human *corpus cavernosum. Life Sci.* **49**:PL195.

103. Segal, S.S., and Duling, B.R. (1986). Flow control among microvessels coordinated by intercellular conduction. *Science* **234**:868.

104. Segal, S.S., and Beny, J.L. (1992). Intracellular recording and dye transfer in arterioles during blood flow control. *Am. J. Physiol.* **263**:1.

105. Moore, L.K., Beyer, E.C., and Burt, J.M. (1991). Characterization of gap junction channels in A7r5 vascular smooth muscle cells. *Am. J. Physiol.* **260**(*Cell Physiol. 29*):C975.

106. Mekata, F. (1981). Electrical current induced contraction in the smooth muscle of the rabbit aorta. *J. Physiol.* **317**:149.

107. Christ, G.J., Spray, D.C., and Brink, P. (1992). Characterization of K currents in cultured human corporeal smooth muscle cells. *J. Androl.*, in press.

108. Larson, D.M., and Sheridan, J.D. (1982). Intercellular junctions and transfer of small molecules in primary vascular endothelial cultures. *J. Cell Biol.* **92**:183.

109. Beny, J.L., and Gribi, F. (1989). Dye and electrical coupling of endothelial cells in situ. *Tissue & Cell* **21**:797.

110. Sheridan, J.D., and Larson, D.M. (1982). Junctional communication in the peripheral vasculature, in *The Functional Integration of Cells in Animal Tissues*, J.D. Pitts and M.E. Finbow, Eds. (Cambridge University Press, Cambridge), British Society for Cell Biology Symposium Series No. 5, p. 263.

111. Davies, P.F., Ganz, P., and Diehl, P.S. (1985). Reversible microcarrier-mediated junctional communication between endothelial and smooth muscle cell monolayers: An in vitro model of vascular cell interactions. *J. Lab Invest.* **53**:710.

112. Asada, Y., and Lee, T.J.-F. (1992). Role of myoendothelial junctions in endothelium dependent vasodilation. *FASEB J. Abstr.* **Part I**:A974.

113. Oh, S.Y., Grupen, C.G., and Murray, A.W. (1991). Phorbol ester induces phosphorylation and down-regulation of connexin43 in WB cells. *Biochem. Biophys. Acta* **1094**:243.

114. Reynhout, J.K., Lampe, P.D., and Johnson, R.G. (1992). An activator of protein kinase C inhibits gap junction communication between cultured bovine lens cells. *Exp. Cell Res.* **198**:337.

PART THREE

Channel Modulation and Autonomic Control

The rate and force of cardiac contraction is profoundly modulated by the autonomic nervous system. Modulation is mediated by adrenergic or cholinergic neurotransmitters acting on cardiac channels, in particular K^+ channels, as discussed by Dr. Giles in Chapter 11, and Ca^{2+} channels as discussed by Dr. Bean in Chapter 12. For cardiac sympathetic nerves the signalling pathway from nerve ending to ion channel involves the neurotransmitter norepinephrine, two classes of membrane receptor proteins, α- and β- adrenoreceptors, and guanine nucleotide binding or "G proteins." G proteins couple a wide range of receptors to different cellular messengers and may act directly or indirectly on ion channels. In the latter case the pathways may include G protein effectors, such as the enzymes adenylyl cyclase and phospholipases C and A_2, protein kinases A and C, cyclic nucleotide phosphodiesterases, and probably a variety of phosphatases. For the parasympathetic cardiac vagal nerve response, the neurotransmitter is acetylcholine (ACh) and the receptors are muscarinic G protein-linked receptors. The inhibitory G protein, G_i, couples the muscarinic cholinergic receptor directly to an inwardly rectifying K^+ channel. Modulation of ion channels by G_i may also occur indirectly. For example, G protein inhibition of adenylyl cyclase may reduce Ca^{2+} currents which have been enhanced previously by β-adrenergic receptor activation.

In Chapter 11, the G protein coupling of α-adrenoreceptors to K^+ channels is dealt with biochemically by measuring the GTPase activity of membrane enriched fractions from cardiac myocytes, and functionally by measuring the effects on K^+ currents. Dr. Giles reports that α-adrenoreceptor stimulation inhibits two distinct K^+ currents, I_t, a transient outward K^+ current, and I_{K1}, an inwardly rectifying K^+ current. This prolongs the cardiac action potential and increases calcium influx resulting in an increase in the force of contraction (i.e. positive inotropic effect). α-adrenoreceptor activation is shown to enhance binding of [γ-^{32}P] GTP to a 75 kDa protein which was not pertussis-toxin sensitive, ruling out the involvement of G_i.

In Chapter 12, Dr. Bean describes in molecular terms the effects of β-adrenoreceptor stimulation on cardiac Ca^{2+} channels. A small component of the stimulation may be due to direct effects of the G protein stimulatory for adenylyl cyclase, G_s, but the predominant effect is evidently due to phosphorylation of the channels via the cAMP, A kinase pathway. At the single channel level, the main effect is an increase in the frequency of channel opening. The effects on channel opening are cyclical and have a period of seconds consistent with phosphorylation-dephosphorylation of the channel protein. There is also a greater probability of opening at more negative potentials indicating that phosphorylation stabilizes the open-state of the channel. The more stable open-state is associated with prolonged open times resembling effects produced by dihydropyridine (DHP) calcium channel agonists.

In Chapter 13, Drs. De Biasi and Brown begin with an examination of the interaction between G_i and the muscarinic atrial K^+ (K^+[ACh]) channel which is a principal target for cholinergic inhibition of heart rate. DeBiasi and Brown end by identifying the ion conduction pathway or pore domain of the delayed rectifier K^+ channels. This work bridges this Part dealing with channel modulation by the autonomic nervous system, and the following Part dealing with the identification of channel domains that determine different channel functions, such as voltage-sensing and ion conduction.

Normally the K^+[ACh] channel is closed and can be opened by G_i following cholinergic activation. Trypsin can also open the channel, although its effects are irreversible. The ion conducting pathway or pore of the K^+ channel protein that is exposed shows sequence homology to the pore of delayed rectifying K^+ channels as noted earlier. This strengthens the relevance of structure-function studies on the pore of delayed rectifier K^+ channels for similar studies on the pore of inwardly rectifying K^+ channels.

Mutational analysis localized about 75% of the pore of delayed rectifier K^+ channels to a stretch of 20 amino acids in the channel protein. This stretch spans the membrane and includes two tetraethylammonium (TEA) binding sites one at the external mouth and one near the internal mouth of the channel pore. In this study not only is the pore domain revealed, but receptor sites for drugs that modulate the channel pore are identified. In Section F below we learn more about domains related to voltage-sensing, gating and modulation in K^+, Na^+, and Ca^+ channels.

Arthur M. Brown & Peter M. Spooner

α₁-Adrenergic Effects on Potassium Currents and Membrane GTPase in Single Rabbit Cardiac Cells

A. P. Braun, M. P. Walsh, R. B. Clark, and W. R. Giles

α-Adrenoceptors are now recognized as part of a large and growing family of cell surface receptors that have an obligatory requirement for guanine nucleotide binding (G) proteins in activating cellular signaling pathways (1–3). Several experimental approaches have provided evidence for interactions of G-proteins with a given hormone receptor. These include demonstrations that (i) GTP and its nonhydrolyzable analogs reduce the high-affinity binding state of the receptor for its natural agonist, or mimic the functional response to a given agonist; (ii) certain bacterial toxins [i.e., pertussis toxin (PTX) and cholera toxin] interfere with the cellular response to agonist; and (iii) receptor activation stimulates GTP binding to, or the intrinsic GTPase activity of, a membrane-associated G-protein. This last approach can provide a direct measure of receptor/G-protein interaction in terms of a quantitative description of hormone-sensitive activation of G-proteins by the receptor molecule (4). Previous studies have shown that GTP analogs reduce the high-affinity binding state of cardiac α₁-adrenoceptors for the agonist, but that this state is insensitive to disruption by PTX (5). It is also known that PTX does not interfere with cellular responses such as PIP₂ metabolism (6, 7), ion channel modulation (3, 8) or the positive inotropic effect (9) resulting from α₁-adrenoceptor activation in the heart. However, recent reports have described α₁-mediated electrophysiological events in the heart that can be blocked by PTX treatment (10, 11).

We have studied α₁-adrenoceptor/G-protein interactions by examining the adrenoceptor stimulation of GTPase activity in plasma membranes prepared from atrial and ventricular myocytes from adult rabbit (4). The effects of α₁-adrenergic agonists and antagonists, nonhydrolyzable derivatives of GTP, and PTX on two time- and voltage-dependent K⁺ currents in rabbit heart have been detailed (4, 12–14). These results demonstrate very similar concentration-dependent response relationships for (i) stimulation of GTPase activity and (ii) inhibition of two different K^+ currents. This observation provides insight into the mechanism of α_1-adrenergic regulation of K^+ channels in rabbit heart.

Experimental Procedures

Atrial and ventricular myocytes were isolated from adult rabbits (2 to 3 kg) as described in our previous publications (4, 12, 14). The following modifications were used for ventricular cell isolations, when large cell yields were needed for biochemical experiments. After perfusion of a whole heart, the left ventricle and septum were incubated for three 10-min periods in ~20 ml of low Ca^{2+}-Tyrodes' solution containing 50 to 75 U/ml collagenase (Yakult Co., Ltd., Japan), but no protease. After each incubation, cells were decanted and the remaining tissue resuspended in fresh collagenase-containing Tyrodes. Following isolation, cells were washed free of enzymes and bovine serum albumin, pelleted, and then stored at $-70°C$. Detailed descriptions of our methods for preparation of myocyte sarcolemmal membranes, assays of membrane-associated GTPase and Na/K-ATPase activities, PTX-catalyzed ADP ribosylation, and covalent affinity labeling of G-proteins were published recently (4).

Whole-cell voltage-clamp techniques were used to record two different K^+ currents from atrial and ventricular myocytes isolated from rabbit hearts. All procedures for electrode fabrication, data acquisition, and analyses were published previously (8, 12–14).

Results

α_1-Adrenergic responses in mammalian heart exhibit pronounced frequency and species dependence (3). We have chosen to study myocardial tissue from rabbit based on the electrophysiological similarities between the atria of rabbit and human (15, 16) and the extensive descriptive literature on adrenergic effects (17–20; cf. ref. 3) and membrane-sarcolemmal biochemistry of rabbit myocardium (21, 22).

Data in Fig. 1 illustrate the electrophysiological effects of the adrenergic neurotransmitter 1-noradrenaline (1-NA) in atrium (Fig. 1A) and the α_1-adrenoceptor agonist methoxamine in ventricle (Fig. 1B) of rabbit heart. Note that in both types of myocytes, there is (i) an increase in plateau height, (ii) an increase in action potential duration, and (iii) a small depolarization in resting potential. Separate experiments, in which changes in cell length were measured in conjunction with action potentials, have shown that effects (i) and (ii) can give rise to a significant increase in cell shortening, that is, to a positive inotropic effect (23). The main goals of the

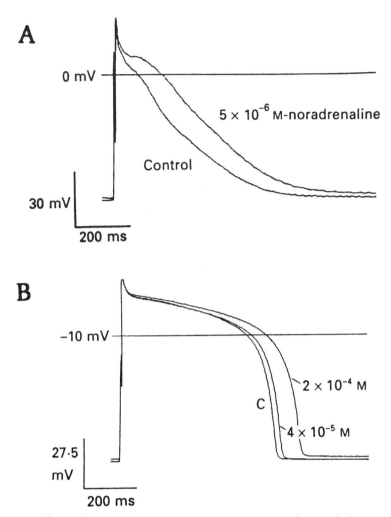

Figure 1. Effects of α_1-adrenergic agonists on action potentials recorded in single myocytes from rabbit atrium and ventricle. **(A)** The effects of 1-NA on action potentials recorded from rabbit atrial myocytes. After recording a control action potential, the cell was superfused with noradrenaline (5×10^{-6} M) and, after a maximal drug effect had been achieved, a second action potential trace was recorded. The broadening of the action potential was almost completely reversible (not shown) and could be blocked by the selective α_1-adrenergic antagonist, prazosin. The horizontal line denotes 0 mV. These recordings were made during constant 0.1 Hz stimulation of the cell in the presence of 10^{-6} M propranolol to block β-adrenergic effects. Temperature was $22 \pm 1°C$. **(B)** The effects of the selective α_1-adrenergic agonist methoxamine on action potentials recorded from rabbit ventricular myocytes. Action potentials were elicited by 2 msec current pulses applied at 0.2 Hz. The control action potential is denoted by **(C)**, and the steady-state effects of two doses of methoxamine are illustrated. 4-Aminopyridine (10^{-3} M) was present in the superfusate. Temperature was 23°C.

experiments described herein were to obtain information concerning the ionic mechanisms of the changes in action potential waveform, and the biochemical pathways mediating these observed effects on ion-selective, time- and voltage-dependent, transmembrane K^+ currents.

We have shown previously that noradrenaline, acting via α_1-adrenoceptors, can significantly reduce a Ca^{2+}-independent, transient outward, K^+ current, I_t, in single cells obtained from rabbit atrium (cf. ref. 3). Similar findings have been reported for the Ca^{2+}-independent transient outward currents in rat ventricle (18–20). Our experiments, which examined the possibility that this α_1-adrenergic response was G-protein–mediated and consistently demonstrated that the reduction of I_t was insensitive to PTX, but could be modulated by nonhydrolyzable GTP analogs (8). Data illustrating the concentration-dependent inhibition of this transient outward current are shown in Fig. 2. In Fig. 2A, the four superimposed current traces demonstrate the inhibitory effects of three doses of norepinephrine (a, control; b, 2×10^{-6} M; c, 10^{-5} M; and d, 5×10^{-5} M). In Fig. 2B, the five traces that are superimposed show a corresponding experiment in which the more selective α_1-agonist, methoxamine, was applied (a, control; b, 10^{-5} M; c, 5×10^{-5} M; d, 2×10^{-4} M; and e, 10^{-3} M). Both the effects of noradrenaline and those of methoxamine could be blocked completely by relatively low concentrations of prazosin. Figure 2C shows the concentration–response relationships for the noradrenaline (open circles) and the methoxamine (closed circles) effects.

The attenuation of I_t induced by α_1-adrenergic agonists in our experiments (8, 14) does not involve activation of protein kinase C (8), because (i) activators of protein kinase C [phorbol 12-myristate-13-acetate (PMA) and 1-oleolyl-2-acetylglycerol] did not decrease I_t—they either had no effect on I_t or, in a few instances, resulted in an increase in I_t; (ii) the protein kinase C inhibitors, staurosporine and H-7, did not block the methoxamine-induced decrease in I_t; and (iii) downregulation of protein kinase C by chronic treatment with PMA had no effect on the methoxamine-induced decrease in I_t. Cell-attached patch experiments demonstrated that the α_1-adrenergic attenuation of I_t involves the production of a diffusible second messenger; its identity, however, remains unclear (cf. ref. 3).

While studying the effects of adrenergic agonists on the transient outward current in rabbit atrium, it became apparent that an additional change in current also occurred quite consistently. Close inspection of the data in Fig. 2, A and B, shows that, in addition to the reduction in size of the transient outward current, the baseline or background current present before the depolarizing voltage-clamp pulse was applied, also changed significantly. With atrial and ventricular myocytes from rabbit heart, we observed that a K^+ current that is present at membrane potentials and that is responsible for the resting potential in ventricle can be reduced significantly by an α_1-adrenergic mechanism. This effect has been studied in detail in ventricular myocytes (14). Inhibition of this inwardly rectifying

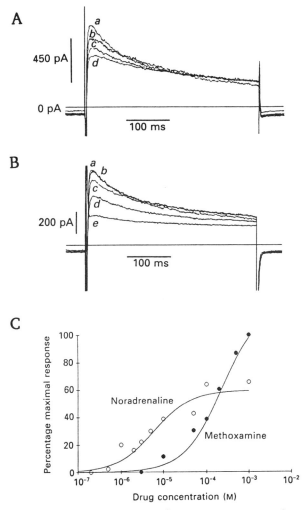

Figure 2. Inhibition of the transient outward potassium current, I_t, by selected concentrations of noradrenaline **(A)** and methoxamine **(B).** Each cell was voltage-clamped near its resting potential (-80 mV) and intermittently depolarized to 20 mV for 400 msec at a frequency of 0.1 Hz. In (A), the four superimposed traces correspond to a, control; b, 2×10^{-6} M; c, 10^{-5} M; and d, 5×10^{-5} M. They illustrate the maximum inhibition of I_t that resulted from each concentration of noradrenaline. A similar experiment is shown in (B) in which the five superimposed traces correspond to a, control; b, 10^{-5} M; c, 5×10^{-5} M; d, 2×10^{-4} M; and e, 10^{-3} M methoxamine. **(C)** The concentration–response relationship corresponding to the noradrenaline and methoxamine effects shown in (A) and (B), respectively. Inhibition of the transient outward current is plotted as a function of the maximal response to 10^{-3} M methoxamine. The open circles denote the inhibitory effects of noradrenaline, and the closed circles denote those due to methoxamine. Continuous curves drawn through the data points yield $K_{0.5}$ values (drug concentrations required for a half-maximal response) of 6.0×10^{-6} M for noradrenaline and 2.3×10^{-4} M for methoxamine.

background K^+ current, I_{K1}, is mediated by α_1-adrenergic receptors, is inhibited by prazosin, is PTX insensitive, and occurs over a concentration range similar to the methoxamine effects on the transient outward K^+ current, I_t (see Fig. 2).

Data describing the voltage dependence of this effect are shown in Fig. 3B. Figure 3C demonstrates its inhibition by prazosin. The concentration dependence of the inhibition of I_{K1} is shown in Fig. 4. Our ability to successfully demonstrate G-protein–mediated, concentration-dependent effects of noradrenaline and methoxamine on K^+ currents that trigger early repolarization, (I_t), late repolarization, and the resting potential (I_{K1}), but our lack of success in identifying the second messengers for these responses led to a series of biochemical experiments in which α_1-adrenergic effects on the first transducing element downstream of the receptor (i.e., the membrane GTPase activity) were studied. Sarcolemmal membranes were prepared from homogenates of atrial and ventricular myocytes by sucrose density gradient centrifugation (4). Sarcolemmal enrichment was verified by a 12- to 15-fold increase in specific activity of ouabain-sensitive Na/K-ATPase. Sarcolemmal GTPase activity was stimulated with the α_1-adrenergic agonists, l-NA and methoxamine, in a concentration-dependent manner (Fig. 5). Half-maximal stimulation occurred at ~5 μM l-NA in both atrial and ventricular sarcolemmal membranes and ~300 μM methoxamine in ventricular membranes. α_1-Adrenergic stimulation had no significant effect on the K_M for GTP (0.14 to 0.21 μM), but caused significant increases in V_{max}: 39% for atrial GTPase and 72% for ventricular GTPase.

Data in Fig. 6 confirm that the effects of 1-NA and methoxamine are mediated via α_1-adrenoceptors: methoxamine stimulation of ventricular sarcolemmal GTPase was blocked by phentolamine, and 1-NA stimulation was blocked by prazosin. The α_2-adrenergic antagonist, yohimbine, on the other hand, had no effect on methoxamine or 1-NA stimulation of the GTPase.

PTX treatment of intact ventricular myocytes had no effect on basal sarcolemmal GTPase activity or methoxamine- or 1-NA–stimulated GTPase activities (4), indicating that the G-protein coupled to the α_1-adrenoceptor is a PTX-insensitive G-protein. Sarcolemmal G-proteins were identified by photoaffinity labeling with [α-^{32}P]GTP (Fig. 7): incubation of ventricular sarcolemmal membranes with [α-^{32}P]GTP followed by exposure to UV light caused almost exclusive labeling of a 75 kDa protein (lane 1). Labeling was enhanced (mean $\pm$ SD = 41.3 $\pm$ 9.7%, N=3) in the presence of α_1-agonist (lane 2) and was prevented in the presence of agonist plus excess nonlabeled GTP (lane 3). Phentolamine prevented the α_1-agonist–stimulated labeling of the 75 kDa protein (4). A similar high-molecular weight G-protein has been observed in rat liver plasma membranes (24, 25).

Discussion

These results reported herein provide the first direct evidence that atrial and ventricular α_1-adrenoceptors can enhance membrane-associated,

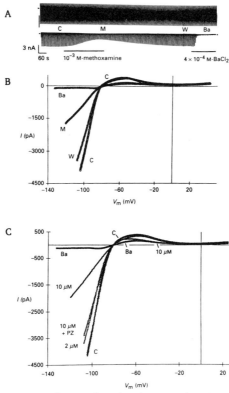

Figure 3. Methoxamine (10^{-3} M)-induced reduction of an inward rectifying potassium current, I_{K1}, in rabbit ventricle. **(A)** A chart record of membrane current changes (lower trace) induced by ramp-shaped voltage-clamp commands (upper traces). The vertical scale bar at the **left of the upper panel** corresponds to 100 mV; the time scale is the same for both panels. This cell was exposed to methoxamine and, thereafter, to $BaCl_2$ (4×10^{-4} M), as depicted by the bars beneath the record. The letters above the current trace mark the times at which the current-voltage relationships shown in **(B)** were recorded. Note that methoxamine (M) resulted in a significant inhibition of the hyperpolarization-activated current and that this current was blocked completely by 4×10^{-4} M $BaCl_2$. (B) Four superimposed current-voltage relations corresponding to the continuous data obtained during the sawtooth-shaped voltage commands applied in (A). Four features of these current traces are noteworthy: (1) the control I–V curve (denoted C) exhibited marked inward rectification; (2) methoxamine significantly reduced this current in both the inward and outward (hump) directions; (3) the methoxamine effect was almost completely reversible; and (4) the entire current change was blocked by $BaCl_2$ providing strong evidence that the methoxamine-sensitive current is the inward rectifying background potassium current, I_{K1}. Data in **(C)** are taken from a different cell. In this experiment, after the control (C) I–V relation was recorded, the cell was exposed to 10 µM noradrenaline and, thereafter, to 2×10^{-6} M prazosin (PZ) that removed a substantial fraction of the noradrenaline-induced inhibition of I_{K1}. Once again, $BaCl_2$ was applied at the end of the experiment to confirm that the current changes seen over the entire voltage range were those due to I_{K1}.

227

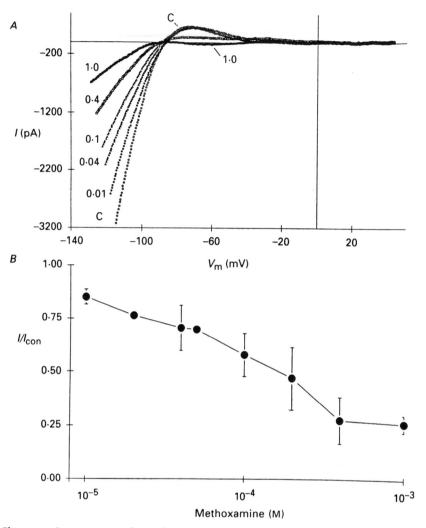

Figure 4. Concentration dependence of the inhibition of I_{K1} by methoxamine. In **(A)** the effects of selected concentrations of methoxamine in a single cell from rabbit ventricle are shown. The trace denoted C corresponds to the control record, and the numerals beside the other traces indicate the concentration of methoxamine (mM). **(B)** Cumulative data describing the mean reduction in I_{K1}, measured as the change in this current at -120 mV in the presence of selected methoxamine concentrations (I), compared with the control level (I_{con}). Data are shown as mean $\pm$ SD ($N = 3$ to 7 at each methoxamine concentration). In this experiment, temperature was maintained at 35°C.

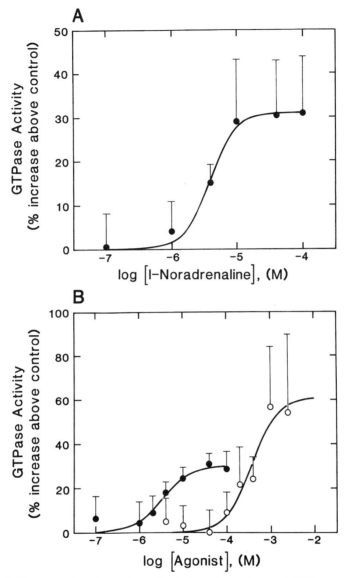

Figure 5. Concentration-dependent stimulation of sarcolemmal GTPase activity by α_1-adrenergic agonists. Sarcolemmal membranes from atrial **(A)** and ventricular myocytes **(B)** were incubated in the presence of increasing concentrations of either 1-NA (●) or methoxamine (○), and GTPase activities were measured as described previously (4). *dl*-Propranolol (10 μM) was present throughout to block β-adrenoceptors. Results are expressed as the percentage increase of agonist-induced GTPase activity above control levels. The points represent the means of three or four determinations; one-sided error bars (± 1 SD) are shown for clarity. Methoxamine-induced activation of atrial membrane GTPase activity was not examined.

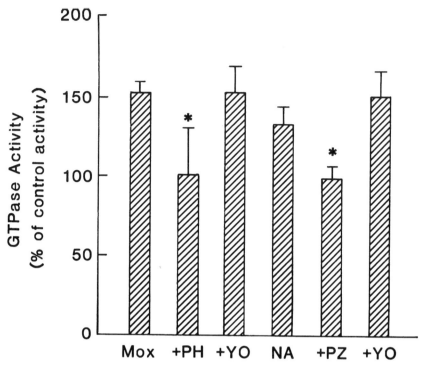

Figure 6. Effects of α-adrenoceptor antagonists on α_1-stimulated GTPase activities in sarcolemmal membranes from ventricular myocytes. After addition of assay reagents, sarcolemmal membranes were incubated for ~20 min at 30°C in the absence or presence of 1 to 5 μM prazosin (PZ), 100 μM phentolamine (PH), or 100 μM yohimbine (YO). Following this incubation, 1-NA (NA, 10 μM final) or methoxamine (Mox, 500 μM final) was quickly added, and the reaction immediately started by addition of $[\gamma\text{-}^{32}P]GTP$ (0.2 μM). Incubation was then performed for an additional 15 min. Prazosin was prepared fresh for each experiment as a stock solution in 95% ethanol, then diluted to give a final alcohol concentration in the assay of #0.1% (by volume), which was present throughout as a vehicle control. Results are presented as means ± SD of three or four experiments. Statistical significance was determined using a paired t test. *$P<0.05$.

high-affinity, GTPase activity. Stimulation of this GTPase by the α_1-adrenergic agonists, noradrenaline and methoxamine, occurs in a concentration-dependent manner and over similar concentration ranges known to produce functional responses in intact cell and tissue preparations. Blockade of this hormone-stimulated GTPase activity by the α_1-adrenoceptor antagonists, phentolamine and prazosin, but not by the α_2-selective antagonist, yohimbine, establish that α_1-adrenoceptors mediate the actions of noradrenaline and methoxamine. The concentrations of noradrenaline and methoxamine required for half-maximal stimulation of sarcolemmal membrane GTPase activity (5 μM and 300 μM, respectively) agree closely with

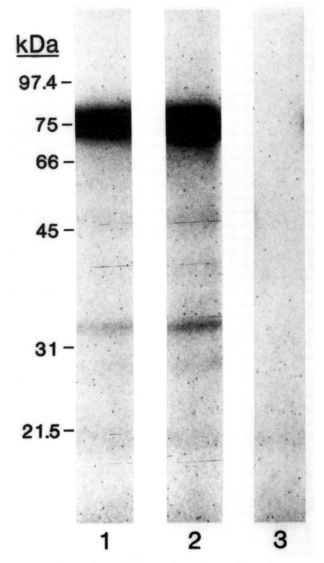

Figure 7. Covalent photoaffinity labeling of sarcolemmal membrane-associated GTP binding protein. Sarcolemmal membranes (25 to 30 μg protein) from ventricular myocytes were incubated as described (4) with 0.2 μM [α-^{32}P]GTP (5 to 8 μCi/tube) in either the absence (lane 1) or presence of 500 μM methoxamine (lane 2), or methoxamine + 1 mM nonlabeled GTP (lane 3). Following UV irradiation, samples were mixed with sodium dodecyl sulfate gel sample buffer and the proteins resolved by sodium dodecyl sulfate-polyacrylamide gel electrophoresis in the presence of 2-mercaptoethanol. Coomassie blue–stained gels were then exposed to x-ray film for 2 days at −70°C. Positions of molecular mass markers are indicated on the **left.** Labeled bands were quantified by scanning laser densitometry.

the EC_{50} for α_1-adrenergic attenuation of K^+ currents in isolated rabbit atrial and ventricular myocytes.

Other recent evidence, however, demonstrates that in rat ventricle the transient outward current elicited by voltage-clamp depolarizations to the plateau range of potentials is generated by two separate K^+ conductances (26); and Wang et al. (27) have shown that these two conductances have different sensitivities to $\alpha_{1\text{-A}}$- and $\alpha_{1\text{-B}}$–antagonists [5-methylurapadil or (+)niguldipine, and chloroethylclonidine, respectively]. Endoh et al. (28) have reported that, in rabbit ventricle, niguldipine, a selective α_1-adrenergic antagonist, can block a small fraction of the α_1-adrenoceptor–mediated positive inotropic effect (29). It will be of interest to determine whether this subtype specificity for inhibition of I_t is significant in rabbit myocytes; and to extend our studies describing the inhibitory effects of α_1-agonists on the inwardly rectifying background K^+ current, I_{K1}, so that new information concerning $\alpha_{1\text{-A}}$–$\alpha_{1\text{-B}}$-specificity, and higher resolution measurements of the decrease in outward current in I_{K1} can be obtained. It is the change in the outward current of the I–V curve that provides the functionally important information (i.e., the small "hump" of outward current controls the late phase of repolarization). Ultimately, effects of α_1-agonists in healthy (30) and ischemic (for review, see ref. 3) human cardiac muscle will also need to be obtained, using combined electrophysiological and biochemical approaches.

The role of protein kinase C in mediating the observed α_1-adrenergic responses will also need to be reexamined after more detailed information is available concerning the subtype of α_1-receptors involved in the inhibition of K^+ currents. In sarcolemmal membranes from rabbit ventricle, α_1-adrenoceptor occupation can augment protein kinase C activity (22); however, the number and types of isozymes that are present, their intracellular localization, and their Ca^{2+} dependence need to be defined before more rigorous electrophysiological tests can be developed (31–33). We have previously shown that α_1-adrenergic attenuation of I_t involves a diffusible second messenger (8), which is not thought to be inositol triphosphate (IP_3), a combination of IP_3 and IP_4, or Ca^{2+}; and which does not involve activation of protein kinase C under the conditions of our whole-cell voltage-clamp experiments. Perhaps ligand occupancy of the α_1-adrenergic receptor with activation of the GTPase activity of the 75 kDa G-protein (24, 25), triggers release of the G-protein from the membrane, followed by diffusion through the cytosol and direct interaction with K^+ channels (34). Alternatively, a distinctly diffusible messenger may be generated as a consequence of α_1-adrenergic stimulation of the GTPase. Elucidation of these mechanisms will require characterization of the functional effects of the isolated G-protein (35).

Our findings suggest that α_1-adrenoceptors in rabbit heart can couple to a G-protein of molecular weight $\approx$75,000. This G-protein, therefore, appears to differ from the G_i and G_0 subclasses of G-proteins associated with cardiac muscarinic acetylcholine receptors (34, 36, 37). However, additional experimental work is needed before we can conclude that cardiac atrial and ventricular α_1-adrenoceptors are coupled to K^+ channels via this type of PTX-insensitive, 75 kDa G-protein. Present data describing the functional coupling between α_1-receptors, G-proteins (in particular G_q), and isozymes of phospholipase C (e.g., β_1 and β_2) will need to be considered (38–41), and attention given to the possible functional role of the $\beta\gamma$-subunits of these G-proteins (42–46).

Acknowledgments

This work was supported by grants from the Medical Research Council of Canada (M.P.W. and W.R.G.) and the Heart & Stroke Foundation of Alberta (M.P.W. and W.R.G.). A.P.B. was a Fellow of the Heart & Stroke Foundation of Canada. M.P.W. and W.R.G. hold Medical Scientist Awards from the Alberta Heritage Foundation for Medical Research.

We gratefully acknowledge the participation of Drs. D. Fedida and Y. Shimoni in many of the electrophysiological experiments in Figs. 1 to 4.

References

1. Harrison, J.K., Pearson, W.R., and Lynch, K.R. (1991). Molecular characterization of α_1- and α_2-adrenoceptors. *Trends Pharmacol. Sci.* **12:**62–67.

2. Dohlman, H.G., Thorner, J., Caron, M.G., and Lefkowitz, R.J. (1991). Model systems for the study of seven-transmembrane-segment receptors. *Annu. Rev. Biochem.* **60:**653–688.

3. Fedida, D., Braun, A.P., and Giles, W.R. (1993). α_1-Adrenoceptors in myocardium. *Physiol. Rev.* **73,** in press.

4. Braun, A.P., and Walsh, M.P. (1993). Cardiac α_1-adrenoceptors stimulate a high-affinity GTPase activity in sarcolemmal membranes from rabbit atrial and ventricular myocytes. *Eur. J. Biochem.,* in press.

5. Buxton, I.L.O., and Brunton, L.L. (1985). Action of the cardiac α_1-adrenergic receptor. *J. Biol. Chem.* **260:**6733–6737.

6. Smitz, W., Scholz, H., Scholz, J., Steinfath, M., Lohse, M., Puurunen, J., and Schwabe, U. (1987). Pertussis toxin does not inhibit the α_1-adrenoceptor-mediated effect on inositol phosphate production in the heart. *Eur. J. Pharmacol.* **134:**377–378.

7. Steinberg, S.F., Kaplan, L.M., Inouye, T., Zhang, J.F., and Robinson, R.B. (1989). Alpha-1 adrenergic stimulation of 1,4,5-inositol trisphosphate formation in ventricular myocytes. *J. Pharmacol. Exp. Ther.* **250:**1141–1148.

8. Braun, A.P., Fedida, D., Clark, R.B., and Giles, W.R. (1990). Intracellular mechanisms for α_1-adrenergic regulation of the transient outward current in rabbit atrial myocytes. *J. Physiol. (Lond.)* **431:**689–712.

9. Bohm, M., Diet, F., Feiler, G., Kemkes, B., and Erdmann, E. (1988). α_1-Adrenoceptors and α_1-adrenoceptor–mediated positive inotropic effects in failing human myocardium. *J. Cardiovasc. Pharmacol.* **12:**357–364.

10. Shah, A., Cohen, I.S., and Rosen, M.R. (1988). Stimulation of cardiac alpha receptors increases Na/K pump current and decreases G_k via a pertussis toxin–sensitive pathway. *Biophys. J.* **54:**219–225.

11. Sen, L., Liang, B.T., Colucci, W.S., and Smith, T.W. (1990). Enhanced α_1-adrenergic responsiveness in cardiomyopathic hamster cardiac myocytes: Relation to the expression of pertussis toxin–sensitive G-protein and α_1-adrenergic receptors. *Circ. Res.* **67:**1182–1192.

12. Fedida, D., Shimoni, Y., and Giles, W.R. (1989). A novel effect of norepinephrine on cardiac cells is mediated by α_1-adrenoceptors. *Am. J. Physiol.* **256:**H-1500–H1504.

13. Fedida, D., Shimoni, Y., and Giles, W.R. (1990). α_1-Adrenergic modulation of the transient outward current in rabbit atrial myocytes. *J. Physiol. (Lond.)* **423:**257–277.

14. Fedida, D., Braun, A.P., and Giles, W.R. (1991). α_1-Adrenoceptors reduce background K^+ current in rabbit ventricular myocytes. *J. Physiol. (Lond).* **441:**673–684.

15. Shibata, E.F., Drury, T., Refsum, H., Aldrete, V., and Giles, W.R. (1989). A transient outward current in human atrium. *Am. J. Physiol.* **257:**H1773–H1781.

16. Giles, W., and Imaizumi, Y. (1988). Comparison of potassium currents in rabbit atrial and ventricular cells. *J. Physiol. (Lond.)* **405:**123–145.

17. Hescheler, J., Nawrath, H., Tang, M., and Trautwein, W. (1988). Adrenoceptor-mediated changes of excitation and contraction in ventricular heart muscle from guinea-pigs and rabbits. *J. Physiol. (Lond.)* **397:**657–670.

18. Apkon, M., and Nerbonne, J.M. (1988). α_1-Adrenergic agonists selectively suppress voltage-dependent K^+ currents in rat ventricular myocytes. *Proc. Natl. Acad. Sci. U.S.A.* **85:**8756–8760.

19. Ravens, U., Wang, X.-L., and Wettwer, E. (1989). Alpha adrenoceptor stimulation reduces outward currents in rat ventricular myocytes. *J. Pharmacol. Exp. Ther.* **250:**364–370.

20. Tohse, N., Nakaya, H., Hattori, Y., Endou, M., and Kanno, M. (1990). Inhibitory effect mediated by α_1-adrenoceptors on transient outward current in isolated rat ventricular cells. *Pflügers Arch.* **415:**575–581.

21. Talosi, L., and Kranias, E.G. (1992). Effect of α_1-adrenergic stimulation on activation of protein kinase C and phosphorylation of proteins in intact rabbit hearts. *Circ. Res.* **70:**670–678.

22. Jones, L.R. (1988). Rapid preparation of cardiac sarcolemmal vesicles by sucrose floatation. *Meth. Enzymol.* **157:**85–91.

23. Fedida, D., and Bouchard, R.A. (1992). Mechanisms for the positive inotropic effect of α_1-adrenoceptor stimulation in rat cardiac myocytes. *Circ. Res.* **71:**673–688.

24. Im, M.-J., and Graham, R.M. (1990). A novel guanine nucleotide-binding protein coupled to the α_1-adrenergic receptor. *J. Biol. Chem.* **265:**18944–18951.

25. Im, M.-J., Riek, R.P., and Graham, R.M. (1990). A novel guanine nucleotide-binding protein coupled to the α_1-adrenergic receptor. *J. Biol. Chem.* **265:**18952–18960.

26. Apkon, M., and Nerbonne, J.M. (1991). Characterization of two distinct depolarization-activated K^+ currents in isolated adult rat ventricular myocytes. *J. Gen. Physiol.* **97**:973–1011.

27. Wang, L.-X., Wettwer, E., Gross, G., and Ravens, U. (1991). Reduction of cardiac outward currents by alpha-1 adrenoceptor stimulation: a subtype-specific effect? *J. Pharmacol. Exp. Ther.* **259**:783–788.

28. Endoh, M., Takanashi, M., and Norota, I. (1992). Effect of (+)-niguldipine on myocardial α_1-adrenoceptors in the rabbit. *Eur. J. Pharmacol.* **223**:143–151.

29. Jahnel, U., Kaufmann, B., Rombusch, M., and Nawrath, H. (1992). Contribution of both α- and β-adrenoceptors to the inotropic effects of catecholamines in the rabbit heart. *Naunyn-Schmiedeberg's Arch. Pharmacol.* **346**:665–672.

30. Jahnel, U., Jakob, H., and Nawrath, H. (1992). Electrophysiologic and inotropic effects of α-adrenoceptor stimulation in human isolated atrial heart muscle. *Naunyn-Schmeideberg's Arch. Pharmacol.* **346**:82–87.

31. Wolf, R.A. (1992). Association of phospholipase C-σ with a highly enriched preparation of canine sarcolemma. *Am. J. Physiol. Soc.* **263**:C1021–C1028.

32. Nishizuka, Y. (1992). Membrane phospholipid degradation and protein kinase C for cell signaling. *Neurosci. Res.* **15**:3–5.

33. Cockcroft, S., and Thomas, G.M.H. (1992). Inositol-lipid-specific phospholipase C isoenzymes and their differential regulation by receptors. *Biochem. J.* **288**:1–14.

34. Brown, A.M. (1993). Membrane-delimited cell signaling complexes: Direct ion channel regulation by G proteins. *J. Membr. Biol.* **131**:93–104.

35. Im, M.-J., Gray, C., and Rim, A.J. (1992). Characterization of a phospholipase C activity regulated by the purified G_h in reconstitution systems. *J. Biol. Chem.* **267**:8887–8894.

36. Hepler, J.R., and Gilman, A.G. (1992). G proteins. *Trends Biochem. Sci.* **17**:383–387.

37. Birnbaumer, L. (1993). Heterotrimeric G proteins molecular diversity and functional correlates. *J. Receptor Res.* **13**:19–26.

38. Sternweis, P.C., and Smrcka, A.V. (1992). Regulation of phospholipase C by G proteins. *Trends Biochem. Sci.* **17**:502–508.

39. Berstein, G., Blank, J.L., Jhon, D.-Y., Exton, J.H., Rhee, S.G., and Ross, E.M. (1992). Phospholipase C-β1 is a GTPase-activating protein for $G_{q/11}$, its physiologic regulator. *Cell* **70**:411-418.

40. Katz, A., Wu, D., and Simon, M.I. (1992). Subunits $\beta\gamma$ of heterotrimeric G protein activate β2 isoform of phospholipase C. *Nature* **360**:686–689.

41. Camps, M., Carozzi, A., Schnabel, P., Scheer, A., Parker, P.J., and Gierschik, P. (1992). Isozyme-selective stimulation of phospholipase C-β2 by G protein $\beta\gamma$-subunits. *Nature* **360**:684–686.

42. Kleuss, C., Scherubl, H., Hescheler, J., Schultz, G., and Wittig, B. (1992). Different β-subunits determine G-protein interaction with transmembrane receptors. *Nature* **358**:424–426.

43. Bourne, H.R., and Stryer, L. (1992). The target sets the temp. *Nature* **358**:541–542.

44. Birnbaumer, L. (1992). Receptor-to-effector signaling through G proteins: Roles for βγ dimers as well as α-subunits. *Cell* **71**:1069–1072.

45. Kleuss, C., Scherubl, H., Hescheler, J., Schultz, G., and Wittig, B. (1993). Selectivity in signal transduction determined by γ subunits of heterotrimeric G-proteins. *Science* **259**:832–834.

46. Wu, D., Katz, A., Lee, C.-H., and Simon, M.I. (1992). Activation of phospholipase C by α_1-adrenergic receptors is mediated by the α-subunits of G_q family. *J. Biol. Chem.* **267**:25798–25802.

12

β-adrenergic Modulation of Cardiac Calcium Channel Gating

Bruce P. Bean

Depolarization-activated calcium (Ca) current in cardiac muscle cells is enhanced by stimulation of β-adrenergic receptors (1). Modulation of Ca current is a major mechanism by which β-adrenergic stimulation produces its positive inotropic effect on heart muscle: the greater entry of Ca triggers more complete Ca release from sarcoplasmic reticulum stores and, in addition, provides more Ca to be taken up into the stores for release during subsequent contractions.

Besides its physiological significance, β-adrenergic enhancement of cardiac Ca current is interesting as a prime example of hormonal modulation of a voltage-dependent ion channel. Enhancement by adrenaline of cardiac Ca current was the first example to be discovered of a voltage-dependent channel whose behavior is modulated by action of a neurotransmitter or hormone, and the process has probably been more thoroughly studied than any other case of channel modulation. Extensive work on this problem has been done at the biochemical as well as the electrophysiological levels. Many of the basic features are known, although details remain unclear.

This chapter focuses on how the gating behavior of cardiac Ca channels is altered by β-adrenergic stimulation. The main goal is to compare the changes in gating described at the single-channel level, with changes in macroscopic currents. All of the experimental results mentioned were obtained in cells possessing only L-type Ca channel current.

Biochemical Pathway and Time Course

There is little doubt that the primary pathway for β-adrenergic control of cardiac Ca channels consists of activation of adenylate cyclase, production of cAMP, and activation of protein kinase A. The effect on Ca channels of β-adrenergic stimulation by adrenaline or isoproterenol can be mimicked by forskolin, activation of adenylate cyclase, by injection of cAMP, or by injection of the catalytic subunit of protein kinase A (for review, see ref.

2). Consistent with such a cascade, the time course of β-adrenergic enhancement has generally been found to be relatively slow (half-time of 5 to 30 sec) and to proceed with a lag of a few seconds after exposure of the cell to agonist. An example is shown in Fig. 1A, from an experiment on a single rabbit ventricular myocyte studied at 34°C. A large concentration (30 μM) of isoproterenol was applied within tens of milliseconds. Despite this high agonist concentration, rapid change, and a warm temperature, it took ~30 sec for the increase in current (2.3-fold) to be completed, and there was a lag of ~2 sec before any increase was evident. This example is representative of many repetitions of the experiment using rabbit ventricular, rabbit atrial, bullfrog ventricular, and bullfrog atrial cells, mostly studied at 22°C. With rabbit and bullfrog cells, the increase in current always occurred only after a delay of several seconds. This result has been previously reported for these and other vertebrate myocytes (3, 4).

In experiments on guinea pig ventricular cells, Yatani and Brown (5) detected a much faster component of Ca channel enhancement, which occurred within hundreds of milliseconds. They have intrepreted this rapid component as reflecting direct modulation of Ca channels by activated glutamyl transpeptidase (GTP)–binding protein. I have seen a similar fast component in a few experiments on rat atrial cells. One such experiment is shown in Fig. 1B. In this experiment, in which current was elicited every 2 sec, there was a 10% enhancement of the current in the first depolarization after the application of isoproterenol. After ~6 sec, a second slow phase of enhancement began that had a half-time of ~50 sec. The rapid phase of enhancement accounted for only a small fraction of the overall increase; in this cell, there was a 20% increase in the fast phase compared with a 450% increase during the slow phase. This result is similar to those of Yatani and Brown (5), who also found that the fast phase was much smaller than the slow phase when isoproterenol concentrations >2 μM were used. Although there is a disagreement over the existence of the fast phase in rat and guinea pig myocytes, all groups nonetheless agree that the large, slowly developing enhancement of current most likely results from the action of protein kinase A. In the subsequent experiments described in this chapter, using rabbit and bullfrog myocytes, channel modifications reflect enhancement of current by this slow pathway.

Single-Channel Experiments

A great deal has been learned from single-channel experiments about how Ca channel gating is modified by β-adrenergic stimulation. At this level, four main effects have been observed when cells are stimulated with β-adrenergic agonists or cAMP derivatives: changes in channel availability; changes in fast gating kinetics; changes in inactivation kinetics; and changes in modal gating behavior.

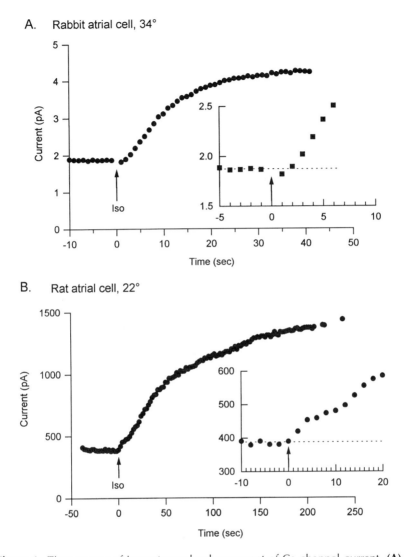

Figure 1. Time course of isoproterenol enhancement of Ca channel current. **(A)** Current recorded at 34° from a rabbit atrial myocyte. Current was elicited every second by a 20 msec step from −80 mV to −10 mV. Leak-corrected current measured at the end of the pulse is plotted versus experimental time. Isoproterenol (30 μM) was applied at the arrow (time 0). (Inset) Detail of early times. External solution (in mM): 5 Ba, 160 tetraethylammonium (TEA) Cl, 0.1 EGTA, 10 HEPES, pH 7.4 with TEA OH. Internal solution (in mM): 108 CsCl, 4.5 MgCl₂, 4 MgATP, 14 creatine phosphate (Tris salt), 0.3 GTP (Tris salt), 9 EGTA, 9 HEPES, pH 7.4 with CsOH. Cell K57G. **(B)** Current recorded at 22° in a rat atrial myocyte. Current was elicited every 2 sec by a 40 msec step from −80 mV to −20 mV. Isoproterenol (30 μM) was applied at time 0. External solution (in mM): 3 Ba, 160 TEA Cl, 10 HEPES, pH 7.4 with TEA OH. Internal solution as in **(A).** Cell B83A.

One major effect of stimulation is an increase in the fraction of time a channel is available for opening. Channels appear to cycle between states from which they can be opened (so that upon depolarization a sweep has some openings) and states from which they cannot be opened (so that depolarization yields a blank or null sweep). Isoproterenol or cAMP derivatives decrease the fraction of null sweeps (6–10). In the most complete study (10) on guinea pig ventricular cells, the fraction of nonnull sweeps was found to increase by about a factor of 2, from ~0.3 in control to ~0.6 with isoproterenol. The average lifetime in each state is a second or so at 30° to 35° (10) and slightly longer at room temperature (11). Ochi and Kawashima (10) found that isoproterenol increased the lifetime of the available state and decreased the lifetime of the nonavailable state. Interestingly, phosphatase inhibitors such as okadaic acid selectively lengthen the available lifetime while having little effect on the nonavailable lifetime (11).

The cycling of channels between available and nonavailable states fits very well with the hypothesis of Reuter and Scholz (12) that Ca channels cyle between phosphorylated and nonphosphorylated states, with channels capable of being opened by depolarization only if they are phosphorylated. However, it is unlikely that the mechanism is as simple as a single phosphorylation site switching availability on and off. Maneuvers that should completely inhibit phosphorylation and promote dephosphorylation do not eliminate Ca current, they depress it by only 20% or so from control (13, 14). More likely, as suggested by Ochi and Kawashima (10), even dephosphorylated channels can enter the available state, but phosphorylation increases the fraction of time a chanel spends in it.

Noise analysis of whole-cell currents shows an increase in the number of functional channels when variance is calculated from the difference of consecutive sweeps elicited every second or so (15). This would be expected if the underlying channels are shifted (on average) into the available state, with cycling occurring with a time scale of seconds. Channels remaining unavailable during two successive sweeps would not count toward the number of functional channels, whereas those remaining available would. If cycling occurred very slowly relative to the time between sweeps, the number of functional channels from noise analysis would reflect the average number of available channels at any given time rather than the total number of channels in the cell (and the estimate for maximum probability of being open during the sweep would reflect the value for channels in the available state). In this case, if there were no gating changes within nonblank sweeps, noise analysis based on comparing pairs of sweeps would yield a change only in the number of functional channels. However, if cycling is on the same time scale as the time between sweeps, an increase in the number of functional channels would be accompanied by an increase in the maximum open probability estimated from the noise data. Increases in both were seen (15), consistent with cycling on a time scale of 1 sec or so.

A second reported effect of isoproterenol is to alter fast gating kinetics of channel gating within nonblank sweeps. Slight increases in mean open times and decreases in closed times were reported in some studies (6, 7), but the effects are small enough that they would contribute only slightly to the overall increase in average current.

A third effect is to slow entry into the inactivated state. This is seen as a slowing of the decay of the averaged current (6, 7, 10).

A fourth effect, recently recognized by Yue et al. (9), is to increase the number of sweeps in which channels show "mode 2" gating, characterized by a high probability of being open and by long open times. This is much like the mode of activity stabilized by dihydropyridine agonist drugs such as Bay K 8644 (16). Yue and colleagues (9) found that enhancement of mode 2 activity could be dramatic in cases where the overall increase in current is especially large. It seems that the enhancement of mode 2 activity may be most noticeable with maximal stimulation of cells. In most of their experiments, stimulation was by 4 mM 8-bromo-cAMP or by isoproterenol given together with the phosphodiesterase inhibitor IBMX, the combination of which results in particularly large increases in current (17). The enhancement of mode 2 activity was not present in the results of Ochi and Kawashima (10), where in experiments with 0.1 µM isoproterenol, the probability of being open in nonblank sweeps was almost unchanged by isoproterenol (after correction for slowing of inactivation). The comparison suggests that the stabilization of the available state and the stabilization of mode 2 represent different processes. In support of this, Ono and Fozzard's (11) data show that the phosphatase inhibitor okadaic acid has two distinguishable effects: a stabilization of the available state, seen with low concentrations of inhibitor, and a stabilization of mode 2 gating, seen with higher concentrations of inhibitor. They suggest that two different phosphorylation sites control the two effects on channel gating.

Whole-Cell Experiments: Voltage-Dependence

It is interesting to consider whole-cell studies of Ca current modulation in light of the single-channel results. Single-channel recordings yield a depth of information about channel gating kinetics that is unmatched by macroscopic current recording. However, single-channel studies can give only a limited view of the voltage-dependence of Ca channels, because single channel currents are large enough to be easily resolved only over a fairly narrow voltage range.

Whole-cell recordings reveal a striking voltage-dependence to the enhancement of Ca channel current (15). The dramatic enhancement of currents elicited by small and moderate depolarizations (often 3- to 15-fold enhancement) is accompanied by far smaller effects on currents elicited by large depolarizations. The contrast is most striking in experiments where currents activated by very large depolarizations can be recorded, using internal cations such as Cesium (Cs) to carry outward current through the Ca channels. An example is shown for isoproterenol applied to a rabbit atrial cell in Fig. 2. Depolarizations beyond 50 mV or so elicit outward current that is carried by the internal Cs. The outward currents, as well as the inward currents, are potently blocked by selective L-type Ca channel blockers such as nitrendipine, leaving little doubt that they flow through the same channels as do the inward currents. In the currents shown in Fig. 2, small currents remaining in nitrendipine (resulting from slightly nonohmic leak) were subtracted to allow comparison of pure L-type currents. Isoproterenol enhanced the current elicited by a step to 0 mV by ~4-fold (155 to 600 pA), but increased the peak current at 150 mV by only 28% (655 to 840 pA).

Another striking effect of isoproterenol is to slow the rate of inactivation at large depolarizations, where inactivation is quite rapid. This effect was consistently seen in both rabbit and bullfrog myocytes. With barium (Ba) as charge carrier, the slowing of inactivation can also be seen if long depolarizations are given to lower voltages, fitting well with the slowing of inactivation reported at the single-channel level. With Ca as charge carrier, however, inactivation can actually become faster (unpublished results), perhaps due to Ca-induced inactivation becoming more rapid.

Figure 3 shows current-voltage curves for Ca channel current before and after modulation by isoproterenol. In this rabbit atrial cell studied with external Ba (10 mM) and internal Cs (135 mM), current at −20 mV was enhanced 6-fold, whereas current at 170 mV was enhanced by 70%. The reversal potential of 70 mV was unchanged.

The difference between large enhancements at small depolarizations and small enhancements at large depolarizations seems to depend on the voltage and not on the difference in ion species carrying the current (Ba for inward current, Cs for outward current). First, when the ratio of currents with and without stimulation are plotted as in Fig. 3B, the voltage dependence of the current ratio is obvious even over voltages where the current is still inward, and the decline of the ratio appears more or less continuous through the reversal potential for the current (although the difficulty in accurately measuring currents near the reversal potential limits the strength of this conclusion). Second, experiments done with monovalent ions carrying inward as well as outward current have shown the same sort of voltage dependence. Lew et al. (18) found that isoproterenol greatly enhanced inward sodium currents through Ca channels when elicited by small depolarizations, but had almost no effect on monovalent ion currents elicited by larger depolarizations.

In a general way, the voltage dependence of the isoproterenol-induced increase in current can be understood as resulting from a shift in channel gating to less depolarized potentials. Such shifts have also been seen with protein kinase A phosphorylation of skeletal muscle L-type Ca channels in planar bilayers (19). If the only effect were a shift in voltage dependence,

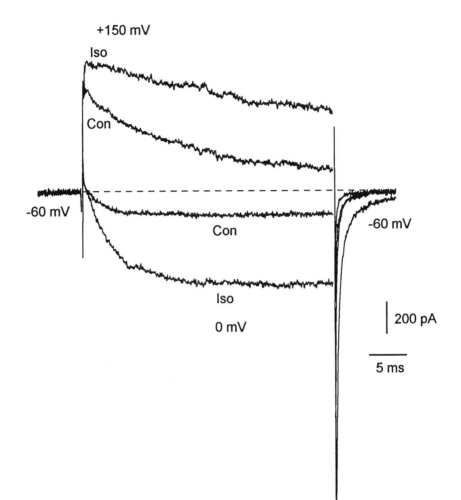

Figure 2. Effect of 30 μM isoproterenol on Ca channel currents elicited by moderate or large depolarizations. Rabbit atrial cell, 22°. External solution: 10 Ba, 154 tetraethylammonium (TEA) Cl, 10 HEPES, 3 μM tetrodotoxin, pH 7.4 with TEA OH. Internal solution: 108 CsCl, 4.5 MgCl2, 4 MgATP, 14 creatinine phosphate (Tris salt), 0.3 GTP (Tris salt), 50 U/ml creatine phosphokinase, 9 EGTA, 9 HEPES, pH 7.4 with CsOH. Traces were corrected for ohmic leak and capacitative transient current using scaled currents elicited by a step from −60 to −70 mV, and the currents remaining after addition of 300 nM nitrendipine (applied at a holding potential of −40 mV to ensure complete block) were subtracted, so that the traces represent nitrendipine-sensitive Ca channel current. Cell E64D.

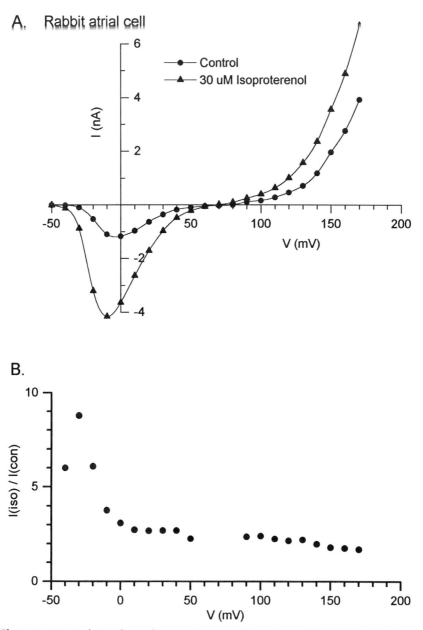

Figure 3. **(A)** Peak Ca channel current versus voltage in a rabbit atrial cell before and after stimulation by 30 μM isoproterenol. Currents were elicited by 60 msec depolarizations from −60 mV. After the recordings in control and with isoproterenol, 300 nM nitrendipine was applied at a holding potential of −40 mV to give complete block, and the small nitrendipine-insensitive currents were subtracted. **(B)** Ratio of current in isoproterenol to control current as a function of test potential. Ionic conditions as in Fig. 2. Cell E73G.

currents at very large depolarizations would be unaffected. Because the current elicited by very large depolarizations is usually enhanced to at least some degree (28% in Fig. 2, 70% in Fig. 3, up to several-fold in rare cases), a change in voltage dependence cannot be the only mechanism. It is possible that the voltage-independent part of the increase, as reflected in the increase in current at large depolarizations, corresponds to the change in the occupancy of the "available" state in single-channel experiments. In the simplest case, a change in availability would produce the same increase in current at all voltages. Based on the single-channel data, such a mechanism could account for increases of up to 2-fold or so. However, because in the single-channel experiments a blank sweep is defined using a fairly small depolarization, there is no guarantee that an apparent "non-available" state would not give openings if a very large depolarization were given. This will be an interesting point to test in future single-channel experiments.

Mode 2 Openings and Tail Currents

How would the enhancement of mode 2 activity reported by Yue et al. (9) be reflected in whole-cell recordings? When mode 2 activity is produced by dihydropyridine agonists, the longer openings during a depolarization are accompanied by dramatically slower closing of channels following repolarization, so that tail current kinetics are greatly slowed (e.g., Fig. 5). Thus, enhancement of mode 2 activity might show up as induction or amplification of slow components in whole-cell tail currents. Figure 4 shows a preliminary attempt to examine this point. Tail currents were measured on repolarization to -50 mV following activation of channels by a 70 msec step to -10 mV (with large enhancement by isoproterenol) or a 10 msec step to 160 mV (with a smaller enhancement by isoproterenol). Particularly with the isoproterenol-enhanced tails, a single exponential did not fit the tail current kinetics well. The currents were, therefore, fit with the sum of two exponentials, with time constants (0.7 and 6 msec) chosen to give the best fit to the isoproterenol-enhanced current following a step to -10 mV. All of the currents could be reasonably well fit by sums of exponentials with these same time constants, with variations in the amplitude of the two components. In all cases, the fast component was much larger than the slow component. Isoproterenol enhanced both the fast and the slow components. Considering the tails after the step to -10 mV, isoproterenol enhanced the amplitude of the fast component 4-fold (1.47 nA to 5.82 pA) and the slow component about 6-fold (0.05 nA to 0.28 nA). After the step to 160 mV, the fast component was enhanced by isoproterenol 3-fold (from 4.52 nA to 13.07 nA) and the slow component ~7-fold (0.05 nA to 0.36 nA). Although there may be a preferential enhancement of the slow component, it is difficult to be sure because of the small amplitude of the slow component (<5% of the total tail) under all conditions. Certainly there

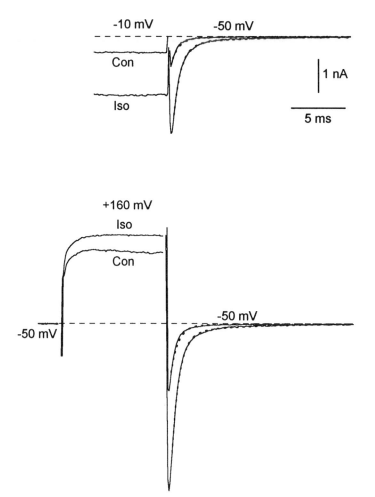

Figure 4. Tail current kinetics before and after modulation by 30 μM isoproterenol. Rabbit atrial cell, 22°. Tail currents were measured on repolarization to −50 mV following a 70 msec step to −10 mV **(top)** or a 10 msec step to 160 mV **(bottom).** Tail currents are fit with a sum of two exponentials with the same two time constants in each case (fast component, 0.7 msec; slow component, 6 msec) with the following amplitudes: −10 mV control—fast, 1.47 nA; slow, 0.05 nA. −10 mV isoproterenol—fast, 5.82 nA; slow, 0.28 nA. +160 mV control—fast, 4.52 nA; slow, 0.05 nA. +160 isoproterenol—fast, 13.07 nA; slow, 0.36 nA. External solution: 10 Ba, 154 tetraethylammonium (TEA) Cl, 10 HEPES, 3 μM tetrodotoxin, pH 7.4 with TEA OH. Internal solution: 108 CsCl, 4.5 $MgCl_2$, 4 MgATP, 14 creatinine phosphate (Tris salt), 0.3 GTP (Tris salt), 50 U/ml creatine phosphokinase, 9 EGTA, 9 HEPES, pH 7.4 with CsOH. Traces corrected for ohmic leak and capacitative transient current using scaled currents elicited by a step from −50 to −73 mV. Spurious transients resulting from imperfect subtraction in the first 400 μsec have been blanked. Con, control; Iso, isoproterenol. Cell E64A.

was not a large-scale conversion of fast-deactivating channels to slow-deactivating channels.

It will be interesting to repeat this experiment using different protocols for stimulating the cell's cAMP/protein kinase A system. As already mentioned, enhancement of mode 2 activity may be most dramatic after especially forceful stimulation using cAMP analogs or isoproterenol applied together with IBMX (9) or phosphatase inhibitors (11).

In principle, the mode 2 openings induced by adrenergic stimulation could differ from those induced by Bay K 8644; opening modes with long openings at 0 mV or so could have short openings (and fast tails) at −50 mV or so. In this case, mode 2 behavior during a test pulse would not necessarily be accompanied by slow tails. However, Yue et al. (9) directly addressed this issue and found that mode 2 activity at 15 mV was in fact accompanied by slow deactivation (time constant about 9 msec), much as for mode 2 activity induced by Bay K 8644. Thus it is likely that the adrenergic-induced mode 2 activity should show up as slow tails at the whole cell level.

Contrast Between β-adrenergic Stimulation and Effects of Dihydropyridine Agonists

The description of phosphorylation-induced mode 2 openings by Yue et al. (9) and by Ono and Fozzard (11) raises anew the question of how similar the effects of dihydropyridine agonists are to enhancement of current induced by phosphorylation. Until recently, the effects seemed quite distinct. The effects of dihydropyridine agonists do not seem to depend on phosphorylation (see ref. 20). The effects of dihydropyridines develop far faster (in less than 1 sec) than those of isoproterenol or cAMP analogs. Isoproterenol can still increase current after enhancement by Bay K 8644 and vice versa (8; unpublished results).

On the other hand, β-adrenergic stimulation and dihydropyridine agonists share the property of shifting the voltage dependence of the channels to less depolarized poetntials. Figure 5 shows the effects of 1 μM (+) − 202-791, a dihdyropyridine agonist, on inward and outward Ca channel currents. The effects may be compared with those of isoproterenol shown in Fig. 2. A similarity is that enhancement is much larger for moderate depolarizations than for very large depolarzations. In the experiment of Fig. 5, the agonist produced an enhancement of 9-fold at 0 mV, and only 1.7-fold at +160 mV.

Unlike β-adrenergic stimulation, dihydropyridine agonists do not slow inactivation. The fairly rapid inactivation at very positive potentials seems unaffected by (+) − 202-791 (Fig. 5, bottom), whereas inactivation at more negative voltages is substantially faster with agonist (top). This may be in part a consequence of the shift in the activation curve. If inactivation proceeds preferentially from the open state of the channel, an enhance-

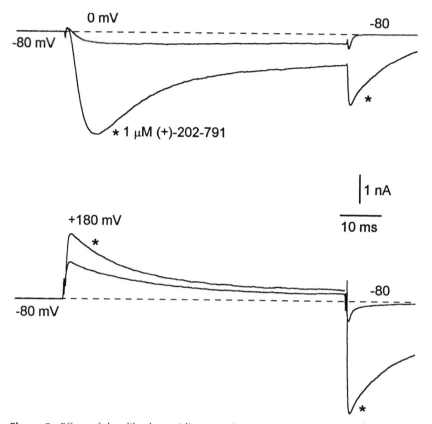

Figure 5. Effect of the dihydropyridine agonist (+)−202-791 on Ca channel currents. Bullfrog ventricular cell, 22°. Traces in the presence of (+)−202-791 are marked by asterisks. External solution: 10 Ba, 160 tetraethylammonium (TEA) Cl, 10 HEPES, 3 μM tetrodotoxin, pH 7.4 with TEA OH. Internal solution: 115 CsCl, 5 MgATP, 5 creatine phosphate (Tris salt), 0.3 GTP (Tris salt), 10 BAPTA, and 10 HEPES, pH 7.4 with CsOH. Traces corrected for ohmic leak and capacitative transient current using scaled currents elicited by a step from −80 to −90 mV. Cell W75G.

ment of the open probability would lead to faster decay of macroscopic current.

The most obvious difference between effects of dihydropyridine agonists and β-adrenergic stimulation is the dramatic effect of dihydropyridines to almost completely convert tail currents into a very slow component of deactivation.

Slow Tail Currents in Rat Cardiac Myocytes

So far our discussion of tail currents has applied to ventricular and atrial cells from bullfrog and rabbit hearts, where (in the absence of dihydropyridine agonists) tail currents are very rapid, with at most a very small slow component. Strikingly different behavior is seen with tail currents in rat ventricular cells. Here, there are very slow components of tail current present under control conditions. Slowly deactivating components (time constants >5 msec) are progressively activated by depolarizations positive to ~0 mV (e.g., ref. 21). These components are due to L-type channels, because they are potently blocked by dihydropyridine antagonists (unpublished observations). An example is shown in Fig. 6. The tail at −80 mV following a step to −20 mV decays relatively quickly (time constant 2.1 msec), although substantially slower than tails in frog or rabbit cells (e.g., Figs. 2, 4, and 5). Following a step to 60 mV, the decay of the tail is much slower, with a time constant of 5.3 msec. At the single-channel level, this behavior shows up as "mode 2" activity following large depolarizations (22). The existence of such activity may be physiologically important; the

Rat ventricular cell

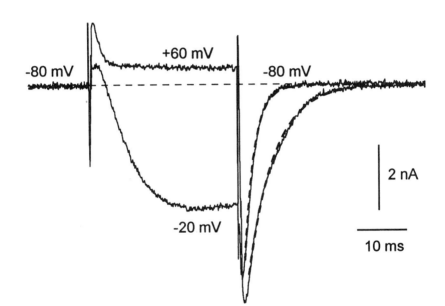

Figure 6. Slow tail following a large depolarization in a rat ventricular myocyte. Current recorded at 22°. Current was elicited by steps from −80 mV to −20 mV or 60 mV. Leak-corrected current is shown. The tail at −80 mV following the step to −20 mV is fit by a single exponential with time constant 2.1 msec (dashed line). The tail at −80 mV following the step to 60 mV is much slower; it is fit by a single exponential of time constant 5.3 msec (dashed line). External solution (in mM): 3 Ba, 160 tetraethylammonium (TEA) Cl, 10 HEPES, pH 7.4 with TEA OH. Internal solution (in mM): 108 CsCl, 4.5 $MgCl_2$, 4 MgATP, 14 creatine phosphate (Tris salt), 0.3 GTP (Tris salt), 9 EGTA, 9 HEPES, pH 7.4 with CsOH. Cell B80C.

persistence of openings for many milliseconds after the repolarization of the action potential provides for large Ca entry following repolarization (when driving force on Ca is especially large). This may be especially significant for the relatively short action potentials in fast-beating rat hearts. A tantalizing possibility is that the long openings induced by large depolarizations are related to phosphorylation. The behavior is at least superficially similar to a form of "facilitation" in adrenal chromaffin cells that apparently results from depolarization-induced phosphorylation controlling mode 2 behavior of L-type Ca channels (23). It will be interesting to see if there is any interaction of this gating behavior with β-adrenergic control of the Ca channels. However, in cardiac cells, this gating behavior seems to be unique to rat (and perhaps chick, see ref. 22).

Summary and Conclusions

Taken together with the earlier single-channel work, the recent work of Yue et al. (9), Ochi and Kawashima (10), and Ono and Fozzard (11) has given new insight into how the gating of cardiac L-type Ca channels is altered by cAMP-dependent phosphorylation processes. There appear to be two separable effects of major importance: an increase in the availability of channels; and an enhancement of a "mode 2" pattern of behavior giving long openings. A set of important questions remains to be answered. (1) How is the change in availability expressed at the whole-cell level? Does this process result in a scaling up of current at all voltages? Do the successive null sweeps used to define availability represent a truly dormant channel or a channel with gating shifted far in the depolarizing direction? Can such channels be opened with very large depolarizations? (2) How does the "mode 2" behavior induced by phosphorylation relate to the mode 2 behavior induced (or stabilized) by Bay K 8644 and other dihydropyridine agonists? Are these modes one and the same or are they two different modes characterized by long openings? How does the activation curve for mode 2 openings compare with that of "normal" gating modes? (3) Does mode 2 behavior induced by phosphorylation always result in slow deactivation of the channels on returning to resting voltages? A figure shown by Yue et al. (9) suggests that there is slow deactivation, but it does not seem prominent at the whole-cell level. This is important to clarify, since slow deactivation of mode 2 openings might be very important physiologically. If channels deactivate slowly, they would be even more effective in supporting large Ca fluxes, because entry would continue after repolarization of the action potential, when the driving force is large. (4) Is the slow deactivation seen in basal conditions in rat myocytes related to the mode 2 activity induced by phosphorylation? Does it represent basal phosphorylation? Can channels in this mode be further altered by phosphorylation? We look forward to answers to these questions with the understanding that they should provide much new information on the function of Ca channels and regulation of cardiac contractility at the single molecule level.

References

1. Reuter, H. (1967). The dependence of slow inward current in Purkinje fibres on the extracellular Ca-concentration. *J. Physiol.* **192:**479–492.

2. Trautwein, W., and Hescheler, J. (1990). Regulation of cardiac L-type calcium channels by phosphorylation and G-proteins. *Ann. Rev. Physiol.* **52:**257–274.

3. Hartzell, H.C., Mery, P.-F., Fischmeister, R., and Szabo, G. (1991). Sympathetic regulation of cardiac calcium current is due exclusively to cAMP-dependent phosphorylation. *Nature* **351:**573–576.

4. Frace, A.M., Mery, P.-F., Fischmeister, R., and Hartzell, H.C. (1993). Rate-limiting steps in the beta-adrenergic stimulation of cardiac calcium current. *J. Gen. Physiol.* **101:**337–353.

5. Yatani, A., and Brown, A.M. (1989). Rapid beta-adrenergic modulation of cardiac calcium channels by a fast G-protein pathway. *Science* **245:**71–74.

6. Brum, G., Osterrieder, W., and Trautwein, W. (1984). Beta-adrenergic increase in the calcium conductance of cardiac myocytes studied with the patch clamp. *Pflügers Arch.* **401:**111–118.

7. Cachelin, A.B., de Peyer, J.E., Kokubun, S., and Reuter, H. (1983). Ca^{2+} channel modulation by 8-bromocyclic AMP in cultured heart cells. *Nature* **304:**462–464.

8. Tsien, R.W., Bean, B.P., Hess, P., Lansman, J.B., Nilius, B., and Nowycky, M.C. (1986). Mechanisms of calcium channel modulation by beta-adrenergic agents and dihydropyridine calcium agonists. *J. Mol. Cell. Cardiol.* **18:**691–710.

9. Yue, D.T., Herzig, S., and Marban E. (1990). Beta-adrenergic stimulation of calcium channels occurs by potentiation of high-activity gating modes. *Proc. Natl. Acad. Sci. U.S.A.* **87:**753–757.

10. Ochi, R., and Kawashima, Y. (1990). Modulation of slow gating process of calcium channels by isoprenaline in guinea-pig ventricular cell. *J. Physiol.* **424:**187–204.

11. Ono, K., and Fozzard, H.A. (1993). Two phosphatase sites on the Ca channel affecting different kinetic functions. *J. Physiol.,* in press.

12. Reuter, H., and Scholz, H. (1977). The regulation of the calcium conductance of cardiac muscle by adrenaline. *J. Physiol.* **264:**49–62.

13. Kameyama, M., Hescheler, J., Hofmann, F., and Trautwein, W. (1986a). Modulation of Ca current during the phosphorylation cycle in the guinea pig heart. *Pflügers Arch.* **407:**123–128.

14. Kameyama, M., Hescheler, J., Mieskes, G., and Trautwein, W. (1986b). The protein-specific phosphatase 1 antagonizes the beta-adrenergic increase of the cardiac Ca current. *Pflügers Arch.* **407:**461–463.

15. Bean, B.P., Nowycky, M.C., and Tsien, R.W. (1984). Beta-adrenergic modulation of calcium channels in frog ventricular heart cells. *Nature* **307:**371–375.

16. Hess, P., Lansman, J.B., and Tsien, R.W. (1984). Different modes of Ca channel gating behavior favoured by dihydropyridine agonists and antagonists. *Nature* **311**:538–544.

17. Cavalie, A., Allen, T.J.A., and Trautwein, W. (1991). Role of the GTP-binding protein G_s in the beta-adrenergic modulation of cardiac calcium channels. *Pflügers Arch.* **419**:433–443.

18. Lew, W.Y.W., Hryshko, L.V., and Bers, D.M. (1991). Dihydropyridine receptors are primarily functional L-type calcium channels in rabbit ventricular myocytes. *Circ. Res.* **69**:1139–1145.

19. Mundina-Weilenmann, C., Ma, J., Rios, E., and Hosey, M.M. (1991). Dihydropyridine-sensitive skeletal muscle Ca channels in polarized planar bilayers: Effects of phosphorylation by cAMP-dependent protein kinase. *Biophys. J.* **60**:902–909.

20. Reuter, H., Kokubun, S., and Prod'hom, B. (1986). Properties and modulation of cardiac calcium channels. *J. Exp. Biol.* **124**:191–201.

21. Bean B.P., and Rios, E. (1989). Nonlinear charge movement in mammalian cardiac ventricular cells. Components from Na and Ca channel gating. *J. Gen. Physiol.* **94**:65–93.

22. Pietrobon, D., and Hess, P. (1990). Novel mechanism of voltage-dependent gating in L-type calcium channels. *Nature* **346**:651–655.

23. Artalejo, C.R., Rossie, S., Perlman, R.L., and Fox, A.P. (1992). Voltage-dependent phosphorylation may recruit Ca current facilitation in chromaffin cells. *Nature* **358**:63–66.

13

Probing Potassium Channel Pores

Mariella De Biasi and Arthur M. Brown

Regulation of K^+ channels, as for all ion channels, has as its final target changes in the ion permeation pathway or pore. The pore of voltage-dependent K^+ channels is highly selective because of a filtering mechanism whose molecular basis is unknown. The property of specific ionic selectivity is responsible for the nomenclature used to designate several voltage-dependent ion channels, such as those for K^+, Na^+, and Ca^{2+}. Furthermore, channels for individual ions, particularly K^+ channels, need not just be activated by changes in membrane potential; there are in fact a large class of channels that are activated or gated by binding of highly specific ligands.

Besides a pore, K^+ channels have two other principal components, a sensor mechanism responsive to changes in membrane potential or to a specific ligand, and a mechanism coupling the sensor to the pore. The moving parts of the coupling mechanism are thought to be "gates." An electromechanical model of voltage-gated K^+ channels depicting these components is shown in Fig. 1.

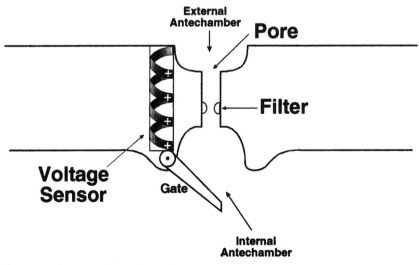

Figure 1. Electromechanical model of K^+ channels.

In this chapter we consider an example of one specific ligand-gated K^+ channel, the muscarinic atrial K^+ ($K^+[ACh]$) channel, and an example of a voltage-gated channel, an outwardly rectifying K^+ channel. With the former example we attempt to illustrate the nature of ligand interactions and how these are coupled to modulate the pore. With the latter we focus attention on what we know of the pore itself.

G-Protein–Gated, $K^+[ACh]$ Channels as an Example of a Ligand-Gated K^+ Channel

The $K^+[ACh]$ channel is regulated via the vagus nerve, which, when stimulated, releases acetylcholine (ACh). ACh binds to the muscarinic membrane acetylcholine receptor (mAChR), which in turn activates the $K^+[ACh]$ channel. As a result, the membrane becomes hyperpolarized, the action potential duration becomes shorter, and propagating currents have a smaller length constant. The unidirectional inward rectification of current is due mainly to Mg^{2+} block, but opening probability is also strongly voltage-dependent, with low values at depolarized potentials (1, 2). The channel is readily distinguished from the inward rectifier channel, I_{K1}, by its brief open time of ~1.0, versus 10 msec, and its unitary conductance of ~40, versus 20 pS when K^+ concentration is symmetrical (i.e., the same) on each side of the membrane at hyperpolarized potentials.

Activation of the mAChR by ACh occurs within ~300 msec, which is much longer than the 1-msec delay following application of ACh to the nicotinic cholinergic receptor (nAChR). Although for the nAChR, the receptor and channel are the same molecule, a second messenger pathway was considered as one explanation for the slower mAChR response (3). The usual second messenger candidates, cAMP and cGMP, had no effect. However, a large number of experiments (4–7) pointed toward the involvement of a pertussis toxin (PTX)–sensitive G-protein, although the mechanism for coupling between G-protein and channel was not known. The possibility that the coupling was membrane-delimited was suggested by patch-clamp experiments (8, 9) and directly confirmed by reconstitution experiments. In these experiments, preactivated PTX-sensitive G-proteins (10–12) were shown to activate $K^+[ACh]$ channels in excised membrane patches.

The PTX-sensitive G-proteins, G_{I-2} or G_{I-3}, when preactivated with GTPγS, stimulated the $K^+[ACh]$ channel in the absence of substrate, proving that the effect was membrane-delimited (Fig. 2) (11). Other G-proteins, such as G_s and G_T, had no effect. The respective α-subunits, when preactivated, mimicked the effects of the holo–G-proteins (12) and activation was ascribed to the α-subunits. The rate at which activation occurred was concentration-dependent and caused by an increased frequency of opening, rather than changes in unitary conductance or mean open time.

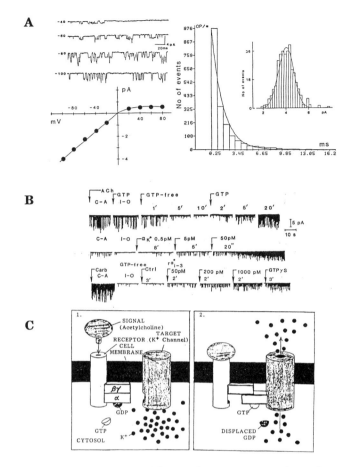

Figure 2. Direct G-protein gating of the atrial muscarinic K$^+$ channel. **(A)** Properties of single muscarinic atrial K$^+$ channel (K$^+$[ACh]) currents. Single-channel recordings were obtained with Carbachol 10 μM in the pipette and symmetrical isotonic K$^+$ solutions. The current-voltage relationship, the open times, and amplitude histograms are shown. At −80 mV, the mean unitary current was ~4 pA, and the mean channel lifetime ~1 msec. **(B)** Three typical records of K$^+$[ACh] channels taken in cell-attached (C-A) mode and after excision of the membrane patch to the inside-out configuration (I-O). GTP and G-proteins were added either by perfusion **(top row)** or directly to the bath **(next two rows)**. ACh or carbachol (Carb) were present in the pipette solution in the first and third record, whereas the second recording was obtained with no agonist present in the pipette. Preactivated Gα$_{i-3}$ (α$_K$*) and a preactivated, recombinant α$_{i-3}$ (rα*$_{i-3}$) were able to reconstitute channel activity either in the absence of receptor stimulation or in the absence of GTP. The α-subunits were preactivated with GTPγS. Results like those in the top row of **(B)** could be repeated many times after patch excision. Thus, G-protein receptor, G-protein, and channel are all well-anchored in the membrane. **(C)** Interactions among the muscarinic M$_2$ receptor, G-protein and subunits, and the K$^+$[ACh] channel to illustrate the GDP, GTP cycle of the coupling G-protein.

Activation of the $K^+[ACh]$ channel may be more complex. Evidence was presented that dimeric $\beta\gamma$-subunits may activate $K^+[ACh]$ channels (12), possibly through a phospholipase A_2 (PLA)–arachidonic acid (AA) pathway. However, a PLA-AA pathway does not seem to be involved in either muscarinic or purinergic stimulation of $K^+[ACh]$ channels (13, 14).

Membrane-delimited activation of K^+ channels by G-proteins is widespread and occurs in brain, heart, muscle, endocrine, and exocrine cells. Other K^+ channels that may be activated by G-proteins in a membrane-delimited manner include ATP-sensitive K^+ channels (15), Ca^{2+}-activated K^+ channels (16), and inwardly and outwardly rectifying K^+ channels (17). In every case preactivated $G\alpha$-subunit was observed to mimic effects produced by the preactivated holo–G-protein, or the effects produced by pharmacological or physiological activation of the cognate G-protein receptor.

Given the possibility of a membrane-delimited intermediary, the question of whether K^+ channels are G-protein effectors, similar to adenylyl cyclase or cGMP phosphodiesterase (PDE), has not been resolved. To do so would require purified K^+ channel proteins, and these are not presently available. The issue has been resolved for Ca^{2+} channels, however. Ca^{2+} channel currents from purified dihydropyridine-binding proteins that had been reconstituted in planar lipid bilayers free of enzymes were shown to be modulated directly by the application of α_s-subunit. The effect was specific for α_s; other G-protein α-subunits were ineffective. Moreover, the α_s effects were asymmetrical; they only occurred with application to the cytoplasmic surface of the Ca^{2+} channel (18).

To examine the mechanism of G-protein activation of $K^+[ACh]$ channels, a known case of effector activation by a G-protein was considered, namely activation of cGMP PDE by G_T. This PDE is inhibited by its γ-subunit and trypsin cleaves the subunit, activating the PDE, thereby simulating activation by G_T (19). Trypsin was applied to $K^+[ACh]$ channels and was found to activate them irreversibly (20). When the channels were activated by trypsin they were no longer responsive to activation by G_I proteins. Trypsin cleaves at Lys and Arg residues but the more Arg-specific reagents glyoxal and phenylglyoxal had no effect, suggesting that a Lys cleavage may be involved. A model was proposed (Fig. 3) in which trypsin cleaves off an inhibitory subunit from the $K^+[ACh]$ channel just as it may for cGMP PDE. In this model the activator G-protein performs its effect in an analogous but reversible manner. In the context of ion channels as effectors, it is interesting that the inactivation gates of Na^+ and K^+ channels are also cleaved by trypsin (21). We speculate that an inhibitory domain keeps the $K^+[ACh]$ channel closed at rest and the block is removed by the activating G-protein ligand. A similar mechanism might apply to all inwardly rectifying K^+ channels, including those that are voltage-dependent. The inhibitory domain might have properties similar to those of the N-terminus "ball and chain" reported for inactivating Shaker K^+ channels (22, 23).

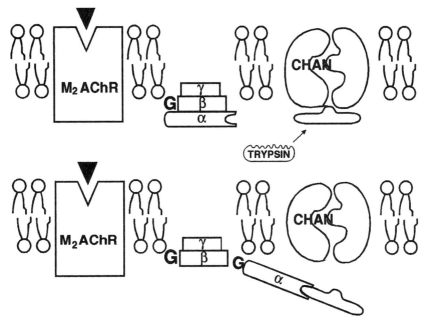

Figure 3. Model of G_K action on K^+[ACh] channel. **Top row** shows the relationship among the M_2 muscarinic cholinergic receptor (M2AChR), a PTX-sensitive G-protein G_K, and the atrial muscarinic K^+ channel (CHAN). G_K is probably $G\alpha_{i-3}$ or $G\alpha_{i-2}$. Trypsin may act by cleavage of an inhibitory domain of the channel in a manner similar to trypsin cleavage of inactivation gates of Na^+ and K^+ channels. **Bottom row** shows how the $Gi\alpha$ subunit may reversibly cleave the inhibitory domain by analogy with $Gt\alpha$ cleavage of the inhibitory α-domain of cGMP PDE.

We speculate that cleaving the inactivation gate of a K^+[ACh] channel leaves a pore that may be continuously conducting ions. The pore has been identified by mutational analysis of voltage-dependent K^+ channels (24–26), and we turn now to a consideration of the ion conduction pathway of the pore of K^+ channels.

The Pore of Voltage-Dependent K^+ Channels

The primary amino acid sequences of voltage-dependent K^+, Ca^{2+}, and Na^+ channels have strong similarities. Hydropathy plots reveal a basic repeat consisting of six or seven hydrophobic stretches of ~20 residues (Fig. 4). From considerations of secondary structure, six of the stretches, S1–S6, are thought to be α-helices. Na^+ and Ca^{2+} channels consist of four similar repeats; K^+ channels consist of a single repeat, but are thought to be assembled in tetramers (27). In the simplest version, the four repeats are thought to be arranged with rotational symmetry or pseudosymmetry, around a central pore (Fig. 4).

A.

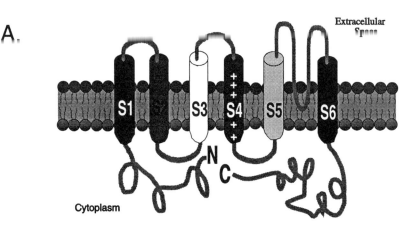

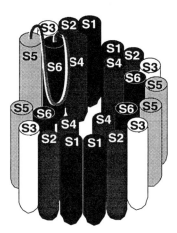

B.

Figure 4. Topography of voltage-dependent K$^+$ channels. **(A)** K$^+$ channels consist of a six-domain single repeat that is believed to assemble in a tetrameric structure around a central pore. **(B)** The arrangements of the six putative transmembrane segments in each subunit, and the arrangement of the subunits around a central pore. S4 is α-helical and is the putative voltage sensor. The loop between S5 and S6 is a β-hairpin and forms a β-barrel channel pore.

One of the α-helices, S4, is highly conserved and has an Arg—X—X—Arg/Lys sequence where X—X are hydrophobic residues that are repeated between four and eight times/helix. Because of its positive charge, S4 is thought to be the voltage sensor or at least an important part of the voltage sensor. Analysis with point mutations supports this view (28–31).

The most conserved region in voltage-dependent K$^+$ channels is the linker between the 5th and 6th transmembrane segments (S5–S6 loop) (32), and the possibility that part of this region forms the channel pore has been raised by Guy and Conti (33). The first functional evidence was the observation that open channel block of a *Shaker* K$^+$ channel by the peptide toxin, charybdotoxin, was modified by point mutations in the S5–S6 loop (34). Subsequently, it was shown for the *Shaker* K$^+$ channel that other point mutations in the linker affected open-channel block by the small quaternary ammonium ion tetraethylammonium (TEA) (35). Then a set of three independent studies simultaneously established this region as the channel pore. Yellen et al. (24) showed that internal TEA block could be changed by a Thr-Ser substitution at a position that occurred almost midway between mutations responsible for changes in external TEA block. Yool and Schwarz (25) showed with the Shaker channel that the same mutation involved in blockade by internal TEA, produced large increases in the relative permeability of NH$_4^+$, as did another specific mutation in the loop (Phe to Ser at position 434). Rather than point mutations, Hartmann et al. (26) took a different approach and used large-scale mutagenesis. A DNA sequence that putatively encoded the pore between two related K$^+$ channels with markedly different pore properties was transplanted from one to the other channel. Thus, a NGK2-like (Kv3.1) (36) K$^+$ channel had a conductance of ~26 pS and was sensitive to external TEA, whereas a delayed rectifier K$^+$ channel DRK1 (Kv2.1) (37) had a conductance of ~8 Ps and was sensitive to internal TEA. When a stretch of DNA that encoded 21 amino acids from the same region studied by Yellen et al. (24) and Yool and Schwarz (25) was transplanted from NGK2 (Kv3.1) to DRK1 (Kv2.1), the chimeric channel, CHM, exhibited the pore behavior of the parental NGK2-like (Kv3.1) phenotype (Fig. 5). In other respects, such as voltage activation and voltage sensitivity, the behavior of the chimeric channel resembled that of the host phenotype, DRK1. The fact that only pore properties were exchanged makes it likely that the channel sensor, gate, and pore complexes are modular structures. From considerations of the length of the sequence involved and the positions for blockade by external and internal TEA, a possible arrangement for the pore or P region is a β-hairpin of 18–20 amino acids (Fig. 6).

The transplanted K$^+$ pore was studied further by mutational analysis taking advantage of the phenotypic and genotypic differences between CHM and DRK1. Point reversions in CHM outside the deep pore between Pro's 361 and 381, and downstream or toward the C-terminus from P381 had either no effect, in the case of the conservative reversions, or had the consequences predicted from a change in side chain charge in this region affecting the local concentration of K$^+$ (38, 39). Thus, Gln 382 → Lys reduced inward and outward current with the reduction in inward current being greater, resulting in a decrease in outward rectification of the single

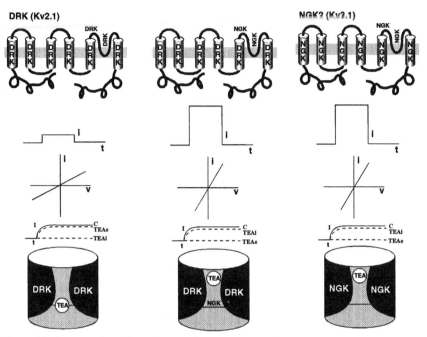

Figure 5. Construction of a K$^+$ pore chimera. **(Top)** The strategy followed to design the chimera between DRK1 and NGK2. Twenty-one amino acids in the loop between S5 and S6 were exchanged between NGK2 (Kv3.1) and DRK1 (Kv2.1). DRK1 consists of 857 amino acids in all. The shape of the current-voltage relationship for DRK1, NGK2, and CHM and their sensitivity to external and internal TEA are also reported.

channel current. Similar, although less marked, results were obtained for Met 387 → Lys.

Within the deep pore there were four differences between CHM and DRK1, three of which were conservative (Fig. 6). Surprisingly, conservative reversions at 369 and 374 introduced novel phenotypes. In both cases, open times were shortened almost 10-fold, but for Val 369 → Ile the shortening was due to stabilization of an inactivated state that was apparent in the whole-cell currents producing the P-type inactivation discussed later. For Leu 374 → Val, the reduction in open time was due to rapid departure from the open state to a proximal closed state, and currents, rather than inactivating, remained steady during standard test pulses. In this mutant, single-channel K$^+$ conductance was greatly reduced. Combined reversions at 369 and 374 restored most of the host pore phenotype. None of the other five possible double reversions had this effect, indicating that positions 369 and 374 interacted with each other. The likelihood of interaction among separate subunits was confirmed when it was established that coinjection of Val 369 → Ile and Leu 374 → Val cRNAs produced channels having the properties of the double reversion (Kirsch et al., manuscript submitted

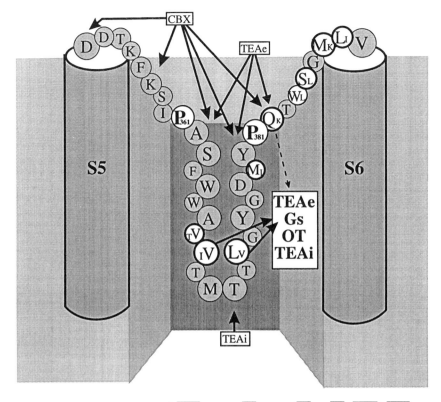

Kv2.1 PASFWWA[TI]TMTT[V]GYGD[I]YP[K]T[LL]G[KI][V]
Kv3.1 -IG----[VV]----[L]----[M]--[Q]-[WS]-[ML]-
CHM   -------[VV]----[L]----[M]--[Q]-[WS]-[ML]-

Figure 6. Model of a K⁺ channel pore. The residues comprise the loop between transmembrane segments 5 and 6 of CHM. Nine residues are boxed and account for the differences between the donor NGK2 and the host DRK1. Arrows at the **top** and **bottom** of the figure indicate the residues that align with *Shaker* residues responsible for blockade by charybdotoxin (CBX) external and internal TEA. Also indicated are the residues at positions 369 and 374 that determine the differences in pore phenotype between DRK1 and NGK2.

for publication). This result has the important implication that different subunits may not simply contribute their recognizable properties to heterotetrameric channel assemblies, but that preexisting differences in pore properties may be canceled by suitable interactions between different subunits.

The substitution Leu 374 → Val in CHM and DRK1 switched K⁺ : Rb⁺ selectivity. To analyze this selectivity filter, extensive amino acid substitutions were introduced at this position (40). The results showed that hydrophobic residues favored Rb^+, whereas polar residues favored K^+. Internal TEA blockade was enhanced by hydrophobic substitutions consistent with a hydrophobic component in the interaction between TEA and the pore. Interactions between preferred ions and TEA blockade, as well as anomalous effects of Leu at this position, led to an interpretation in which both the side chains at 374 and the peptide backbone were involved in selectivity and internal TEA blockade.

Pore or P-Type Inactivation

The S6 residue responsible for C-type inactivation with the Shaker channel was thought to reside near the external mouth of the pore (41). In lymphocytes, a His at a corresponding position in Shaker forms part of the external TEA receptor, and when protonated, produced large changes in inactivation (42). Thus, residues near the pore appear to contribute to inactivation of the non-"ball" type mechanism. A study involving point reversions of a chimeric K^+ channel showed that a Val → Ile reversion at a position in the tunnel or deep part of the pore (38, 39) produced a novel phenotype with the unique property of rapid inactivation. Unitary conductance was unchanged, however. Subsequently, a Val → Ser substitution at the same position produced more complete inactivation and marked reduction in conductance, confirming that this position was in the pore (43).

P-type inactivation differed markedly from C-type inactivation, because external TEA rather than slowing inactivation, increased channel availability. Only at higher concentrations did external TEA actually produce blockade. For this reason and because of other differences, pore- or P-type inactivation is thought to be distinct from C-type inactivation. It was considered unlikely that these pore mutations introduced a receptor for N-terminus inactivation, because internal TEA scaled the currents downward, but did not slow inactivation.

The enhanced currents produced by external TEA may be compared with the observation that extracellular K^+ increased availability of RCK_3 (Kv1.3) and RCK_4 (Kv1.4) channels (44). The external concentration increase, or K_0-induced increase, in availability was blocked by a Thr → Lys substitution, which also abolished block by external TEA. However, changes in sensitivity to external TEA and K_0 were not accompanied by changes in the rate of inactivation, single-channel conductance, mean open time, or gating charge displacement. Apparently it is the coupling between gating charge and channel opening that is modulated by K_0.

On the other hand, with inactivation experiments involving amino acid substitution of specific pore residues, increasingly external K^+ slowed inactivation and increased recovery from inactivation. These results indicate a highly complex situation in which TEA and K^+ receptors near the external mouth of the pore couple to an inactivation process within the pore. There appears to be an external site at which TEA produces blockade; there is another site at which TEA has an enhancing effect on K^+ currents, possibly the same site as the one responsible for the enhancing effect of K_0. In addition, there may be a site at which increased K_0 slows inactivation.

The effects of external TEA can be qualitatively accounted for by extending a closed-closed-open-block model to include transitions between C_1 and I_4. A 5th state, B, is the blocked state produced by higher concentrations of TEA. Thus, we have:

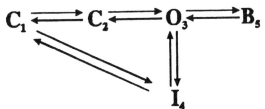

The $I_4C_1O_3$ transitions are stabilized by lower concentrations of TEA to enhance currents, and the O_3B_5 transition is stabilized by higher concentrations to produce blockade. The experimental data of P-type inactivation were well-fitted by this extended model. The potentiating effects of increased K_0 were accounted for in the same way, but omitting B_5.

P-type inactivation can be compared with N-type inactivation by testing the effects of internal TEA injected into oocytes using the method described by Taglialatela et al. (45). For N-type inactivation, internal TEA prolongs currents, whereas for P-type inactivation internal TEA simply reduces the currents at all test potentials (43).

Despite the differences noted, both P- and C- types of inactivation involve residues in or near the pores and both may share similar mechanisms. They should be distinguished from the N-terminus "ball"type of activation (22) and from deletions of the C-terminus in which Kv2.1 showed an increased rate of inactivation (46). If the distinction lies between inactivation mechanisms involving the nonconserved cytoplasmic N- and C-termini and inactivation mechanisms involving the conserved, hydrophobic core, a more suitable nomenclature might be to use the terms "core" and "noncore inactivation."

Acknowledgments

This work was supported in part by the National Institutes of Health Grants HL-37044, HL-39262, HL-36930, and NS-23877.

We thank our collaborators, Maurizio Taglialatela, Glenn Kirsch, John Drewe, and Hali Hartmann. We thank Judy Breedlove and Marianne Anderson for their secretarial assistance, and Brooke Summers for her graphics design.

References

1. Horie, M., and Irisawa, H. (1987). Rectification of muscarinic K^+ current by magnesium ion in guinea pig atrial cells. *Am. J. Physiol.* **253**:H210–H214.

2. Yatani, A., and Brown, A.M. (1991). Voltage-gated ionic channels: Diversity and modulation by Mg^{2+}, in *Mg^{2+} and Excitable Membranes*, P. Strata and E. Carbone, Eds. (Springer-Verlag, Berlin), pp. 21–31.

3. Pott, L. (1979). On the time course of the acetylcholine-induced hyperpolarization in quiescent guinea-pig atria. *Pflügers Arch.* **380**:71–77.

4. Sorota, S., Tsuji, T., Tajima, T., and Pappano, A.J. (1985). Pertussis toxin treatment blocks hyperpolarization by muscarinic agonists in chick atrium. *Circ. Res.* **57**:748–758.

5. Endoh, M., Manyama, M., and Tajima, T. (1985). Attenuation of muscarinic cholinergic inhibition by islet-activating protein in the heart. *Am. J. Physiol.* **249**:H309–H320.

6. Pfaffinger, P.J., Martin, J.M., Hunter, D.D., Nathanson, N.M., and Hille, B. (1985). GTP-binding proteins couple cardiac muscarinic receptors to a K channel. *Nature* **317**:536–538.

7. Breitweiser, G.E., and Szabo, G. (1985). Uncoupling of cardiac muscarinic and β-adrenergic receptors from ion channels by a guanine nucleotide analogue. *Nature* **317**:538–540.

8. Soejima, M., and Noma, A. (1984). Mode of regulation of the ACh-sensitive K^+ channel by the muscarinic receptor in rabbit atrial cells. *Pflügers Arch.* **400**:424–431.

9. Kurachi, Y., Nakajima, T., and Sugimoto, T. (1986). On the mechanism of activation of muscarinic K^+ channels by adenosine in isolated atrial cells: involvement of GTP-binding proteins. *Pflügers Arch.* **407**:264–274.

10. Yatani, A., Codina, J., Brown, A.M., and Birnbaumer, L. (1987). Direct activation of mammalian atrial muscarinic potassium channels by GTP regulatory protein G_k. *Science* **235**:207–211.

11. Codina, J., Yatani, A., Grenet, D., Brown, A.M., and Birnbaumer, L. (1987). The *alpha* subunit of the GTP binding protein G_k opens atrial potassium channels. *Science* **236**:442–445.

12. Logothetis, D.E., Kurachi, Y., Galper, J., Neer, E.J., and Clapham, D.E. (1987). β subunits of GTP-binding proteins activate the muscarinic K^+ channel in heart. *Nature* **325**:321–326.

13. Kurachi, Y., Itoh, H., Sugimoto, T., Shimizu, T., Miki, I., and Ui, M. (1989). Arachidonic acid metabolites as intracellular modulators of the G protein-gated cardiac K^+ channel. *Nature* **337**:555–557.

14. Kim, D., Lewis, D.L., Graziadei, L., Neer, E.J., Bar-Sagi, D., and Clapham, D.E. (1989). G-protein beta gamma subunits activate the cardiac muscarinic K^+ channel via phospholipase A2. *Nature* **337**:557–560.

15. Kirsch, G.E., Codina, J., Birnbaumer, L., and Brown, A.M. (1990). Coupling of ATP-sensitive K^+ channels to A_1 receptors by G proteins in rat ventricular myocytes. *Am. J. Physiol.* **259**:H820–826.

16. Toro, L., Ramos-Franco, J., and Stefani, E. (1990). GTP-dependent regulation of myometrial KCa channels incorporated into lipid bilayers. *J. Gen. Physiol.* **96**:373–394.

17. VanDongen, T., Codina, J., Olate, J., Mattera, R., Joho, R., Birnbaumer, L., and Brown, A.M. (1988). Newly identified brain potassium channels gated by the guanine nucleotide binding protein G_0. *Science* **242**:1433–1437.

18. Hamilton, S.L., Codina, J., Hawkes, M.J., Yatani, A., Sawada, T., Strickland, F.M., Froehner, S.C., Spiegel, A.M., Toro, L., Stefani, E., Birnbaumer, L., and Brown, A.M. (1991). Evidence for direct interaction of $G_s\alpha$ with the Ca^{2+} channel of skeletal muscle. *J. Biol. Chem.* **266:**19528–19535.

19. Stryer, L. (1986). Cyclic GMP cascade of vision. *Ann. Rev. Neurosci.* **9:**87–119.

20. Kirsch, G.E., and Brown, A.M. (1989). Trypsin activation of atrial muscarinic K^+ channels. *Am. J. Physiol.* **257:**H334–H338.

21. Armstrong, C.M. (1981). Sodium channels and gating currents. *Physiol. Rev.* **61:**644–683.

22. Hoshi, T., Zagotta, W.N., and Aldrich, R.W. (1990). Biophysical and molecular mechanisms of *Shaker* potassium channel inactivation. *Science* **250:**533–538.

23. Zagotta, W.N., Hoshi, T., and Aldrich, R.W. (1990). Restoration of inactivation in mutants of *Shaker* potassium channels by a peptide derived from ShB. *Science* **250:**568–571.

24. Yellen, G., Jurman, M., Abramson, T., and MacKinnon, R. (1991). Mutations affecting internal TEA blockade identify the probable pore-forming region of a K^+ channel. *Science* **251:**939–942.

25. Yool, A.J., and Schwarz, T.L. (1991). Alteration of ionic selectivity of a K^+ channel by mutation of the H5 region. *Nature* **349:**700–704.

26. Hartmann, H.A., Kirsch, G.E., Drewe, J.A., Taglialatela, M., Joho, R.H., and Brown, A.M. (1991). Exchange of conduction pathways between two related K^+ channels. *Science* **251:**942–944.

27. MacKinnon, R. (1991). Determination of the subunit stoichiometry of a voltage-activated potassium channel. *Nature* **350:**232–235.

28. Stühmer, W., Conti, F., Suzuki, H., Wang, X., Noda, M., Yahagi, N., Kubo, H., and Numa, S. (1989). Structural parts involved in activation and inactivation of the sodium channel. *Nature* **339:**597–603.

29. Liman, E.R., Hess, P., Weaver, F., and Koren, G. (1991). Voltage-sensing residues in the S4 region of a mammalian K^+ channel. *Nature* **353:**752–756.

30. Bezanilla, F., Perozo, E., Papazian, D.M., and Stefani, E. (1991). Molecular basis of gating charge immobilization in Shaker potassium channels. *Science* **254:**679–683.

31. Logothetis, D.E., Movahedi, S., Satler, C., Lindpaintner, K., and Nadal-Ginard, B. (1992). Incremental reductions of positive charge within the S4 region of a voltage-gated K^+ channel result in corresponding decreases in gating charge. *Neuron* **8:**531–540.

32. Tempel, B.L., Papazian, D.M., Schwarz, T.L., Jan, Y.N., and Jan, L.Y. (1987). Sequence of a probable potassium channel component encoded at the *Shaker* locus of *Drosophila*. *Science* **237:**770–775.

33. Guy, H.R., and Conti, F. (1990). AChR structure: a new twist in the story. *Trends Neurosci.* **13:**201–206.

34. MacKinnon, R., and Miller, C. (1989). Mutant potassium channels with altered binding of charybdotoxin, a pore-blocking peptide inhibitor. *Science* **245:**1382–1385.

35. MacKinnon, R., and Yellen, G. (1990). Mutations affecting TEA blockade and ion permeation in voltage-activated K^+ channels. *Science* **250:**276–279.

36. Yokoyama, S., Imoto, K., Kawamura, T., Higashida, H., Iwabe, N., Miyata, T., and Numa, S. (1989). Potassium channels from NG108-15 neuroblastoma-glioma hybrid cells. *FEBS Lett.* **259**:37–42.

37. Frech, G.C., VanDongen, A.M.J., Schuster, G., Brown, A.M., and Joho, R.H. (1989). A novel potassium channel with delayed rectifier properties isolated from rat brain by expression cloning. *Nature* **340**:642–645.

38. Kirsch, G.E., Drewe, J.A., De Biasi, M., Hartmann, H.A., and Brown, A.M. (1992). Emergent properties produced by the interaction of pore residues located in separate K$^+$ channel subunits. *J. Gen. Physiol.*, manuscript submitted for publication.

39. Kirsch, G.E., Drewe, J.A., Hartmann, H., Taglialatela, M., De Biasi, M., Brown, A.M., and Joho, R.H. (1992). Differences between the deep pores of K$^+$ channels determined by an interacting pair of non-polar amino acids. *Neuron* **8**:499–505.

40. Taglialatela, M., Drewe, J.A., Kirsch, G.E., De Biasi, M., Hartmann, H., and Brown, A.M. (1992). Regulation of K$^+$/Rb$^+$ selectivity and internal TEA blockade by mutations at a single site in K$^+$ pores. *Pflügers Arch.*, in press.

41. Hoshi, T., Zagotta, W.N., and Aldrich, R.W. (1991). Two types of inactivation in *Shaker* K$^+$ channels: Effects of alterations in the carboxy-terminal region. *Neuron* **7**:547–556.

42. Busch, A.E., Hurst, R.S., North, R.A., Adelman, J.P., and Kavanaugh, M.P. (1991). Current inactivation involves a histidine residue in the pore of the rat lymphocyte potassium channel RGK5. *Biochem. Biophys. Res. Comm.* **179**:1384–1390.

43. De Biasi, M., Hartmann, H.A., Drewe, J.A., Taglialatela, M., Brown, A.M., and Kirsch, G.E. (1992). Inactivation determined by a single site in K$^+$ pores. *Pflügers Arch.*, in press.

44. Pardo, L.A., Heinemann, S.H., Terlau, H., Ludewig, U., Lorra, C., Pongs, O., and Stühmer, W. (1992). Extracellular K$^+$ specifically modulates a rat brain K$^+$ channel. *Proc. Natl. Acad. Sci. U.S.A.* **89**:2466–2470.

45. Taglialatela, M., VanDongen, A.M.J., Drewe, J.A., Joho, R.H., Brown, A.M., and Kirsch, G.E. (1991). Patterns of internal and external tetraethylammonium block in four homologous K$^+$ channels. *Mol. Pharmacol.* **40**:299–307.

46. VanDongen, A.M.J., Frech, G.C., Drewe, J.A., Joho, R.H., and Brown, A.M. (1990). Alteration and restoration of K$^+$ channel function by deletions at the N- and C-termini. *Neuron* **5**:433–443.

PART FOUR

Structure and Function
of Ion Channels

In this Part the relationship between structure and function in ion channels is the central issue. Numerous studies, mainly electrophysiological, have established three major functional domains in voltage-dependent Na^+, K^+ and Ca^{2+} channels, a voltage sensor, an ion conduction pathway or pore and activation and inactivation gates which couple the voltage sensor to the pore. The present challenge is to identify where these domains are located within the amino acid sequence of the proteins. This is not easy because ion channels are large containing about 2,000 amino acids, and are relatively sparse in plasma membranes. Consequently isolation of large quantities of material required for structural analyses, has for the moment not been achieved. Based on similarities in their primary amino acid sequences ion channels are clearly related to each other as a gene superfamily. Na^+ and Ca^{2+} channels are encoded by genes having four similar repeats while the K^+ channel gene encodes a single repeat, four of which are thought to be assembled to give a final tetrameric K^+ channel structure. The channel topologies thus show four-fold symmetry in the case of homo-tetrameric K^+ channels or pseudo-symmetry in the case of Na^+ and Ca^{2+} channels around a central pore.

The topology of a single repeat has been modelled as six membrane-spanning α-helices (S1-S6) having about 20 residues per helix. Linkers connect each helix and as we learned in Chapter 13, the linker between S5 and S6 also spans the membrane and forms a good part of the channel pore.

The fourth transmembrane segment, S4, of all voltage-gated channels examined has a repetitive pattern of a positively charged lysine or arginine separated by two usually hydrophobic residues. The extreme conservation of this charged segment has lead to the suggestion that it acts as the voltage sensor. In Chapter 14, Drs. Tytgat and Hess use mutational analysis to test whether S4 is the voltage sensor of K^+ channels. To examine voltage sensitivity, the charge on S4 was reduced systematically using some clever protein engineering. The results show that the voltage sensitivity was reduced as expected if S4 were the voltage sensor. This type of imaginative experimentation typified Peter Hess' many important contributions to ion channel physiology and his premature death is a great loss to the field.

In Chapter 15, the present status of K^+ and Na^+ channel cDNA's that have been cloned from the cardiovascular system, primarily the heart, is reviewed by Dr. Tamkun. Six of the cardiac K^+ channels belong to the Drosophila Shaker family and one belongs to a completely different class of K^+ channels which has only a single transmembrane segment. Of the six Shaker-related clones three are expressed primarily in heart, whereas the other three are expressed primarily in brain and their function in heart remains problematical. One of the cloned channels expresses currents similar, but not identical, to I_t, the main difference being a marked slowing in the recovery from inactivation. Interestingly, co-expression with another cardiac K^+ channel clone corrects this feature while retaining the other properties of I_t.

Dr. Catterall discusses structure-function relationships of Na^+ channels in Chapter 16. Besides the main voltage-dependent protein α subunit, neural Na^+ channels have two associated subunit proteins. Co-expression of the subunits has clear effects on the rate of inactivation. The primary sequence of the 1 subunit has a large extracellular domain, one transmembrane segment, and a small intracellular domain.

Evidence from mutational experiments that S4 is the voltage sensor of Na^+ channels is reviewed. Another important functional domain in Na^+ channels, the inactivation gate, is localized to the linker between repeats III and IV. Furthermore, a stretch of three hydrophobic residues are the major determinants of inactivation. In contrast to the charged ball and chain model for the inactivation gate in K^+ channels, charged residues have no role in Na^+ channel inactivation. Instead, a hinged-lid model of inactivation is postulated, rather like the hinged-lids that cover the active sites of allosteric enzymes.

In addition to acute regulation by phosphorylation mechanisms, long-term regulation of Na^+ channels was demonstrated following chronic treatment with the antiarrhythmic drug mexilitene. An increase in mRNA for the cardiac Na^+ channel followed chronic administration and was also observed after chronic administration of the Ca^{2+} channel blocker verapamil. The extent to which these mechanisms may play an actual role in human therapeutics is as yet an unanswered question, but one of obvious importance.

Based on electrochemical considerations, K^+ currents should be reduced when extracellular K^+ ($[K_o]$) is increased and increased when $[K_o]$ is reduced. In Chapter 17 Drs. Pardo and Stühmer show that this is not the case for the current expressed by a K^+ channel clone that has most of the properties of I_t. The current expressed by this clone is markedly reduced when $[K_o]$ is lowered. Likewise, I_t is reduced in atrial myocytes when $[K_o]$ is lowered. For the cloned channel, a single residue near the outer mouth of the pore appears to be an important determinant of the phenomenon. The mechanism for the K_o effect is unknown, but is associated with an enhanced recovery from inactivation. For clinical situations in which $[K_o]$ is altered, changes in this current could change the cardiac action potential.

None of the channels described up to this point in this work are directly involved in initiating excitation-contraction coupling which is essential for cardiac contraction. In Chapter 18 Drs. Garcia and Beam deal with the nature of the contact between the dihydropyridine receptor (DHPR) or Ca^{2+} channel of skeletal muscle and the Ca^{2+} release channel of the sarcoplasmic reticulum. This is important because the nature of this contact is central to the issue of the coupling between excitation and contraction in cardiac and skeletal muscle. In skeletal muscle it is believed that entry of Ca^{2+} is unimportant; by contrast, Ca^{2+} entry is essential for release in cardiac muscle. Using dysgenic myoblasts as a readout and chimeric constructs between skeletal and cardiac α_1 subunits, it is shown that the loop between repeats II and III determines whether the release of Ca^{2+} is typical for skeletal or cardiac muscle. For skeletal release to occur, the II-III loop must be skeletal, although the rest of the protein may be cardiac.

Ca^{2+} channels have the most complex quaternary structure of all voltage-dependent ion channels as discussed by Dr. Hofmann in Chapter 19. Ca^{2+} channels are pentameric proteins having α_1, α_2-δ, β and γ subunits. In Chapter 19, the quaternary structure of cardiac and smooth muscle Ca^{2+} channels is compared using Northern blots to detect the presence of the different subunit mRNAs. The α_1 subunits embody the Ca^{2+} channel properties of gating, ion conduction and contain the binding sites for Ca^{2+} channel ligands such as dihydropyridines, phenylalkylamines and benzothiazepines. Co-expression of α_1 subunits with α_2-δ and β subunits changed either current kinetics or amplitudes indicating that the interactions between subunits have functional consequences.

The structure-function relationships described in this Section represent the beginnings of a more complete analysis of this major issue in channel biology. Among the more important considerations for the future will be the determination of receptor sites for drugs that act upon ion channels. In subsequent chapters drug actions on Na^+, K_+ and Ca^{2+} channels are examined.

Arthur M. Brown & Peter M. Spooner

14

Mechanisms of Potassium Channel Gating Probed by Site-directed Mutagenesis

Jan Tytgat and Peter Hess

$\mathbf{V}$oltage-dependent opening and closing of transmembrane ion channels underlies the generation and propagation of action potentials in nerve, muscle, and heart cells. The mechanism for opening and closing these channels involves controlling molecular conformation by the voltage across the cellular membrane. Long before the identity of channels was known, Hodgkin and Huxley (1) observed K^+ and Na^+ currents induced by membrane depolarization in the squid giant axon, and developed an empirical model to describe the sigmoidal kinetics and voltage dependence of the observed conductances (1). Hodgkin and Huxley (1) viewed channel gating as the result of a number of charged gating particles moving independently in response to a change of the transmembrane electric field. They also supposed that the steepness of the relationship between the probability of a channel being open and membrane voltage would depend on the number of charges that move across the membrane for the channel to open. Gating currents corresponding to charge movement were then observed with K^+ channels (2, 3) and Na^+ channels (4) in the squid giant axon, supporting the first predictions by Hodgkin and Huxley (1). The physical correlate to these charge movements, however, and the molecular mechanism of ion channel gating remained uncertain. It is only with the cloning of K^+, Na^+, and Ca^{2+} channels in recent years that ion channel gating has become more accessible to investigate (5–7). Unlike Na^+ and Ca^{2+} channels, which consist of four homologous, but distinct, internal repeating subunits (8, 9), voltage-dependent K^+ channels, first cloned from *Drosophila* (10–15), contain only a single repeat. The hydropathy profile of this repeating sequence of amino acids is similar to those of each of the internal repeating of Na^+ and Ca^{2+} channels, suggesting a similar transmembrane topology for each of the three voltage-dependent channels (5, 6). Several topological models have been proposed for the homologous domains of Na^+ and Ca^{2+} channels and for the single K^+ channel subunit.

The prevailing model proposes six transmembrane segments, designated S1 through S6 with cytoplasmic amino- and carboxy-terminals (8, 12, 16). Based on primary structure analysis of voltage-dependent Na^+ channels, it was proposed that the putative fourth transmembrane region (S4), characterized by a motif of 4 to 7 of the positively charged residues arginine (R) and lysine (K) spaced three residues apart, represents the channel voltage sensor (8, 17). It has been hypothesized that the positive charged residues form ion pairs with negative charges in other transmembrane regions, thereby stabilizing the channel in the nonconducting, closed conformation (18). With a change in the electric field across the cellular membrane, these ion pairs would break as the S4 charges move, and new ion pairs would form to stabilize the conducting, open conformation. The sequential, voltage-induced conformational change of four domains of Na^+ and Ca^{2+} channels, or four subunits of K^+ channels, each containing a voltage sensor with 4 to 7 moving charges in the S4 segment, could account for the gating charge of six proposed in the Hodgkin–Huxley model. Experimental evidence attributing voltage sensing properties to the S4 region is the finding that mutation of positively charged amino acids present in S4, in both the Na^+ (18) and the *Shaker* K^+ channel (19), alter the voltage dependence of channel activation. A first step toward defining the movement of the entire S4 region was to assess the individual contribution of each charge to the overall charge movement and to investigate whether basic amino acids in S4 contribute equally to total charge movement. For the *Shaker* K^+ channel, it was found that neutralization of the third arginine in S4 (R368Q) reduces the channel's sensitivity to voltage much more than would be expected if the seven S4 charges contribute equally to the total gating charge. However, neutralization of four other basic residues in S4 do not reduce the estimated total gating charge (R362Q, R365Q, R371Q and K380Q). By contrast, some mutations can reduce channel sensitivity to voltage without reducing the charge on the S4 sequence (R377K) (19). For the delayed rectifier K^+ channel, RCK1, only some charge neutralizations in S4 correlate with the change in total gating valence (i.e., R295, the second arginine in S4) (20, 21). These findings cannot be explained by simple models based on electrostatic interactions, and illustrate contributions from chemical interactions between basic residues and the surrounding protein in channel gating behavior (19–21). The findings showing that gating charge movement is not equally distributed over the charged amino acids in S4 are not congruent with the original helical screw model of S4 voltage sensing (5).

Influences on the voltage dependence of activation are not simply limited to charged residues in the S4 region. Recent studies have also demonstrated shifts of the activation process along the voltage axis, with mutations of noncharged residues, most likely because of changes in the relative stability of the closed and open conformations of the channel (6, 22–24).

The slowly, or noninactivating, delayed recitifier K^+ channels provide an ideal model system for studying voltage-dependent channel gating, because the activation process can be considered in isolation. Such channels have recently been cloned from mammalian brain and expressed in *Xenopus* oocytes (25–30). Expression of the delayed rectifier K^+ channel, RCK1, in a mammalian cell line allowed the recording of single channels, and thereby facilitated the development of a preliminary kinetic model for the channel's gating mechanism (25). Because voltage-activated K^+ channels are composed of four identical subunits (31), the model assumes that each of four subunits undergoes a voltage-induced conformational change before the channel can open. This assumption predicts five closed conformations, of which four are linked by voltage-dependent transitions, followed by a voltage-independent transition leading to the open state of the channel. This is because the single-channel data suggest that the direct transition into and out of the open conformation is not voltage-dependent (25, 32).

We have constructed cDNAs encoding four RCK1 subunits on a single polypeptide chain, enabling us to specify the subunit stoichiometry of the resulting K^+ channels. We then designed K^+ channels composed of different subunits with distinct voltage sensitivities to test whether each subunit gates independently, as originally proposed by Hodgkin and Huxley (1), or whether the gating of a single subunit is influenced by its neighbors (i.e., exhibits cooperative behavior). Nonindependent subunit gating would be more in line with the widespread subunit cooperativity observed in multisubunit proteins such as enzymes and receptors (33) and would also be more consistent with measurements of the kinetics of K^+ channel gating currents (34–38).

Methodology

All our cDNAs were cloned into a 3-kb high-expression vector based on pGEM3Z (Promega) containing 5′- and 3′-nontranslated sequences of a *Xenopus* β-globin gene flanking the channel cDNA (39). For in vitro transcription, the plasmid was linearized 3′- to the 3′-nontranslated β-globin sequence.

Dimeric cDNA

Monomeric RCK1 cDNA was flanked by an *Eco*RI (5′) and a *Hind*III site (3′). For the construction of dimeric cDNA, the *Eco*RI site was mutated to a *Bam*HI site and a new *Eco*RI site was created before the stop codon, 5′ to the *Hind*III site. After digestion of this cDNA (channel A) and of an original RCK1 channel (channel B) with *Eco*RI (5′) and *Hind*III (3′), channel B could be ligated in frame after channel A, creating a dimeric cDNA. The link between the two channels thus contained the entire C-terminus of channel A, the entire N-terminus of channel B, plus 17 new amino acids derived from the 5′-nontranslated region of the RCK1 clone of channel B between the *Eco*RI site and the normal initiation codon. The sequence of the 17 amino acids was LHPGLSPGLLPLHPASI.

Tetrameric cDNA

Dimeric cDNA was cut with KpnI (single site at 5′ end of nontranslated β-globin sequence) and DraI (single site after first base of stop codon in channel B), yielding a 3-kb fragment containing channels A and B. A plasmid containing channel C was cut with XmaI (single site at bases coding for first PG amino acids of link listed previously), blunted with Klenow fragment of DNA polymerase and recut with KpnI, yielding a 4.5-kb fragment containing the vector and channel C. Ligation of the two fragments (A,B + C) produced trimeric cDNA (channels A, B, and C), with a single remaining DraI site at the end of channel C. In an iterative way, channels A, B, and C were then excised as a 4.5-kb fragment with KpnI and DraI and ligated to a 4.5-kb fragment (KpnI to blunted XmaI) containing the vector and channel D to yield tetrameric cDNA (channels A, B, C, and D). The links between the C- and N-termini of channels B and C, and C and D contained the last 15 of the 17 amino acids listed previously.

For site-directed mutagenesis, the "Altered Sites" system (Promega) was used. Single-stranded template was produced by a helper phage in a phagemid vector containing a tetracycline resistance gene and an inactivated (four-base deletion) ampicillin resistance gene. The single-stranded template was annealed with the mutagenic oligonucleotide and a second oligonucleotide designed to repair the ampicilline resistance gene in the vector. Second strand synthesis was conducted in vitro, and two successive rounds of transformation under ampicillin selection were used to separate the wild-type (WT) template strand from the mutant strand. Mutations were verified by dideoxy DNA sequencing. For each construct, several independent clones were sequenced, transcribed, and expressed.

Two microelectrode voltage-clamp recordings of K$^+$ currents through *Xenopus*-expressed RCK1 channels were made as previously described (20, 25). Linear components of capacity and leak currents were subtracted digitally. To increase resolution at low values of channel activation, we measured currents through RCK1 channels with 50 mM external RbCl as charge carrier to obtain large inward tail currents upon repolarization. Rb slows the rate of channel closure (deactivation) and thus facilitates measurement of tail currents (40). The bathing solution (in mM) uses 50 mM RbCl, 70 mM NaCl, 0.3 CaCl$_2$, 1 MgCl$_2$, 10 HEPES, pH 7.2. Currents were recorded by a Dagan 8,500 voltage-clamp amplifier, filtered (1 to 10 kHz, 3 dB), digitized, and analyzed on a PDP11/73 computer.

Monomeric, Dimeric, and Tetrameric K⁺ Channel Constructs

In order to specify subunit stoichiometry and to manipulate subunit composition of the RCK1 K⁺ channel (20, 25, 27, 29), we constructed cDNAs that code for two RCK1 subunits, also called dimers (41–43) or four RCK1 subunits, also called tetramers (44–46) on a single cDNA (Fig. 1). In an initial series of control experiments we found that gating phenotypes of RCK1 K channels expressed in *Xenopus* oocytes from cDNAs encoding either WT monomers, WT dimers, or WT tetramers are indistinguishable (Fig. 2a).

In a second series of control experiments, we obtained strong evidence that the vast majority of channels expressed from a cDNA encoding all four subunits are composed of the subunits specified on that cDNA, and that formation of heteromultimeric channels from subunits coming together from different polypeptide chains was negligible. This conclusion was based on five major findings. (1) Dose-response curves for tetraethylammonium in tetramers that contain either 1, 2, or 3 tetraethylammonium-insensitive mutant subunits demonstrate single and distinct inhibition constants (42, 47). (2) The rate of tail current deactivation in tetramers contain-

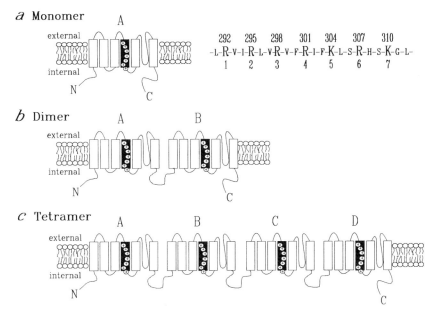

Figure 1. Construction of cDNAs. **(a)** Putative transmembrane folding scheme for a monomeric subunit of voltage-dependent K⁺ channels **(left)** with the S4 sequence for RCK1 **(right)**. Residue numbers are indicated **above** Arg (R) and Lys (K) residues. For simplicity we refer to the residues by the numbers indicated **below** the sequence (1 to 7). The complete sequence of RCK1 can be found in Baumann et al. (29) and Christie et al. (27). **(b, c)** Scheme for dimeric and tetrameric constructs. [From Tytgat and Hess (46).]

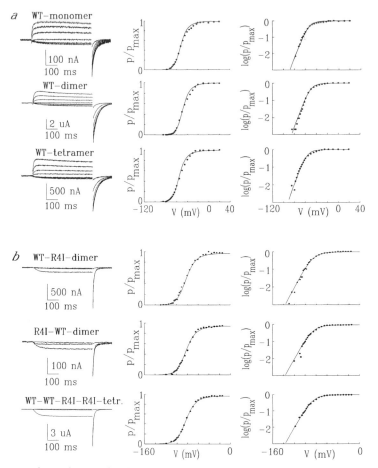

Figure 2. Channels encoded by monomeric, dimeric, or tetrameric RCK1 cDNAs. Current records **(left column)** and steady-state activation curves **(middle column:** linear scale and **right column:** semilogarithmic scale) from oocytes injected with RNA in vitro transcribed. **(a)** WT monomeric, WT dimeric, and WT tetrameric cDNA. Holding potentials: −100 mV (monomer) and −110 mV (dimer and tetramer). Test potentials for WT currents shown ranged from −60 to 0 mV in 10 mV increments. Steady-state activation curves were obtained as relative amplitudes of the tail currents elicited by repolarization from the test potentials indicated on the x-axis. Mean voltages (±SEM) for 10% and 50% activation: −65 ± 1 and −53 ± 1 mV (monomer, $N = 10$), −65.1 ± 2 and −52.5 ± 2 mV (dimer, $N = 5$), −69.5 ± 3.1 and −56.6 ± 2.4 mV (tetramer, N = 5). Mean equivalent gating valences z: respectively, 6.7 ± 0.2, 6.8 ± 0.2, and 6.7 ± 0.5. **(b)** WT-R4I dimeric, R4I-WT dimeric, and WT-WT-R4I-R4I tetrameric cDNA. Holding potential: −140 mV. Test potentials were −110, −60, and −40 mV. Mean voltages for 10% and 50% activation: −102.4 ± 2 and −82 ± 2 mV (WT-R4I dimer, $N = 42$), −99.3 ± 1.9 and −78.7 ± 2.3 mV (R4I-WT dimer, $N = 14$), and −100.4 ± 1.4 and −81.3 ± 2 mV (WT-WT-R4I-R4I tetramer, N = 12). Mean z values: respectively, 4.2 ± 0.3, 4.3 ± 0.3, and 4.7 ± 0.4. [From Tytgat and Hess (46)].

ing WT subunits can differ substantially from that of tetramers composed of mixtures of WT and mutant subunits. Interestingly, the time course of deactivation is always monoexponential, which implies the expression of a single population of channels from each construct. (3) cDNAs coding for WT-X dimers, where X is one of a number of nonexpressing subunits [e.g., R3I, K5I, R6N; see Liman et al. (20)], give no functional expression. This implies that assembly of WT subunits from different polypeptide chains into functional homotetramers does not take place if WT and mutant subunits are present on the same polypeptide chain. Additional support for this conclusion is that the corresponding tetramers WT-X-WT-X do not express functional channels either. (4) The order in which different subunits are encoded on dimeric cDNA is of no consequence for its phenotype (Fig. 2b). (5) All channel cDNAs reported in this work are cloned into a high-expression vector in which the channel cDNAs are flanked by 5'- and 3'-untranslated regions from a *Xenopus* β-globin gene (39). This construct enhances expression by a factor of 100 to 1,000. The 3'-untranslated region by itself enhances expression by a factor of 4 to 10, thus favoring the translation of full-length mRNAs over RNAs that might have been degraded and would have encoded fewer than the four subunits specified on the full-length cDNA (47).

Voltage Dependence of "R2-mutated" Channels

Hodgkin and Huxley (1) considered that voltage sensing of channels requires charge movement through the cell membrane. Because four K^+ channel peptides are needed to form a functional K^+ channel (31), S4 charges in each of the four subunits were thought to move in response to a change in electric field. To test for interactions between charges in S4 of individual subunits during the process of channel activation, dimeric and tetrameric cDNAs encoding combinations of two kinds of subunits with very different gating phenotypes were constructed. Steady-state activation curves for combinations of WT subunits and subunits in which the second Arg residue in S4 has been replaced by Asn (R2N) are shown in Fig. 3. The R2N mutant was chosen because of its very pronounced gating phenotype: WT channels activate at ~80 mV more positive potential than R2N mutant channels (20). We then replaced WT subunits by mutant R2N subunits, resulting in constructs containing a different combination of WT and R2N subunits. Distinct phenotypes were observed with activation curves shifted toward progressively more negative potentials as more WT subunits were replaced by mutant R2N subunits. The smooth curves superimposed on the data points in Fig. 3a are predictions from a model of steady-state activation in which each subunit gates independently (see legend to Fig. 3 for details of the model). Once parameters are chosen to fit activation curves for all WT and all R2N channels separately, no further adjustable parameters are needed to predict the activation curves of channels with

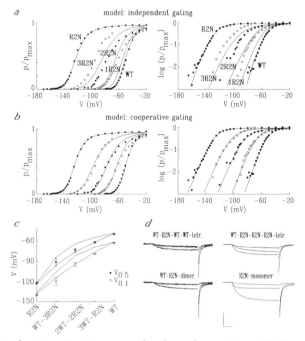

Figure 3. Steady-state activation curves for channels consisting of WT and mutant subunits suggest cooperative gating. **(a, b)** Steady-state activation curves for WT and R2N channels, WT-R2N dimers (2R2N), or tetrameric combinations in which either 1 (1R2N, R2N in position B) or 3 (3R2N, WT in position A) WT subunits were substituted by an R2N subunit. Experimental conditions as in Fig. 2. Solid curves are model predictions for independent (a) or cooperative gating (b). Model: each subunit can assume a nonpermissive and a permissive state, with voltage-dependent rate constants for the forward (k_f) and backward (k_b) transitions. $k_f = k_{f0} * \exp(z_f VF/RT)$ and $k_b = k_{b0} * \exp(-z_b VF/RT)$, where $k_{f0} = k_f$ at V = 0, $k_{b0} = k_b$ at V = 0, z_f and z_b are the valences of the forward and backward gating transitions, and R, F, and T have their usual thermodynamic meaning. The model has 16 closed states, corresponding to all possible permutations of four subunits. The closed state with all subunits in the permissive conformation is linked to a single open state via voltage-independent rate constants (opening rate constant $k_o = 30,000$/sec, closing rate constant $k_c = 2,200$/sec; see refs. 20 and 25). Parameters for independent model: WT: $k_{f0} = 2,447$/sec, $k_{b0} = 94$/sec, $z_t = z_f + z_b = 1.7$ electronic charges (*e*) per sensor. R2N: $k_{f0} = 18,100$/sec, $k_{b0} = 12$/sec, $z_t = 1.5$ *e*. Cooperative model: WT: $k_{f0} = 376$/sec, $k_{b0} = 645$/sec, $z_t = 1.3$ *e*. R2N: $k_{f0} = 1,507$/sec, $k_{b0} = 153$/sec, $z_t = 1.1$ *e*. In the cooperative model, a factor k_{coop} was defined such that for the transition of a subunit with a neighboring subunit in the permissive state, k_f was set to $k_{f*}k_{coop}$ and k_b to k_b/k_{coop}. The curves in b were obtained with $k_{coop} = 6$. **(c)** Voltages of 50% activation ($V_{0.5}$, filled symbols) and 10% activation ($V_{0.1}$, open symbols) for the indicated channel constructs. Symbols are mean + SEM of 6, 4, 6, 4, and 35 measurements (**left** to **right**). Curves are model fits with same parameters as in (a) and (b). The more positive voltages are those predicted by the independent model. **(d)** Current traces: WT-R2N-WT-WT with holding potential (h.p.) −140 mV and test potentials (t.p.) −80, −60, and −40 mV; WT-R2N (h.p. −160 mV; t.p. −100, −70, and −40 mV); WT-R2N-R2N-R2N (h.p. −160 mV; t.p. −120, −100, and −80 mV); and R2N (h.p. −180 mV; t.p. −140, −100, and −60 mV). Scale bars: 100 msec and 200 nA (**left traces**), 2 µA (**right**). [From Tytgat and Hess (46).]

combinations of WT and R2N subunits. As can be concluded from Fig. 3a, the model that assumes independent gating of subunits cannot account for the gating phenotypes observed with the three different combinations of WT and R2N subunits. The observed shifts in the activation curves are substantially larger than the shifts predicted by the model with independent gating, and this applies to each of the WT-R2N combinations. Qualitatively, this is the result expected if subunits were gating in a cooperative way: in this case, the presence of an R2N subunit that gates at more negative potentials will tend to promote the conformational change of a neighboring WT subunit, thus shifting the activation curve to more negative potentials than would be observed with independent movement of individual subunits. A quantitative fit of the same data to a model that incorporates positive cooperativity is shown in Fig. 3b. Herein, the forward (opening) transition rate constant for each subunit is multiplied by a cooperativity factor k_{coop} ($= 6$), and the backward rate constant divided by k_{coop} ($= 6$), if a neighboring subunit has already undergone the voltage-dependent forward transition. The observed activation curves for all WT-R2N combinations are predicted nicely with an equilibrium cooperativity factor $= 36$. Mean values of voltage shifts observed in 4 to 10 oocytes for each of the five combinations of WT-R2N constructs confirm the greatly superior fit to the data by the cooperative versus the noncooperative model (Fig. 3c).

Voltage Dependence of "R4-mutated" Channels

To date no functional expression of RCK1 K⁺ channel has been observed, when the fourth positive residue, (R4), in the S4 segment is neutralized (20, 21). However, the construction of heteromultimeric tetramers containing WT and mutant R4I subunits has allowed us to obtain functional expression for the first time. This is an interesting result, because it helps to elucidate why mutant homomultimeric R4I channels do not express K⁺ currents in RCK1. Steady-state activation curves obtained with tetramers made of combinations of WT subunits and mutant subunits in which the fourth Arg residue in S4 has been mutated to Ile (R4I) are shown in Fig. 4. The activation curves shift toward more negative potentials and the steepness of activation decreases with each substitution of a WT subunit by an R4I mutant. The voltage dependence of activation, expressed in mV/e-fold change, is nearly inversely proportional to the number of WT subunits present in each tetramer, as can be concluded from a plot of the limiting slope of activation for each WT-R4I combination (Fig. 4c). This result suggests that over the testable voltage range, the voltage dependence observed for activation is primarily determined by gating of the WT subunits. This implies that R4I subunits are stuck in a "permissive" conformation, even at potentials negative to -180 mV. That is, the voltage dependence of activation for R4I mutant subunits appears shifted to extremely negative potentials. mRNA coding for R4I subunits alone failed to produce

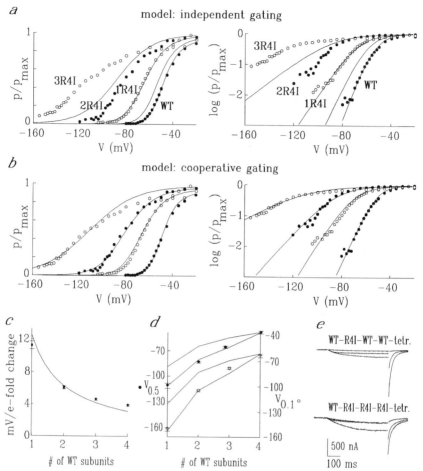

Figure 4. Tetramers containing combinations of WT and R4I mutant subunits. (**a, b**) Steady-state activation curves from WT channels and tetrameric cDNAs in which either 1 (1R4I), 2 (2R4I), or 3 (3R4I) WT subunits were substituted with mutant subunits R4I. Solid lines: model predictions for independent (a) or cooperative gating (b). Model parameters for WT subunits as in Fig. 3. For R4I subunits, $k_{b0} = 0$ (i.e., the activation of R4I subunits is assumed to be shifted to infinitely negative potentials). In b, $k_{coop} = 6$, as in Fig. 3b. (**c**) Exponential slopes of steady-state activation curves at low values of P, expressed as mV/e-fold change of fractional activation. Values are means + SEM from 24, 70, 9, and 35 oocytes (**left** to **right**). The solid line indicates the expected slopes for the case the observed voltage dependence of activation was contributed by the WT subunits. (**d**) Voltages of 50% activation ($V_{0.5}$, filled symbols) and 10% activation ($V_{0.1}$, open symbols) for WT-R4I combinations. Symbols are means ± SEM of 24, 70, 9, and 35 measurements (**left** to **right**). Curves are model fits with same parameters as in (a) and (b). The more positive voltages are those predicted by the independent model. (**e**) Current traces: WT-R4I-WT-WT ([holding potential (h.p.) −120 mV; testing potential (t.p.) −90, −70, and −40 mV)]; WT-R4I-R4I-R4I (h.p. −180 mV; t.p. −150, −120, and −80 mV). [From Tytgat and Hess (46).]

measurable time-dependent currents in oocytes, consistent with the expectation that channels should be permanently inactivated at holding potentials much more positive than the voltage range of activation (48). If we make the assumption that R4I channels are never in the closed state (i.e., their voltage dependence of activation is shifted to infinitely negative potentials), the maximal shift in activation the model with independent subunit gating is capable of producing becomes as shown in Fig. 4a. Clearly, the observed voltage shifts considerably exceed those predicted by the noncooperative model, as was the case with WT-R2N tetramers. However, the cooperative model, with the same k_{coop} (= 6) and equilibrium cooperativity factor (= 36) used to fit the WT-R2N combinations, nicely fits the activation curves of the WT-R4I mixtures (Fig. 4b). Mean values of voltage shifts observed in 9 to 35 oocytes for each of the four combinations of WT-R4I constructs confirm the superior fit to the data by the cooperative versus the noncooperative model (Fig. 4d).

Conclusions

The gating of heterotetramers strongly suggests that individual K⁺ channel subunits do not gate independently, but show positive cooperativity. Our conclusions about cooperative gating of individual voltage sensors are based on a modeling of steady-state activation curves. We do not propose that this model, with a single voltage-dependent gating transition for each subunit, is mechanistically correct; other gating schemes with more transitions can equally well be made to fit a particular activation curve. However, cooperativity among individual voltage sensors seems to provide a simpler explanation for these observed gating phenotypes (19, 34–36, 38). Positive cooperativity among individual subunits appears to be a useful mechanism for voltage-activated ion channels, because it allows the channel to maximize the voltage sensitivity of gating for any given number of intramembrane gating charges contained in a voltage sensing segment.

Our findings also demonstrate that the subunit composition of RCK1 K⁺ channels can reproducibly be manipulated by constructing homo- and heteromultimeric tetrameric cDNAs. In addition to revealing information on subunit interactions, such tetrameric constructs permit obtaining functional expression on channels containing mutated subunits that by themselves do not produce measurable currents (e.g., R4I; see refs. 20 and 21, and unpublished results). In addition, our findings with WT-R4I tetramers illustrates an important point concerning interpretation of changes in the steepness of activation. This parameter cannot be used to estimate the total equivalent gating charge of a channel in which a mutation confined to a single domain or subunit has caused a voltage shift of that voltage sensor (18). Thus we cannot assess whether charge neutralization of the fourth Arg in S4 (R4I) had an effect on the gating valence of its voltage sensor. On the contrary, the apparent large negative voltage shift produced by the mutation at R4 has simply removed its voltage sensor from the testable voltage range, and the steepness of activation in the WT-R4I tetramers is dominated by the fewer remaining WT subunits in these constructs.

Acknowledgments

This work was supported by a grant from the National Heart, Lung, and Blood Institute, NIH (HL-37124), and fellowships to J.T. from BAEF (Francqui-Fund), Fulbright, and NATO. P.H. is an Established Investigator of the American Heart Association.

We thank Drs. G. Koren, B. Nadal-Ginard, F. Weaver, and D. Melton for critical materials. Drs. R. MacKinnon, F. McKeon, D. Finley, and I. Wefes provided technical advice. Drs. K. Chua, K. Nakazawa, A. Gross, A. Rittenhouse, E. Liman, D. Slish, and C. Kuo provided helpful suggestions.

References

1. Hodgkin, A.L., and Huxley, A.F. (1952). A quantitative description of membrane current and its application to conduction and excitation in nerve. *J. Physiol. (Lond.)* **117:**500–544.

2. Gilly, W.F., and Armstrong, C.M. (1980). Gating current and potassium channels in the giant axon of the squid. *Biophys. J.* **29:**485–492.

3. Bezanilla, F., White, M.M., and Taylor, R.E. (1982). Gating currents associated with potassium channel activation. *Nature* **296:**657–659.

4. Armstrong, C.M. (1981). Sodium channels and gating currents. *Physiol. Rev.* **61:**644–683.

5. Catterall, W.A. (1988). Structure and function of voltage-sensitive ion channels. *Science* **242:**50–61.

6. Jan, L.Y., and Jan, Y.N. (1989). Voltage-sensitive ion channels. *Cell* **56:**13–25.

7. Miller, C. (1989). Genetic manipulation of ion channels: A new approach to structure and mechanism. *Neuron* **2:**1195–1205.

8. Noda, M., Shimizu, S., Tanabe, T., Takai, T., Kayano, T., Ikeda, T., Takahashi, H., Nakayama, H., Kanaoka, Y., Minamino, N., Kangawa, K., Matsuo, H., Raftery, M.A., Hirose, T., Inayama, S., Hayashida, H. Miyata, T., and Numa, S. (1984). Primary structure of *Electrophorus electricus* sodium channel deduced from cDNA sequence. *Nature* **312:**121–127.

9. Tanabe, T., Takeshima, H., Mikami, A., Flockerzi, V., Takahashi, H., Kangawa, K., Kojima, M., Matsuo, H., Hirose, T., and Numa, S. (1987). Primary structure of the receptor for calcium channel blockers from skeletal muscle. *Nature* **328:**313–318.

10. Papazian, D.M., Schwarz, T.L., Tempel, B.L., Jan, Y.N., and Jan, L.Y. (1987). Cloning of genomic and complementary DNA from *Shaker*, a putative potassium channel gene from *Drosophila*. *Science* **237:**749–753.

11. Kamb, A., Iverson, L.E., and Tanouye, M.A. (1987). Molecular characterization of *Shaker*, a *Drosophila* gene that encodes a potassium channel. *Cell* **50:**405–413.

12. Pongs, O., Kecskemethy, N., Müller, R., Krah-Jentgens, I., Baumann, A., Kiltz, II.II., Canal, I., Llamazares, S., and Ferrus, A. (1988). *Shaker* encodes a

family of putative potassium channel proteins in the nervous system of *Drosophila*. *EMBO J.* **7**:1087–1096.

13. Timpe, L.C., Schwarz, T.L., Tempel, B.L., Papazian, D.M., Jan, Y.N., and Jan, L.Y. (1988). Expression of functional potassium channels from *Shaker* cDNA in *Xenopus* oocytes. *Nature* **331**:143–145.

14. Iverson, L.E., Tanouye, M.A., Lester, H.A., Davidson, N., and Rudy, B. (1988). A-type potassium channels expressed from *Shaker* locus cDNA. *Proc. Natl. Acad. Sci. U.S.A.* **85**:5723–5727.

15. Butler, A., Wei, A., Baker, K., and Salkoff, L. (1989). A family of putative potassium channel genes in *Drosophila*. *Science* **243**:943–947.

16. Greenblatt, R.E., Blatt, Y., and Montal, M. (1985). The structure of the voltage-sensitive sodium channel. *FEBS Lett.* **193**:125–134.

17. Noda, M., Ikeda, T., Kayano, T., Suzuki, H., Takeshima, H., Kurasaki, M., Takahashi, H., and Numa, S. (1986). Existence of distinct sodium channel messenger RNAs in rat brain. *Nature* **320**:188–192.

18. Stühmer, W., Conti, F., Suzuki, H., Wang, X., Noda, M., Yahagi, N., Kubo, H., and Numa, S. (1989a). Structural parts involved in activation and inactivation of the sodium channel. *Nature* **339**:597–603.

19. Papazian, D.M., Timpe, L.C., Jan, Y.N., and Jan, L.Y. (1991). Alteration of voltage-dependence of *Shaker* potassium channel by mutations in the S4 sequence. *Nature* **349**:305–310.

20. Liman, E.R., Hess, P., Weaver, F., and Koren, G. (1991). Voltage-sensing residues in the S4 region of a mammalian K+ channel. *Nature* **353**:752–756.

21. Logothetis, D.E., Movahedi, S., Satler, C., Lindpaintner, K., and Nadal-Ginard, B. (1992). Incremental reductions of positive charge within the S4 region of a voltage-gated K+ channel result in corresponding decreases in gating charge. *Neuron* **8**:531–540.

22. Auld, V.J., Goldin, A.L., Krafte, D.S., Catterall, W.A., Lester, H.A., Davidson, N., and Dunn, R.J. (1990). A neutral amino acid change in segment IIS4 dramatically alters gating properties of the voltage-dependent sodium channel. *Proc. Natl. Acad. Sci. U.S.A.* **87**:323–327.

23. McCormack, K., Tanouye, M.A., Iverson, L.E., Lin, J.-W., Ramaswami, M., McCormack, T., Campanelli, J.T., Mathew, M.K., and Rudy, B. (1991). A role for hydrophobic residues in the voltage-dependent gating of *Shaker* K+ channels. *Proc. Natl. Acad. Sci. U.S.A.* **88**:2931–2935.

24. Lopez, G.A., Jan, Y.N., and Jan, L.Y. (1991). Hydrophobic substitution mutations in the S4 sequence alter voltage-dependent gating in *Shaker* K+ channels. *Neuron* **7**:327–336.

25. Koren, G., Liman, E.R., Logothetis, D.E., Nadal-Ginard, B., and Hess, P. (1990). Gating mechanism of a cloned potassium channel expressed in frog oocytes and mammalian cells. *Neuron* **2**:39–51.

26. Frech, G.C., VanDongen, A.M.J., Schuster, G., Brown, A.M., and Joho, R.H. (1989). A novel potassium channel with delayed rectifier properties isolated from rat brain by expression cloning. *Nature* **340**:642–645.

27. Christie, M.J., Adelman, J.P., Douglass, J., and North, R.A. (1989). Expression of a cloned rat brain potassium channel in *Xenopus* oocytes. *Science* **244**:221–224.

28. Stühmer, W., Ruppersberg, J.P., Schröter, K.H., Sakmann, B., Stocker, M., Giese, K.P., Perschke, A., Baumann, A., and Pongs, O. (1989b). Molecular basis of functional diversity of voltage-gated potassium channels in mammalian brain. *EMBO J.* **8:**3235–3244.

29. Baumann, A., Grupe, A., Ackermann, A., and Pongs, O. (1988). Structure of the voltage-dependent potassium channel is highly conserved from *Drosophila* to vertebrate central nervous systems. *EMBO J.* **7:**2457–2463.

30. Grupe, A., Schröter, K.H., Ruppersberg, J.P., Stocker, M., Drewes, T., Beckh, S., and Pongs, O. (1990). Cloning and expression of a human voltage-gated potassium channel. A novel member of the RCK potassium channel family. *EMBO J.* **9:**1749–1756.

31. MacKinnon, R. (1991). Determination of the subunit stoichiometry of a voltage-activated potassium channel. *Nature* **350:**232–235.

32. Zagotta, W.N., and Aldrich, R.W. (1990). Voltage-dependent gating of *Shaker* A-type potassium channels in *Drosophila* muscle. *J. Gen. Physiol.* **95:**29–60.

33. Monod, J., Wyman, J., and Changeux, J.-P. (1965). On the nature of allosteric transitions: a plausible model. *J. Mol. Biol.* **12:**88–118.

34. Gilly, W.F., and Armstrong, C.M. (1982). Divalent cations and the activation kinetics of potassium channels in squid giant axons. *J. Gen. Physiol.* **79:**965–996.

35. Stühmer, W., Conti, F., Stocker, M., Pongs, O., and Heinemann, S.H. (1991). Gating currents of inactivating and non-inactivating potassium channels expressed in *Xenopus* oocytes. *Pflügers Arch.* **418:**423–429.

36. Bezanilla, F., Perozo, E., Papazian, D.M., and Stefani, E. (1991). Molecular basis of gating charge immobilization in *Shaker* potassium channels. *Science* **254:**679–683.

37. Vandenberg, C.A., and Bezanilla, F. (1991). A sodium channel gating model based on single-channel, macroscopic ionic, and gating currents in the squid giant axon. *Biophys. J.* **60:**1511–1533.

38. Schoppa, N.E., McCormack, K., Tanouye, M.A., and Sigworth, F.J. (1992). The size of gating charge in wild-type and mutant *Shaker* potassium channels. *Science* **255:**1712–1715.

39. Krieg, P.A., and Melton, D.A. (1984). Functional messenger RNAs are produced by SP6 in vitro transcription of cloned cDNAs. *Nucleic Acids Res.* **12:**7057–7070.

40. Swenson, R.P., and Armstrong, C.M. (1981). K^+ channels close more slowly in the presence of external K^+ and Rb^+. *Nature* **291:**427–429.

41. Isacoff, E.Y., Jan, Y.N., and Jan, L.Y. (1990). Evidence for the formation of heteromultimeric potassium channels in *Xenopus* oocytes. *Nature* **345:**530–534.

42. Heginbotham, L., and MacKinnon, R. (1992). The aromatic binding site for tetraethylammonium ion on potassium channels. *Neuron* **8:**483–491.

43. Kavanaugh, M.P., Hurst, R.S., Yakel, J., Varnum, M.D., Adelman, J.P., and North, R.A. (1992). Multiple subunits of a voltage-dependent potassium channel contribute to the binding site for tetraethylammonium. *Neuron* **8:**493–497.

44. Hurst, R.S., Kavanaugh, M.P., North, R.A., and Adelman, J.P. (1992). Construction of functional potassium channel from four covalently linked subunits. *Biophys. J.* **61**:A425.

45. Tytgat, J., and Hess, P. (1992a). Dimeric and tetrameric channels made from wildtype and mutant RCK1-K channels. *Biophys. J.* **61**:A426.

46. Tytgat, J., and Hess, P. (1992b). Evidence for cooperative interactions in potassium channel gating. *Nature* **359**:420–423.

47. Liman, E.R., Tytgat, J., and Hess, P. (1992). Subunit stoichiometry of a mammalian K⁺ channel determined by construction of multimeric cDNAs. *Neuron* **9**:861–871.

48. Hille, B. (1992). *Ionic Channels of Excitable Membranes* (Sinauer Associates, Inc., Sunderland, MA).

15

Molecular Physiology of Voltage-Gated Potassium and Sodium Channels: Ion Channel Diversity within the Cardiovascular System

Michael M. Tamkun, Timothy J. Knittle, Karen K. Deal,
Melissa H. House, Steven L. Roberds, Sunny Po,
Paul B. Bennett, Alfred L. George, Jr.,
and Dirk J. Snyders

Electrically excitable cells of the heart display a complex and unique action potential. The depolarizing phase is mediated by a rapid influx of Na^+ ions via voltage-sensitive Na^+ channels and is followed by a rapid, but incomplete early repolarization due to K^+ efflux through transiently active K^+ channels. This transient outward current in part determines action potential duration. The plateau phase follows and is dominated by Ca^{2+} influx that inactivates and a rising K^+ permeability that ultimately repolarizes the cell. Not only is the cardiac action potential interesting from a basic science standpoint, but its modification is an important mode of therapeutic intervention. Both presently used antiarrhythmic drugs, as well as agents under development, modify action potential characteristics. Because the voltage-gated channels of the cardiac sarcolemma are the pharmacological targets of these agents, ion channel proteins are of tremendous clinical importance. Clearly, our knowledge of the structure, function, regulation, and molecular pharmacology of these channels must be increased to achieve important clinical goals.

This chapter reviews the progress that our laboratories have made over the past 3 years in understanding the structural and functional diversity of the voltage-gated K^+ and Na^+ channels in mammalian myocardium. The Na^+ and K^+ channel field has grown tremendously over the past several years. Thus this chapter makes no attempt to review this vast literature. Rather, the findings of our research group, as they pertain to cardiac ion channel diversity, are presented. Data discussed represent our first attempts to understand the physiological and pharmacological roles cloned ion channels play within the heart.

Cardiac K⁺ Channel Diversity

It was once generally accepted that voltage-dependent K^+ currents in the heart could be divided between a slowly activating delayed rectifier, I_K, the inward rectifier, I_{K1}, and the transient outward current, I_{to} (1). However, recent whole-cell voltage clamp (2, 3) and patch-clamp (4, 5) studies indicate that the number of functionally distinct K^+ channels in heart is greater than once perceived. As shown in Table 1, at least seven voltage-gated K^+ channels have been described thus far in mammalian heart, and more channels will likely be discovered. The inward rectifier (I_{K1}) opens at relatively negative membrane potentials (6) and is mainly responsible for maintaining the resting potential in atrial (7, 8) and ventricular cells (6, 7). At least two components of the delayed rectifier, I_{Kr} and I_{Ks}, exist in the guinea pig atrium (2) and ventricle (5, 9). An additional noninactivating K^+ current in guinea pig ventricular myocytes, which is detected only with the patch-clamp technique, has been termed the plateau current (I_{Kp}) (4). Boyle and Nerbonne (10) have observed a depolarization-activated, noninactivating K^+ current in adult rat atrial myocytes that is distinct from I_{Kr}. Two subtypes of the transient outward current may exist in mouse (5) and dog (11)

Table 1. Voltage-gated K^+ currents in the heart

Name	Description	Location	Blockers or Inhibitors
I_{to1}	Inactivating	V	4-AP, quinidine
I_{to2}*	Inactivating	V	Mg^{2+}, caffeine
I_{Kr}	Rapidly activating Noninactivating	A & V	E-4031, sotalol, quinidine, UK-68,798
I_{Ks}	Slowly activating Noninactivating	A & V	Clofilium, quinidine, amiodarone
I_{Kp}	Rapidly activating Noninactivating	V	Ba^{2+}
Boyle	Rapidly activating Noninactivating	A	4-AP
I_{K1}	Inward rectifier Open at hyperpolarizing voltages	A & V	TEA, Cs^{2+}

A, atrium; V, ventricle.
*Recent evidence suggests that a 4-AP insensitive I_{to} current in rabbit ventricle may be carried by Cl^- ions (13).

ventricles and in human atrium (12), although it is possible the I_{to2} current is carried by Cl^- ions (13). In addition, the shape of the action potential changes during cardiac development, in part caused by changes in K^+ currents. A transient outward current increases 4-fold during the first 10 days after birth, whereas the inward rectifier decreases 3-fold over the same period (14, 15). It is reasonable to assume that the diversity and developmental regulation of cardiac K^+ channels is much more complex than previously thought.

Some native myocyte K^+ currents may be masked by larger currents during whole-cell voltage-clamp recordings. This does not mean they are physiologically or pharmacologically insignificant, for these currents can have important effects on the action potential. The plateau phase of the action potential is a delicate balance of inward and outward currents with little net ion flow, so components such as I_{Kr} and I_{Kp} can have a significant effect. For example, the agent E-4031 blocks I_{Kr}, only one component of I_K, but results in action potential prolongation (2). Another reason for suspecting that additional cardiac K^+ channels remain to be discovered is that native myocyte voltage-clamp studies are performed only on those cells that survive enzymatic dissociation. Perhaps physiologically important myocytes, with unique K^+ channels, do not dissociate or survive dissociation. Because the heart is an electrical syncytium, a few cells with unique electrical properties could influence large regions of myocardium. Also, the disaggregation process using enzyme treatments may inactivate some channels, while leaving others unaltered.

The presence of multiple overlapping currents in cardiac myocytes complicates the study of individual K^+ channels. A traditional approach uses a combination of holding potential modulation, ion substitution, and pharmacological dissection to eliminate all but the current of interest. However, these approaches have limitations. For example, divalent cations used to block Ca^{2+} currents may modify gating properties of K^+ channels (16). Therefore, it is desirable to study individual channels in a system without contaminating currents and in physiological solutions. One method to achieve this would be to purify individual K^+ channels from the heart and study their function in reconstituted membranes, as has been done for brain Na^+ channels (17). However, purification of K^+ channels has been frustrated by a lack of high-affinity, channel-specific ligands with which to purify the protein following membrane solubilization. Although several neurotoxins have recently been used for this purpose, these toxins are unlikely to be specific for one K^+ channel isoform. Thus, multiple isoforms are expected within any purified K^+ channel sample. Another problem is the low number of K^+ channels present in cardiac myocytes. Electrophysiological experiments indicate that as few as 1,000 to 5,000 copies of some K^+ channels are present in the membrane of a typical cardiac myocyte (unpublished data). Biochemical purification of protein present at such a low level is difficult. The problems of isoform diversity and low abundance are circumvented by the use of molecular cloning and cDNA expression technologies, allowing the study of a single cloned isoform in the expression system of choice. However, as discussed later, this approach poses a new challenge in terms of correlating cloned channels with endogenous currents.

Cardiac Sodium Channel Diversity

Although the functional diversity of voltage-gated Na^+ channels in excitable membranes is not as extensive as that for voltage-dependent K^+ channels, there is evidence for the existence of functional phenotypes not clearly represented by previously identified Na^+ channel isoforms. Specifically, a class of Na^+ channels exhibiting activation and inactivation kinetics significantly slower than those responsible for the fast inward Na^+ current of the action potential have been described in heart (18–22), glia (23), and in some neuronal preparations (24). These channels may be important physiologically and may also participate in the pathogenesis of certain diseases. Recent work suggests functionally distinct Na^+ channels exist in the cardiac sarcolemma that are easily masked by larger currents as previously discussed (22).

The predominant Na^+ channel isoform in adult heart is resistant (K_D = 5 μM) to tetrodotoxin (TTX), and this channel is responsible for most of the Na^+ current observed in mammalian cardiac myocytes (25). This TTX-resistant Na^+ channel is also expressed in skeletal muscle during early development and following denervation (26). In addition, two other structurally defined Na^+ channel isoforms have been found in heart. There is evidence that both the rat brain I isoform (27) and another partially characterized Na^+ channel cDNA sequence (28) are also present in heart, but their exact cellular location is unknown. The presence of other functional Na^+ channels in heart is supported by both pharmacological and electrophysiological studies. In rat heart homogenates, ~20% of the binding sites for saxitoxin exhibit high affinity, and these data may indicate the presence of a Na^+ channel isoform other than the predominant TTX-resistant channel (26). One group has described a TTX- and Mn^{2+}-insensitive slow Na^+ channel in the myocardial membranes of genetically cardiomyopathic hamsters (29) and in skeletal muscle fibers excised from patients with Duchenne muscular dystrophy (30). The functional attributes of this type of Na^+ channel are quite distinct from channels that have been expressed from cDNA and indicate the existence of a distinct class of Na^+ channels. In addition, voltage-clamp recordings of normal heart cells from a variety of species have demonstrated the existence of a class of low-amplitude, Na^+- and voltage-dependent, slow inward currents that may contribute to the plateau phase of the cardiac action potential (18, 19, 21, 30). Noninactivating inward currents are often attributed to Ca^{2+} channels but the discovery of such a current that is TTX-sensitive suggests some of these noninactivating inward currents are caused by unusual Na^+ channels (22). Taken together, these observations suggest the existence of a class of voltage-dependent, Na^+ conducting channels that exhibit very distinct functional properties from the predominant cardiac Na^+ channel.

At the present time, only a limited number of highly related mammalian Na^+ channel isoforms have been characterized by the molecular cloning approach. One partial and five full-length Na^+ channel cDNA sequences have been cloned from rat brain or rat cardiac and skeletal muscle (27, 28, 31–34). All of these reported mammalian cDNA sequences predict proteins that exhibit striking similarity to one another ($>80\%$ overall amino acid sequence identity) and appear to comprise a single multigene family. There is evidence that this Na^+ channel gene family has related members in such diverse species as eel (35), *Drosophila* (36, 37), and man (38–40).

Na^+ channels are thought to have a common ancestry with other voltage-dependent ion channels and appear to have most recently evolved from K^+ channels via two rounds of gene duplication (41). In view of the extensive structural diversity that exists among members of the voltage-dependent K^+ channel family, it is surprising that a greater variety of mammalian Na^+ channel isoforms has not been identified by the molecular cloning approach.

Cardiac K^+ Channel Cloning

The rapid advances that have occurred in K^+ channel molecular biology are primarily due to a *Drosophila* mutant strain, *Shaker*, which has altered K^+ channel activity. Several laboratories identified the *Shaker* locus (42, 43), leading to the cloning of the first voltage-gated K^+ channel. The *Shaker* K^+ channel cDNA encodes a protein with a molecular weight of 70,200 (42). This protein has six potential membrane-spanning domains. The fourth such domain is an arginine- and lysine-rich region (the S4 domain), which is thought to be involved in the voltage-sensing function of the protein (44, 45). Expression studies in *Xenopus* oocytes have confirmed that additional proteins are not required for voltage-sensitive K^+ transport (46) and that a tetramer of channel subunits is the likely structure (47, 48).

The original *Shaker* clone was used to screen mouse brain cDNA libraries and isolate the first mammalian K^+ channel with homology to *Shaker* (42, 48a). The amino acid sequence that was conserved between the *Drosophila* and mouse brain channels, and therefore assumed to be functionally important, was used by our laboratory to screen for homologous K^+ channels in mammalian heart. By first using degenerate primers with the polymerase chain reaction to clone fragments of new channels, and then using these fragments to screen unamplified libraries, our laboratory cloned five distinct voltage-gated K^+ channel cDNAs from rat and human heart as summarized in Table 2. Two additional channels present in heart [Kv2.1 (49) and I_{sk} (50)], but not originally cloned by our laboratory, are also listed. Several of these channels were cloned simultaneously by multiple laboratories, causing near identical clones to be given different names. Hence a universal nomenclature has been proposed (51). The "Kv" designates a voltage-gated K^+ channel, the first number designates the *Drosophila* subfamily to which the clone is most homologous, and the second number indicates the order in which a given clone was identified. Kv1 family members are homologues of the *Drosophila Shaker* K^+ channel. Human Kv1.4 is 98% identical to rat Kv1.4, whereas what appears to be human Kv1.5 is only 86% identical to rat Kv1.5. Most of the nonidentity occurs in the amino- and carboxyl-terminal regions, which have 64% and 75% identity, respectively. Whether such amino acid differences represent interspecies variation or indicate that human and rat Kv1.5 represent different K^+ channel isoforms is still in question.

As summarized in Table 2, none of the K^+ channels cloned from heart are specific to cardiac tissue and Kv1.1, Kv1.2, and Kv4.2 mRNAs are much more abundant in brain than they are in heart. In contrast, Kv1.4 and Kv1.5 are expressed at higher levels in heart than in brain, whereas Kv2.1 transcripts are present at equivalent levels in brain and heart. Interestingly, rat Kv1.5 mRNA is equally expressed between rat atrium and ventricle (52), whereas human Kv1.5 transcripts are at least 10- to 20-fold more abundant in human atrium than in ventricle (53). The question remains as to whether these channels are present in cells other than cardiac myocytes, such as endothelial or smooth muscle cells, because RNA blots, from which these data were derived, do not indicate which cells in each tissue express each mRNA. Arguing against the channels being present only in a ubiquitous cell type, such as vascular smooth muscle or endothelial cells, is the absence of channel mRNA in liver and the varied levels of expression within atrium, ventricle, aorta, and skeletal muscle. If these channels were simply of endothelial or smooth muscle origin, mRNA expression would be expected to be less tissue-specific. However, this statement assumes that endothelial and smooth muscle cells express the same K^+ channel isoforms regardless of the tissue location of the vascular bed, an assumption that may be incorrect.

The developmental expression of Kv1.1, 1.2, 1.4, and 1.5; Kv4.2; and Kv2.1 was examined using RNA blot analysis (54). Kv1.4 mRNA is detected at low levels at embryonic day 14, but it reaches ~10- to 20-fold higher levels at embryonic day 20 and remains high. Kv1.5 mRNA is present at high, relatively equal levels at all four time points examined. Kv2.1 is somewhat intermediate, being absent at embryonic day 14, but detectable at embryonic day 20 and abundant at day 10 and 20 postbirth. Continuous expression from embryonic day 14 suggests that Kv1.4 and Kv1.5 are essential to cardiac function throughout development. In contrast, Kv1.1, Kv1.2, and Kv4.2 are absent or extremely low during early cardiac development but increase

Table 2. Cloned K⁺ Channels from Rat and Human Heart

Universal Name	Original Designation	Relative Tissue Distribution
Shaker-related		
rKv1.1	RK1, RBK1, RCHK1	Brain » Atrium > Skeletal Muscle > Aorta
rKv1.2	RK2, RBK2, RCK5	Brain > Atrium > Aorta = Ventricle
rKv1.4/hKv1.4	RK3, RCK4, RHK1, hPCN2	Atrium > Brain > Aorta > Ventricle = Skeletal Muscle
rKv1.5/hKv1.5	RK4, Kv1, hPCN1	Atrium > Ventricle = Aorta > Skeletal Muscle > Brain
Shab-related		
rKv2.1	drk1, MShab	Brain = Atrium = Aorta > Ventricle
Shal-related		
rKv4.2	RK5, MShal, Rat Shal	Brain » Ventricle = Atrium
Non-*Drosophila*-related		
I_{sk}	minK	Heart = Kidney = Diethylstilbestrol-Primed Uterus = Pancreas > Stomach

dramatically between days 10 and 20 following birth. Therefore, these channels may play a modulatory role as the heart develops further. These changes may partially explain the shortening of the cardiac action potential in the rat during maturation of the heart after birth (14, 15) and may provide clues as to which native currents the clones represent.

The deduced amino acid sequences of rat Kv 1.1, 1.2, 1.4, and 1.5, and Kv4.2 are shown in Fig. 1. The likely transmembrane regions are underlined and the putative N-linked glycosylation sites indicated by bold-face type. Potential protein kinase A phosphorylation sites are circled and protein kinase C sites are boxed. Two distinct clones of the Kv4.2 channel were sequenced and found to differ by the deletion of two nucleotides in the C-terminal encoding region, thereby shifting the reading frame and resulting in two channels with differing C-terminal amino acid number and sequence. The Kv4.2 sequence presented in Fig. 1 represents the longer clone and that published earlier (54) represents the clone with the two deleted bases. Because both versions of Kv4.2 express in both oocytes and L-cells at the same level and with identical kinetics, the role of the C-terminal sequence is not clear (55–57). Given this lack of functional difference between the versions, it is possible that they represent allelic polymorphisms as opposed to a simple cloning artifact.

Functional Expression of Cloned Cardiovascular K$^+$ Channels

The K$^+$ channel clones previously described have been expressed either transiently in *Xenopus* oocytes (49, 50, 56, 58–64) or in tissue culture as stable cell lines (65, 66; Fig. 2). Both systems produce similar currents for a given isoform, indicating that observed properties accurately reflect channel function (unpublished data). Figure 2 shows currents generated by expression of Kv1.1, 1.2, 1.4, 1.5, and 4.2 clones in mouse L-cells. The channel phenotypes were clearly clone-specific, and sham-transfected cells expressed no voltage-dependent currents under the conditions used. All currents shown activate within 20 msec. Among these five channels, the time to peak ranges from 3 to 20 msec at a 20 mV test potential, with Kv1.1 and Kv4.2 activating most rapidly and Kv1.2 most slowly. In contrast to the currents in Fig. 2, I$_{sK}$ expressed in oocytes is not maximally activated even after 20 sec at a test potential of 50 mV (50, 67–69). Kv1.4 and Kv4.2 display nearly complete inactivation, Kv1.1 shows little inactivation, and Kv1.2 and Kv1.5 show varying degrees of slow inactivation. The activation and inactivation observed with these channels increases markedly with temperature in the L-cell expression system (unpublished data). This suggests that cloned channels characterized at or near room temperature will behave very differently at more physiological temperatures.

The pharmacological sensitivities of the cloned K$^+$ channels are summarized in Table 3. This pharmacology aids in the correlation of cloned channels with endogenous currents as described. We have observed no

```
Kv4.2    1                                              MTVmsGenaDEA
Kv1.1    1                                              MTVatGdpvDEA
Kv1.2    1
Kv1.5    1 ME                            islvplengsAmtlrGGG  EAgascvQT
Kv1.4    1 MEvamvsaessgcnshmpygyaaqararererlahsraaaaaavaaatAavegtGGsgggphhhhQTr

Kv4.2    1                maagvaawlpfaraAA
Kv1.1   13                           sAA    P    GHPQ           D
Kv1.2   13                           aA    LP    GHPQ           D           ty
Kv1.5   30    prgecgcpptsglnnqskeTllrgrttledanqggrpLPPmaqElPQpRrLS  aEDEE      gEg
Kv1.4   69  gaysshdpqgsrgsrrrrqrTpkkklhhrqssfphcsdLmPsgsEekilReLSeeeEDEEeeeeeEe

Kv4.2   17                     igwmpvasgpmpapprqerkrCgdaliVlNvSGtRFqTwqdTLeryPdTLLG
Kv1.1   22                         gsyprQadhdDHECCERVVINISGLRFETQLKTLAQFPnTLLG
Kv1.2   24 DP                          eADHECCERVVINISGLRFETQLKTLAQFPeTLLG
Kv1.5   90 DPglgtvEED          qaPQD      AgSlhhqRVlINISGLRFETQLgTLAQFPnTLLG
Kv1.4  137 egrfyysEEDhgdgcsytdllPQDdgggggysSvrySdCCERVVINvSGLRFETQmKTLAQFPeTLLG

Kv4.2   69  sseRdffyhPetqqYFFDRdpdiFrhILnfYrGklhyprhecisaydeElaffFglipEiigdccyE
Kv1.1   65  nPKKRMRYFDPLRNEYFFDRNRPSFDAILYYYQSGGRLRRPVNVPLDmFSEEIkFYELGEEAMEkFRE
Kv1.2   61  DPKKRMRYFDPLRNEYFFDRNRPSFDgILYYYQSGGRLRRPVNVsLDvFadEIRYQLGdEAMErFRE
Kv1.5  139  DPaKRlhYFDPLRNEYFFDRNRPSFDAILYYYQSGGRLkRPVNVPfDiFtEEvkFYQLGEEAllkFRE
Kv1.4  205  DPeKRtqYFDPLRNEYFFDRNRPSFDAILYYYQSGGRLkRPVNVPfDiFtEEvkFYQLGEEAllkFRE

Kv4.2  136  eykdrrrE naerlqddadtdntgesalPtmtarqRVwrafenphtstmalvfyyvtgffiavsvia
Kv1.1  133  DEGFIKEEE RPLPEkEyQRQVWLLFEYPESSGPARVIAIVSVMVILISIVifCLETLP
Kv1.2  129  DEGyIKEEE RPLPENEFQRQVWLLFEYPESSGPARiIAIVSVMVILISIVsFCLETLPiFRDE
Kv1.5  207  DEGFIKEEE kPLPrNEFQRQVWLiFEYPESSGSAraIAIVSVLVILISIitFCLETLPEFRDErell
Kv1.4  273  DEGFvrEEEdRaLPENEFkkQiWLiFEYPESSsPARgIAIVSVLVILISIViFCLETLPEFRD    dr
                                                        S1
Kv4.2  182                nvvetVpcgsspGhikelpcgeryavaFFcldTaCvmiFtvEyLlRlaAaPSry
Kv1.1  191  elkddkdftgtihridNTtviytSniFTDPFFIVETLCIIWFSFElvVRRFACPSKt
Kv1.2  192  nedmhgGgVtfhtySNsTigyqqStsFTDPFFIVETLCIIWFSFEfLVRRFACPSKA
Kv1.5  274  rhppvppqpppapapgiNGSVsgalsSGpTvapllprtlaDPFFIVETtCvIWFtFElvVRcFACPSqA
Kv1.4  338  dlimalsagghsrllNdtSaphlenSG    htiFnDPFFIVETvCIvWFSFEfvVRcFACPSqA
                                                   S2
Kv4.2  250  rFvrsvMsIIDvVAIlPYyIgLvmtdnE     dvsgafvtLRV   fRVFRIFKfSRHSqGL
Kv1.1  248  dFFkNIMNfIDIVAIIPYFITLGTEiAE   qEgnQkGeQAtSLAILRVIRLVRVFRIFKLSRHSKGL
Kv1.2  249  gFFtNIMNIIDIVAIIPYFITLGTELAE   kpEdaQqGQQAMSLAILRVIRLVRVFRIFKLSRHSKGL
Kv1.5  342  eFSrNIMNIIDvVAIfPYFITLGTELAEQQpGGGgQnGQQAMSLAILRVIRLVRVFRIFKLSRHSKGL
Kv1.4  399  lFFkNIMNIIDVsIlPYFITLGTdLA  QQqGGGnqqqQQAMSfAILRiIRLVRVFRIFKLSRHSKGL
                      S3                                S4
Kv4.2  311  rILGytLKscasELGfLlFsLtmaiIiFatvmfyAEkgssaSkFtSIPaAFWytiVTMTTlGYGDMvP
Kv1.1  313  QILGQTLKASMRELGLLIFFLFIGVILFSSAVYFAEADErdSqFpSIPDAFWWAVVSMTTVGYGDMvP
Kv1.2  315  QILGQTLKASMRELGLLIFFLFIGVILFSSAVYFAEADErdSqFpSIPDAFWWAVVSMTTVGYGDMvP
Kv1.5  410  QILGkTLqASMRELGLLIFFLFIGVILFSSAVYFAEADnhgSHFsSIPDAFWWAVVTMTTVGYGDMrP
Kv1.4  466  QILGhTLrASMRELGLLIFFLFIGVILFSSAVYFAEADEpttHFqSIPDAFWWAVVTMTTVGYGDMkP
                  S5
Kv4.2  379  kTIaGKIfGSiCslsGVLvIALPVPVIVSNFsriYHqnqradkrrA     Q   kkarLA rira
Kv1.1  381  vTIGGKIVGSLCAIAGVLTIALPVPVIVSNFNYFYH RETEGEEQA   Q LlhvSsPnLASdsDL
Kv1.2  383  tTIGGKIVGSLCAIAGVLTIALPVPVIVSNFNYFYH RETEGEEQA     QyLQvtScPkipSspDL
Kv1.5  478  ITVGGKIVGSLCAIAGVLTIALPVPVIVSNFNYFYH RETdhEEQAalkeeQgnQrreSldtggqrk
Kv1.4  534  ITVGGKIVGSLCAIAGVLTIALPVPVIVSNFNYFYH RETEnEEQ tqltqnavscpylPsnllkkfr
                   S6
Kv4.2  436  aksgSAnaymqSkrngllsnqlqS    sedepafvsksGssfeTqhhhllhclekTtnhefvdeqvfe
Kv1.1  442  SrRSQQTISKSeYMEIeEdmNNSiahyRqaN    irTGNCTaTdqNcVNksKlLTDV
Kv1.2  445  kksREASTISKSdYMEIqEgvNNSnedfReeNLK    TaNCTlantNyVNiTKmLTDV
Kv1.5  545  vSrSkASfsKtggslEssdSirrgScplEKChLKaksnvDlrrslyalcldTsrETDl
Kv1.4  600  SStSSslgdKseylemeegvkeslcgkeEKC    qgkgdDsetHknNcsNakavETDV

Kv4.2  501  escmevatvnrpsshspslssqqgvtstccSrrhkkTfripnanvsgSrgsvqelstiqircvertp

Kv4.2  569  lsnsrsslnakmeecvklnceqpyvttaiisiptppvttpegddrpespeysggnivrvsal
```

Figure 1. Deduced amino acid sequence of cloned cardiovascular K$^+$ channels. **(A)** Amino acid sequence comparison of the *Shaker*- and *Shal*-like K$^+$ channels. Gaps were inserted to maximize alignment. Identical residues are indicated by capital letters, and the six membrane spanning regions (S1–S6) are indicated by bold lines. Consensus sites for *N*-linked glycosylation sites are boldfaced, potential cAMP-dependent protein kinase phosphorylation sites are circled, and consensus sites for protein kinase C phosphorylation sites are boxed.

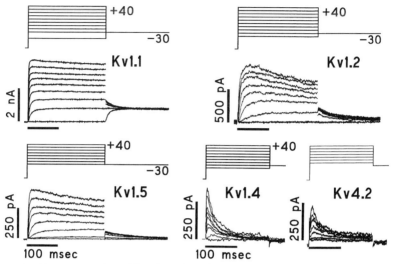

Figure 2. Currents produced by cloned cardiovascular K⁺ channels expressed in mouse L-cells. cDNA encoding each channel was subcloned into pCMV4 (Kv1.2) or pMSVneo (all others) and transfected into mouse L-cells by calcium phosphate precipitation. Stable clonal cell lines were obtained following selection in G418. Whole-cell voltage-clamp tracings were obtained from cell lines expressing isoform-specific mRNA as determined by RNA blot analysis. Extracellular solutions contained 140 mM NaCl, 4 mM KCl, 1.8 mM CaCl₂, 1 mM MgCl₂, 10 mM HEPES, and 10 mM glucose. Intracellular solutions contained 110 mM KCl, 5 mM K₄BAPTA, 5 mM K₂ATP, 1 mM MgCl₂, and 10 mM HEPES. Currents were elicited by depolarization in 10 mV steps as indicated. Cells transfected without K⁺ channel cDNA did not display voltage-gated currents under these recording conditions. Horizontal calibration is 100 msec in all panels.

differences in sensitivity to various agents as a function of the expression system used, with the exception of the widely prescribed antiarrhythmic agent quinidine. This drug blocks human Kv1.5 expressed in mouse L-cells in a voltage- and state-dependent manner with a $K_{0.5}$ of 6 μM, a clinically relevant concentration (66).

However, in the oocyte the $K_{0.5}$ is closer to 100 μM. This discrepancy may be caused by drug equilibration problems, for the yolk within the oocyte may interfere with the equilibration of internally binding antiarrhythmic drugs, because most of these agents are positively charged and contain a hydrophobic domain. Yolk is both negative and hydrophobic. Alternatively, this discrepancy could be caused by differences in membrane composition or channel protein processing between the two expression systems.

Analysis of Quinidine Block of the Human Kv1.5 K⁺ Channel

Because one goal of our K⁺ channel cloning project was to improve understanding of antiarrhythmic drug action, we have characterized the

Table 3. Summary of cloned cardiovascular K$^+$ channels

Clone	Current	IC$_{50}$ of Blockers and Inhibitors						Possible Endogenous Current
		4-AP (mM)	TEA (mM)	DTX (nM)	Quin (μM)	Clof (μM)	Ba^{2+} (mM)	
Kv1.1	Noninactivating	0.2	2	0.96	ND	ND	0.8	—
Kv1.2	Noninactivating	0.6	65	0.38	ND	ND	10	Atrial noninactivating
Kv1.4	Inactivating	1.2	[20]	[200]	ND	ND	0.8	I$_{to}$
Kv1.5	Noninactivating	0.1	40*	[200]	6	<1	ND	Atrial noninactivating
Kv4.2	Inactivating	5.0	[100]	[1000]	ND	ND	ND	I$_{to}$
I$_{sk}$	Noninactivating	[3.0]	40*	ND	ND	100	1	I$_{Ks}$

*This concentration blocked <50% of current. Numbers in brackets refer to concentrations that had no effect. DTX, dendrotoxin; Quin, quinidine; Clof, clofilium; ND, not determined.

block of the human Kv1.5 (hKv1.5) channel by quinidine in detail. This analysis of the mechanism of quinidine block of hKv1.5 is the first pharmacological study of a cloned human cardiac K^+ channel expressed in permanently transfected mammalian tissue culture cells (66). This tissue culture system has several advantages over the commonly used oocyte expression system: (1) a clonal cell line ensures reproducible results and avoids problems with seasonal variations in oocyte quality, (2) the L-cell plasma membrane more closely resembles that of the cardiac myocyte, and (3) the oocyte expression system may be inappropriate for quinidine pharmacology as previously described.

Quinidine displayed interesting state-, voltage-, and time-dependent interactions with the hKv1.5 K^+ channel. The initial time course of activation was not modified in the presence of quinidine, suggesting block mainly occurred after channel opening (Fig. 3A). In addition, block increased sharply in the voltage range of channel activation. Thus, prior to channel activation the quinidine binding site is either in a low-affinity state or inaccessible to the drug. The binding rates can be derived from the EC_{50} (6.2 μM = l/k) and the time constant of block ($\tau_b = 1/(k[D] + l$, 8 msec at 50 mV), thus yielding $k = 4.5 \times 10^6$ sec^{-1} M^{-1} and $l = 34$ sec^{-1}.

Drugs that interact predominantly with the open state of a channel can do so by moving into the ion-conducting pore. If a positively charged drug moves into the membrane field from the inside, block should increase upon depolarization. With a pK_a of 8.9, quinidine is charged at physiological pH. Figure 3B shows that Kv1.5 block by quinidine was indeed voltage-dependent. The voltage dependence of the K_D ($\delta = 0.18$) can therefore be interpreted to indicate that quinidine moves 18% into the membrane field from the inside to reach the receptor and block ion current (or more precisely, that the positively charged amine senses that fraction of the membrane field). An alternative explanation for the voltage dependence of quinidine block is that the drug binding site is allosterically linked to the channel voltage-sensing apparatus. This alternative explanation is unlikely for two reasons. The observed voltage dependence of block was measured over a voltage range where the channels are maximally activated. Second, the magnitude of the voltage dependence is similar to that measured for tetraethylammonium (TEA), a compound likely to bind in the ion pore (70).

As shown in Fig. 3C the deactivating tail current observed in the presence of 20 mM quinidine crosses over the tail current observed in the absence of drug when the two tracings are superimposed. This cross-over, indicating that quinidine block slows channel closing, suggests that the channel must unblock before it can close (i.e., that unblock occurs through the open state). Therefore, upon repolarization in the presence of quinidine, the open state unblocks and then either closes or binds drug again to repeat the process; thus giving rise to a current increase followed by a slowing of the rate of current decay and the observed crossover. This open

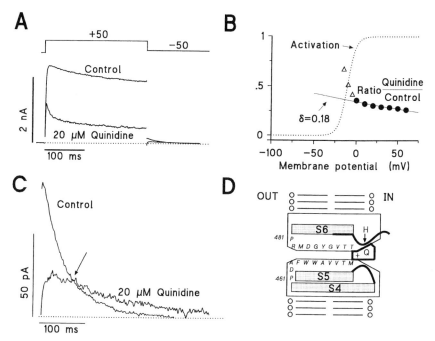

Figure 3. Block of the human Kv1.5 channel by quinidine. **(A)** Block of depolarization-induced current by 20 mM quinidine. Currents are shown in response to depolariaztion from −80 mV to 50 mV in the absence or presence of 20 μM quinidine. **(B)** Voltage-dependence of quinidine block. Relative current in the presence of 20 μM quinidine ($I_{quinidine}/I_{control}$) observed at 250 msec is plotted against membrane potential. The dashed line represents the voltage-activation curve for this experiment. The voltage dependence of block between 0 and 60 mV yielded δ = 0.18 (63). **(C)** Analysis of tail currents during quinidine block. Tail currents were obtained at −50 mV after a 250-msec depolarization to 50 mV. The tail current in control decays more rapidly and crosses over the tail current recorded in the presence of 20 μM quinidine. **(D)** Model of the quinidine binding site. The quinidine binding site is postulated to exist at the inner mouth of the channel pore and involve charge binding residues ~20% within the plane of the membrane. Residues involved in hydrophobic binding are located on the sequence linearly removed from the ion pore.

channel block model is similar to the one originally proposed by Armstrong (71) for the interaction of TEA derivatives with neuronal K^+ channels.

The interaction of the ammonium group of quinidine with hKv1.5 is expected to occur near the membrane spanning or intramembrane segments of the channel. hKv1.5 displays a high degree of homology with *Drosophila Shaker (ShA)*, especially in the transmembrane segments (95% identity in S4–S6). In the *Shaker* K^+ channels, the ion conducting pore has been localized to amino acids 431–449 (70, 72). The amino acid sequence 462–480 of hKv1.5 is identical to this "pore" sequence of *Shaker*, with the exception of the last amino acid (R in hKv1.5, T in *Sh*). Mutations on either end of the ion pore in *Shaker* alter the affinity for TEA (T441S for internal and T449Y external TEA). Interestingly, internal TEA block of *ShB* has a voltage dependence described by a fractional electrical distance of 0.15. This suggests that internal TEA moves ~15% into the membrane field. The T441S mutation in *Shaker* reduces affinity for internal TEA, and is therefore assumed to be located near or at the TEA binding site 15% into the membrane field. The similarities between quinidine block of the hKv1.5 channel and the quaternary ammonium block of *Shaker* channels, and the high structural similarity of the ion pore, suggests that the T472 residue (equivalent of T441 *Sh*) in HK2 is involved in quinidine binding.

Although mutations of the neighboring amino acids of *ShB* did not alter internal TEA sensitivity (70), these residues may be involved in binding the hydrophobic domains of quinidine (the log P is 2.4), and thus be responsible for the enhanced affinity of quinidine relative to TEA, 6 vs. 700 μM, respectively. The Kv1.5 channel has higher affinity for quaternary ammonium compounds with longer alkyl side chains or aromatic rings (data not shown). For example, the affinity for tetrapentyl ammonium is 10-fold higher than that of TEA and the affinity for the class III agent clofilium is below 1 μM. The increase in affinity with more hydrophobic side chains suggests that binding of these agents is stabilized by hydrophobic interactions. These data suggest that the receptor consists of an area for electrostatic interactions, and one or more domains for hydrophobic interactions (Fig. 3D).

Comparison of Cloned K⁺ Channels with Endogenous Cardiac Currents

Now that several cDNAs have been cloned from mammalian heart and shown to encode functional K⁺ channels, the challenge is to establish in which cells these proteins are expressed. The mere resemblance between some properties of a cloned channel with a native current is insufficient to this end. Afterall, most K⁺ channels cloned to date resemble either an inactivating I_{to}-type current or a delayer rectifier current. To test the hypothesis that a specific clone encodes the channel responsible for a specific myocyte current, the following criteria should be met.

1. The channel kinetics at both the whole-cell and single-channel level must be in reasonable agreement. Comparison of single-channel records will not always be possible because, in several cases, single-channel measurements have not been feasible in the heart. The rate constants for activation, inactivation, and recovery from inactivation should agree well as should the ion selectivity. Minor differences in voltage dependence may not be important because of the contribution of factors such as surface charge that are potentially different between the native myocyte and the heterologous expression system. A potential problem involves possible regulation of channel kinetics by phosphorylation. If channel kinetics are altered

by phosphorylation and the basal level of channel phosphorylation varies between native myocytes and the heterologous expression system, different currents may be recorded from essentially the same channel.

2. The pharmacology of compounds known to interact directly with the channel pore (e.g., dendrotoxin, charybdotoxin, TEA, and quinidine) should be similar.

3. Immunohistochemistry with isoform-specific antibodies made against the cloned channel subunits must confirm that the channel protein is present in the expected cardiac cells.

4. Isoform-specific antibodies that alter channel function must confirm the identity of the current being studied under voltage-clamp. This "immunoelectrophysiological" approach is in principle reasonable with a native myocyte preparation.

5. Affinity-purification from native tissue must be performed to confirm the protein composition of the native channel in terms of accessory subunits and heterotetramer formation.

6. Deletion of the cloned channel gene via homologous recombination from a transgenic animal should confirm the identity of the current that this gene supports.

As previously discussed, characterization of the functional and pharmacological properties of expressed K^+ channel clones has been accomplished. Both the Kv1.2 and Kv1.5 channels resemble a noninactivating current recently described in rat atrium (10) and in 23% of neonatal canine ventricular myocytes (73). Paulmichl and coworkers (60) suggested that the Kv1.2 channel represents this atrial current, because the activation kinetics are similar and the Kv1.2 mRNA is more abundant in atrium relative to ventricle. Both the endogenous current and Kv1.2 are sensitive to 1 to 5 mM 4-aminopyridine (4-AP) and are relatively insensitive to TEA. However, the Kv1.5 clone is also similar to the endogenous current with respect to activation kinetics and it has similar 4-AP sensitivity (63). Human Kv1.5 is much more abundant in human atrium than ventricle, although rat Kv1.5 mRNA is equally abundant in atrium and ventricle. Kv1.5 mRNA is detected in embryonic rat heart, whereas Kv1.2 mRNA does not appear until 10 to 20 days after birth (54). Thus, the presence or absence of the noninactivating current described by Boyle and Nerbonne (10) in embryonic or neonatal rat heart would suggest whether Kv1.5 or Kv1.2 is more likely to encode a component of this current. Also the Kv1.2 and 1.5 channels have differing affinities for dendrotoxin, but the dendrotoxin sensitivity of the native current has not been reported.

The Kv1.4 and Kv4.2 clones are candidates for the I_{to} current due to their rapidly inactivating currents. The Kv1.4 channel has the predicted voltage dependence for activation and the expected sensitivity to 4-AP (EC_{50} = 0.7 mM) (62, 74, 75). However, Kv1.4 expressed in oocytes recovers from inactivation much more slowly than I_{to}. The Kv4.2 clone is blocked by 4-AP, but current is reduced only by 50% in 5 mM 4-AP (57). In contrast, rat I_{to} is completely blocked by 2 to 4 mM 4-AP (74). It is important to note that rat brain Kv1.4 (RCK4) has a reported EC_{50} of 12 mM (76). Whether these discrepancies in 4-AP sensitivity are meaningful or whether they result from the experimental system remains a question. The time constant for Kv4.2 recovery from inactivation is ~200 msec at 20° in the L-cells (unpublished data). A 1-Hz pulse train does not produce large use-dependent inactivation in the L-cells as it does with Kv1.4, making Kv4.2 a good candidate for an I_{to} component.

Despite the slow recovery from inactivation, Kv1.4 may still be a component of I_{to}. K^+ channel isoforms that belong to the same gene subfamily can assemble with each other to form heterotetramers (47, 77, 78). The heterotetramers have properties that are intermediate between those observed with each isoform alone, rather than the sum of separate channels (77, 78). Kv1.2 alone shows little inactivation, but that portion which does inactivate recovers rapidly. Kv1.4 inactivates rapidly but recovers from inactivation slowly. When Kv1.4 is coexpressed with Kv1.2, a hybrid, I_{to}-like channel is formed that inactivates like Kv1.4 but recovers from inactivation much faster (Fig. 4). This result illustrates an additional challenge in correlating cloned channels with endogenous cardiac currents, for several endogenous currents may result from heterotetrameric channels. Even if isoform combinations that mimic the endogenous channels with respect to kinetics, ion selectivity, and pharmacology are achieved in the laboratory, it is challenging to prove that such a combination exists in the native myocyte.

Cloning of Voltage-Gated Na$^+$ Channels from Human Myocardium

Our laboratory initiated the cloning of human cardiac Na$^+$ channels with the goal of finding unique Na$^+$ channels that may be responsible for one of the unusual inward cardiac currents described at the beginning of this chapter. Because great genetic diversity had already been demonstrated with K^+ channels, and given that Na$^+$ channels are postulated to have evolved from K^+ channels, Na$^+$ channel diversity might be predicted to approach that seen with K^+ channels. Until recently it appeared as though mammalian Na$^+$ channel diversity was much less complicated than that observed with K^+ channels.

Screening of a human left ventricular cDNA library with polymerase chain reaction–generated fragments encoding a human ventricular Na$^+$ channel yielded six positive clones that could be identified by sequence analysis as members of the Na$^+$ channel gene family. The deduced peptide sequence of three of these clones was found to be nearly identical to either the rat heart I [RH-I (27)] or rat brain I [(RB-I) (31)]. Na$^+$ channel isoforms most likely represent the human homologs of these previously described channels. The remaining three cDNAs encoded a unique protein with <50% sequence identity with its closest Na$^+$ channel relative. This

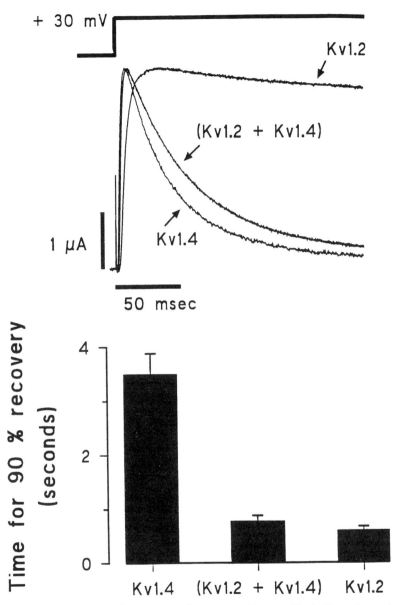

Figure 4. Heterotetramer formation with Kv1.2 and Kv1.4. **(Top)** Two-electrode voltage clamp of K$^+$ channel clones expressed in *Xenopus* oocytes. Oocytes were injected with mRNA transcribed in vitro from Kv1.2 or Kv1.4, or with a mixture of the two mRNAs. **(Bottom)** Recovery from inactivation of Kv1.2, Kv1.4, and channels resulting from coexpression of both mRNAs. The bath solution contained 96 mM NaCl, 2 mM KCl, 1.8 mM CaCl$_2$, 1 mM MgCl$_2$, and 5 mM HEPES (pH 7.5) at 22°C.

new Na$^+$ channel candidate was designated hNav2.1, adopting the nomenclature developed for K$^+$ channels (51). The 2.1 refers to the first member of a second gene subfamily of Na$^+$ channels. According to this classification scheme, all previously described mammalian Na$^+$ channels are placed in subfamily 1.

The deduced primary structure of hNa$_V$2.1 consists of 1682 amino acids and has a calculated molecular weight of 193,472 Da. Figure 5 shows the primary sequence of hNa$_V$2.1 aligned with the RB-II and RH-I Na$^+$ channels. Prediction of transmembrane topology by hydropathy analysis reveals a profile similar to other Na$^+$ channels, with four large (229–280 residues each) hydrophobic domains, each composed of at least six potential membrane spanning segments, including a positively charged amphipathic segment designated S4. Comparison of hNa$_V$2.1 to each of the five complete rat Na$^+$ channel sequences reveals a uniform pattern of overall primary structure homology [overall amino acid identity is 52% for RB-II (31); 51% for both RB-I and RB-III (31, 32); 49% for rat skeletal muscle (33); and 46% for RH-I (27)], indicating a high degree of relatedness to this family of ion channel proteins (Table 4). Significant homology is also evident from comparisons of hNa$_V$2.1 to Na$^+$ channels from the eel electric organ (35) (44% amino acid identity) and the *Drosophila* para locus (22%) (37). A search of available protein and nucleic acid data bases also revealed significant homology between hNa$_V$2.1 and the α_1-subunit of L-type voltage-dependent Ca^{2+} channels (79), although the extent of primary sequence identity (9% to 14%) was less than that found for Na$^+$ channels. hNa$_V$2.1 shares no significant overall amino acid identity with voltage-dependent K$^+$ channels or other known protein sequences.

The highest degree of amino acid sequence identity with other Na$^+$ channels is found within two short segments (SS1 and SS2) of the S5–S6 interhelical region (Fig. 6) that are believed to form membrane-penetrating hairpin structures that contribute to the formation of the ion pore (80) and various neurotoxin-binding sites (81–83). The primary sequence in this region is much more homologous to the Na$^+$ channel gene family than to the α_1-subunit of voltage-dependent Ca^{2+} channels (Fig. 6). The aspartic and glutamic acid residues boxed with the solid line in domains 1, 2, and 4 represent negative charge that is required for high-affinity TTX binding (81). The arrow indicates residues also involved in TTX and Cd^{2+} block (83). The rat heart channel (RH-1) is insensitive to TTX presumably because of the substitution of the aromatic tyrosine or phenylalanine with a cysteine. The rat brain and eel channels are TTX-sensitive. The residues boxed with a stippled line represent amino acids involved in ion selectivity. These lysine or alanine residues in domains 3 and 4 of the Na$^+$ channels, when converted to the glutamic acid found at the same position in the Ca^{2+} channel convert the Na$^+$ channel into a Ca^{2+} selective channel (84). The amino acid sequence within this pore region suggests that the hNa$_V$2.1

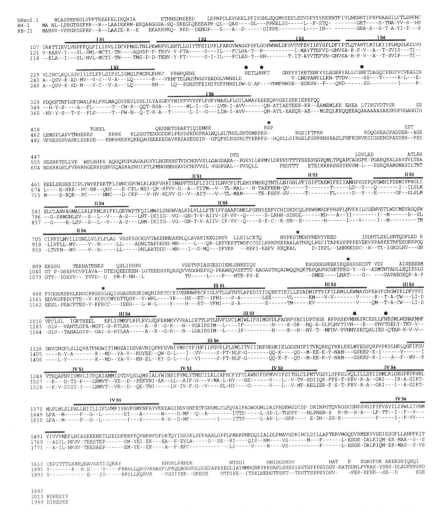

Figure 5. Amino acid sequence of hNa$_V$2.1. The channel sequence, deduced from its cloned cDNA, is compared with the sequences of RH-I and RB-II. Translation starts from the first in-frame methionine found in an open reading frame of 5,046 nucleotides. Identical amino acid residues are represented as dashes, and gaps were inserted to maximize the alignment. The suggested locations of the 24 putative membrane spanning regions are indicated with bold lines above the sequence. Potential extracellular consensus *N*-linked glycosylation sites are indicated by filled circles. Potential sites for phosphorylation by protein kinase A are indicated by the asterisks.

Table 4. Comparison of hNa$_v$2.1 to other NaCh isoforms

NaCh Isoform	% Amino Acid Identity with hNa$_v$2.1*								
	N	D1	ID1-2	D2	ID2-3	D3	ID3-4	D4	C
RB-I	43	53	20	59	16	58	50	57	43
RB-II	43	52	18	60	33	57	50	59	46
RB-III	33	52	18	59	28	56	50	59	46
SkM1	40	51	14	60	4	58	50	54	41
RH-I	37	48	13	56	7	56	54	54	41
CSC-1	—	—	—	—	—	—	—	—	41
Eel	32	45	16	58	9	54	41	49	26
Drosophila para	21	38	5	39	4	43	17	40	—

*Only exact matches were considered. Gaps were considered as a single nonidentity independent of length. N, amino terminus; D, domain; ID, interdomain region; C, carboxy terminus; SkM1, adult rat skeletal muscle NaCh; RH-I, rat heart NaCh I; CSC-1, rat cardiac Na$^+$ channel (partial cDNA sequence); RB-I, rat brain NaCh I; RB-II, rat brain NaCh II; RB-III, rat brain NaCh III; Eel, *Electrophorus electricus* electric organ NaCh.

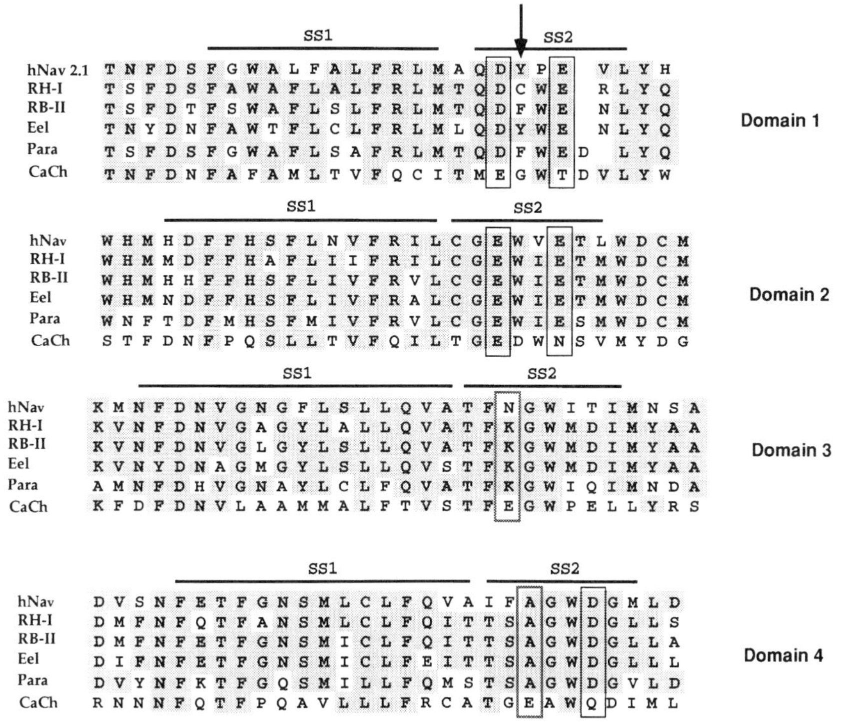

Figure 6. Comparison of S5–S6 interhelical regions of hNa$_V$2.1 to other voltage-dependent ion channels. Identical amino acid residues are shaded. Suggested locations of the putative ion pore forming segments SS1 and SS2 are indicated by horizontal lines. The arrow indicates Na$^+$ channel amino acids involved in TTX and Cd^{2+} block; the residues boxed with solid lines indicate amino acids involved TTX block; and the residues boxed with the stippled line are involved in cation selectivity. RH-I, rat heart I Na$^+$ channel; RB-II, rat brain II Na$^+$ channel; Eel, *Electrophorus electricus* electric organ Na$^+$ channel; Para, *Drosophila* para locus Na$^+$ channel; CaCh, rabbit heart dihydropyridine receptor α1-subunit.

channel is TTX-sensitive, but the substitution of the positive lysine with a neutral asparagine in domain 3 may predict altered ion selectivity.

The hNa$_V$2.1 Na$^+$ Channel Has Unusual Amino Acid Sequence in Functionally Important Regions

Structural features of the hNa$_V$2.1 channel are consistent with novel functional properties. The length of hNa$_V$2.1 (1682 residues) is significantly less than other Na$^+$ channels (1819–2018 residues) and the basis for this difference is not limited to an isolated region of the sequence. The length of the ID1-2 region (104 intracellular residues linking domains 1 and 2) is slightly smaller than that for rat SkM1 (121 residues) and eel (154 residues) Na$^+$ channels. The greatest segmental length difference between hNa$_V$2.1 and other Na$^+$ channels exists in the carboxy-terminus, where hNa$_V$2.1 (184 residues) is 38–67 amino acids shorter than other Na$^+$ channels. The reduced size of hNa$_V$2.1 is also reflected in the size of the corresponding mRNA transcript (7.8 kb), which is slightly smaller than observed for other Na$^+$ channels (8.5 to 9.0 kb).

The primary sequence of hNa$_V$2.1 has distinct features in regions known to be important in voltage-dependent activation and inactivation. The most striking difference between hNa$_V$2.1 and other Na$^+$ channels exists in the S4 segments. The S4 segments, which are believed to function as voltage sensors, collectively exhibit fewer positive charges than is typical of other Na$^+$ channels (Figs. 5 and 7). The greatest differences occur in domain 4, where there are only 4 arginine or lysine residues as compared with 8 for other Na$^+$ channels. Histidines (residues 1,355 and 1,367) replace arginines at two positions in the S4 segment of domain 4. Other S4 segment variations include the substitution of glutamines (residues 207 and 1,346) for arginines in domains 1 and 4, and aliphatic residues (Ile, 1,028; Leu, 1,349) for arginines in domains 3 and 4. Only the S4 segment in domain 2 has the same number of positively charged residues as do other Na$^+$ channels.

The electrostatic charge present on histidine at physiological pH (pK$_a$ ~6.0) is expected to be highly dependent on the environment and it is difficult to predict precisely the effect this amino acid substitution will have on voltage-sensing. The functional consequences of replacing arginine residues by glutamine in the S4 segment of domain 1 has been previously

Domain 4 S4

```
                          +          +     +     +
hNav    L V Q L I L L S R I I H M L R L G K G P K V F H N L M
RH-I    L F R V I R L A R I G R I L R L I R G A K G I R T L L
RB-II   L F R V I R L A R I G R I L R L I K G A K G I R T L L
Eel     L F R V I R L A R I A R V L R L I R A A K G I R T L L
Para    L L R V V R V A K V G R V L R L V K G A K G I R T L L
          +     +     +     +     +     +     +     +
```

Interdomain 3-4

```
hNav   N F N K H K I K L G G S N   I F I T V K Q R K Q Y R R L K K L M Y E D S Q R P V P
RH-I   N F N Q Q K K K L G G Q D   I F M T E E Q K K Y Y N A M K K L G S K K P Q K P I P
RB-II  N F N Q Q K K K F G G Q D   I F M T E E Q K K Y Y N A M K K L G S K K P Q K P I P
Eel    N F N R Q K Q K L G G E D   L F M T E E Q K K Y Y N A M K K L G S K K A A K C I P
Para   N F N E Q K K K A G G S L E M F M T E D Q K K Y Y S A M K K M G S K K P L K A I P
```

Figure 7. Comparison of primary sequence of structures involved in activation and inactivation. **(Top)** Alignment of domain 4 S4 segments for hNa$_V$2.1 and other Na$^+$ channels. Identical amino acid residues are shaded. Positively charged residues are indicated by +. **(Bottom)** Alignment of the interdomain 3–4 region for hNa$_V$2.1 and other Na$^+$ channels. Identical amino acid residues are shaded. The rectangle indicates the position of a highly conserved site for phosphorylation by protein kinase C that is absent in hNa$_V$2.1. RH-I, rat heart I Na$^+$ channel; RB-II, rat brain II Na$^+$ channel; Eel, *Electrophorus electricus* electric organ Na$^+$ channel; Para, *Drosophila* para locus Na$^+$ channel.

examined by Stühmer et al. (76) by site-directed mutagenesis of the RB-II Na$^+$ channel (61). Neutralizations of S4 segment positive charge in domain 1 result in decreased steepness in the voltage dependence of activation and cause a shift in the current-voltage relationship toward more positive potentials. These findings suggest that hNa$_V$2.1 may encode a Na$^+$ channel with altered activation kinetics.

Significant structural variations are also present in the ID3-4 region of hNa$_V$2.1 (Figs. 5 and 7). The role of the ID3-4 region in Na$^+$ channel inactivation has been demonstrated by the use of site-directed antibodies and by mutagenesis (61, 85). The extent of sequence conservation in this region of hNa$_V$2.1 is less than has been determined for other Na$^+$ channels. The most apparent structural differences that exist in hNa$_V$2.1 are the absence of a highly conserved site for phosphorylation by protein kinase C and a variation in the number and position of charged residues. The protein kinase C target sequence (as indicated by the boxed serine residues) is found in all other cloned Na$^+$ channels ranging from *Drosophila* to man and appears to affect inactivation kinetics. These differences suggest that hNa$_V$2.1 may have distinct inactivation kinetics.

There are five potential sites for *N*-linked glycosylation in regions of hNa$_V$2.1 predicted to be extracellular. Like other Na$^+$ channels, these potential sites are clustered in the S5–S6 interhelical regions of domains 1 and 3. Potential sites for cyclic nucleotide-dependent phosphorylation are present in the ID1-2 (Ser-442) and ID2-3 (Thr-777, Ser-869, and Ser-905) regions of hNa$_V$2.1. The density of these sites in the ID1-2 region is much less than in rat brain Na$^+$ channels (85).

The tissue distribution of hNa$_V$2.1 mRNA transcripts suggests that this Na$^+$ channel is prominently expressed in adult human heart and uterus with moderate expression in skeletal muscle (39, 40). Tissues in which the Na$_v$2.1 channel is absent or expressed at a very low level include cerebral cortex, kidney, liver, spleen, and vascular smooth muscle. The finding of a Na$^+$ channel mRNA transcript in uterus was unexpected. The existence of functional Na$^+$ channels in uterine smooth muscle has been demonstrated electrophysiologically (86), but the structural nature of these channels has not been determined. There is evidence that the density of active voltage-dependent Na$^+$ channels in gravid rat uterine smooth muscle increases during gestation with a peak immediately preceding parturition (87). These changes may affect myometrial excitation and the force of uterine contractions at term. Additional studies are needed to define the role of hNa$_v$2.1 in these events. Interestingly, cardiac muscle and myometrium also share the voltage-dependent K$^+$ channel Isk (50).

Our current hypothesis is that the Na$_v$2.1 channel represents the first member of a new Na$^+$ channel gene subfamily. Therefore, we predict that additional members of this subfamily will be cloned from human and other mammalian sources. Interestingly, a partial cDNA sequence has been reported (88) from rat glial cells that encodes a protein with 78% amino acid identity to the hNa$_v$2.1 channel. Although only 435 amino acids of sequence have been reported, it appears this clone represents the first member of this new Na$^+$ channel subfamily in the rat.

Summary

Molecular cloning technology has greatly expanded our knowledge of cardiovascular ion channel diversity. Both voltage-gated K$^+$ and Na$^+$ channel diversity is greater than previously anticipated in the heart. Seven K$^+$ channels cDNAs have thus far been cloned from cardiovascular tissue. With the cloning of the Na$_v$2.1 channel, we now know that at least four structurally distinct Na$^+$ channels are present in the heart.

Although it is too early to correlate positively the K$^+$ channels cloned to date with native cardiac currents, it is certain that the K$^+$ channels responsible for several myocyte currents still await cloning. These include a rapid component of delayed rectifier current in guinea pig and other species, I$_{kr}$, and the inward rectifier, I$_{k1}$. Channels cloned thus far from the heart are also expressed in other tissues. It is possible that voltage-gated channels play diverse physiological roles depending on the tissue in which they are expressed (e.g., regulating the action potential in one cell type while modulating cell volume in another). Such a duality of function could explain toxic side effects of antiarrhythmic drug therapy. Predicting whether such a problem will occur depends on determining the exact physiological role of the channels cloned thus far.

Acknowledgments

This research was supported by the National Institutes of Health Grants GM-41325 (M.M.T.), HL-47599 (D.J.S.), HL-40608 (P.B.B.), and PO1-HL-46681 (M.M.T., D.J.S., P.B.B.), and by a Grant-in-Aid (M.M.T.) from the America Heart Association (National Chapter). M.M.T. and P.B.B. are Established Investigators of the American Heart Association. A.L.G. is a Lucille P. Markey Scholar, and this work was supported in part by a grant from the Lucille P. Markey Charitable Trust.

References

1. Colatsky, T.J., Follmer, C.H., and Starmer, C.F. (1990). Channel specificity in antiarrhythmic drug action: Mechanism of potassium channel block and its role in suppressing and aggravating cardiac arrhythmias. *Circulation* **82**:2235–2242.

2. Sanguinetti, M.C., and Jurkiewicz, N.K. (1991). Delayed rectifier outward potassium current is composed of two currents in guinea pig atrial cells. *Am. J. Physiol.* **260**:H393–H399.

3. Balser, J.R., Bennett, P.B., and Roden, D.M. (1990). Time-dependent outward current in guinea pig ventricular myocytes. Gating kinetics of the delayed rectifier *J. Gen. Physiol.* **96**:835–863.

4. Yue, D.T., and Marban, E. (1988). A novel cardiac potassium channel that is active and conductive at depolarized potentials. *Pflügers Arch.* **413**:127–133.

5. Benndorf, K., Markwardt, F., and Nilius, B. (1987). Two types of transient outward currents in cardiac ventricular cells of mice. *Pflügers Arch.* **409**:641–643.

6. Sakmann, B., and Trube, G. (1984). Conductance properties of single inwardly rectifying potassium channels in ventricular cells from guinea pig heart. *J. Physiol. (Lond.)* **347**:641–657.

7. Hume, J.R., and Uehara, A. (1985). Ionic basis of the different action potential configurations of single guinea pig atrial and ventricular myocytes. *J. Physiol. (Lond.)* **368**:525–544.

8. Heidbüchel, H., Vereecke, J., and Carmeliet, E. (1990). Three different potassium channels in human atrium. Contribution to the basal potassium conductance. *Circ. Res.* **66**:1277–1286.

9. Sanguinetti, M.C., and Jurkiewicz, N.K. (1990). Two components of cardiac delayed rectifer K^+ current. *J. Gen. Physiol.* **96**:195–215.

10. Boyle, W.A., and Nerbonne, J.M. (1991). A novel type of depolarization-activated K^+ current in isolated adult rat atrial myocytes. *Am. J. Physiol.* **260**:H1236–H1247.

11. Tseng, G.-N., and Hoffman, B.F. (1989). Two components of transient outward current in canine ventricular myocytes. *Circ. Res.* **64**:633–647.

12. Escanade, D., Coulombe, A., Faivre, J.F., Deroubaix, E., and Coraboeuf, E. (1987). Two types of transient outward currents in adult human atrial cells. *Am. J. Physiol.* **252**:H142–H148.

13. Zygmunt, A.C., and Gibbons, W.R. (1991). Calcium activated chloride current in rabbit ventriclar myocytes. *Circ. Res.* **68**:424–437.

14. Kilborn, M.J., and Fedida, D. (1990). A study of developmental changes of outward currents in rat ventricular myocytes. *J. Physiol. (Lond.)* **430**:37–60.

15. Jeck, C.D., and Boyden, P.A. (1992). Age-related appearance of outward currents may contribute to developmental differences in ventricular repolarization. *Circ. Res.* **71**:1390–1403.

16. Fan, Z., and Hiraoka, M. (1991). Depression of delayed outward K^+ current by Co^{++} in guinea pig ventricular myocytes. *Am. J. Physiol.* **261**:C23–C31.

17. Tamkun, M.M., Talvenheimo, J.A., and Catterall, W.A. (1984). The sodium channel from rat brain. Reconstitution of neurotoxin-activated ion flux and scorpion toxin binding from purified components. *J. Biol. Chem.* **259**:1676–1688.

18. Bkaily, G., Jacques, D., Yamamoto, T., Sculptoreanu, A., and Payet, M.D. (1988). Three types of slow inward currents as distinguished by melittin in 3-day-old embryonic heart. *Can. J. Physiol. Pharmacol.* **66**:1017–1022.

19. Coraboeuf, E. (1980). *The Slow Inward Current and Caridac Arrhythmias*, D.P. Zipes, J.C. Bailey, and V. Elharrar, Eds. (Martinus Nijhoff Publishers, The Hague, The Netherlands), pp. 25–95.

20. Bkaily, G., Jacques, D., Sculptoreanu, A., Yamamoto, T., Carrier, D., Vigneault, D., and Sperelakis, N. (1991). Apamin, a highly potent blocker of the TTX- and Mn^{2+}-insensitive fast transient Na^+ current in young embryonic heart. *J. Mol. Cell. Cardiol.* **23**:25–39.

21. Lee, K.S. (1990). A novel slow inward Na$^+$ current at the plateau potential of guinea pig and monkey ventricular cell action potentials *J. Mol. Cell. Cardiol.* (Suppl. I) **22**:S.15.

22. Saint, D.A., Ju, Y.K., and Gage, P.W. (1992). A persistent sodium current in rat ventricular myocytes. *J. Physiol. (Lond.)* **453**:219–231.

23. Barres, B.A., Chun, L.L.Y., and Corey, D.P. (1989). Glial and neuronal forms of the voltage-dependent sodium channel: Characteristics and cell type distribution. *Neuron* **2**:1375–1388.

24. Llinas, R.R. (1988). The intrinsic electrical properties of mammalian neurons: Insights into central nervous system function. *Science* **242**:1654–1664.

25. Brown, A.M., Lee, K.S., and Powell, T. (1981). Voltage clamp and internal perfusion of single rat heart muscle cells. *J. Physiol. (Lond.)* **318**:455–477.

26. Rogart, R.B. (1986). High STX affinity vs. low STX affinity Na$^+$ channel subtypes in nerve, heart, and skeletal muscle. *Ann. N.Y. Acad. Sci.* **479**:402–430.

27. Rogart, R.B., Cribbs, L.L., Muglia, L.K., Kephart, D.D., and Kaiser, M.W. (1989). Molecular cloning of a putative tetrodotoxin-resistant rat heart Na$^+$ channel isoform. *Proc. Natl. Acad. Sci. U.S.A.* **86**:8170–8174.

28. Sills, M.N., Xu, Y.C., Baracchini, E., Goodman, R.H., Cooperman, S.S., Mandel, G., and Chien, K.R. (1989). Expression of diverse Na$^+$ channel messenger RNAs in rat myocardium. Evidence for a cardiac specific Na$^+$ channel. *J. Clin. Invest.* **84**:331–336.

29. Jacques, D., and Bkaily, G. (1991). Presence of early embryonic slow Na$^+$ channels in cardiomyopathic hamster. *Biophys. J.* **59**:259a.

30. Bkaily, G., Jasmin, G., Tautu, C., Prochek, L., Yamamoto, T., Sculptoreanu, A., Peyrow, M., and Jacques, D. (1990). A tetrodotoxin and Mn^{2+}-insensitive Na$^+$ current in Duchenne muscular dystrophy *Muscle Nerve* **13**:939–948.

31. Noda, M., Ikeda, T., Kayano, T., Suzuki, H., Takeshima, H., Kurasaki, M., Takahashi, H., and Numa, S. (1986). Existence of distinct sodium channel messenger RNAs in rat brain. *Nature (Lond.)* **320**:188–192.

32. Kayano, T., Noda, M., Flockerzi, V., Takahashi, H., and Numa, S. (1988). Primary structure of rat brain Na$^+$ channel III deduced from the cDNA sequence. *FEBS. Lett.* **228**:187–194.

33. Trimmer, J.S., Cooperman, S.S., Tomiko, S.A., Zhou, J., Crean, S.M., Boyle, M.B., Kallen, R.G., Sheng, Z., Barchi, R.L., Sigworth, F.J., Goodman, R.H., Agnew, W.S., and Mandel, G. (1989). Primary structure and functional expression of a mammalian skeletal muscle sodium channel. *Neuron* **3**:33–49.

34. Kallen, R.G., Sheng, Z., Yang, J., Chen, L., Rogart, R.B., and Barchi, R.L. (1990). Primary structure and expression of a sodium channel characteristic of denervated and immature rat skeletal muscle. *Neuron* **4**:233–242.

35. Noda, M., Shimizu, S., Tanabe, T., Takai, T., Kayano, T., Ikeda, T., Takahashi, H., Nakayama, H., Kaknaoka, Y., Minamino, N., Kkangawa, K., Matsuo, H., Raftery, M.A., Hirose, T., Inayama, S., Hayashida, H., Miyata, T., and Numa, S. (1984). Primary structure of *Electrophorus electricus* sodium channel deduced from cDNA sequence. *Nature (Lond.)* **312**:121–127.

36. Salkoff, L., Butler, A., Wei, A., Scavarda, N., Giffen, K., Ifune, C., Goodman, R., and Mandel, G. (1987). Genomic organization and deduced amino acid sequence of a putative sodium channel gene in *Drosophila. Science* **237:**744–749.

37. Loughney, K., Kreber, R., and Ganetzky, B. (1989). Molecular analysis of the para locus, a sodium channel gene in *Drosophila. Cell* **58:**1143–1154.

38. Gellens, M.E., George, A.L., Chen, L., Chahine, M., Horn, R., Barchi, R.L., and Kallen, R.G. (1992). Primary structure and functional expression of the human cardiac tetrodotoxin-insensitive voltage-dependent sodium channel. *Proc. Natl. Acad. Sci. U.S.A.* **89:**554–558.

39. George, A.L., Komisarof, J., Kallen, R.G., and Barchi, R.L. (1992a). Primary structure of the adult human skeletal muscle voltage-dependent sodium channel. *Ann. Neurol.* **31:**131–137.

40. George, A.L., Knittle, T.J., and Tamkun, M.M. (1992b). Molecular cloning of an atypical voltage-gated sodium channel expressed in human heart and uterus: Evidence for a distinct gene family. *Proc. Natl. Acad. Sci. U.S.A.* **89:**4893–4897.

41. Hille, B. (1992). *Ionic Channels of Excitable Membranes* (Sinauer Associates, Inc., Sunderland, MA), pp. 525–544.

42. Tempel, B.L., Papazian, D.M., Schwarz, T.L., Jan, Y.N., and Jan, L.Y. (1987). Sequence of a probable potassium channel component encoded at *Shaker* locus of *Drosophila. Science* **237:**770–775.

43. Pongs, O., Kecskemethy, N., Muller, R., Krah-Jentgens, I., Baumann, A., Kiltz, H.H., Canal, I., Llamazares, S., and Ferrus, A. (1988). Shaker encodes a family of putative potassium channel proteins in the nervous system of *Drosophila. EMBO J.* **7:**1087–1096.

44. Papazian, D.M., Timpe, L.C., Jan, Y.N., and Jan, L.Y. (1991). Alteration of voltage-dependence of Shaker potassium channels by mutations in the S4 sequence. *Nature (Lond.)* **349:**305–310.

45. Liman, E.R., Hess, P., Weaver, F., and Koren, G. (1991). Voltage-sensing residues in the S4 region of a mammalian K$^+$ channel. *Nature (Lond.)* **353:**752–756.

46. Timpe, L.C., Schwarz, T.L., Tempel, B.L., Papazian, D.M., Jan, Y.N., and Jan, L.Y. (1988). Expression of functional potassium channels from Shaker cDNA in *Xenopus* oocytes. *Nature (Lond.)* **331:**143–145.

47. MacKinnon, R. (1991). Determination of the subunit stoichiometry of a voltage-activated potassium channel. *Nature (Lond.)* **350:**232–235.

48. Liman, E.R., Tytgat, J., and Hess, P. (1992). Subunit stoichiometry of a mammalian K$^+$ channel determined by construction of multimeric cDNAs. *Neuron* **9:**861–871.

48a. Tempel, B.L., Jan, Y.N., and Jan, L.Y. (1988). Cloning of a probable potassium channel from mouse brain. *Nature* **332:**837–839.

49. Frech, G.C., VanDongen, A.M.J., Schuster, G., Brown, A.M., and Joho, R.H. (1989). A novel potassium channel with delayed rectifier properties isolated from rat brain by expression cloning. *Nature (Lond.)* **340:**642–645.

50. Folander, K., Smith, J.S., Antanavage, J., Bennett, C., Stein, R.B., and Swanson, R. (1990). Cloning and expression of the delayed rectifier IsK

channel from neonatal rat heart and diethylstilbestrol-primed rat uterus. *Proc. Natl. Acad. Sci. U.S.A.* **87:**2975–2979.

51. Chandy, K.G. (1991). Simplified gene nomenclature. *Nature (Lond.)* **352:**26 (Letter).

52. Roberds, S.L., and Tamkun, M.M. (1991). Developmental expression of cloned cardiac potassium channels. *FEBS Lett.* **284:**152–154.

53. Tamkun, M.M., Knoth, K., Walbridge, J., Kroemer, H., Roden, D., and Glover, D. (1991). Molecular cloning and characterization of two voltage-gated K$^+$ channel cDNAs from human ventricle. *FASEB. J.* **5:**331–337.

54. Roberds, S.L., and Tamkun, M.M. (1991). Cloning and tissue-specific expression of five voltage-gated potassium channel cDNAs expressed in rat heart. *Proc. Natl. Acad. Sci. U.S.A.* **88:**1798–1802.

55. Blair, T.A., Roberds, S.L., Tamkun, M.M., and Hartshorne, R.P. (1991). Functional expression of RK5, a voltage-gated K$^+$ channel isolated from the rat cardiovascular system. *FEBS Lett.* **295:**211–213.

56. Roberds, S.L. (1992). Voltage-gated cardiac potassium channels: Structure, function, and tissue-specific expression. Ph.D. Dissertation, Vanderbilt University.

57. Baldwin, T.J., Tsaur, M.-L., Lopez, G.A., Jan, Y.N., and Jan, L.Y. (1991). Characterization of a mammalian cDNA for an inactivating voltage-sensitive K$^+$ channel. *Neuron* **7:**471–483.

58. Christie, M.J., Adelman, J.P., Douglass, J., and North, R.A. (1989). Expression of a cloned rat brain potassium channel in *Xenopus* oocytes. *Science* **244:**221–224.

59. Baumann, A., Grupe, A., Ackermann, A., and Pongs, O. (1988). Structure of the voltage dependent potassium channel is highly conserved from *Drosophila* to vertebrate central nervous systems. *EMBO J.* **7:**2457–2463.

60. Paulmichl, M., Nasmith, P., Hellmiss, R., Reed, K., Boyle, W.A., Nerbonne, J.M., Peralta, E.G., and Clapham, D.E. (1991). Cloning and expression of a rat cardiac delayed rectifier potassium channel. *Proc. Natl. Acad. Sci. U.S.A.* **88:**7892–7895.

61. Stühmer, W., Conti, F., Suzuki, H., Wang, X., Noda, M., Yahagi, N., Kubo, H., and Numa, S. (1989). Structural parts involved in activation and inactivation of the sodium channel. *Nature (Lond.)* **339:**597–603.

62. Tseng-Crank, J.C.L., Tseng, G.-N., Schwartz, A., and Tanouye, M.A. (1990). Molecular cloning and functional expression of a potassium channel cDNA isolated from a rat cardiac library. *FEBS Lett.* **268:**63–68.

63. Swanson, R., Marshall, J., Smith, J.S., Williams, J.B., Boyle, M.B., Folander, K., Luneau, C.J., Antanavage, J., Oliva, C., Buhrow, S.A., Bennett, C., Stein, R.B., and Kaczmarek, L.K. (1990). Cloning and expression of cDNA and genomic clones encoding three delayed rectifier potassium channels in rat brain. *Neuron* **4:**929–939.

64. Philipson, L.H., Hice, R.E., Schaefer, K., LaMendola, J., Bell, G.I., Nelson, D.J., and Steiner, D.F. (1991). Sequence and functional expression in *Xenopus* oocytes of a human insulinoma and islet potassium channel. *Proc. Natl. Acad. Sci. U.S.A.* **88:**53–57.

65. Koren, G., Liman, E.R., Logothetis, Nadal-Ginard, B., and Hess, P. (1990). Gating mechanism of a cloned potassium channel expressed in frog oocytes and mammalian cells. *Neuron* **4:**39–51.

66. Snyders, D.J., Knoth, K.M., Roberds, S.L., and Tamkun, M.M. (1992). State, time, and voltage-dependent block by quinidine of a cloned human cardiac potassium channel. *Mol. Pharmacol.* **41:**322–330.

67. Murai, T., Kakizuka, A., Takumi, T., Ohkubo, H., and Nakanishi, S. (1989). Molecular cloning and sequence analysis of human genomic DNA encoding a novel membrane protein which exhibits a slowly activating potassium channel activity. *Biochem. Biophys. Res. Comm.* **161:**176–181.

68. Takumi, T., Moriyoshi, K., Aramori, I., Ishii, T., Oiki, S., Okada, Y., Ohkubo, H., and Nakanishi, S. (1991). Alteration of channel activities and gating by mutation of slow-IsK potassium channel. *J. Biol. Chem.* **266:**22192–22198.

69. Takumi, T., Ohkubo, H., and Nakanishi, S. (1988). Cloning of a membrane protein that induces a slow voltage-gated potassium current. *Science* **242:**1042–1045.

70. MacKinnon, R., and Yellen, G. (1990). Mutations affecting TEA blockade and ion permeation in voltage-activated K$^+$ channels. *Science* **250:**276–279.

71. Armstrong, C.M. (1971). Interaction of tetraethylammonium ion derivatives with the potassium channels of giant axons. *J. Gen. Physiol.* **58:**413–437.

72. MacKinnon, R., and Miller, C. (1989). Mutant potassium channels with altered binding of charybdotoxin, a pore-blocking peptide inhibitor. *Science* **245:**1382–1385.

73. Jeck, C.D., Ebihara, L., and Boyden, P.A. (1991). A unique outward current in neonatal myocytes. *Biophys. J.* **59:**267a.

74. Josephson, I.R., Sanchez-Chapula, J., and Brown, A.M. (1984). Early outward current in rat single ventricular cells. *Circ. Res.* **54:**157–162.

75. Po, S., Snyders, D., Baker, R., Tamkun, M.M., and Bennett, P.B. (1992). Functional expression of inactivating K$^+$ channels cloned from human heart. *Circ. Res.* **71:**732–736.

76. Stühmer, W., Ruppersberg, J.P., Schröter, K.H., Sakmann, B., Stocker, M., Giese, K.P., Perschke, A., Baumann, A., and Pongs, O. (1989). Molecular basis of functional diversity of voltage-gated potassium channels in mammalian brain. *EMBO J.* **8:**3235–3244.

77. Christie, M.J., North, R.A., Osborne, P.B., Douglas, J., and Adelman, J.P. (1990). Heteropolymeric potassium channels expressed in *Xenopus* oocytes from cloned subunits. *Neuron* **4:**405–411.

78. Covarrubias, M., Wei, A., and Salkoff, L. (1991). Shaker, Shal, Shab, and Shaw express independent K$^+$ current systems. *Neuron* **7:**763–773.

79. Mikami, A., Imoto, K., Tanabe, T., Niidome, T., Mori, Y., Takeshima, H., Narumiya, S., and Numa, S. (1989). Primary structure and functional expression of the cardiac dihydropyridine-sensitive calcium channel. *Nature (Lond.)* **340:**230–233.

80. Guy, H.R., and Conti, F. (1990). Pursuing the structure and function of voltage-gated channels. *Trends Neurosci.* **13:**201–206.

81. Terlau, H., Heinemann, S.H., Stühmer, W., Pusch, M., Conti, F., Imoto, K., and Numa, S. (1991). Mapping the site of block by tetrodotoxin and saxitoxin of sodium channel II. *FEBS. Lett.* **293:**93–96.

82. Satin, J., Kyle, J.W., Chen, M., Bell, P., Cribbs, L.L., Fozzard, H.A., and Rogart, R.B. (1992). A mutant of TTX-resistant cardiac sodium channels with TTX-sensitive properties. *Science* **256**:1202–1205.

83. Backx, P.H., Yue, D.T., Lawrence, J.H., Marban, E., and Tomaselli, G.F. (1992). Molecular localization of an ion binding site within the pore of mammalian sodium channels. *Science* **257**:248–251.

84. Heinemann, S.H., Terlau, H., Stuhmer, W., Imoto, K., and Numa, S. (1992). Calcium channel characteristics conferred on the sodium channel by single mutations. *Nature (Lond.)* **356**:441–443.

85. Catterall, W.A. (1988). Structure and function of voltage-sensitive ion channels. *Science* **242**:50–61.

86. Ohya, Y., and Sperelakis, N. (1989). Fast Na^+ and slow Ca^{++} channels in single uterine muscle cells from pregnant rats. *Am. J. Physiol.* **257**:C408–C41.

87. Inoue, Y., and Sperelakis, N. (1991). Gestational change in Na^+ and Ca^{++} channel current densities in rat myometrial smooth muscle cells. *Am. J. Physiol.* **260**:C658–C663.

88. Gautron, S., Dos Santos, G., Pinto-Henrique, D., Koulakoff, A., Gros, F., and Berwald-Netter, Y. (1992). The glial voltage-gated sodium channel: Cell and tissue specific mRNA expression. *Proc. Natl. Acad. Sci. U.S.A.* **89**:7272–7276.

16

Structure and Modulation of Voltage-Gated Sodium Channels

William A. Catterall, Todd Scheuer, James W. West,
Randal Numann, D. Earl Patton, Henry J. Duff, and
Alan L. Goldin

$\mathbf{E}$lectrical excitation and action potential conduction in the heart depend on the ion conductance activity of voltage-gated ion channels in the cardiac sarcolemma. Their activity is controlled on the millisecond time scale by two experimentally separable processes: (i) *voltage-dependent activation*, which controls the time- and voltage dependence of ion channel openings in response to changes in membrane potential; and (ii) *inactivation*, which controls the rate and extent of ion channel closure during a maintained depolarization. These two processes ensure a rapid, but transient, activation of ion channels in response to membrane potential changes. In addition, ion conductance activity of voltage-sensitive ion channels is modulated over longer time periods by protein phosphorylation and interactions with guanine nucleotide-binding regulatory proteins (G-proteins). These processes play an essential role in the regulation of cardiac function by hormones and neurotransmitters.

Recent research has shown that voltage-gated ion channels are members of a closely related gene family and have revealed aspects of their structure that are important for their physiological function. This chapter focuses on three related questions concerning the molecular mechanisms of Na^+ channel function in these voltage-dependent membrane signaling processes in the heart. (i) What are the subunit components of voltage-sensitive Na^+ channels in the heart? (ii) What are the primary structural characteristics of the principal subunits of the Na^+ channel? (iii) How do the structural features of the Na^+ channel subunits relate to mechanisms of voltage-dependent activation, inactivation, selective ion conductance, and long-term modulation?

Subunit Structures of Voltage-sensitive Na^+ Channels

Direct experimental work on the protein components of each of the voltage-gated ion channels began with studies of pharmacologically active agents, such as neurotoxins and drugs, that modify their properties. These compounds were used as molecular probes to identify and isolate the protein components of the ion channels. Protein components of Na^+ channels were first identified by photoaffinity labeling with photoreactive derivatives of α-scorpion toxins that act at neurotoxin receptor site 3 (1). The first two polypeptides found are now designated the α- and β_1-subunits of the Na^+ channel (Fig. 1). Na^+ channels can be solubilized from excitable membranes by treatment with nonionic detergents, detected in solubilized form by high-affinity binding of tetrodotoxin or saxitoxin at neurotoxin receptor site 1, and purified by a combination of conventional methods

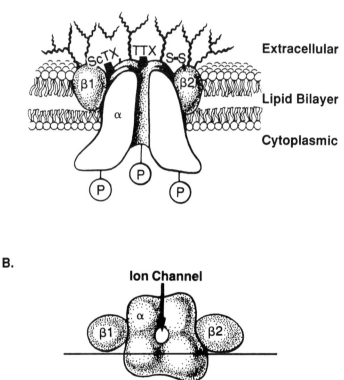

A.

B.

Figure 1. Subunit structure of the sodium channel. **(A)** A view of a cross-section of a hypothetical Na^+ channel consisting of a single transmembrane α-subunit of 260 kDa in association with a β_1-subunit of 36 kDa and a β_2-subunit of 33 kDa. The β_1-subunit is associated noncovalently, whereas the β_2-subunit is linked through disulfide bonds. All three subunits are heavily glycosylated on their extracellular surfaces and the α-subunit has receptor sites for α-scorpion toxins (ScTx) and tetrodotoxin (TTX). The intracellular surface of the α-subunit is phosphorylated by multiple protein kinases (P). **(B)** A view of the Na^+ channel from the extracellular side illustrating the formation of the transmembrane pore in the center of the α-subunit.

including ion exchange chromatography, lectin-Sepharose chromatography, and sucrose gradient sedimentation (1–3). Highly purified, functional preparations with well-defined subunit composition have been obtained from mammalian brain and skeletal muscle and electric eel electroplax. The Na^+ channel from mammalian brain has been found to consist of a heterotrimeric complex of α- (260 kDa), β_1- (36 kDa), and β_2- (33 kDa) subunits. The β_2-subunit is attached to the α-subunit by disulfide bonds. The Na^+ channel from mammalian skeletal muscle contains subunits of 260 kDa and 38 kDa analogous to the α- and β_1-subunits of the brain Na^+ channel, whereas the Na^+ channel purified from eel electroplax contains only a single 260 kDa subunit. These results show that the large α-subunits contain the binding site for tetrodotoxin and saxitoxin and argue that these subunits are the main functional components of Na^+ channels. Reconstitution and expression of functional Na^+ channel activity confirms this conclusion (1–3). In the heart, specific antibodies against the Na^+ channel subunits recognize related α-subunits (4, 5; Fig. 2, lane 2) and β_1-subunits (Fig. 2, lanes 7 and 8). In contrast to results with rat brain Na^+ channels, the α-subunits have the same apparent mass before and after reduction of disulfide bonds (Fig. 2, lanes 3 and 4), indicating that there is no disulfide-linked β_2-subunit. Therefore, it appears that the principal α-subunits of Na^+ channels are expressed in association with a variable number of smaller subunits in different excitable tissues and that cardiac Na^+ channels are a complex of α- and β_1-subunits.

The overall arrangement of α-, β_1-, and β_2-subunits in the membrane has been inferred from biochemical experiments (Fig. 1). The α- and β_1-subunits are covalently labeled by neurotoxins that act from outside the cell, and all three subunits are heavily glycosylated with up to 30% of their apparent mass due to carbohydrate, suggesting that they are all exposed to the extracellular surface. Removal of sialic acid residues from the α-subunit of the cardiac Na^+ channel has only a small effect on its apparent mass (Fig. 2, lanes 5 and 6), indicating that the α-subunit of the cardiac Na^+ channel is less heavily glycosylated than its counterpart in brain.

The α-subunit of rat brain Na^+ channels is phosphorylated by a cAMP-dependent protein kinase in intact cells or synaptosomes (1), indicating that it is exposed at the intracellular surface and therefore is a transmembrane protein. The α-subunit of cardiac Na^+ channels is also rapidly phosphorylated by cAMP-dependent protein kinase in vitro (Fig. 2, lanes 3 and 4). The β_1- and β_2-subunits are also intrinsic membrane proteins that have substantial hydrophobic domains labeled by hydrophobic photoaffinity probes and are preferentially extracted into hydrophobic detergent phases.

Structure and Function of Na⁺ Channel Subunits

Primary Structures of Na⁺ Channel α-Subunits

Availability of purified and functionally characterized Na^+ channel preparations provided the necessary starting material for identification of

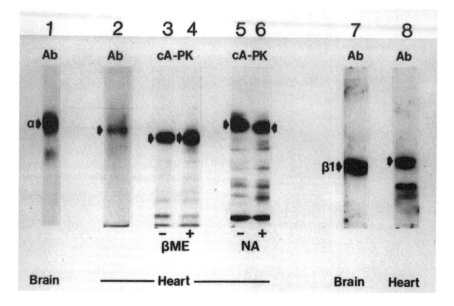

Figure 2. Na$^+$ channel subunits expressed in the heart. Na$^+$ channels were solubilized from rat brain or rat heart membranes with Triton X-100, immunoprecipitated with the generally reactive antipeptide antibody anti-SP19, and analyzed for several different biochemical properties as described previously (4). (Lanes 1 and 2) The immunoprecipitated cardiac and brain Na$^+$ channels were analyzed by sodium dodecyl sulfate-polyacrylamide gel electrophoresis (SDS-PAGE) on 3% to 10% gradient gels and immunoblotting with anti-SP19 to reveal the α-subunits of the Na$^+$ channels. (Lanes 3 and 4) The immunoprecipitated cardiac Na$^+$ channels were phosphorylated by incubation with cAMP-dependent protein kinase and [γ-^{32}P]ATP and analyzed by SDS-PAGE and autoradiography to detect the phosphorylation of the α-subunits of the cardiac Na$^+$ channels. The sample in lane 3 was analyzed without reduction of disulfide bonds, whereas the sample in lane 4 was incubated with β-mercaptoethanol to reduce disulfide bonds. The similarity in apparent molecular mass before and after reduction of disulfide bonds indicates that cardiac Na$^+$ channels have no disulfide-linked β$_2$-subunit in contrast to brain Na$^+$ channels. (Lanes 5 and 6) The immunoprecipitated cardiac Na$^+$ channels in lane 5 were incubated under control conditions, and those in lane 6 were incubated with neuraminidase from *Clostridium perfringens* to remove sialic acid residues. The reduction in apparent molecular mass from 230 kDa to 222 kDa indicates a low level of glycosylation and sialation of the cardiac α-subunit compared with the brain Na$^+$ channel. (Lanes 7 and 8) Na$^+$ channels from brain and heart were immunoprecipitated with antibodies against the β$_1$-subunits and analyzed by SDS-PAGE on 12% acrylamide gels and immunoblotting with anti–β1-antibodies as described previously (5).

the genes encoding the Na⁺ channel subunits and determination of their primary structures. Using oligonucleotides encoding short segments of the electric eel electroplax Na⁺ channel and antibodies directed against it, Noda et al. (6) isolated cDNAs encoding the entire polypeptide from expression libraries of electroplax mRNA. The deduced amino acid sequence revealed a protein with four internally homologous domains, each containing multiple potential α-helical transmembrane segments (Fig. 3). The wealth of information contained in this deduced primary structure has revolutionized research on Na⁺ channels.

The cDNAs encoding the electroplax Na⁺ channel were used to isolate cDNAs encoding three distinct, but highly homologous, rat brain Na⁺ channels (types I, II, and III; refs. 7 and 8). cDNAs encoding the alternatively spliced type IIA Na⁺ channel were isolated independently by screening

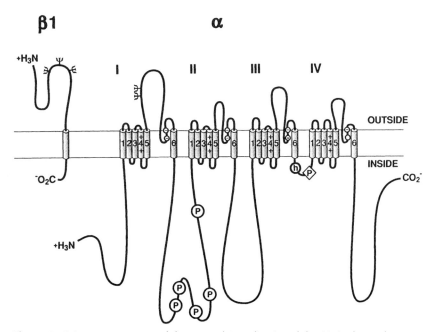

Figure 3. Primary structures of the α- and β₁-subunits of the Na⁺ channel illustrated as transmembrane folding diagrams. The bold line represents the polypeptide chains of the α- and β₁-subunits with the length of each segment approximately proportional to its true length in the rat brain Na⁺ channel. Cylinders represent probable transmembrane α-helices. Other probable membrane-associated segments are drawn as loops in extended conformation like the remainder of the sequence. Sites of experimentally demonstrated gylcosylation (Ψ), cAMP-dependent phosphorylation (P in a circle), protein kinase C phosphorylation (P in a diamond), amino acid residues required for tetrodotoxin binding (small circles with +, −, or open fields depict positively charged, negatively charged, or neutral residues), and amino acid residues that form the inactivation particle (h in a circle) are illustrated.

expression libraries with antibodies against the rat brain Na^+ channel α-subunit (9). cDNAs encoding the type II/IIA Na^+ channel were used as probes to isolate cDNAs encoding Na^+ channel α-subunits expressed in skeletal muscle and heart by low-stringency hybridization (10–12). The μ_1 Na^+ channel α-subunit is expressed primarily in adult skeletal muscle (10); the h_1 Na^+ channel α-subunit is expressed primarily in heart and also in uninnervated or denervated skeletal muscle (11, 12). These Na^+ channels have a close structural relationship to the three brain Na^+ channel α-subunits. In general, the similarity in amino acid sequence is greatest in the homologous domains from transmembrane segment S1 through S6, whereas the intracellular connecting loops are not highly conserved.

Primary Structures of Na+ Channel β-Subunits

The primary structures of Na^+ channel $β_1$-subunits have been determined only recently (13). The $β_1$-subunit cloned from rat brain is a small protein of 218 amino acids (22,821 Da), with a substantial extracellular domain having four potential sites of N-linked glycosylation, a single α-helical membrane-spanning segment, and a very small intracellular domain. Experiments with anti–$β_1$-subunit antibodies (5) and isolation of cross-hybridizing cDNA clones by low-stringency screening of cDNA libraries (Isom et al., unpublished observations) indicate that there is a small family of $β_1$-subunits. These distinct $β_1$-subunits may form specific associations with different α-subunits and contribute to the diversity of Na^+ channel structure and function. $β_2$-Subunits have not yet been cloned, but it may be anticipated that they may also add to the potential diversity of Na^+ channel structure and function.

Functional Expression of Na+ Channel Subunits

α-Subunit mRNAs isolated from rat brain by specific hybrid selection with type IIA cDNAs (14) and RNAs transcribed from cloned cDNAs encoding α-subunits of rat brain (9, 15–17), skeletal muscle (10), or heart (18, 19) Na^+ channels are sufficient to direct the synthesis of functional Na^+ channels when injected into Xenopus oocytes. These results establish that the protein structures necessary for voltage-dependent gating and ion conductance are contained within the α-subunit itself, as suggested from the work on purified and reconstituted Na^+ channels.

Although α-subunits alone are sufficient to encode functional Na^+ channels, their properties are not normal. Inactivation is slow relative to that observed in intact neurons or muscle cells and its voltage dependence is shifted to more positive membrane potentials. Coexpression of low-molecular weight RNA from brain or skeletal muscle can accelerate inactivation, shift its voltage dependence to more negative membrane potentials, and increase the level of expressed Na$^+$ current (9, 20). These results suggested that the low-molecular weight β_1- or β_2-subunits may modulate functional expression of the α-subunit. Coexpression of RNA transcribed from cloned β_1-subunits directly demonstrates this modulation (13). Coexpression of β_1-subunits in *Xenopus* oocytes accelerates the decay of the Na$^+$ current 5-fold, shifts the voltage-dependence of Na$^+$ channel inactivation 20 mV in the negative direction, and increases the level of Na$^+$ current 2.5-fold. Evidently, β_1-subunits are essential for normal functional expression of rat brain Na$^+$ channels.

Na$^+$ channel α-subunits can also be functionally expressed in mammalian cells in culture. Stable lines of Chinese hamster ovary (CHO) cells expressing the type IIA Na$^+$ channels generate Na$^+$ currents with normal time course and voltage dependence, even though there is no evidence that these cells express an endogenous β_1-subunit that complexes with the transfected α-subunit (21, 22). Evidently, β_1-subunits do not have as important a functional impact when the α-subunit is expressed in the genetic background of a mammalian somatic cell. The α-subunits expressed in CHO cells have normal pharmacological properties as well. They have high-affinity receptor sites for saxitoxin and tetrodotoxin and are inhibited by low concentrations of tetrodotoxin. The voltage dependence of their activation is shifted in the negative direction, and they are persistently activated by veratridine in a stimulus-dependent manner. Their inactivation is slowed by α-scorpion toxins. In addition, they are inhibited in a strongly frequency- and voltage-dependent manner by local anesthetic, antiarrhythmic, and anticonvulsant drugs (23). Thus, the receptor sites for all of these diverse pharmacological agents are located on the α-subunits.

Structural Basis of Na$^+$ Channel Function

A major goal of current research on the voltage-gated Na$^+$ channels is to define the structural components that are responsible for specific aspects of channel function. Two main experimental approaches have proven valuable in these studies. Antibodies against short, $\sim$20-residue, peptide segments of the principal α-subunits of the Na$^+$ channels have been used to probe domains required for specific channel functions or can be covalently labeled by neurotoxins or protein phosphorylation. Alternatively, mutations have been introduced into cDNAs encoding the principal α-subunits by oligonucleotide-directed mutagenesis and subsequently expressed in recipient cells analyzed by electrophysiological recordings.

Voltage-Dependent Activation

The steep voltage dependence of activation of the voltage-sensitive ion channels is their most unique characteristic. It requires that they have charged amino acid residues or strongly oriented dipoles within the electric field of the membrane phospholipid bilayer. The steepness of voltage-dependent activation of Na^+ channels requires the movement of the equivalent of six protein-bound positive charges from the inner surface of the bilayer membrane to the outer surface during activation, or movement of a larger number of charges a proportionally smaller distance across the membrane (24). Movement of these gating charges or voltage sensors under the force of the electric field is believed to initiate a conformational change in the channel protein resulting in activation. Because activation of the Na^+ channel is rapid, the movement of its gating charges causes a measurable capacitive gating current that has been detected in voltage-clamp experiments. This movement of gating charge begins immediately upon depolarization of the membrane, is largely complete before movement of ionic current through the open channel is detected, and is blocked if the Na^+ channel is first inactivated before depolarization.

The requirement for transmembrane movement of multiple charges during Na^+ channel activation has focused attention on the S4 segments of the voltage-sensitive ion channels that are both positively charged and hydrophobic. These unique structures, which consist of repeated motifs of a positively charged amino acid residue, usually arginine, followed by two hydrophobic residues (Fig. 3), were first observed in the amino acid sequence of the electroplax Na^+ channel (6). Conservation of this amino acid sequence among different voltage-sensitive ion channels, first noted for Na^+ channels from electroplax and brain, is striking across this broad range of ion channels from diverse species.

Several authors have independently proposed that these S4 segments have a transmembrane orientation and are the gating charges or voltage sensors of the Na^+ channel. In the "sliding helix" model of voltage-dependent gating (1), the S4 segments are proposed to adopt an α-helical conformation. In this conformation, the arginine residues form a spiral ribbon of positive charge around the core of the helix. They are stabilized in their transmembrane position by formation of ion pairs between the positive charges of the S4 segments and negatively charged amino acid residues from the surrounding transmembrane segments. This ion pairing arrangement is metastable, held in place by the force of the electric field drawing the positive charges into the cell and repelling the negative charges outward at a typical resting membrane potential of -80 mV. Upon depolarization, this force is relieved, and the S4 segment is released to slide outward along a spiral path and form a new set of ion pairs. This sliding motion of the S4 helix transfers the equivalent of a full positive charge across the membrane with only a 5 Å outward movement and a 60° rotation. Sequential, voltage-driven movements of the S4 helices are proposed to initiate sequential conformational changes in the four domains of the Na^+ channel resulting in the transfer of at least four gating charges across the membrane and, finally, in activation of the ion channel.

Direct experimental support for designation of the S4 segments as the voltage sensors for activation of the voltage-gated Na$^+$ channels has been provided by site-directed mutagenesis experiments (9, 25) as described for K$^+$ channels by Tytgat and Hess (see Chapter 14). Neutralization of the 1 to 3 positively charged amino acid residues in the S4 segment in domain I of the Na$^+$ channel α-subunit causes a progressive reduction in the steepness of the voltage-dependent activation of Na$^+$ channels as expected if these positively charged amino acid residues serve as gating charges. The effect of neutralization of different charged residues is not equivalent, indicating that they do not all move through a comparable fraction of the membrane electric field. Because the electric field is not expected to be strictly uniform through the membrane, the relative distance moved by the gating charges cannot be directly inferred from the fraction of the field through which they move, so this value cannot be used to define a detailed molecular mechanism. If the S4 helices must move through the protein structure of the Na$^+$ channel as the channel activates, the size and shape of the amino acid side chains might affect the voltage dependence of gating by making it easier or more difficult for the gating segments to move. In fact, mutation of positively charged amino acid residues in S4 helices from arginine to lysine, which retains positive charge, can cause a large shift in the voltage dependence of channel activation (25). Moreover, the shifts in voltage dependence of activation caused by mutation of arginine residues to uncharged glutamine residues are not precisely correlated with the number of charges neutralized, suggesting that size and shape of the residues may also be important (25). In addition, mutation of a hydrophobic residue in the S4 segment in domain II from leucine to phenylalanine causes a 20 mV shift in the voltage dependence of gating to more positive membrane potentials (9). These effects would be expected if these segments must move through the channel structure. Overall, these mutational analyses provide strong evidence that the S4 segments are indeed the voltage sensors of the voltage-gated ion channels, but do not yet prove either mechanism.

Inactivation Gate

Depolarization of the membrane of excitable cells results in a transient inward Na$^+$ current that is terminated within a few milliseconds by the process of inactivation. Perfusion of the intracellular surface of the Na$^+$ channel with proteolytic enzymes prevents inactivation, implicating intracellular structures in the inactivation process (24). The α-subunit of Na$^+$ channels consists of four homologous domains connected by cytoplasmic linker sequences (Fig. 3). Antibodies directed against the intracellular linker between homologous domains III and IV (L$_{III/IV}$, Fig. 3) completely block fast inactivation of affected single Na$^+$ channels (25–27). Expression of the Na$^+$ channel as two polypeptides with a cut between domains III and IV slows inactivation ~20-fold (25), and small insertions in this loop also slow inactivation (28). Phosphorylation of a single serine residue in $L_{III/IV}$ by protein kinase C slows inactivation (29). The amino acid sequence of LIII–IV contains several clustered positively and negatively charged residues (Fig. 4). Surprisingly, these highly conserved residues are not essential for fast Na$^+$ channel inactivation (30, 31). However, deletions of 10 amino acid segments within LIII–IV can completely block fast Na$^+$ channel inactivation supporting an essential role for this segment in the inactivation process (31). To assess the role of hydrophobic amino acids within $L_{III/IV}$ in inactivation, site-directed mutants were constructed in which conserved hydrophobic residues were altered, expressed in *Xenopus* oocytes or transfected CHO cells, and analyzed by whole-cell voltage clamp and single-channel recording.

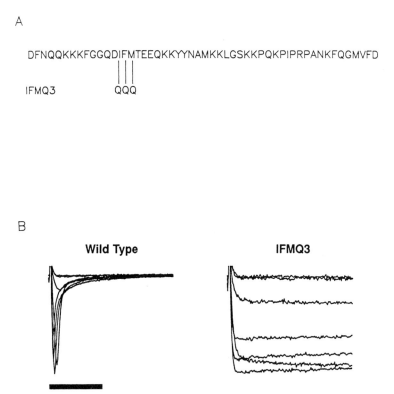

Figure 4. Inactivation of wild-type and mutant Na$^+$ channels. **(A)** The amino acid sequence of the intracellular loop connecting domains III and IV. **(B)** RNA encoding wild-type or IFMQ3 Na$^+$ channel α-subunits was transcribed in vitro and injected into *Xenopus* oocytes together with RNA encoding β_1-subunits. Na$^+$ currents expressed in the oocytes were recorded by whole-cell voltage clamp using two-microelectrode voltage clamp procedure. Na$^+$ currents were elicited by voltage steps from a holding potential of -100 mV to test potentials of -50 to 0 mV in 10 mV increments. Calibration bar is 20 msec.

Effects of Mutations of Hydrophobic Amino Acids on Na⁺ Channel Inactivation

The amino acid sequence of $L_{III/IV}$ is shown in Fig. 4A. The contiguous hydrophobic residues ile1488, phe1489, and met1490 (IFMQ3) were substituted with glutamine, and RNA encoding mutant Na⁺ channel α-subunits was coinjected into *Xenopus* oocytes with RNA encoding the β_1-subunit (13). The expressed channels were analyzed by two-microelectrode voltage clamp recording. Na⁺ currents from oocytes injected with RNA encoding Na⁺ channel α-subunit IFMQ3 show a dramatic removal of fast inactivation (Fig. 4B). Whereas wild-type Na⁺ channels inactivate within 1 to 2 msec at − 10 mV, currents resulting from IFMQ3 last for over 5 sec at this membrane potential. Only a minor shift (about 6 mV) was observed in the voltage dependence of peak Na⁺ conductance. Thus, the mutation IFMQ3 results in a specific and potent inhibition of the fast inactivation process.

We examined the role of each amino acid in the cluster IFM in Na⁺ channel inactivation by substitution of each individually with glutamine (I1488Q, F1489Q, and M1490Q)and expression in mammalian cells. Chinese hamster R-1610 cells were transfected with the expression plasmid ZemRVSP6 (22) containing the wild-type IIA Na⁺ channel α-subunit cDNA or I1488Q, F1489Q, or M1490Q cDNAs. Clonal cell lines were picked for resistance to the antibiotic G418 and screened for expression of transfected Na⁺ channel α-subunit mRNA by high-stringency Northern blot analysis. Small Na⁺ currents (<100 pA) were recorded in only two of >30 untransfected cells analyzed by voltage clamp, whereas the remainder had no detectable Na⁺ currents. In contrast, whole-cell Na⁺ currents were recorded in all cells expressing wild-type or mutant Na⁺ channels. The mutant channels activate rapidly, but display altered inactivation kinetics (Fig. 5). Mutant M1490Q inactivates more slowly than wild-type, but inactivation is essentially complete (Fig. 5B). Mutant I1488Q also inactivates more slowly than wild-type, but its inactivation is incomplete (Fig. 5B). Inactivation of mutant F1489Q is dramatically slowed, and most of the Na⁺ current remains at the end of a 20-msec test pulse (Fig. 5C). Depolarization to − 40 mV or − 30 mV produces Na⁺ currents that do not decay appreciably during the 20-msec test pulse, whereas depolarization to more positive voltages yields Na⁺ currents with a small component that decays within 5 msec and a large component that remains at the end of the test pulse. The large noninactivating component of Na⁺ current for mutant F1489Q suggests almost complete loss of fast inactivation of this mutant Na⁺ channel.

Representative traces of single Na⁺ channel currents recorded during pulses to − 20 mV from F1489Q cells are shown in Fig. 5D. Single wild-type Na⁺ channels expressed in CHO cells open once or twice early in a depolarization and then inactivate and remain silent for the remainder of the pulse (32). Single F1489Q channels open early in the pulse, but continue to reopen for the duration of the pulse instead of inactivating. The

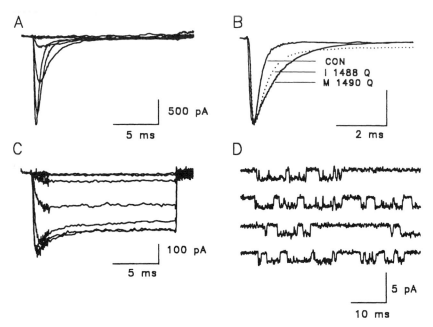

Figure 5. Na$^+$ currents recorded in CHO cells expressing wild-type IIA and mutant Na$^+$ channels. **(A)** Whole-cell currents from an R-1610 cell expressing wild-type Na$^+$ channels elicited by test depolarizations ranging from -60 mV to 0 mV in 10 mV steps. The holding potential was -100 mV. **(B)** Comparison of normalized whole-cell currents recorded during test depolarizations to 20 mV for wild-type and the mutants indicated. **(C)** Whole-cell currents recorded from mutant F1489Q during test depolarizations ranging from -60 mV to 0 mV in 10 mV steps. **(D)** Representative cell-attached single-channel current recordings from mutant F1489Q during pulses to -20 mV. Records were filtered at 2.5 kHz.

increased probability of reopening of single channels evidently causes the noninactivating component of Na$^+$ current observed at the macroscopic level.

An Essential Cluster of Hydrophobic Residues in the Inactivation Gate of Na$^+$ Channels

In contrast to the nonessential role of positively charged amino acids in L$_{III/IV}$ (17, 30, 31), substitution of three contiguous hydrophobic amino terminal region of L$_{III/IV}$, ile1488, phe1489, and met1490 with glutamine (mutant IFMQ3), completely removes fast inactivation (29). Substitution of phe1489 alone with glutamine (mutant F1489Q) removes fast inactivation nearly completely, and substitution of glutamine for ile1488 (I1488Q) and met1490 (M1490Q) results in slowed Na$^+$ current inactivation with a significant sustained component in the case of I1488Q. These results identify the cluster of hydrophobic amino acid residues at positions 1488–1490 as a critical structural component for fast inactivation, possibly forming the fast inactivation gate itself.

Comparison to the Predictions of the Ball-and-Chain Model of Inactivation

The original ball-and-chain model of Na^+ channel inactivation (24) has three essential structural features: a positively charged inactivation particle (the ball), a polypeptide tether (the chain), and a negatively charged receptor site at the intracellular mouth of the Na^+ channel that develops a high affinity for the inactivation ball when the channel is activated. The process of inactivation in the ball-and-chain model then involves binding of the loosely tethered ball to its receptor site at the intracellular mouth of the pore and occlusion of the pore.

Molecular analyses of potassium channel inactivation by Aldrich and coworkers show that it conforms closely to a ball-and-chain model. In contrast, our results on Na^+ channels are consistent with some, but not all, of the features of the original ball-and-chain formulation. As for a ball-and-chain model, we propose that the hydrophobic cluster, IFM, serves as an essential component of the inactivation particle that occludes the intracellular mouth of the activated Na^+ channel. However, in contrast to the original formulation of the ball-and-chain model, positively charged residues are not required, and hydrophobic forces rather than electrostatic interactions seem to mediate the interaction of the inactivation particle with its receptor. In addition, the primary structure of $L_{III/IV}$—which positions the IFM hydrophobic cluster only 14 amino acid residues from transmembrane segment IIIS6 in a loop that is predicted to have an ordered, partially α-helical structure and is tethered at both ends—is most consistent with an ordered conformational transition that folds $L_{III/IV}$ into the intracellular mouth of the transmembrane pore. A conformational change of this kind is consistent with previous results (26, 27), showing that antibodies against $L_{III/IV}$ that block inactivation can only do so by binding to the noninactivated state of the channel, as if their binding site is made inaccessible by the process of inactivation.

A Hinged-Lid Model of Na⁺ Channel Inactivation

The loop structure of the Na^+ channel inactivation gate differs from that of the K^+ channel, but closely resembles the hinged-lid structures of allosteric enzymes (33). Hinged lids have been defined structurally by x-ray crystallography and molecular modeling and provide a model for the unknown structure of the Na^+ channel inactivation gate. These structures consist of structured loops of 10 to 20 residues between two hinge points and serve as rigid lids that fold over the active sites of allosteric enzymes to control substrate access. Binding of allosteric ligands causes a conformational change of the lid to open or close the active site. By analogy, $L_{III/IV}$ may function as a rigid lid to control Na^+ entry to, and exit from, the intracellular mouth of the pore of the Na^+ channel (Fig. 6). This hinged lid may be held in the closed position during inactivation by a hydrophobic latch formed by the hydrophobic cluster, IFM. Glycine and proline residues on either side of the IFM domain (Fig. 4A) that are conserved in all five cloned rat Na^+ channels that have been functionally expressed may function as hinge points allowing the inactivation gate region of $L_{III/IV}$ to move in and out of the channel pore. Simultaneous mutation of the paired glycines at positions 1484 and 1485 or all four prolines at positions 1509 through 1516 to alanine prevents expression of functional Na^+ channels as might be expected if these residues play a critical structural role as hinge points.

Modulation of Na^+ Channel Function by Protein Kinase C

α-Subunits of purified Na^+ channels from rat brain are also phosphorylated by protein kinase C (34, 35), suggesting that they may be modulated by the calcium/diacylglycerol signaling pathway. In agreement with this suggestion, Na^+ currents in neuroblastoma cells are reduced by treatment with fatty acids that can activate protein kinase C (36), and sodium currents in *Xenopus* oocytes injected with rat brain mRNA are reduced by treatment with phorbol esters that activate protein kinase C (37, 38). Activation of protein kinase C in rat brain neurons (32), rat ventricular myocytes (Fig. 7), skeletal muscle myocytes, or in CHO cells transfected with cDNA encoding the type IIA Na^+ channel α-subunit by treatment with diacylglycerols causes two functional effects: slowing of inactivation and reduction of peak current. Both of these actions are prevented by prior injection of the pseudosubstrate inhibitory domain of protein kinase C into the cells, indicating that they reflect phosphorylation by protein kinase C. Moreover, both effects can be observed by phosphorylating Na^+ channels in excised, inside-out membrane patches, directly with purified protein kinase C (32). These results support the conclusion that protein kinase C can modulate Na^+ channel function by phosphorylation of the α-subunit of the Na^+ channel protein itself as observed with purified Na^+ channels (34, 35).

The intracellular loop connecting domains III and IV has been implicated in Na^+ channel inactivation. This segment has a consensus sequence for phosphorylation by protein kinase C centered at serine 1506 (Fig. 4). Mutagenesis of this serine residue to alanine blocks both of the modulatory effects of protein kinase C (39). Evidently, phosphorylation of this site is required for both slowing of Na^+ channel inactivation and reduction of peak Na^+ current by protein kinase C.

Treatment of neurons or cardiac myocytes with increasing concentrations of diacylglycerol reveals a biphasic modulation; low concentrations slow Na^+ channel inactivation, whereas higher concentrations are required

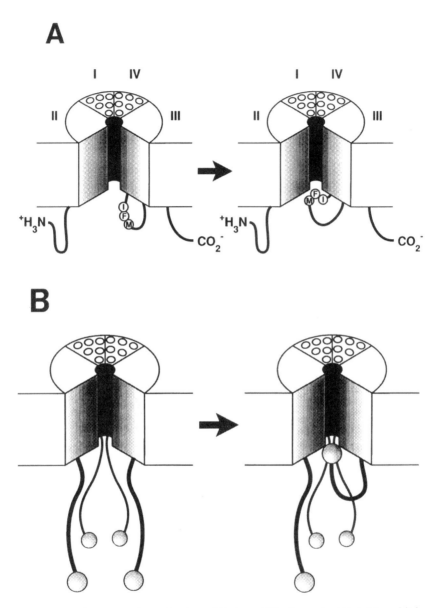

Figure 6. Mechanisms of inactivation of Na^+ and K^+ channels. **(A)** A hinged-lid model for Na^+ channel inactivation illustrating the inactivation gate formed by the intracellular segment connecting domains III and IV and the critical cluster of hydrophobic residues (IFM, isoleucine—phenylalanine—methionine) that forms a latch holding the inactivation gate closed. **(B)** A ball-and-chain model of K^+ channel inactivation. Each of the four subunits of a K^+ channel has a ball-and-chain structure at its *N*-terminal. Any one of the four can bind to the intracellular mouth of the open channel and inactivate it.

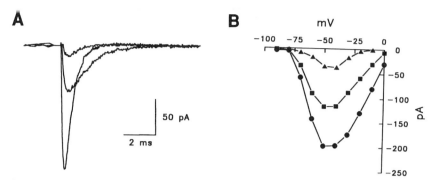

Figure 7. Modulation of Na$^+$ currents by protein phosphorylation in a neonatal rat ventricular cell. **(A)** Na$^+$ currents were recorded in the cell-attached patch configuration during depolarizations from a holding potential of -110 mV to a test potential of -40 mV. Ensemble average currents were calculated from macropatches containing up to 30 active Na$^+$ channels. Current traces are illustrated under control conditions and after activation of protein kinase C by treatment with the synthetic diacylglycerol oleylacetylglycerol for 37.5 min at 60 μM followed by an additional 20 min at 100 μM. **(B)** Na$^+$ currents recorded during test pulses to the indicated voltages are plotted versus membrane potential.

to cause reduction of peak Na$^+$ currents. These results suggest that a second site of phosphorylation is required for reduction of peak Na$^+$ currents. Because cAMP-dependent phosphorylation of sites in the intracellular loop between domains I and II causes reduction of peak Na$^+$ currents, mutant Na$^+$ channels with alterations in consensus sequences for protein kinase C phosphorylation in that region of the channel were examined for modulation by protein kinase C. Mutation of serine 554 located in a protein kinase consensus sequence toward the amino terminal end of this intracellular loop (Fig. 3) prevented the reduction in Na$^+$ current by protein kinase C (40). These results implicate phosphorylation of this residue in the reduction in peak Na$^+$ current caused by protein kinase C and suggest that this effect of protein kinase C phosphorylation has the same underlying molecular mechanism as reduction of peak Na$^+$ current by cAMP-dependent protein phosphorylation of this same region.

Modulation of Expression of Na$^+$ Channels in the Heart by Antiarrhythmic Drugs

Class I antiarrhythmic drugs prevent arrhythmias by inhibiting cardiac Na$^+$ channels in a complex voltage- and frequency-dependent manner. Chronic in vivo treatment with the class I antiarrhythmic drug mexiletine produced an increase in cardiac Na$^+$ channel number as measured by high-affinity binding of batrachotoxin benzoate (41). Na$^+$ channel number, as measured by high-affinity binding of saxitoxin, was also increased in skeletal muscle cells in culture, during chronic treatment with bupivacaine, another

Na$^+$ channel blocker (42, 43). These results show that reduction of the electrical activity of cardiac and skeletal muscle cells causes a compensatory increase in Na$^+$ channel number, and they imply that the normal level of electrical activity of these cells is sufficient to cause a chronic decrease in Na$^+$ channel number.

The decrease in Na$^+$ channel number in skeletal muscle cells caused by the normal level of electrical activity may be mediated by calcium entering the cell during each action potential because chronic elevation of cytosolic calcium by treatment of myocytes in the calcium ionophore A23187, or the calcium-releasing agent ryanodine, substantially reduces Na$^+$ channel number (42, 43). The changes in Na$^+$ channel number in skeletal muscle cells in culture are correlated with comparable changes in the level of mRNA encoding sodium channel α-subunits (44), indicating that regulation of transcription of mRNA or its processing and stability is primarily responsible for regulation of channel number.

Effects of Mexiletine and Verapamil Treatment on Level of mRNA Encoding the α-Subunit of the Na$^+$ Channel

Adult rats were treated with mexiletine or placebo, and cardiac mRNA was isolated and probed with a cRNA complementary to domain I of the Na$^+$ channel. Figure 8 shows a representative Northern blot hybridization of rat heart mRNA encoding the cardiac Na$^+$ channel in animals treated with placebo and mexiletine at doses of 50 mg/kg/day for 24, 48, and 72 hr. Mexiletine (50 mg/kg/day) produced a significant (3-fold) increase in mRNA levels encoding the cardiac Na$^+$ channel ($P < 0.01$), but had no effect on mRNA encoding brain Na$^+$ channels (Fig. 8). The mRNA levels were not further increased at doses of mexiletine of 75 mg/kg/day. If the effect of normal cardiac electrical activity to reduce Na$^+$ channel mRNA level is mediated by calcium entry during the action potential, treatment with a calcium channel blocker like the class IV antiarrhythmic drug verapamil should mimic the effect of mexiletine. Verapamil (3 to 16 mg/kg) produced a significant increase in mRNA levels encoding the cardiac Na$^+$ channel in a dose-dependent fashion (Fig. 8). The mRNA levels encoding the α-subunit of the Na$^+$ channel were substantially increased by 24 hr of treatment and increased little thereafter. Densitometric assessment of levels of mRNA during treatment with placebo and verapamil (3 mg/kg/day) indicate a 3-fold increase in Na$^+$ channel mRNA in heart, with no increase in brain as observed for mexiletine.

Effect of Increased Cytosolic Calcium on Na$^+$ Channel mRNA on Cardiac Myocytes in Cell Culture

To examine whether changes in cytosolic calcium concentrations modulate Na$^+$ channel mRNA levels, neonatal myocytes in dissociated cell

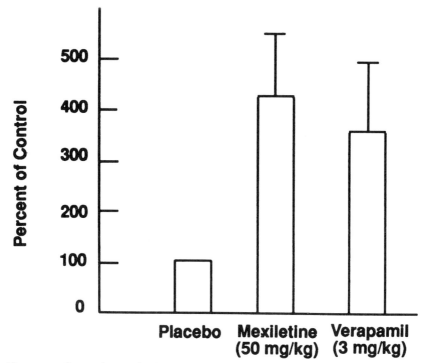

Figure 8. Effects of antiarrhythmic drugs on levels of Na$^+$ channel mRNA in the heart. **(Top)** Adult Sprague–Dawley rats were treated with placebo (lanes 1 to 3), 50 mg/kg mexiletine (lanes 4 to 6), or 3 mg/kg verapamil (lanes 7 to 9). Total RNA was isolated, and the level of RNA encoding the sodium channel α-subunit was determined by Northern blotting, autoradiography, and quantitative densitometry. **(Bottom)** The level of Na$^+$ channel mRNA was normalized to the level of RNA for elongation factor 1α to correct for variation in sample recovery, and the mean values were calculated. Results are presented as a percentage of the values for placebo-treated animals.

culture were treated for 3 days with placebo, verapamil, or A23187. Treatment with verapamil produced only a small increase in the level of mRNA encoding Na$^+$ channel α-subunits that was not statistically significant (Fig. 9). This may indicate that the asynchronous action potentials and contractions of cardiac myocytes in culture are insufficient to cause a substantial chronic reduction in Na$^+$ channel mRNA level that can be reversed by verapamil treatment. Nevertheless, the cell culture system allows chronic elevation of cytosolic calcium by treatment with a calcium ionophore. Treatment with A23187 produced a substantial decrease in the Na$^+$ channel mRNA level (Fig. 9) without effect on the level of mRNA for elongation factor 1 - α used as a control (not shown). Densitometric assessment of mRNA levels in autoradiograms during treatment with placebo and A23187 indicates at least a five-fold reduction due to treatment with ionophore.

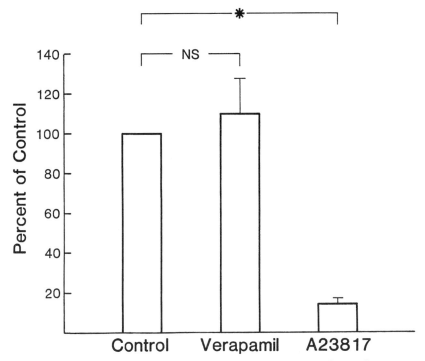

Figure 9. Effects of verapamil and A23187 on mRNA encoding the cardiac Na⁺ channel in cultured neonatal myocytes. Neonatal cultured rat myocytes were treated with verapamil (500 μg/L) and A23817 (1 μM) for 3 days. Total RNA was prepared and the level of mRNA encoding cardiac Na⁺ channel α-subunits was determined by Northern blotting and quantitative densitometry. Na⁺ channel mRNA was normalized to the level of the mRNA for elongation factor 1α to control for differences in sample recovery.

These results are consistent with previous studies, suggesting that calcium mediates the regulation of Na⁺ channel mRNA by electrical activity in skeletal muscle cells.

Regulatory Mechanism

Treatment with other Na⁺ channel blockers, such as bupivacaine, has also been reported to increase Na⁺ channel receptor number in skeletal muscle cells and to produce a concomitant increase in messenger RNA levels encoding the α-subunit of the Na⁺ channel (42–44). Calcium iono-phores and calcium-releasing agents reduce the level of Na⁺ channels and the mRNA encoding them consistent with a primary role for calcium as a second messenger regulating Na⁺ channel expression in response to changes in electrical activity. These data suggest a common regulation system in skeletal muscle and cardiac muscle for mRNA levels encoding the α-subunit of the Na$^+$ channel. The finding that the calcium channel blocker verapamil and the calcium ionophore A23187 produced opposite effects on levels of mRNA encoding the cardiac Na$^+$ channel suggest that the cytosolic calcium concentration is involved in the regulation of mRNA levels in cardiac cells as well as in skeletal muscle cells. Based on the results of the present and past studies, we propose a pathway of regulation of the level of mRNA encoding the α-subunit of the Na$^+$ channel, wherein changes in cytosolic calcium concentration modulate its transcription rate or its processing and stability.

Clinical Relevance

Some patients who respond to an acute intravenous class I antiarrhythmic drug develop resistance to that same drug at nearly identical concentrations when the class I drug is given chronically (45). One possible mechanism for this drug resistance is that chronic Na$^+$ channel blocker treatment produces an increase in the Na$^+$ channel number that decreases the pharmacodynamic response to these class I drugs. A testable prediction from the current study is that pretreatment of animals with the class IV antiarrhythmic verapamil will increase Na$^+$ channel number and result in a lesser response to acute intravenous class I drug therapy. The increased number of Na$^+$ channels caused by chronic treatment with these drugs may itself cause arrhythmias as a secondary consequence of therapy. Such arrhythmias would be particularly likely on withdrawal of treatment.

References

1. Catterall, W.A. (1986). Molecular properties of voltage-sensitive sodium channels. *Ann. Rev. Biochem.* **55**:953–985.

2. Agnew, W.S. (1984). Voltage-regulated sodium channel molecules. *Ann. Rev. Physiol.* **46**:517–530.

3. Barchi, R.L. (1988). Probing the molecular structure of the voltage-dependent sodium channel. *Ann. Rev. Neurosci.* **11**:455–495.

4. Gordon, D., Merrick, D., Wollner, D.A., and Catterall, W.A. (1988). Biochemical properties of sodium channels in a wide range of excitable tissues studied with site-directed antibodies. *Biochemistry* **27**:7032–7038.

5. McHugh-Sutkowski, E., and Catterall, W.A. (1990). β$_1$ subunits of sodium channels. Studies with subunit-specific antibodies. *J. Biol. Chem.* **265**:12393–12399.

6. Noda, M., Shimizu, S., Tanabe, T., Takai, T., Kayano, T., Ikeda, T. Takahashi, H., Nakayama, H., Kanaoka, Y., Minamino, N., Kangawa, K., Matsuo, H., Raftery, M., Hirose, T., Inayama, S., Hayashida, H., Miyata, T., and Numa, S. (1984). Primary structure of *Electrophorus electricus* sodium channel deduced from cDNA sequence. *Nature* **312**:121–127.

7. Noda, M., Ikeda, T., Kayano, T., Suzuki, H., Takeshima, H., Kurasaki, M., Takahashi, H., and Numa, S. (1986). Existence of distinct sodium channel messenger RNAs in rat brain. *Nature* **320**:188–192.

8. Kayano, T., Noda, M., Flockerzi, V., Takahashi, H., and Numa, S. (1988). Primary structure of rat brain sodium channel III deduced from the cDNA sequence. *FEBS Lett.* **228:**187–194.

9. Auld, V.J., Goldin, A.L., Krafte, D.S., Catterall, W.A., Lester, H.A., Davidson, N., and Dunn, R.J. (1990). A neutral amino acid change in segment IIS4 dramatically alters the gating properties of the voltage-dependent sodium channel. *Proc. Natl. Acad. Sci. U.S.A.* **87:**323–327.

10. Trimmer, J.S., Cooperman, S.S., Tomiko, S.A., Zhou, J.Y., Crean, S.M., Boyle, M.B., Kallen, R.G., Sheng, Z.H., Barchi, R.L., Sigworth, F.J., Goodman, R.H., Agnew, W.S., and Mandel, G. (1989). Primary structure and function expression of a mammalian skeletal muscle sodium channel. *Neuron* **3:**33–49.

11. Rogart, R.B., Cribbs, L.L., Muglia, L.K., Kephart, D.D., and Kaiser, M.W. (1989). Molecular cloning of a putative tetrodotoxin-resistant rat heart sodium channel isoform. *Proc. Natl. Acad. Sci. U.S.A.* **86:**8170–8174.

12. Kallen, R.G., Sheng, Z.H., Yang, J., Chen, L.Q., Rogart, R.B., and Barchi, R.L. (1990). Primary structure and expression of a sodium channel characteristic of denervated and immature rat skeletal muscle. *Neuron* **4:**233–242.

13. Isom, L.L., DeJongh, K.S., Patton, D.E., Reber, B.F., Offord, J., Charbonneau, H., Walsh, K., Goldin, A.L., and Catterall, W.A. (1992). Primary structure and functional expression of the β_1 subunit of the rat brain sodium channel. *Science* **256:**839–842.

14. Goldin, A.L., Snutch, T., Lubbert, H., Dowsett, A., Marshall, J., Auld, V., Downey, W., Fritz, L.C., Lester, H.A., Dunn, R., Catterall, W.A., and Davidson, N. (1986). Messenger RNA coding for only the α-subunit of the rat brain Na channel is sufficient for expression of functional channels in *Xenopus* oocytes. *Proc. Natl. Acad. Sci. U.S.A.* **83:**7503–7507.

15. Noda, M., Ikeda, T., Suzuki, T., Takeshima, H., Takahashi, Kuno, M., and Numa, S. (1986). Expression of functional sodium channels from cloned cDNA. *Nature* **322:**826–828.

16. Suzuki, H., Beckh, S., Kubo, H., Yahagi, N., Isha, H., Kayano, T., Noda, M., and Numa, S. (1988). Functional expression of cloned cDNA encoding sodium channel III. *FEBS Lett.* **228:**195–200.

17. Moorman, J.R., Kirsch, G.E., Vandongen, A.M., Joho, R.H., and Brown, A.M. (1990). Fast and slow gating of sodium channels encoded by a single mRNA. *Neuron* **4:**243–252.

18. Cribbs, L.L., Satin, J., Fozzard, H.A., and Rogart, R.B. (1990). Functional expression of the rat heart. I. Na⁺ channel isoform. Demonstration of properties characteristic of native cardiac Na⁺ channels. *FEBS Lett.* **275:**195–200.

19. White, M.M., Chen, L., Kleinfield, R., Kallen, R.G., and Barchi, R.L. (1991). SkM2, a Na⁺ channel cDNA clone from denervated skeletal muscle, encodes a tetrodotoxin-insensitive Na⁺ channel. *Mol. Pharmacol.* **39:**604–608.

20. Krafte, D.S., Goldin. A.L., Auld, V.J., Dunn, R.J., Davidson, N., and Lester, H.A. (1990). Inactivation of cloned Na channels expressed in *Xenopus* oocytes. *J. Gen. Physiol.* **96:**689–706.

21. Scheuer, T., Auld, V.J., Boyd, S., Offord, J., Dunn, R., and Catterall, W.A. (1990). Functional properties of rat brain sodium channels expressed in a somatic cell line. *Science* **247:**854–858.

22. West, J.W., Scheuer, T., Maechler, L., and Catterall, W.A. (1992). Efficient expression of rat brain type IIA Na$^+$ channel α-subunits in a somatic cell line. *Neuron* **8:**59–70.

23. Ragsdale, D.S., Scheuer, T., and Catterall, W.A. (1991). Frequency and voltage-dependent inhibition of type IIA sodium channels expressed in a mammalian cell line by local anesthetic, antiarrhythmic, and anticonvulsant drugs. *Mol. Pharmacol.* **40:**756–765.

24. Armstrong, C.M. (1981). Sodium channels and gating currents. *Physiol. Rev.* **61:**644–682.

25. Stühmer, W., Conti, F., Suzuki, H., Wang, X., Noda, M., Yahagi, N., Kubo, H., and Numa, S. (1989). Structural parts involved in activation and inactivation of the sodium channel. *Nature* **339:**597–603.

26. Vassilev, P., Scheuer, T., and Catterall, W. A. (1988). Identification of an intracellular peptide segment involved in sodium channel inactivation. *Science* **241:**1658–1661.

27. Vassilev, P., Scheuer, T., and Catterall, W. A. (1989). Inhibition of inactivation of single sodium channels by a site-directed antibody. *Proc. Natl. Acad. Sci. U.S.A.* **86:**8147–8151.

28. Patton, D.E., and Goldin, A.L. (1991). A voltage-dependent gating transition induces use-dependent block by tetrodotoxin of rat IIA sodium channels expressed in *Xenopus* oocytes. *Neuron* **7:**637–647.

29. West, J.W., Patton, D.E., Scheuer, T., Wang, Y.-L., Goldin, A.L., and Catterall, W.A. (1992). A cluster of hydrophobic amino acid residues required for fast Na$^+$ channel inactivation. *Proc. Natl. Acad. Sci. U.S.A.* **89:**10910–10914.

30. Moorman, J.R., Kirsch, G.E., Brown, A.M., and Joho, R.H. (1990). Changes in sodium channel gating produced by point mutations in a cytoplasmic linker. *Science* **250:**688–691.

31. Patton, D.E., West, J.W., Catterall, W.A., and Goldin, A.L. (1992). Amino acid residues required for fast sodium channel inactivation. Charge neutralizations and deletions in the III–IV linker. *Proc. Natl. Acad. Sci. U.S.A.* **89:**10905–10909.

32. Numann, R., Catterall, W.A., and Scheuer, T. (1991). Functional modulation of brain sodium channels by protein kinase C phosphorylation. *Science* **254:**115–118.

33. Joseph, D., Petsko, G.A., and Karplus, M. (1990). Anatomy of a conformational change: Hinged "lid" motion of the triosephosphate isomerase loop. *Science* **249:**1425–1428.

34. Costa, M.R., and Catterall, W.A. (1984). Phosphorylation of the α-subunit of the sodium channel by protein kinases. *Cell Mol. Neurobiol.* **4:**291–297.

35. Murphy, B.J., and Catterall, W.A. (1992). Phosphorylation of purified rat brain Na$^+$ channel reconstituted into phospholipid vesicles by protein kinase C. *J. Biol. Chem.* **267:**16129–16134.

338

36. Linden, D.J., and Routtenberg, A. (1989). Cis-fatty acids, which activate protein kinase C, attenuate Na^+ and Ca^{2+} currents in mouse neuroblastoma cells. *J. Physiol.* **419**:95–119.

37. Sigel, E., and Baur, R. (1988). Activation of protein kinase C differentially modulates neuronal Na^+, Ca^{2+}, and γ-aminobutyrate type A channels. *Proc. Natl. Acad. Sci. U.S.A.* **85**:6192–6196.

38. Dascal, N., and Lotan, I. (1991). Activation of protein kinase C alters voltage dependence of a Na^+ channel. *Neuron* **6**:165–175.

39. West, J.W., Numann, R., Murphy, B.M., Scheuer, T., and Catterall, W.A. (1991). Identification of a phosphorylation site in a conserved intracellular loop that is required for modulation of sodium channels by protein kinase C. *Science* **254**:866–868.

40. Numann, R., West, J.W., Li, M., Smith, R.D., Goldin, A.L., Scheuer, T., and Catterall, W.A. (1992). Biphasic modulation of sodium channels by phosphorylation at two different sites. *Soc. Neurosci. Abstr.* **18**:1133.

41. Taouis, M., Sheldon, R.S., and Duff, H.J. (1991). Unregulation of the rat cardiac sodium channel by in vivo treatment with a class I antiarrhythmic drug. *J. Clin. Invest.* **88**:375–378.

42. Sherman, S.J., and Catterall, W.A. (1984). Electrical activity and cytosolic calcium regulate levels of tetrodotoxin-sensitive sodium channels in cultured rat muscle cells. *Proc. Natl. Acad. Sci. U.S.A.* **81**:262–266.

43. Sherman, S.J., Chrivia, J., and Catterall, W.A. (1985). Cyclic adenosine 3′:5′ monophosphate and cytosolic calcium exert opposing effects on biosynthesis of tetrodotoxin-sensitive sodium channels in rat muscle cells. *J. Neurosci.* **5**:1570–1576.

44. Offord, J., and Catterall, W.A. (1989). Electrical activity, cAMP, and cytosolic calcium regulate mRNA encoding sodium channel α-subunits in rat muscle cells. *Neuron* **2**:1447–1452.

45. Duff, H.J., Wyse, D.G., Manyari, D., and Mitchell, L.B. (1985). Intravenous quinidine: Relations among concentration, tachyarrhythmia suppression, and electrophysiologic actions with inducible sustained ventricular tachycardia. *Am. J. Cardiol.* **55**:92–97.

17

Extracellular Potassium Modulates a Transient Potassium Current in Rat Atrial Cells

L. A. Pardo and W. Stühmer

Among ion channels, Na^+ and Ca^+ channels are the usual targets for drugs used to treat various cardiac diseases, because in heart cells much of the action potential current is carried by Na^+ and Ca^+. There is, however, a theoretical alternative to this concept, because K^+ channels could also act as regulators of the electrical activity of the heart. K^+ channels are responsible for such processes as rhythmogenesis, maintenance of resting potential, and repolarization of the action potential (1). Heart cells show a large variety of K^+ channels, which can be modulated by both voltage and second messengers (2). Despite extensive studies on the electrophysiology of heart cells using the patch-clamp technique, little has been found concerning the molecular mechanisms of channel function. The recent possibility of using patch clamp methods in parallel with molecular biology techniques has greatly increased our ability to explore this topic.

The voltage-gated channels are well characterized because several members of this group have been cloned and studied in expression systems. These channels belong to a family, as demonstrated by the high homology among its members. The major structural parts in these channels have been deduced based on primary sequence comparison and verified by site-directed mutagenesis. Of course, if an heterologous expression system is used, not all the properties of the channel are necessarily identical to those found in situ.

Multiple K+ Channels

Rat heart contains at least five mRNAs coding for different voltage-gated K^+ channel types. All of them have homologous counterparts to 1 of the 4 families of channels found in *Drosophila*. These families (called *Shaker, Shab, Shal,* and *Shaw* in the insect) are grouped according to sequence homologies into four types (Kv1 to Kv4) in mammals. Different laboratories have cloned and sequenced essentially identical channels, and each one has used its own nomenclature for them. For clarity, we will use the standard notation (3). Some of the channels mentioned herein may therefore appear under a different name elsewhere in the volume.

Three of the rat heart K^+ channels express noninactivating currents in *Xenopus* oocytes: Kv1.1 (RCK1, ref. 4; RK1, refs. 6 and 7), Kv1.2 (RCK5, ref. 5; RK2, refs 6 and 7), and Kv1.5 (RK4, refs. 6 and 7). The other two show fast-inactivating (A-type) currents: Kv1.4 (RCK4, ref. 5; RHK1, ref. 8; RK3, refs. 6 and 7) and Kv4.1 (RShal, ref. 8). These five appear to be the most abundant messages in heart, but not necessarily the only ones. In addition, heterooligomers formed between different channels from a given family can be an important added source for variability (9). Therefore, functionally different heart cells may be expressing either different types or different combinations of channels. As an example, the expression of different populations of channels seems to be developmentally controlled: Kv1.1, Kv1.2, and Kv1.4 are increasingly expressed during the first two postnatal weeks, whereas Kv1.5 is constitutively expressed (6, 7). This might explain several of the physiological differences between young and adult hearts.

Two different channels homologous to Kv1.4 (HK1) and Kv1.5 (HK2) have been identified in human heart (10). Although the similarities between the sequences from the two species are striking, the distribution patterns of these channels seem to differ. In humans Kv1.4 is equally abundant in atria and ventricle, whereas in rat it seems to be restricted to atrium. The opposite is true for Kv1.5, which is more specific for atria in humans while ubiquitous in rat. These differences are specially important for our purpose, because we will focus on the properties of Kv1.4. The exact role for this channel in human heart remains to be clarified, but we will assume a strong functional similarity between rat and human Kv1.4 channels because the two are 98% identical in primary structure; virtually all the different residues are located in the N-terminus of the protein. A mutant rat channel whose N-terminus is deleted is virtually identical to the wild type with regard to the aspects discussed herein. Therefore we will assume that the human and rat channels behave in a similar way.

It is well known that heart cells are extremely sensitive to the composition of the extracellular milieu. One of the parameters most frequently related to the generation of severe arrhythmias is the extracellular K^+ concentration, $[K^+]_0$ (see ref. 11 for a review). These alterations can quickly lead to ventricular fibrillation, a rhythm disturbance that essentially consists of erratic ventricular contraction. The result is a compromise of the ability of the heart to pump, frequently having fatal consequences. General alterations of serum K^+ levels are relatively infrequent. However, local K^+ concentration increase is an early event during heart ischemia. The K^+ concentration in extracellular heart tissue has been measured with K^+-sensitive electrodes during heart surgery and shown to rise shortly after the reduction in blood supply. This rise is dramatic, reaching 10 to 15 mM within minutes (12). In addition, these changes in $[K^+]_0$ are not homogeneous within the tissue, so that the conduction is strongly altered, a fact contributing to rhythm alteration (13). Even after an ischemic episode, heart behavior is abnormal, and this facilitates induction of new arrythmias upon reperfusion. For example, the transient outward current (I_{to}) density is decreased for prolonged times after an ischemic event (14).

KV1.4 and External K+

Changes in $[K^+]_0$ are bound to alter the resting potential in cells, but this is only one of the effects observed when the $[K^+]_0$ is manipulated in different preparations. $[K^+]_0$ seems to affect the macroscopic conductance of at least three different currents: a delayed rectifier (15), a transient outward current (16), and an inwardly rectifying current (17). One of these currents, I_{to}, matches the properties of the current carried through Kv1.4, a channel that has been cloned and characterized in detail.

Because the mRNA for Kv1.4 can be detected in rat atria after the 14th postnatal day (6, 7), we isolated atrial myocytes from rats aged 3 to 4 weeks. The heart was perfused with a collagenase-containing solution in situ, after which the atria were removed and the digestion completed. Electrophysiological studies were performed 6 to 8 hr after plating cells. Recording conditions were designed to isolate rapidly inactivating K^+ currents having a slow recovery from inactivation and that were insensitive to both tetraethylammonium (TEA) and charybdotoxin (CTX). A standard extracellular medium containing 2.8 mM KCl was used. In some experiments NaCl was replaced with Tris-Cl to abolish Na^+ currents. A double-pulse protocol was used to isolate the currents that were both rapidly inactivating and slowly reactivating: a first depolarizing pulse was applied from a holding potential of -70 mV, followed by an identical second depolarization after a 40-msec interval at the holding potential. The second pulse evoked noninactivating currents, as well as those currents that inactivate but are able to recover during the 40-msec interpulse interval. These currents were subtracted from those flowing during the first pulse. With this protocol, most of the outward current through a fast-inactivating, slowly recovering (A-type) channel is isolated (Fig. 1, trace 1). As previously described, this current closely matches both kinetically and pharmacologically the properties found in Kv1.4 channels that are expressed in *Xenopus* oocytes (5): it activates rapidly at room temperature; inactivates with a time constant of ~50 msec; and reactivates (recovery from inactivation) very slowly with a time constant of >100 msec. This last property means that only a small fraction of the current is recovered within 40 msec. The current is not reduced by external application of 5 mM TEA or CTX, but is sensitive to TEA applied from the cytoplasmic side. In addition, we did not detect

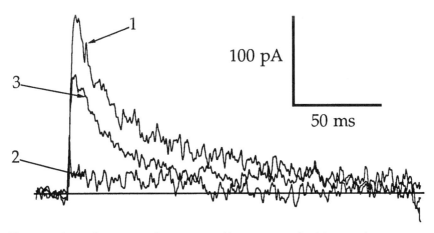

Figure 1. A transient outward current sensitive to external K^+ in acutely dissociated rat atrial cells. Trace 1: Control in 2.8 mM K^+. Trace 2: Perfusion with K^+-free solution. Trace 3: Recovery. Data were obtained as described in the text and digitally filtered off-line at 3 kHz.

any comparable current in very young hearts (1 to 3 postnatal day), in good agreement with the developmental regulation of Kv1.4 expression.

If a heart preparation is perfused with a solution nearly identical to the control one, lacking only K^+, an increase in the amplitude of the current is expected, because the displacement of the K^+ equilibrium potential to more negative values increases the driving force for the cation. Surprisingly, however, this transient outward current is heavily reduced (Fig. 1, trace 2). The control amplitude is readily recovered when the K^+ is reintroduced into the bath solution (trace 3).

Kv1.4 also shows a strong modulation by extracellular K^+ in *Xenopus* oocytes. Interestingly, Kv1.4 is expressed in only a few tissues, mainly heart and brain. We have localized a very similar current also in rat hippocampal cells, that also express Kv1.4 (18). All these observations suggest that the currents detected in situ are in fact caused by Kv1.4 channels.

In addition, it has been mentioned that K^+ channels can form heterooligomers between subunits coded by different genes. Heterooligomeric channels formed by Kv1.1–Kv1.4 subunits inherit most properties from the Kv1.4 channel, in particular their sensitivity to $[K^+]_0$, although to a lesser extent. Therefore, we cannot exclude the possibility that the native channels both in rat hippocampus and heart are heterooligomeric channels having as one component the Kv1.4 subunit (or a subunit with similar properties), even when the almost complete abolition of the current in heart cells suggests the presence of homooligomers.

The oocyte system allows the expression of high densities of virtually pure heterologous channels, and this makes it possible to perform measurements in macropatches (i.e., membrane patches that contain enough channels to measure macroscopic currents). This combines two technical advantages. First, they are relatively small areas of membrane so that the voltage clamp is more efficient, second, they produce macroscopic current so that it is easier to follow kinetic parameters of the channel population. Hence, we have characterized the properties of this channel in outside-out patches obtained from *Xenopus* oocytes injected with Kv1.4 mRNA (16). Provided that $[K^+]_0$ is properly controlled, the Kv1.4 current disappears completely when external K^+ is removed. This kind of experiment requires a very careful control of the $[K^+]_0$, because the K^+ ions flowing through active channels can be sufficient to maintain the activity of other channels. To achieve this, we usually remove the oocyte from the chamber after obtaining the patch, because it contains K^+ concentrations in the range of 0.1 M, and we use fast flow of K^+-free solution directly onto the patch to avoid accumulation of the cation in the immediate vicinity of the channels.

The modulation of Kv1.4 by a $[K^+]_0$ is not a general feature of K^+ channels. In fact, it is quite specific for Kv1.4. In oocytes, no other exogenously expressed channels showed a comparable behavior. Channels from the same family, like *Shaker* A2, Kv1.1, Kv1.2, Kv1.3, Kv1.5, and Kv1.6 were tested, and only Kv1.5 (also expressed in heart at high levels) showed a similar effect, although to a lesser extent; some current flowing through this channel is detected even at 0 $[K^+]_0$. We also tested a channel from the *Shaw* family, Kv3.4 (19), with negative results. On the other hand, many K^+ channels show effects of very high or very low $[K^+]_0$, but in the case of Kv1.4 the effects are significant within the physiological range of $[K^+]_0$. In oocytes expressing Kv1.4, and at 20° to 22°, the dose-response relationship fits to a Boltzmann distribution, with a half-maximal effect at 2.2 mM, a concentration that matches the physiological value of $[K^+]_0$. This means that, under physiological conditions, the $[K^+]_0$ falls on the steepest part of the dose-response curve, and is then most sensitive to any change.

Not only K^+, but also Rb^+, Cs^+, and NH_4^+ can to some extent modulate the macroscopic conductance of the channel. This implies that the effect of the cations must be exerted acting from the outside of the cell, because Cs^+ ions are virtually nonpermeant through the Kv1.4 channel. It has also been shown that $[K^+]_0$ does not change either the single channel conductance or the mean open time; the gating charge displacement upon depolarization is also unaltered by the $[K^+]_0$. Taken together, these observations indicate that the channels keep most of their properties unaltered, but K^+ is not able to permeate. If both the conductance and the mean open time are constant, the number of channels available for opening is the remaining factor that can change the amplitude of Kv1.4 current responding to changes in $[K^+]_0$. This can be achieved in different ways from a molecular point of view. The simplest scheme implies that the channel is either in a closed or in an inactivated state.

If K^+ ions need not permeate to be effective in increasing the amplitude, a site located on the outer part of the channel, and closely related to conduction, should be involved. External K^+ is known to compete with TEA (20), a widely used K^+ channel blocker. The site responsible for the sensitivity to TEA is known, and is located close to what is thought to be the external mouth of the channel (21). Kv1.4 is highly resistant to external TEA, because it has a lysine residue in the position 533, instead of the uncharged residues that TEA-sensitive channels have in the equivalent position (Thr in *Shaker*, and Tyr in Kv1.1, Kv1.6, and Kv3.4). Substituting that residue for Tyr in Kv1.4 confers TEA sensitivity to the channel and also removes the K^+ dependence.

There is some correlation between the charge in that position (positive for Kv1.4) and the sensitivity to $[K^+]_0$. In this sense, the mutant where the lysine residue has been replaced by histidine shows dependence on $[K^+]_0$ when the external pH is lowered to 5 (most of the histidine residues are then charged), but is insensitive at neutral pH (Fig. 2). When the tyrosine in the equivalent position of Kv1.6 is replaced by lysine or arginine, the mutant channel is very sensitive to external K^+.

Thus, the general tendency is that those channels that show a charged residue are resistant to TEA and sensitive to $[K^+]_0$. However, the relationship is not unequivocal, because there are several exceptions. Kv1.2 shows an uncharged residue, valine, and is insensitive to K^+, but also to TEA; in addition, the conservative mutation Y430Q for Kv1.6 renders a channel strongly sensitive to external K^+.

Mechanism of the $[K^+]_0$ Effect

We have tried to elucidate the molecular mechanisms underlying the dependence of the channel on the $[K^+]_0$. For that reason, we have studied kinetic parameters of Kv1.4 influenced by $[K^+]_0$, especially ones related to inactivation and recovery from inactivation.

Some evidence against inactivation having a decisive role in the generation of $[K^+]_0$ sensitivity arises from gating charge measurements (16). Inactivation of the channel should immobilize the gating charge, so that if inactivation is involved, the gating charge displacement at low $[K^+]_0$ should be smaller than at high $[K^+]_0$, but this is not the case. However, this evidence cannot definitively exclude inactivation as the mechanism for the reduction in current when $[K^+]_0$ is decreased. As with other inactivating K^+ channels, inactivation of Kv1.4 depends on the N-teminal region of the protein (22). Although our preliminary data indicate that a deletion mutant that lacks the first 110 residues is also sensitive to modulation by $[K^+]_0$, it is unlikely that the inactivation mechanism is essential for this modulation.

Recovery from inactivation is the most strongly influenced parameter of the channels when $[K^+]_0$ is changed. This is known for several inactivating K^+ channels, but it is most dramatic in this case, because of the extremely slow kinetics of this process in Kv1.4 under normal $[K^+]_0$. The time constant

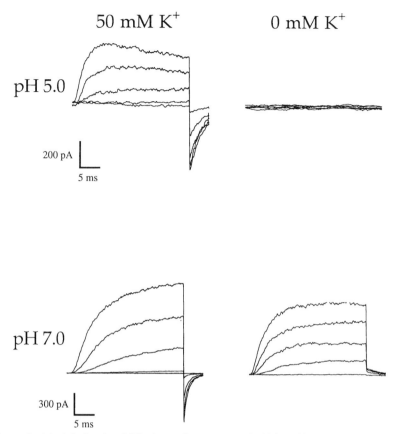

Figure 2. Modulation by $[K^+]_0$ depends on external pH in a Kv1.4 mutant carrying a His residue at position 533. The upper traces show the effect of lowering $[K^+]_0$ at a pH below the expected pK of the His residue, whereas the lower traces were obtained at pH 7.

for the recovery from inactivation can be of tens of milliseconds with 50 mM external K^+, whereas it is in the range of seconds in 1 mM $[K^+]_0$ (Fig. 3).

Why does external K^+ accelerate the recovery from inactivation? A-type currents have an inactivation mechanism that involves the N-terminal part of the molecule (20). This end binds to the internal part of the pore and blocks ion flow. Intuitively, it is easy to imagine that the outward flow of K^+ will facilitate this process, whereas K^+ flowing inward will tend to displace the inactivation particle and reactivate the channel. A mechanism similar to this "knock-off" effect has been shown to exist in K^+ channels (23).

Several lines of evidence support this mechanism, and most experiments have been done on channels like *Shaker* that show a time constant

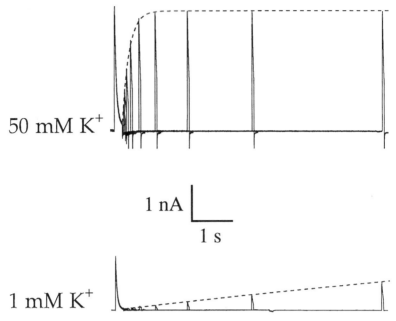

Figure 3. The recovery from inactivation is strongly influenced by $[K^+]_0$ in Kv1.4. A long pulse was applied in order to inactivate the channels, and the fraction already reactivated was determined after a variable interpulse interval. At 1 mM $[K^+]_0$, the time constant of the process is over one order of magnitude slower than at 50 mM $[K^+]_0$.

for this process in the range of milliseconds. However, because of the slower kinetics of Kv1.4, we now have the opportunity to study this effect in greater detail, because manipulation of the external medium can be done during reactivation. Such an experiment is shown in Fig. 4. There the channels are completely inactivated by a long pulse, and $[K^+]_0$ is suddenly raised at the beginning of the reactivation period. It can be seen that the reactivation process is accelerated. $[K^+]_0$ is effective on channels that are already inactivated. Moreover, during the period at high K^+, an inward current flows through the membrane patch. In principle, there should not be open channels at -80 mV, and if there were many channels in the closed state, they should show up during the second depolarizing pulse. This means that most of the channels are in the inactivated state and that the inward current induced by increasing $[K^+]_0$ is flowing through them. The upper trace in Fig. 4 shows that if a high concentration of Cs^+ is applied during the recovery period, no inward current is induced, and the recovery is not accelerated. Hence, there is probably a causal relation between inward flow of ions and accelerated recovery from inactivation, so that the inward current is responsible for knocking off the inactivation particle.

This effect could explain why fewer channels are active at low $[K^+]_0$: they might remain for a very long time in an inactivated state. However,

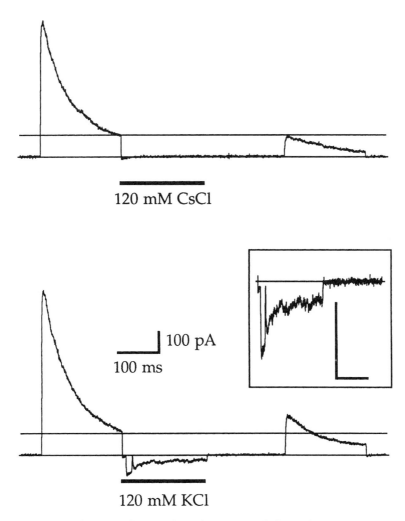

Figure 4. Inward current flowing through inactivated channels. Upper trace: Cs⁺ was applied after an inactivating pulse and the test pulse showed no recovery from inactivation. In the lower trace, K⁺ was applied, which led to an inward current and to an accelerated recovery from inactivation, as evidenced from the larger currents during the test pulse. The inset shows the inward current flowing through inactivated channels at a higher magnification. The numerical values of the scale bars outside the inset apply.

we have several pieces of evidence against this possibility. The main one is that Cs⁺, which as mentioned is not permeant, is able to maintain the current, but not to accelerate its recovery. This was shown in experiments like the one depicted in Fig. 5. The same patch was subjected to two identical pulses separated by 1 sec at holding potential, while exposed to three different solutions. In 1 mM $[K^+]_0$, the amplitude of the current is

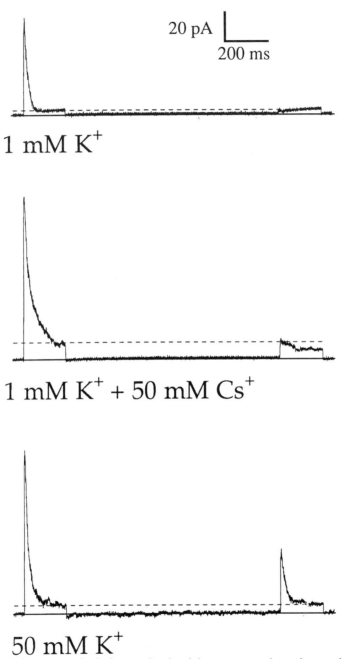

20 pA

200 ms

1 mM K$^+$

1 mM K$^+$ + 50 mM Cs$^+$

50 mM K$^+$

Figure 5. K$^+$ increases both the amplitude of the current and accelerates the reactivation, whereas Cs$^+$ only increases the amplitude. The three traces were obtained from the same patch, perfused with different solutions.

small in the first pulse, and very little current is recovered during the second pulse. In 50 mM Cs^+ plus 1 mM K^+, the first pulse elicits bigger amplitude, but the fraction recovered after 1 sec is virtually the same. In 50 mM K^+, however, both the current amplitude and the recovery are affected. This difference already suggests that, although the amplitude modulation is exerted from the outside, the acceleration of the recovery requires permeation to be completed. On the other hand, the inactivation itself seems to be independent of the flow of ions, as shown by experiments like the one depicted in Fig. 6. The membrane patch containing Kv1.4 channels was perfused with K^+-free solution until isoosmolar K^+ was added by fast application (i.e., in a few milliseconds). After 300 msec in this solution, a test pulse was applied; if the patch had been maintained at the holding potential while in K^+-free solution, a fraction of current was recovered as assayed during a test depolarization. However, if a depolarizing pulse was applied while the patch was in K^+-free solution, the response to the test pulse was much smaller. The latter result indicates that channels are able to inactivate even if (since at 0 $[K^+]_0$ the current is abolished) no current flows through them.

Summary

In conclusion, although many kinetic parameters are strongly influenced by $[K^+]_0$, we have not been able, up to now, to determine any correlation between these variations in Kv1.4 channel function and modulation by $[K^+]_0$. The remaining possibility, now under study, is that the link between the voltage sensor and the gate of the channel, or even the gate itself, is altered by reducing $[K^+]_0$.

The physiological relevance of the presence of K^+-sensitive K^+ channels is not well known, but several hypotheses can be proposed. During increased activity in any excitable cell, K^+ concentrations in the immediate

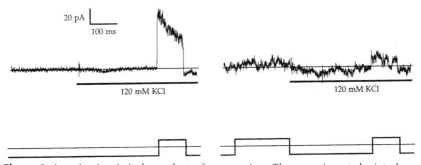

Figure 6. Inactivation is independent of permeation. The experiment depicted herein shows how inactivation occurs in channels that are not permeable. When the patch was depolarized in 0 $[K^+]_0$ the current present during a depolarization in high $[K^+]_0$ is much smaller than when the patch was maintained at holding potential while in low $[K^+]_0$.

vicinity of the cell rise. This would, by two different mechanisms, change the behavior of Kv1.4. First, it would increase its current amplitude. A-currents are thought to control the duration of the action potentials (24, 25) so that with a bigger A-current shorter action potentials would be generated. Second, recovery from inactivation would be much faster, and this would allow it to resist any tendency toward depolarization, clamping the membrane potential effectively.

Channel function can also be compromised by this mechanism, however; for example, during ischemia, when the $[K^+]_0$ rise is not correlated with increased activity, but has a pathological origin. In response to the increase in $[K^+]_0$, action potentials would be shorter, and the contraction less effective; on the other hand, faster repolarization would then shorten the effective refractory period and allow reentry, thus contributing to the tendency to ventricular fibrillation.

We have concentrated on cardiac tissue from rat because most of the results on cloned K^+ channels have been acquired from this species, although many classical physiological and physiopathological experiments have been mostly done with different animals, such as rabbit, guinea pig, cat, or dog (all of them with much bigger hearts). The reason for choosing rat tissue is that all the K^+ channels cloned from heart have been isolated by homology with other channels, and were first available from rat. Rat heart does not express high levels of Kv1.4 in ventricle; this is not surprising if one thinks that the channel would be always inactivated in a heart beating with such a high frequency (300 strokes/min). In any case, this specificity in location would argue against Kv1.4 being a candidate for the generation of postinfarction arrhythmias in humans. This tissue distribution of the channel, however, seems to be a peculiarity of rat heart. Human heart does show high levels of this channel in ventricle, and herein the kinetics would allow it to be active. We have already mentioned that human and rat Kv1.4 channels share 98% homology, and that the differences between them are concentrated in the N-terminal part of the channel, whereas an N-terminal deleted Kv1.4 is still sensitive to external K^+. Thus, it is very likely that the human channel is also strongly modulated by $[K^+]_0$. This makes it a good candidate for being the origin of K^+-induced rhythm disturbances, and suggests direction for future physiological and pharmacological studies.

Acknowledgments

We thank Professor Olaf Pongs for providing the mRNAs used throughout this work, and Dr. Anant B. Parekh for critical reading of the manuscript.

References

1. Rudy, B. (1988). Diversity and ubiquity of K channels. *J. Neurosci.* **25**:729–750.

2. Hille, B. (1992). *Ionic Channels of Excitable Membranes* (Sinauer Associates, Inc., Sunderland, MA), 2nd ed.

3. Chandy, K.G. (1992). Simplified gene nomenclature. *Nature* **352**:26.

4. Stühmer, W., Stocker, M., Sakmann, B., Seeburg, P., Baumann, A., Grupe, A., and Pongs, O. (1988). Potassium channels expressed from rat brain cDNA have delayed rectifier properties. *FEBS Lett.* **242**:199–206.

5. Stühmer, W., Ruppersberg, J.P., Schröter, K.H., Sakmann, B., Stocker, M., Giese, K.P., Perschke, A., Baumann, A., and Pongs, O. (1989). Molecular basis of functional diversity of voltage-gated potassium channels in mammalian brain. *EMBO J.* **8**:3235–3244.

6. Roberds, S.L., and Tamkun, M.M. (1991a). Developmental expression of cloned cardiac potassium channels. *FEBS Lett.* **284**:152–154.

7. Roberds, S.L., and Tamkun, M.M. (1991b). Cloning and tissue-specific expression of five voltage-gated potassium channel cDNAs expressed in rat heart. *Proc. Natl. Acad. Sci. U.S.A.* **88**:1798–1802.

8. Tseng-Cranck, J.C.L., Tseng, G.-N., Schwartz, A., and Tanouye, M.A. (1990). Molecular cloning and functional expression of a potassium channel cDNA isolated from a rat cardiac library. *FEBS Lett.* **268**:63–68.

9. Ruppesberg, J.P., Schröter, K.H., Sakmann, B., Stocker, M., Sewing, S., and Pongs, O. (1990). Heteromultimeric channels formed by rat brain potassium-channel proteins. *Nature* **345**:535–537.

10. Tamkun, M.M., Knoth, K.M., Walbridge, J.A., Kroemer, H., Roden, D.M., and Glover, D.M. (1991). Molecular cloning and characterization of two voltage-gated K⁺ channel cDNAs from human ventricle. *FASEB J.* **5**:331–337.

11. Ten Eick, R.E., Whalley, D.W., and Rasmussen, H.H. (1992). Connections: Heart disease, cellular electrophysiology, and ion channels. *FASEB J.* **6**:2568–2580.

12. Fozzard, H.A., and Makielski, J.C. (1985). The electrophysiology of acute myocardial ischemia. *Ann. Rev. Med.* **36**:275–284.

13. Müller, A., Klaus, W., and Dhein, S. (1991). Heterogeneously distributed sensitivities to potassium as a cause of hypokalemic arrhythmias in isolated rabbit hearts. *J. Cardiovasc. Electrophysiol.* **2**:145–155.

14. McCullog, J., Chua, W., Rasmussen, H., Ten Eick, R.E., and Singer, D. (1990). Effects of potassium on the diastolic potential of partially depolarized cells in human ventricular myocardium. *Circ. Res.* **66**:191–201.

15. Carmeliet, E. (1989). K⁺ channels in cardiac cells: Mechanisms of activation, inactivation, rectification and K⁺ₑ sensitivity. *Pflügers Arch.* **414**:S88–S92.

16. Pardo, L.A., Heinemann, S.H., Terlau, H., Ludewig, U., Lorra, C., Pongs, O., and Stühmer, W. (1992). Extracellular K⁺ specifically modulates a rat brain potassium channel. *Proc. Natl. Acad. Sci. U.S.A.* **89**:2466–2470.

17. Leu, W.M., and Boyden, P.A. (1989). The transient outward current is markedly decreased in canine myocytes from the epicardial border zone of the infarcted heart. *Circulation* **80**:II–500.

18. Beckh, S., and Pongs, O. (1990). Members of the RCK potassium channel family are differentially expressed in the rat nervous system. *EMBO J.* **9**:777–782.

19. Schröter, K.H., Ruppesberg, J.P., Wunder, F., Rettig, J., Stocker, M., and Pongs, O.(1991). Cloning and functional expression of a TEA-sensitive A-type potassium channel from rat brain. *FEBS Lett.* **278**:211–216.

20. Armstrong, C.M. (1971). Interaction of tetraethylammonium ion derivatives with the potassium channels of giant axons. *J. Physiol. (Lond.)* **58**:413–437.

21. MacKinnon, R., and Yellen, G. (1990). Mutations affecting TEA blockade and ion permeation in voltage-activated K^+ channels. *Science* **250**:276–279.

22. Hoshi, T., Zagotta, W.N., and Aldrich, R.W. (1991). Biophysical and molecular mechanisms of *Shaker* potassium channel inactivation. *Science* **250**:533–538.

23. Demo, S.D., and Yellen, G. (1991). Ion effects on gating of the Ca^{2+}-activated K^+ channel correlate with occupancy of the pore. *Neuron* **7**:743–753.

24. Segal, M., Rogawaski, M.A., and Barker J.L. (1984). A transient potassium conductance regulates the excitability of cultures hippocampal and spinal neurons. *J. Neurosci.* **4**:604–609.

25. Wu, R.-L., and Barish, M.E. (1992). Two pharmacologically and kinetically distinct transient potassium currents in cultured embryonic mouse hippocampal neurons. *J. Neurosci.* **12**:2235–2246.

18

Physiological and Molecular Insights into Excitation-Contraction Coupling in Cardiac and Skeletal Muscle

Jesús García and Kurt G. Beam

Contraction of a skeletal muscle cell is initiated by an action potential, which propagates both longitudinally and radially. The radial propagation of this electrical signal occurs via infoldings of the surface membrane, termed the transverse tubular system or T-tubules. Depolarization of the T-tubular membrane triggers calcium release from a specialized, intracellular, membrane-bound organelle, the sarcoplasmic reticulum (SR), which comes into close apposition to the T-tubule membrane. The released calcium causes a sudden increase in cytosolic-free calcium, which in turn causes the muscle to contract. A key protein involved in the excitation-contraction (E-C) coupling mechanism is the dihydropyridine (DHP) receptor, which is embedded in the T-tubular membrane and is activated by depolarization of this membrane. The DHP receptor is thought to serve a dual role as an L-type calcium channel in the T-tubular membrane and as the voltage sensor responsible for controlling the opening and closing of the calcium release channel of the SR (1, 2). This chapter briefly discusses experiments to characterize physiological interactions of the DHP receptor in the T-tubular membrane and the calcium release channel in the SR, with special emphasis on recent molecular studies.

Structures Involved in E-C Coupling

The primary morphological structure at which coupling of excitation to contraction occurs is termed a triad (Fig. 1, A and B), a region of close association between a T-tubule and the SR. The triad consists of a T-tubule flanked by two SR terminal cisternae. Electron microscopy has revealed the presence of regularly spaced structures in the gap between the T-tubule and the SR, commonly known as feet (3). The feet are integral proteins

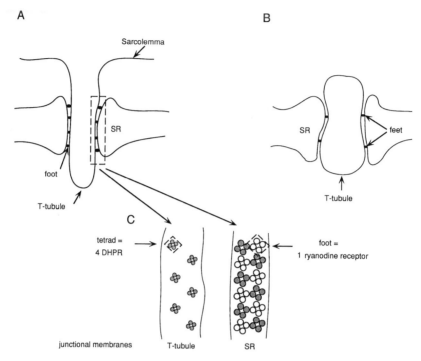

Figure 1. Representation of structures at the triad involved in E-C coupling. **(A)** Diagram representing a lateral view of the elements that constitute a triad in skeletal muscle. A triad is formed by a T-tubule that is flanked by two terminal cisternae of the SR. The T-tubules are invaginations of the sarcolemma. The structures between the T-tubule and the SR are termed feet and correspond to the cytoplasmic regions of the ryanodine receptor/SR calcium release channel. **(B)** Transverse section of the triad showing the T-tubule and its relation with the SR cisternae. **(C)** Representation of the structures found in the junctional membrane of the SR and the T-tubule corresponding to the area enclosed by the dashed-line box in (A). Both membranes are illustrated as seen from the lumen of the T-tubule. The structures corresponding to the feet are shown on the cytoplasmic face of the junctional membrane of the SR. The feet are arranged in two rows. One individual foot (enclosed by the diamond) is formed by four identical subunits. The illustration of the T-tubular junctional membrane represents a freeze-fracture replica. The T-tubular junctional membrane contains particle arrays termed tetrads. One tetrad (delimited by the diamond) is thought to be composed of four individual DHP receptors. The tetrads are arranged in two rows such that every other ryanodine receptor lies opposite to a tetrad. This is indicated by the shading of every other ryanodine receptor.

of the SR membrane composed of four identical subunits (4, 5) and have been characterized as the high-affinity receptor for the plant alkaloid ryanodine (6, 7). The idea that the ryanodine receptor serves as the SR calcium release channel for E-C coupling has emerged from experiments in which the purified receptor has been incorporated into lipid bilayers and demonstrated to function as a high conductance calcium channel (8, 9). Thus, the feet structures, the ryanodine receptor, and the SR calcium release channel are evidently different terms for the same structure. Recently, a 106 kDa protein labeled by disulfide reagents has been identified as another kind of SR calcium channel (10).

Electron microscopic analyses suggest that feet interact directly with a molecular component of the transverse tubule (11). In the swimbladder muscle of the toadfish, a face-on view of the cytoplasmic aspect of the terminal cisternae of the SR reveals that the feet are arrayed in two rows, within which the individual feet are regularly spaced (Fig. 1C). Freeze-fracture replicas of T-tubule junctional membrane also reveal regularly spaced particles, arranged in groups of four, termed junctional tetrads. Like feet, junctional tetrads are regularly arranged within two rows, and the spacing of the individual particles within a tetrad is such that each lies opposite to 1 of the 4 subunits of a foot (Fig. 1C). The individual particles of a junctional tetrad have dimensions similar to those of biochemically purified DHP receptors. Interestingly, the junctional tetrads are spaced such that only every other foot is apposed by a junctional tetrad (Fig. 1C). On the basis of these results, Block et al. (11) have suggested that a junctional tetrad in the T-tubule represents a group of four DHP receptors and that every other foot protein of the SR is in direct contact with the four DHP receptors of a junctional tetrad. Further evidence relating to the identity between junctional tetrads and DHP receptors is presented in the section entitled "Dysgenic Skeletal Muscle."

Calcium Release from the SR

A physiological explanation for the morphological findings has been suggested by electrophysiological and optical studies. Depolarization of the T-tubular membrane activates a voltage sensor, the DHP receptor (1, 12), which in turn transmits this information (via an unknown mechanism in skeletal muscle) to the ryanodine receptor causing the ryanodine receptor to open and release calcium. The transient increase in free myoplasmic calcium has been monitored with both absorbance and fluorescence optical indicators (13–16). The change in free myoplasmic calcium can be used to calculate the rate of release from the SR. In order to calculate the rate of release, one must consider the calcium binding to myoplasmic buffers and the optical indicator as well as the contribution of the systems that remove calcium from the myoplasm (14, 17, 18). By using this approach, it has been demonstrated that the calcium release from the SR consists of a fast initial peak that decays toward a lower sustained level (17). It has been proposed that the early decline of the rate of release is caused by a calcium-dependent inactivation mechanism (19, 20). However, as previously mentioned, only every other ryanodine receptor has a corresponding DHP receptor and these "free" ryanodine receptors may not be directly controlled by the T-tubular voltage change. This led Ríos and Pizarro (21) to propose that the ryanodine receptors that are voltage-gated give rise to the sustained level of SR calcium release, and that the calcium leaving the SR activates the neighboring free ryanodine receptors producing the fast initial peak component of the release. This idea is supported by experiments of Jacquemond et al. (22), who have found that the early peak of release is selectively eliminated and the maintained release unaltered when strong calcium buffers (BAPTA at 3.8 mM or Fura2 at 2.2 to 2.8 mM) are injected into frog cut skeletal muscle fibers. A similar phenomenon has been observed in isolated SR vesicles (23), with purified and reconstituted calcium release channel (8), and in isolated skinned muscle fibers (24). However, Hollingworth et al. (25) observed that the total amount and rate of calcium release in response to an action potential were increased when Fura2 was injected into intact fibers at concentrations of 2 to 3 mM. A number of differences in preparation and experimental conditions may account for the discrepancy between Jacquemond et al. (22) and Hollingworth et al. (25).

The DHP receptor

Skeletal Muscle

The T-tubular membrane of skeletal muscle is a rich source of DHP receptors (26, 27). The DHP receptor is formed of 5 subunits, termed α_1, α_2, β, γ, and δ (28). The α_1-subunit is the site of DHP binding and by itself can function as a voltage-gated calcium channel (29, 30). Based on cloned cDNA, the α_1-subunit of the skeletal muscle DHP receptor and the voltage-dependent sodium channel show a surprisingly high similarity in their primary amino acid sequences, predicted tertiary structures, and hydropathicity profiles (12). For both proteins the amino and carboxy terminals are predicted to be cytoplasmic, and the primary sequence shows four homology repeats (designated I–IV) linked by putative cytoplasmic loops; in turn, each repeat consists of six putative transmembrane spanning α-helices, designated as S1–S6 (Fig. 2A). Striessnig et al. (31), using (+)-PN200-110 and azidopine have localized the DHP binding region within the α_1-subunit to the connecting loop between segments S5 and S6 of repeat III and the segment S6 of both repeats III and IV; they propose, based on physiological studies, that these sites interact to form a receptor on the external side of the channel.

Interestingly, the S4 segment in each repeat of the DHP receptor contains regularly spaced positively charged amino acids that are thought to confer the voltage-sensing property to the protein. When a voltage change occurs across the membrane, charged amino acids (putatively in S4 and perhaps others) are translocated and thereby generate an intramem-

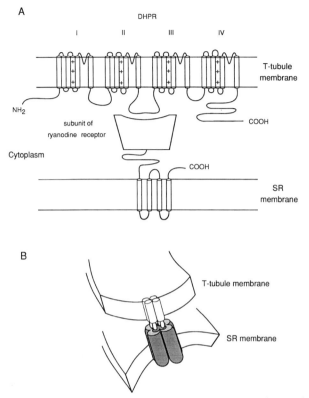

Figure 2. **(A)** Hypothetical arrangement of the DHP receptor in the T-tubular junctional membrane and the ryanodine receptor in the SR membrane. The illustration gives a schematic representation of the α_1-subunit of the DHP receptor. This α_1-subunit consists of four homologous repeats labeled I–IV; within each repeat, there are six putative transmembrane spanning regions, designated as segments S1–S6. The S4 segment contains positively charged amino acids (indicated by plus signs) that are thought to confer the voltage-sensing property to the DHP receptor. The amino- and carboxy-terminals, as well as the loops connecting the four repeats, are thought to be cytoplasmic. For clarity, repeats I–IV are illustrated side by side, but in actuality they are likely arranged like barrel staves around a central pore. The loop connecting repeats II and III is shown here as having close contact with the ryanodine receptor, because it has been shown that this loop is a critical determinant of the type of E-C coupling. In the polypeptide comprising 1 of the 4 identical subunits of the ryanodine receptor, only a small portion near the carboxy-terminal is believed to contribute to the formation of the transmembrane calcium release channel; the bulk of the protein, including the amino-terminal, is cytoplasmic and contributes to the formation of the foot structure (63, 64) visualized by microscopy. **(B)** Representation of the three-dimensional relationship between four DHP receptors and one ryanodine receptor. Within the T-tubule membrane, each cylinder represents a single DHP receptor; whereas within the SR membrane each cylinder represents 1 of the 4 subunits of a single ryanodine receptor. For each DHP receptor, only the II–III loop is indicated as approaching a subunit of the ryanodine receptor.

brane current (32) that represents conformational changes necessary for channel opening or for E-C coupling. Assuming that all the intramembrane charge in skeletal muscle is involved in E-C coupling, Simon and Hill (33) have related the charge movement and SR calcium release in frog muscle following a Hodgkin–Huxley model. In their model, each of n identical and independent gating particles must make a transition between a resting and an activated state, and the SR release channel can open only when all n particles are in the activated state. By comparing charge movement and the steady-state rate of calcium release, these authors found that both the time course of the rate of release, and its dependence on voltage, could be fit by the fourth power of charge movement, as would be predicted by a Hodgkin–Huxley model with four independent gating particles. Similar results were obtained by Melzer et al. (18) studying the voltage dependencies of charge movement and the peak rate of release. They found that they could fit their data with a Hodgkin–Huxley model having three gating particles. These results agree well with the morphological studies that suggest that four DHP receptors are associated with an individual ryanodine receptor. It is attractive to equate the four DHP receptors to the four gating particles in the model of Simon and Hill (33).

The role of the other subunits of the DHP receptors is less well known. Experiments in which the α_1-subunit is coexpressed with a combination of the other subunits have suggested that the amplitude, kinetics, and voltage dependence of activation and inactivation of the calcium current are modified, thus suggesting a regulatory role to these other subunits (34, 35a–c).

Dysgenic Skeletal Muscle

A system that has proven valuable for the analysis of the function of DHP receptors is skeletal muscle obtained from mice with the muscular dysgenesis *(mdg)* mutation. Skeletal muscle from mice homozygous for the *mdg* mutation fails to contract in response to membrane depolarization (36). This failure of E-C coupling in dysgenic muscle cannot be ascribed to an obvious defect in the SR, because both ryanodine receptors and $(Ca^{2+} + Mg^{2+})$ ATPase are present (37), and both are evidently functional because caffeine, an activator of SR calcium release, causes dysgenic muscle to contract (38, 39). Rather, the failure of E-C coupling can be ascribed to a mutation of the gene encoding the α_1-subunit of the skeletal muscle DHP receptor (2, 40). The mutant mRNA is very labile (40), and the translation product is not detectably present by immunoblotting (37). Consistent with the hypothesis that the DHP receptor has dual functions as calcium channel and voltage sensor, dysgenic muscle lacks the DHP-sensitive slow calcium current (I_{slow}) that is characteristic of normal muscle (41), and has a significantly reduced amount of intramembrane charge movement (42, 43). Importantly, E-C coupling, I_{slow}, and charge movement can all be restored by microinjection of dysgenic myotubes with an expression plasmid carrying the cDNA for the rabbit skeletal muscle DHP receptor α_1-subunit (2, 42).

In the course of early development of skeletal muscle fibers, functional E-C coupling appears prior to the formation of T-tubules. Although triadic contacts between the SR and T-tubules are lacking in these developing muscle fibers, peripheral couplings between the SR and surface membrane do occur. In the SR of developing mouse diaphragm, foot structures are present at sites of peripheral coupling; within the surface membrane are found clusters of particles arrayed in tetrads like those found in the T-tubular membrane at triads in fish muscle (44). These junctional tetrads are absent from the surface membrane of developing dysgenic skeletal muscle both in vivo (44) and in vitro (45). Moreover, junctional tetrads reappear in dysgenic myotubes injected with cDNA encoding the rabbit skeletal muscle DHP receptor (45). Taken together, results obtained from dysgenic muscle provide strong support for the idea that the skeletal muscle DHP receptor functions as the slow calcium channel, as the voltage sensor for E-C coupling, and is the particle that forms junctional tetrads.

Although dysgenic muscle lacks the normal skeletal muscle DHP receptor, it does express an unidentified DHP receptor that is manifested as a small, DHP-sensitive calcium current (46, 47). This current, I_{dys}, is distinguishable from I_{slow} in that it activates at more negative potentials, is more sensitive to DHPs, and has much faster activation kinetics (47). Based both on the rapid activation kinetics observed, and the recent demonstration that mRNA for the cardiac DHP receptor is present in skeletal muscle tissue of normal and dysgenic embryonic mice (48), it is tempting to hypothesize that I_{dys} reflects a low-level expression of the cardiac DHP receptor.

Cardiac Muscle

Cardiac muscle membrane also contains DHP receptors whose α_1-subunit is encoded by a different gene from that of skeletal muscle (29). Nevertheless, it has ~66% amino acid sequence identity with the skeletal muscle DHP receptor, as well as a similar predicted transmembrane structure. The main differences from the skeletal DHP receptor reside in the amino and carboxy terminals and the putative cytoplasmic loops that link the four repeats. For E-C coupling, probably the most important structural difference between the two DHP receptors is in the loop that links repeats II and III (29).

Skeletal and Cardiac E-C Coupling

Contraction of both skeletal muscle cells and most cardiac cells is due to calcium release from the SR (24), but different mechanisms control the response of the SR in these two tissues. Cardiac muscle DHP receptors function as calcium channels which, upon depolarization of the plasma membrane, activate with a fast time course allowing a large influx of calcium ions into the cell; this calcium triggers the opening of the SR calcium release channel causing a large further increase in intracellular calcium (49). Contraction of a cardiac cell is abolished if calcium entry is prevented by blocking the channels or by removing calcium from the external solution. By contrast, the entry of calcium is not required to elicit contraction in skeletal muscle. Although skeletal muscle contains calcium channels, their activation is so slow that negligible influx of calcium occurs during an action potential (50). Moreover, when calcium is withdrawn from the external solution and replaced by magnesium, E-C coupling is still operative (51). These findings indicate that calcium entry is unlikely to play a role in initiating calcium release from the SR. Although the function of the skeletal muscle DHP receptor as a calcium channel is not important for E-C coupling, considerable evidence has accumulated that indicates that the DHP receptor does function as the voltage sensor in the T-tubular membrane to regulate SR calcium release in response to changes of potential (1, 2).

Chimeric DHP Receptors and E-C Coupling

Because skeletal muscle of dysgenic mice lacks the normal α_1-subunit of the DHP receptor it provides an excellent environment for the expression of this receptor and a model system for the study of its interaction with the SR release channel. In dysgenic muscle, expression of the cDNA encoding the DHP receptor of rabbit skeletal muscle was demonstrated to restore I_{slow}, immobilization-resistant charge movement, and E-C coupling (2, 42). The restored E-C coupling resembled that of normal skeletal muscle in that it did not require influx of extracellular calcium. On the contrary, when the cardiac DHP receptor cDNA was injected into dysgenic myotubes in a separate set of experiments, a fast (cardiac-like) calcium current and cardiac-type E-C coupling were produced. This E-C coupling required entry of extracellular calcium (52, 53).

A series of experiments has been conducted in an effort to identify regions that are responsible for the important functional differences between skeletal and cardiac muscle DHP receptors. The morphological studies described suggest the possibility that cytoplasmic regions of the skeletal muscle DHP receptor might be important for the interaction of the voltage sensor with the SR calcium release channel (see Fig. 2). In order to examine this idea, various chimeric DHP receptor cDNAs were constructed and expressed in dysgenic myotubes (52, 53). In these chimeric constructs, the four membrane repeats were of cardiac origin, whereas one or more of the putative cytoplasmic regions were of skeletal muscle origin. Expression of these chimeric DHP receptors resulted in the appearance of calcium current that activated rapidly like that in heart. Thus, the putative cytoplasmic regions do not appear to have a strong influence on the channel's activation kinetics. However, it was determined that if the loop linking repeats II and III in an entirely cardiac DHP receptor were substituted by the II–III loop of skeletal muscle, the resulting chimeric DHP receptor could support skeletal muscle type E-C coupling in which calcium entry is unnecessary. This result suggests the possibility that the II–III loop of the skeletal muscle DHP receptor interacts with the SR calcium release channel (Fig. 2). Another possibility is that there is an intervening protein (54) that mediates the interaction between the II–III loop and the SR calcium release channel. Because putative cytoplasmic regions were found not to be important in channel activation kinetics, a separate set of chimeric constructs were made in which one or more of the four repeats of the cardiac DHP receptor were replaced by their skeletal muscle counterparts. It was determined that activation was slow for all chimeras in which the first repeating homology unit is of skeletal muscle sequence (55).

The results from expression of cDNAs in dysgenic myotubes support the hypothesis that the DHP receptor in skeletal muscle functions as both the slow calcium channel and as the essential voltage sensor for E-C coupling. However, it is not known whether a single DHP receptor molecule can simultaneously perform both roles. Whereas only a single form of mRNA encoding the α_1-subunit has been found (12, 30, 56), two differently sized forms of the DHP receptor α_1-subunit have been detected (57–59). The larger form is recognized by peptide-specific antibodies directed against the carboxy-terminal predicted from the cDNA, whereas the smaller form appears to arise by posttranslational cleavage of the carboxy-terminal from the larger form (58). For convenience we will refer to these two forms as $\alpha_{1\text{-full}}$, which is a polypeptide of 1,873 residues, and $\alpha_{1\text{-trunc}}$, which site-directed antibodies indicate is truncated between residues 1,685 and 1,699 (58). $\alpha_{1\text{-trunc}}$ and $\alpha_{1\text{-full}}$ represent ~95% and 5%, respectively, of total DHP receptor α_1 in skeletal muscle. The existence of these two forms of α_1, together with other results (60), led to the hypothesis (57, 61) that only $\alpha_{1\text{-full}}$ could function as a calcium channel and that $\alpha_{1\text{-trunc}}$ could function as a voltage sensor for E-C coupling, but not as a calcium channel. To examine this hypothesis, Beam et al. (62) constructed a plasmid (designated as pC6Δ1) that encoded a skeletal muscle α_1-subunit truncated after residue 1,662. When expressed in dysgenic myotubes, pC6Δ1 was found to function fully as both the voltage sensor for E-C coupling and the slow calcium channel. This result is consistent with the idea that an individual DHP receptor can simultaneously carry out both functions, although it does not exclude the possibility that the two functions are carried out by separate populations of the same form of the protein.

In summary, at the junction between T-tubules and SR, each junctional tetrad within the T-tubular membrane is in close apposition to a single ryanodine receptor within the SR membrane. This appears to represent the morphological site at which E-C coupling takes place in skeletal muscle. A single particle of a junctional tetrad appears to represent one DHP receptor. In skeletal muscle the DHP receptor operates both as a calcium channel and as the voltage sensor that triggers calcium release from the SR, whereas in cardiac muscle it functions only as a calcium channel. The role of the DHP receptor as a calcium channel can be performed by the α_1-subunit alone, whereas the other subunits of the DHP receptor complex seem to modulate the properties of the calcium current. The intracellular loops of the DHP receptor appear to be important for its interaction with the SR release channel, whereas the first membrane repeat is important in determining the kinetics of the calcium channel activation. An important goal of future experiments will be to determine which amino acids within the first membrane repeat affect calcium channel activation kinetics, which amino acids of the intracellular loops are most important for the interaction with the SR release channel, and whether this interaction is direct or involves other proteins.

References

1. Ríos, E., and Brum, G. (1987). Involvement of dihydropyridine receptors in excitation-contraction coupling in skeletal muscle. *Nature (Lond.)* **325**:717–720.

2. Tanabe, T., Beam, K.G., Powell, J.A., and Numa, S. (1988). Restoration of excitation-contraction coupling and slow calcium current in dysgenic muscle by dihydropyridine receptor complementary DNA. *Nature (Lond.)* **336**:134–139.

3. Franzini-Armstrong, C., and Nunzi, G. (1983). Junctional feet and particles in the triads of a fast-twitch muscle fibre. *J. Mus. Res. Cell Motil.* **4**:233–252.

4. Ferguson, D.G., Schwartz, H.W., and Franzini-Armstrong, C. (1984). Subunit structure of junctional feet in triads of skeletal muscle: A freeze-drying, rotary-shadowing study. *J. Cell Biol.* **99**:1735–1742.

5. Saito, A., Seiler, S., Chu, A., and Fleischer, S. (1988). Preparation and morphology of sarcoplasmic reticulum terminal cisternae from rabbit skeletal muscle. *J. Cell Biol.* **99**:875–885.

6. Imagawa, T., Smith, J.S., Coronado, R., and Campbell, K.P. (1987). Purified ryanodine receptor from skeletal muscle sarcoplasmic reticulum is the Ca^{2+}-permeable pore of the calcium release channel. *J. Biol. Chem.* **262**:16636–16643.

7. Inui, M., Saito, A., and Fleischer, S. (1987). Purification of the ryanodine receptor and identity with feet structures of junctional terminal cisternae of sarcoplasmic reticulum from fast skeletal muscle. *J. Biol. Chem.* **262**:1740.

8. Smith, J.S., Coronado, R., and Meissner, G. (1986). Single channel measurements of the calcium release channel from skeletal muscle sarcoplasmic reticulum. Activation by Ca^{2+} and ATP and modulation of Mg^{2+}. *J. Gen. Physiol.* **88**:573–588.

9. Lai, F.A., Erickson, H.P., Rosseau, E., Liu, Q.Y., and Meissner, G. (1988). Purification and reconstitution of the calcium release channel from skeletal muscle. *Nature (Lond.)* **331**:315–319.

10. Zaidi, N.F., Lagenaur, C.F., Hilkert, R.J., Abramson, J.J., and Salama, G. (1989). Disulfide linkage of biotin identifies a 106-kDa Ca^{2+} release channel in sarcoplasmic reticulum. *J. Biol. Chem.* **264:**21737–21747.

11. Block, B.A., Imagawa, T., Campbell, K.P., and Franzini-Armstrong, C. (1988). Structural evidence for direct interaction between the molecular components of the transverse tubule/sarcoplasmic reticulum junction in skeletal muscle. *J. Cell Biol.* **107:**2587–2600.

12. Tanabe, T., Takeshima, H., Mikami, A., Flockerzi, V., Takahashi, H., Kangawa, K., Kojima, M., Matsuo, H., Hirose, T., and Nima, S. (1987). Primary structure of the receptor for calcium channel blockers from skeletal muscle. *Nature (Lond.)* **328:**313–318.

13. Baylor, S.M., Chandler, W.K., and Marshall, M.W. (1982). Use of metallochromic dyes to measure changes in myoplasmic calcium during activity in frog skeletal muscle fibres. *J. Physiol. (Lond.)* **331:**139–177.

14. Baylor, S.M., Chandler, W.K., and Marshall, M.W. (1983). Sarcoplasmic reticulum calcium release in frog skeletal muscle fibres estimated fron Arsenazo III calcium transients. *J. Physiol. (Lond.)* **344:**625–666.

15. Klein, M.G., Simon, B.J., Szucs, G., and Schneider, M.F. (1988). Simultaneous recording of calcium transients in skeletal muscle using high and low affinity calcium indicators. *Biophys. J.* **55:**971–988.

16. García, J., and Schneider, M.F. (1993). Calcium transients and calcium release in rat fast-twitch skeletal muscle fibres. *J. Physiol. (Lond.),* in press.

17. Melzer, W., Ríos, E., and Schneider, M.F. (1984). Time course of calcium release and removal in skeletal muscle fibers. *Biophys. J.* **45:**637–641.

18. Melzer, W., Schneider, M.F., Simon, B., and Szücs, G. (1986). Intermembrane charge movement and Ca relase in frog skeletal muscle. *J. Physiol. (Lond.)* **373:**481–511.

19. Schneider, M.F., and Simon, B. (1988). Inactivation of calcium release from the SR in frog skeletal muscle. *J. Physiol. (Lond.)* **405:**727–745.

20. Simon, B.J., Klein, M.G., and Schneider, M.F. (1991). Calcium dependence of inactivation of calcium release from the sarcoplasmic reticulum in skeletal muscle fibers. *J. Gen. Physiol.* **97:**437–471.

21. Ríos, E., and Pizarro, G. (1988). Voltage sensors and calcium channels of excitation contraction coupling. *News Physiol. Sci.* **3:**223–228.

22. Jacquemond, V., Csernoch, L., Klein, M.G., and Schneider, M.F. (1991). Voltage-gated and calcium-gated calcium release during depolarization of skeletal muscle. *Biophys. J.* **60:**867–873.

23. Meissner, G., Darling, E., and Eveleth, J. (1986). Kinetics of rapid Ca^{2+}, Mg^{2+}, and adenine nucleotides. *Biochemistry* **25:**236–244.

24. Endo, M. (1985). Calcium release from sarcoplasmic reticulum. *Curr. Top. Membr. Transport* **25:**181–230.

25. Hollingworth, S., Harkins, A.B., Kurebayashi, N., Konishi, M., and Baylor, S.M. (1992). Excitation-contraction coupling in intact frog skeletal muscle fibers injected with m molar concentrations of fura-2. *Biophys. J.* **63:**224–234.

26. Fosset, M., Jaimovich, E., Delpont, E., and Lazdunski, M. (1983). (^{3}H)-nitrendipine receptors in skeletal muscle: Properties and preferential localizations in transverse tubules. *J. Biol. Chem.* **258:**6086–6092.

27. Galizzi, J.-P., Fosset, M., and Lazdunski, M. (1984). [^{3}H]Verapamil binding sites in skeletal muscle transverse tubule membranes. *Biochem. Biophys. Res. Commun.* **118**:239–245.

28. Campbell, K.P., Leung, A.T., and Sharp, A. H. (1988). The biochemistry and molecular biology of the dihydropyridine-sensitive calcium channel. *Trends Nucl. Sci.* **11**:425–430.

29. Mikami, A., Imoto, K., Tanabe, T., Niidome, T., Mori, Y., Takeshima, H., Narumiya, S., and Numa, S. (1989). Primary structure and functional expression of the cardiac dihydropyridine-sensitive calcium channel. *Nature (Lond.)* **340**:230–233.

30. Perez-Reyes, E., Kim, H.S., Lacerda, A.E., Horne, W., Wei, X., Rampe, D., Campbell, K.P., Brown, A.M., and Birnbaumer, L. (1989). Induction of calcium currents by the expression of the alpha$_1$ subunit of the dihydropyridine receptor from skeletal muscle. *Nature (Lond.)* **340**:233–236.

31. Striessnig, J., Murphy, B.J., and Catterall, W.A. (1991). Dihydropyridine receptor of L-type Ca^{2+} channels: Identification of binding domains for [^{3}H](+)-PN200-110 and [^{3}H]azidopine within the α1 subunit. *Proc. Natl. Acad. Sci. U.S.A.* **88**:10769–10773.

32. Schneider, M.F., and Chandler, W.K. (1973). Voltage-dependent charge movement in skeletal muscle: A possible step in excitation-contraction coupling. *Nature (Lond.)* **242**:244–246.

33. Simon, B.J., and Hill, D.A. (1992). Charge movement and SR calcium release in frog skeletal muscle can be related by a Hodgkin–Huxley model with four gating particles. *Biophys. J.* **61**:1109–1116.

34. Lacerda, A.E., Kim, H.S., Ruth, P., Perez-Reyes, E., Flockerzi, V., Hofmann, F., Birnbaumer, L., and Brown, A. M. (1991). Normalization of current kinetics by interaction between the α1- and β-subunits of the skeletal muscle dihydropyridine-sensitive Ca^{2+} channel. *Nature* **352**:527–530.

35a. Singer, D., Biel, M., Lotan, I., Flockerzi, V., Hofmann, F., and Dascal, N. (1991). The roles of the subunits in the function of the calcium channel. *Science* **253**:1553–1557.

35b. Varadi, G., Lory, P., Schultz, D., Varadi, M., and Schwartz, A. (1991). Acceleration of activation and inactivation by the β-subunit of the skeletal muscle calcium channel. *Nature (Lond.)* **352**:159–162.

35c. Perez-Reyes, E., Castellano, A., Kim, H.S., Bertrand, P., Baggstrom, E., Lacerda, A.E., Wei, X., and Birnbaumer, L. (1992). Cloning and expression of a cardiac/brain β-subunit of the L-type calcium channel. *J. Biol. Chem.* **267**:1792–1797.

36. Powell, J.A., and Frambrough, D.M. (1973). Fine structure of mutants (muscular dysgenesis) embryonic muscular dysgenesis. *Dev. Biol.* **112**:458–466.

37. Knudson, C.M., Chaudhari, N., Sharp, A.H., Powell, J.A., Beam, K.G., and Campbell, K.P. (1989). Specific absence of the alpha-subunit of the dihydropyridine receptor in mice with muscular dysgenesis. *J. Biol. Chem.* **264**:1345–1348.

38. Bowden-Eissen, F. (1972). An in vitro study of normal and mutant myogenesis in the mouse. *Dev. Biol.* **27**:351–364.

39. Bournaud, R., and Mallart, A. (1987). An electrophysiological study of skeletal muscle fibers in the "muscular dysgenesis" mutation of the mouse. *Pflügers Arch.* **409:**468–476.

40. Chaudhari, N. (1992). A single nucleotide deletion in the skeletal muscle-specific calcium channel transcript of muscular dysgenesis *(mdg)* mice. *J. Biol. Chem.* **267:**25636–25639.

41. Beam, K.G., Knudson, C.M., and Powell, J.A. (1986). A lethal mutation in mice eliminates the slow calcium current in skeletal muscle cells. *Nature (Lond.)* **320:**168–170.

42. Adams, B.A., Tanabe, T., Mikami, A., Numa, S., and Beam, K.G. (1990). Intramembrane charge movement restored in dysgenic skeletal muscle by injection of dihydropyridine receptor complementary DNAs. *Nature* **346:**569–572.

43. Shimahara, T., Bournaud, R., Inoue, I., and Strube, C. (1990). Reduced intramembrane charge movement in the dysgenic skeletal muscle cell. *Pflügers Arch.* **417:**111–113.

44. Franzini-Armstrong, C., Pinçon-Raymond, M., and Rieger, F. (1991). Muscle fibers from dysgenic mouse in vivo lack a surface component of peripheral couplings. *Dev. Biol.* **146:**364–376.

45. Takekure, H., Bennett, L., Tanabe, T., Beam, K., and Franzini-Armstrong, C. (1993). Tetrads are restored in dysgenic myotubes transfected with cDNA for skeletal muscle DHPR. *Biophys. J.,* in press.

46. Bournaud, R., Shimahara, T., García, L., and Rieger, F. (1989). Appearance of the slow Ca conductance in myotubes from mutant mice with "muscular dysgenesis." *Pflügers Arch.* **414:**410–415.

47. Adams, B.A., and Beam, K.G. (1989). A novel calcium current in dysgenic skeletal muscle. *J. Gen. Physiol.* **94:**429–444.

48. Chaudhari, N., and Beam, K.G. (1993). mRNA for cardiac calcium channel is expressed during development of skeletal muscle. *Dev. Biol.,* in press.

49. Nabauer, M., Callewaert, G., Cleeman, L., and Morad, M. (1989). Regulation of calcium release is gated by calcium current, not gating charge, in cardiac myocytes. *Science* **244:**800–803.

50. Sánchez, J.A., and Stefani, E. (1978). Inward calcium current in twitch muscle fibres of the frog. *J. Physiol. (Lond.)* **283:**197–209.

51. Armstrong, C.M., Bezanilla, F.M., and Horowicz, P. (1972). Twitches in the presence of ethylene glycol bis(β-aminoethyl ether)-N-N′-tetraacetic acid. *Biochim. Biophys. Acta* **267:**605–608.

52. Tanabe, T., Beam, K.G., Adams, B.A., Niidome, T., and Numa, S. (1990a). Regions of the skeletal muscle dihydropyridine receptor critical for excitation-contraction coupling. *Nature (Lond.)* **346:**567–568.

53. Tanabe, T., Mikami, A., Numa, S., and Beam, K.G. (1990b). Cardiac-type excitation-contraction coupling in dysgenic skeletal muscle injected with cardiac dihydropyridine receptor cDNA. *Nature (Lond.)* **344:**451–453.

54. Kim, K.C., Caswell, A.H., Talvenheimo, J.A., and Brandt, N.R. (1990). Isolation of a terminal cisternae protein which may link the dihydropyridine receptor to the junctional foot protein in skeletal muscle. *Biochemistry* **29:**9281–9289.

55. Tanabe, T., Adams, B.A., Numa, S., and Beam, K.G. (1991). Repeat I of the dihydropyridine receptor is critical in determining calcium channel activation kinetics. *Nature (Lond.)* **352**:800–803.

56. Ellis, S.B., Williams, M.E., Ways, N.R., Brenner, R., Sharp, A.H., Leung, A.T., Campbell, K.P., McKenna, E., Koch, W.J., Hui, A., Schwartz, A., and Harpold, M.M. (1988). Sequence and expression of mRNAs encoding the alpha1- and alpha2-subunits of a DHP-sensitive calcium channel. *Science* **241**:1661–1664.

57. De Jongh, K.S., Merrick, D.K., and Catterall, W.A. (1989). Subunits of purified calcium channels: A 212-kDa form of α_1 and partial amino acid sequence of a phosphorylation site of an independent β-subunit. *Proc. Natl. Acad. Sci. U.S.A.* **86**: 8585–8589.

58. De Jongh, K.S., Warner, C., Colvin, A.A., and Catterall, W.A. (1991). Characterization of the two size forms of the α_1-subunit of skeletal muscle L-type calcium channels. *Proc. Natl. Acad. Sci. U.S.A.* **88**:10778–10782.

59. Lai, Y., Seagar, M.J., Takahashi, M., and Catterall, W.A. (1990). Cyclic AMP-dependent phosphorylation of two size forms of α1-subunits of L-type calcium channels in rat skeletal muscle cells. *J. Biol. Chem.* **265**:20839–20848.

60. Schwartz, L.M., McCleskey, E.W., and Almers, W. (1985). Dihydropyridine receptors in muscle are voltage-dependent but most are not functional calcium channels. *Nature (Lond.)* **314**:747–750.

61. Catterall, W.A. (1991). Excitation-contraction coupling in vertebrate skeletal muscle: A tale of two calcium channels. *Cell* **64**:871–874.

62. Beam, K.G., Adams, B.A., Niidome, T., Numa, S., and Tanabe, T. (1992). Function of a truncated dihydropyridine receptor as both voltage sensor and calcium channel. *Nature (Lond.)* **360**:169–171.

63. Takeshima, H., Nishimura, S., Matsumoto, T., Ishida, H., Kangawa, K., Minamino, N., Matsuo, H., Ueda, M., Hanaoka, M., Hirose, T., and Numa, S. (1989). Primary structure and expression from complementary DNA of skeletal muscle ryanodine receptor. *Nature (Lond.)* **339**:439–445.

64. Zorzato, F., Fujii, J., Otsu, K., Phillips, M., Green, N.M., Lai, F.A., Meissner, G., and MacLennan, D.H. (1990). Molecular cloning of cDNA encoding human and rabbit forms of the Ca^{2+} release channel (ryanodine receptor) of skeletal muscle sarcoplasmic reticulum. *J. Biol. Chem.* **265**:2244–2256.

19

Functional Expression of Cardiac and Smooth Muscle Calcium Channels

F. Hofmann, M. Biel, E. Bosse, V. Flockerzi,
P. Ruth, and A. Welling

Hormones and neurotransmitters play an important role in regulating the force of contraction in heart and smooth muscle. The force of contraction of the heart is primarily controlled by the calcium influx across the cell membrane during the action potential, whereas that of smooth muscle is initially controlled by the release of calcium from intracellular stores followed by a calcium influx from the extracellular space through voltage-dependent calcium channels. The best-characterized pathway for calcium entry in both cell types are voltage-dependent L-type calcium channels, which activate at membrane potential around -30 mV, inactivate slowly, and are expressed in many different cell tissue (1). These channels are readily blocked by classical organic calcium channel blockers (CaCBs) nifedipine [a 1,4-dihydropyridine (DHP)], verapamil [a phenylalkylamine (PAA)], and diltiazem (a benzothiazepine) (2–4).

Cardiac and smooth muscle calcium channels have common electrophysiological characteristics, yet they are regulated distinctly by CaCBs and hormones. The β-adrenergic receptor agonist isoproterenol increases cardiac calcium current 3- to 7-fold either by cAMP-dependent phosphorylation of the channel (5, 6), or through the activated α-subunit of the trimeric glutamyl transpeptidase (GTP) binding protein G_s (7, 8), or by the combined action of $G\alpha_s$ and the catalytic subunit of cAMP kinase (9). The L-type calcium current of isolated tracheal smooth muscle cells is stimulated also by the activation of the β-adrenergic receptor (10). This β-receptor effect is not mediated by cAMP kinase, but by the direct effect of a G-protein. These and further results (11) lead to the conclusion that the smooth and cardiac muscle calcium channels may be regulated in vivo by the α-subunit of a G-protein, but only the cardiac channel by cAMP-dependent phosphorylation. The primary sequences of the cardiac and a putative smooth muscle calcium channel have been identified by cloning their cDNAs. The sequences of these clones are very similar, and they direct the expression of L-type calcium channels of very similar properties.

Molecular Identity of Cardiac and Smooth Muscle Calcium Channels

General Composition of the Calcium Channel

Initially, the L-type calcium channel was purified from skeletal muscle. The purified complex contains four proteins (Fig. 1): the α_1-subunit (212,018 Da), which contains the binding sites for all known CaCBs and the calcium conducting pore; the intracellular located β-subunit (57,868 Da); the transmembrane γ-subunit (25,058 Da); and the α_2-/δ-subunit, a disulfide-linked dimer of 125,018 Da (2–4 and references cited there). Reconstitution of the purified complex into phospholipid bilayers resulted in functional calcium channels that are reversibly blocked by CaCBs and

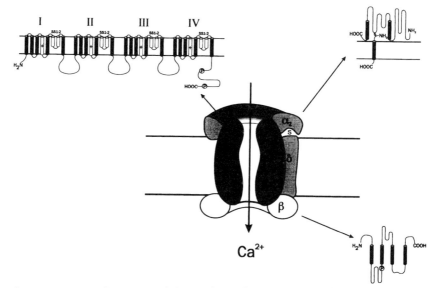

Figure 1. Proposed structure of the cardiac calcium channel. The putative transmembrane configuration of individual subunits is based on hydropathicity analysis of the deduced primary sequences, I, II, III, and IV, proposed repeats of calcium channel α_1-subunit; +, transmembrane amphipathic α-helix, respectively, the proposed voltage-sensing helix of the channel; Ⓟ, putative cAMP kinase phosphorylation sites; only two of several phosphorylation sites are shown in the sequence of the α_1-subunit; s, disulfide bridge between the transmembrane δ and the extracellular-located α_2-subunit; SS1–SS2, suggested part of the channel pore. The extracellular space is above the horizontal lines. Note that a γ-subunit that is present in the skeletal muscle calcium channel has not been identified in cardiac tissue.

are modulated by cAMP-dependent phosphorylation (12–15). The primary sequences of these proteins have been deduced by cloning their corresponding cDNAs from rabbit skeletal muscle (16–20). Using these cDNAs as probes, different α_1- and β-subunits have been cloned from heart and smooth muscle.

The Calcium Conducting α_1-Subunit

The L-type calcium channel α_1-subunits are encoded by three different genes (CaCh1–3) (see refs. 21 and 22 for nomenclature, and Fig. 2). The product of the CaCh1 gene occurs in skeletal muscle; the product of the CaCh2 gene is expressed in heart, smooth muscle, endocrine, and neuronal cells, and that of the CaCh3 gene is present in neuroendocrine and neuronal cells. The α_1-subunits from cardiac (CaCh2a) (23) and smooth muscle

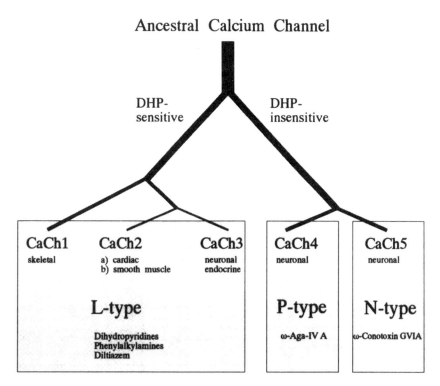

Figure 2. Developmental tree of cloned and functionally expressed calcium channel α_1-subunits. The identification of the calcium channel α_1-subunits follows the order of publication and includes only those clones that have been expressed functionally (21, 22, 25). The Snutch nomenclature (52) for the brain calcium channels does not include the CaCh1 gene. The CaCh2, CaCh3, CaCh4, and CaCh5 genes correspond to Snutch genes C, D, A, and B, respectively.

(CaCh2b) (24) are splice products of the second gene (CaCh2) (Fig. 3). The CaCh2b sequence is 95% identical with the CaCh2a sequence and differs only at four sites. The use of alternative exons (25) results in different IVS3 segments (Fig. 3, site D). Diebold and coworkers (26) reported that the two exons are differentially expressed during cardiac development. Northern blots using the CaCh2a and CaCh2b specific 5'-sequences as probes, and polymerase chain reaction analysis of the nonidentical sequences, showed that the sequence of cardiac site A is present only in cardiac muscle polyA$^+$ mRNA, whereas the sequences of the smooth muscle sites A, B, and C are present in tracheal, lung, and cardiac polyA$^+$ mRNA (27). This distribution of the CaCh2a and CaCh2b sequences strongly favors the conclusion that the CaCh2a protein is a cardiac muscle-specific α_1-subunit, whereas the CaCh2b protein is a smooth muscle-specific α_1-subunit (27).

cDNA of the third gene (CaCh3) was isolated from neuronal and endocrine tissues and represents a neuroendocrine specific L-type calcium channel (28, 29), whereas the gene products of the fourth and fifth gene (CaCh4 and CaCh5) have been found exclusively in neuronal tissues. Calcium channels transiently expressed from cRNA of CaCh4 induce high-voltage–activated, calcium currents insensitive to nifedipine and ω-cono-toxin, but inhibited by a mixture of toxins from the funnel web spider, thus characterizing this channel as a P-type calcium channel (30). The gene product of CaCh5 binds and is irreversibly blocked by picomolar concentrations of ω-conotoxin identifying the CaCh5 protein as a neuronal N-type calcium channel (31, 32).

Additional Subunits

α_2-/δ-Subunit

The skeletal muscle α_2-/δ-subunit is a glycosylated membrane protein of 125,018 Da (17) that is apparently high conserved in most tissues. In

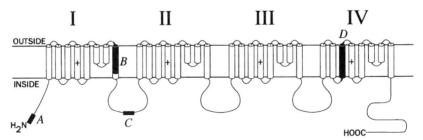

Figure 3. Sequence differences between the CaCh2a (cardiac) and CaCh2b (smooth muscle) α_1-subunit. The sequences that are different in the smooth muscle clone are shown in black and are identified by A, B, C, and D.

skeletal muscle the primary protein product of the α_2-/δ-gene is processed post-translationally by proteolysis resulting in an α_2-protein containing amino acids 1 through 934, and a δ-protein containing amino acids 935 through 1080 (33) (see Fig. 1). The transmembrane δ-subunit anchors the extracellular located α_2-protein by disulfide bridges to the plasma membrane (34). Immunoblot (35) and Northern blot (17, 27) show that similar or identical α_2-/δ-subunits exist in skeletal muscle, heart, brain, vascular, and intestinal smooth muscle. Coexpression of the cardiac α_1-subunit with the skeletal muscle α_2-/δ-protein in *Xenopus* oocytes increases slightly the current density (23, 26) and decreases 2-fold channel activation time (36). It is not clear whether these modulatory effects are physiologically relevant properties of the α_2-/δ-protein or restricted to the *Xenopus* oocyte expression system.

γ-Subunit

Northern blots and screening of cardiac cDNA libraries failed to identify the presence of the γ-subunit in cardiac or smooth muscle polyA$^+$ mRNA, suggesting that this protein may be specific for skeletal muscle.

β-Subunit

The skeletal muscle β-subunit (CaB1) is an intracellular located membrane protein consisting of 524 amino acids (18). Its deduced amino acid sequence contains stretches of heptad repeat structure that are characteristic of cytoskeletal proteins. Two other genes (CaB2 and CaB3) encoding β-proteins different from the skeletal muscle β-subunit have been isolated from a cardiac cDNA library (37). Their deduced amino acid sequences show an overall homology to CaB1 of 71% (CaB2) and 66.6% (CaB3). Differential splicing of the primary transcript of CaB1 results in at least four isoforms: CaB1a through CaB1d (18, 32, 38). CaB1a is expressed in skeletal muscle, whereas the other isoforms are expressed in brain. Four different splice variants have been characterized for the CaB2 gene (CaB2a through CaB2d); CaB2a and CaB2b have been isolated from a rabbit cardiac cDNA library, whereas CaB2c and CaB2d have been cloned from rabbit and rat brain libraries (37, 39). Like the CaB1 gene, the CaB2 and CaB3 genes are expressed tissue specifically, with transcripts of CaB2 existing abundantly in heart and to a lower degree in aorta, trachea, and lung. Transcripts of CaB3 genes are expressed in brain and smooth muscle-containing tissues, such as aorta, trachea, and lung (37). This suggests that the CaB3 gene product may be expressed predominantly in neuronal and smooth muscle cells. The deduced amino acid sequence of the skeletal muscle β-subunit (CaB1) contains several phosphorylation sites. Two of these sites, Ser-182 and Thr-205, are phosphorylated in vitro by cAMP-dependent protein kinase (18, 40). The equivalent to Thr-205 is conserved in the "cardiac" β-subunit (Thr-165 in CaB2a and Thr-191 in CaB2b), but is not present in the "smooth muscle" β-subunit, CaB3. The sequence following this potential phosphorylation site is highly variable and determines several splice variants (37). The absence of a putative cAMP kinase phosphorylation site in the variable region of the "smooth" muscle β-subunit and its presence in the "cardiac" muscle β-subunit may be responsible for the tissue-specific regulation the L-type calcium currents by cAMP kinase.

Expression of the Cloned Cardiac and Smooth Muscle Calcium Channel α_1-Subunits

The two alternative splice variants CaCh2a and CaCh2b have been expressed transiently in *Xenopus* oocytes (23, 24, 36) and stably in Chinese hamster ovary (CHO) cells (41, 42). In either system they direct the synthesis of functional L-type calcium channels. CHO cells transfected with either CaCh2a or CaCh2b cDNA express 1,4-dihydropyridine binding sites that bind isradipine stereospecifically with an affinity of 0.1 nM (Table 1). Binding of isradipine is modulated allosterically by *d-cis*-diltiazem (41). Nontransfected cells, or CHO cells transfected with a cDNA unrelated to

Table 1. Electrophysiological properties of the expressed cardiac (CaCh2a) and smooth (CaCh2b) muscle α_1-subunit of the calcium channel.

cell line	CaCh2a (heart)	CaCh2b (smooth muscle)
DHP binding sites (fmol/mg)	73.5 ± 5.4 (3)	141 ± 3 (3)
Affinity (nM)	0.2	0.1 ± 0.04 (3)
Current density (μA/cm^2)		
− Bay K 8644	− 15.2 ± 4.4 (9)	− 13.3 ± 1.9 (11)
+ Bay K 8644	− 68.2 ± 16.6 (8)	− 46.7 ± 5.4 (14)
Increase with Bay K 8644 at 10 mV (fold)	9.3 ± 2.6 (8)	5.5 ± 0.8 (11)
90% ttp (msec)	7.9 ± 0.8 (9)	12.5 ± 1.5 (12)*
dec$_{100}$ (%)	87.1 ± 2.7 (9)	84.7 ± 1.8 (11)
$V_{0.5}$inact (mV)	+ 5.2 ± 3.6 (9)	+ 5.1 ± 4.0 (5)
$V_{0.5}$act (mV)	+ 8.3 ± 0.8 (9)	+ 9.5 ± 0.8 (5)

CHO cells were stably transfected and inward currents were measured as described in Fig. 4 legend. The current is the maximum current from the current−voltage relation divided by the cell capacitance. The increase in I_{Ba} caused by Bay K 8644 was calculated for each cell at a membrane potential of 10 mV. 90% ttp, time for I_{Ba} to reach 90% of its peak amplitude at 10 mV; dec$_{100}$, decrease in I_{Ba} from peak to the level observed 100 msec after the beginning of depolarization to 10 mV; $V_{0.5}$inact, half-maximal inactivation voltage, $V_{0.5}$act, half-maximal activation voltage. Values are given as mean ± SEM, with the number of cells in parentheses. The DHP binding sites were determined with (^{3}H)isradipine.
*Significantly different from the CaCh2a value at $P< 0.05$.

the calcium channel, do not possess DHP binding sites or L-type calcium current, whereas cells expressing the cardiac or smooth muscle α_1-subunit have L-type calcium current (Fig. 4). The basic electrophysiological characteristics of these two splice variants of the CaCh2 gene are almost identical (Table 1). Both channels are blocked by isradipine and are stimulated 5- to 10-fold by Bay K 8644 at 10mV (Table 1). Activation of the channel by Bay K 8644 shifts the maximal inward current by 10 mV to 10 mV. In the presence of Bay K 8644 and 30 mM $BaCl_2$, half-maximal activation ($V_{0.5act}$) occurred at 9.5 and 8.3 mV for the smooth and cardiac muscle, respectively. Under the same conditions, half-maximal steady-state inactivation ($V_{0.5inact}$) occurred at 5.1 and 5.2 mV, respectively. Both channels inactivate faster in the presence of Ca^{2+} than Ba^{2+} (i.e., inactivation of the CaCh2 channel is voltage- and calcium-dependent as known for the native L-type calcium channel). The only difference noted was faster activation for cardiac than for smooth muscle channels in the absence and presence of the Bay K 8644. Functional expression of chimeras of the skeletal and the cardiac muscle α_1-subunit showed that repeat I determines the activation time of the chimeric channel; that is, a slow activation upon membrane depolarization with the repeat from skeletal muscle, and rapid activation with that from cardiac muscle (43). It is possible that the difference in activation times between the cardiac and smooth muscle channels is caused by the difference in the IS6 sequence (site B in Fig. 3). The open probability of the expressed smooth muscle channel increases with membrane depolarization. The channel has a single-channel conductance of 26 pS in 80 mM $BaCl_2$ (41). These data show that the α_1-subunit alone is sufficient to form a physiologically relevant calcium channel that has the properties of a smooth or cardiac muscle L-type calcium channel.

Stable expression of the CaCh2b channel with the skeletal muscle β-gene (CaB1), increased in parallel the number of DHP binding sites and the amplitude of whole-cell barium current suggesting that the amplitude of the inward current is directly related to the density of expressed α_1-protein (35). In addition the coexpression of the β-subunit decreased channel activation time 2-fold and shifted the voltage dependence of steady-state inactivation by 18 mV, to -13 mV, without affecting sensitivity to the calcium channel agonist Bay K 8644.

Modulation of the Expressed Calcium Channel

In heart, β-adrenergic stimulation leads to activation of cAMP kinase and an increase in L-type calcium current. Two subunits of the purified skeletal muscle calcium channel, the α_1- and β-subunits, are substrates for cAMP-kinase in vitro (4, 18, 40, 44–46). Similar potential cAMP kinase phosphorylation sites are present in the CaCh2 calcium channel sequence of both splice variants. The potential importance of these phosphorylation sites is supported by experiments that showed that the L-type calcium

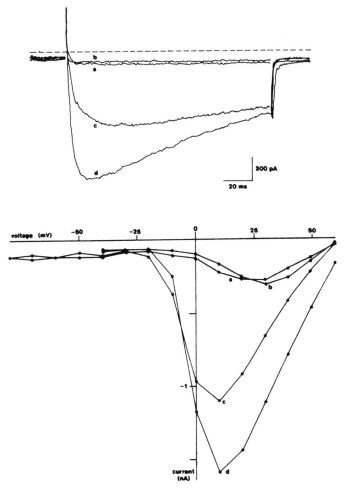

Figure 4. Electrophysiology of expressed smooth **(a, c)** and cardiac **(b, d)** muscle α_1-subunit of the calcium channel. **(Top)** Barium currents (I_{Ba}) were elicited by a 140-msec depolarization pulse from a holding potential of -80 mV to 10 mV before (a, b) and during the exposure to 2 µM Bay K 8644 (c, d). The dashed line represents the 0 current level. **(Bottom)** Current-voltage relationships were determined by stepping the membrane potential from -80 mV to the potentials indicated. I_{Ba} was measured in the absence (a, b) and presence (c, d) of 2 µM Bay K 8644. CHO cells were stably transfected (41) with the cDNA of the smooth muscle α_1-subunit of the calcium channel (24) in a p91023(B) expression vector or with the cDNA of the cardiac α_1-subunit (23) in a pKNH expression vector (53). Positive clones were selected for the expression of dihydrofolate reductase or with the neomycine derivative G418. Whole-cell current was recorded at room temperature in a solution containing (in mM) 82 NaCl, 20 tetraethylommonium-chloride, 30 BaCl$_2$, 5.4 CsCl, 1 MgCl$_2$, 5 HEPES, and 10 glucose, pH 7.4 (NaOH), with a pipette solution containing (in mM) 112 CsCl, 1 MgCl$_2$, 3 Na$_2$ATP, 10 EGTA, and 5 HEPES, pH 7.4 (CsOH).

current expressed in *Xenopus* oocytes after the injection of rat cardiac poly(A$^+$) RNA is modulated by cAMP-dependent phosphorylation (47). However, perfusion of a CHO cell expressing the CaCh2b gene with 8Br-cAMP for 5 min did not increase significantly the inward current (Fig. 5), although CHO cells contain a functional adenylyl cyclase, G$_S$, and cAMP-dependent protein kinase. The inward barium current was not affected significantly when the pipette solution contained 3mM ATPγSalme; 3 mM ATPγS + 10; or 100 μM 8Br-cAMP or 3 mM ATPγS + 10 μM GTPγS. Isoproterenol failed to increase the barium current in a CHO cell line that expressed the β$_2$-adrenergic receptor at a concentration of 1 pmol/mg protein and the CaCh2b calcium channel. These negative findings suggest that the α$_1$-subunit alone is not sufficient to restore hormonal regulation of the native calcium channel. Similar conclusions were reached by Klöckner et al. (48), who injected the cardiac α$_1$-subunit alone or together with the skeletal muscle β-subunit into *Xenopus* oocyctes. These authors reported

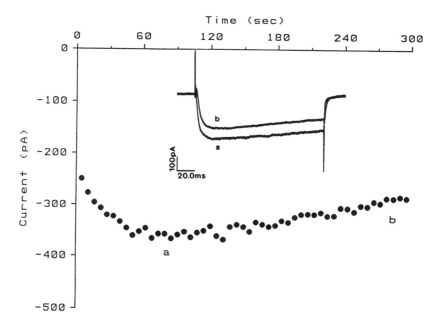

Figure 5. 8Br-cAMP has no effect on the barium current. The cell was transfected stably with the CaCh2b clone. The barium inward current was measured as described in Table 1 footnote. Cells were superfused with (in mM) 79.0 NaCl, 20 tetraethylammonium, 30 BaCl$_2$, 5.4 CsCl, 1 MgCl$_2$, 10 glucose, and 10 HEPES, pH 7.4. The pipette solution contained (in mM) 107 CsCl, 3 MgCl$_2$, 10 EGTA, and 10 HEPES, pH 7.4, 3 mM ATPγS, and 10μM 8Br-cAMP. The inward current at 10 mV is shown. The inset shows two current traces taken at time points a and b. The small increase in inward current occurring within the first minute was observed also in all cells perfused in the absence of ATPγS and 8Br-cAMP and is caused most likely by the chelation of calcium by EGTA.

that cAMP increased barium currents only in *Xenopus* oocytes expressing the cardiac α_1- and the skeletal muscle β-subunit (48). However, the reported inward currents were small and their sensitivity toward Bay K 8644 or a 1,4-dihydropyridine blocker was not tested. Therefore, these authors did not exclude the possibility that the β-subunit associated with the endogenous *Xenopus* oocyte calcium channel (36, 49), which is insensitive to the 1,4-dihydropyridines, is stimulated by cAMP in the presence of the skeletal muscle subunits (50). Perfusion of CHO cells expressing the CaCh2 α_1-subunit and the skeletal muscle β-subunit with cAMP or 8Br-cAMP had no effect on the size of the inward current, suggesting that at least in CHO cells the combination of these two subunits, which are not expressed in vivo in the same tissue, does not restore hormonal control of the cardiac calcium channel. These negative results are unexplained, so far. The cAMP kinase activity of *Xenopus* oocytes is higher than in most cells and could phosphorylate constantly the α_1-subunit in vivo.

Different results were obtained with protein kinase C. The cardiac L-type calcium current is enhanced and subsequently inhibited by the activation of protein kinase C (51). Activation of protein kinase C has been proposed to mediate the potential effects of angiotensin II on the calcium current in heart. The skeletal muscle α_1-subunit is rapidly phosphorylated by protein kinase C (44). Currents through the CaCh2a α_1-subunit expressed in *Xenopus* oocytes were biphasically modulated by activation of protein kinase C (49). Initially the current increased followed by a marked inhibition. The biphasic modulation was not modified significantly by coexpression of the cardiac α_1-subunit with the α_2-/δ-, β-, and γ-subunits from skeletal muscle, suggesting that protein kinase C affected the current by phosphorylation of the α_1-subunit.

Conclusions

The cardiac and the smooth muscle, high-voltage–activated, L-type calcium channels are oligomeric complexes of three different subunits: α_1, α_2/δ, and β. The α_1-subunits are splice products of the CaCh2 gene. The α_2-/δ-subunit may be identical with the skeletal muscle subunit. The β-subunits are encoded by different genes. The expression of a tissue-specific subunit combination most likely results in the differences in pharmacology and function of the channel. This genetic polymorphism may explain also the different regulatory mechanisms and possibly offers a chance for refined drug therapy in the future.

Acknowledgment

The results obtained in the authors' laboratory were supported by grants from Deutsche Forschungsgemeinschaft and Fond der Chemie.

References

1. Tsien, R.W., Ellinor, P.T., and Horne, W.A. (1991). *Trends Pharmacol. Sci.* **12:**349.

2. Glossmann, H., and Striessnig, J. (1988). *Vit. Horm.* **44:**155.

3. Catterall, W.A., Seagar, M.J., and Takahashi, M. (1988). *J. Biol. Chem.* **263:**3533.

4. Hofmann, F., Flockerzi, V., Nastainczyk, W., Ruth, P., and Schneider, T. (1990). *Curr. Top. Cell Regul.* **31:**223.

5. Osterrieder, W., Brum, G., Hescheler, J., Trautwein, W., Flockerzi, V., and Hofmann, F. (1982). *Nature* **298:**576.

6. Hartzell, H.C., Mery, P.F., Fischmeister, R., and Szabo, G. (1991). *Nature* **351:**573.

7. Yatani, A., and Brown, A.M. (1989). *Science* **245:**71.

8. Pelzer, S., Shuba, Y.M., Asai, T., Codina, J., Birnbaumer, L., McDonald, T.F., and Pelzer, D. (1990). *Am. J. Physiol.* **259:**H264.

9. Cavalié, A., Allen, T.J.A., and Trautwein, W. (1991). *Pflügers Arch.* **419:**433.

10. Welling, A., Felbel, J., Peper, K., and Hofmann, F. (1992). *Am. J. Physiol.* **262:**L351.

11. Hamilton, S.L., Codina, J., Hawkes, M.J., Yatani, A., Sawada, T., Strickland, F.M., Froehner, S.C., Spiegel, A.M., Toro, L., Stefani, E., Birnbaumer, L., and Brown, A.M. (1991). *J. Biol. Chem.* **266:**19528.

12. Flockerzi, V., Oeken, H.J., Hofmann, F., Pelzer, D., Cavalié, A., and Trautwein, W. (1986). *Nature* **323:**66.

13. Hymel, L., Striessnig, J., Glossmann, H., and Schindler, H. (1988). *Proc. Natl. Acad. Sci. U.S.A.* **85:**4290.

14. Nunoki, K., Florio, V., and Catterall, W.A. (1989). *Proc. Natl. Acad. Sci. U.S.A.* **86:**6816.

15. Mundina-Weilenmann, C., Chang, Ch.F., Gutierrez, L.M., and Hosey, M.M. (1991). *J. Biol. Chem.* **266:**4067.

16. Tanabe, T., Takeshima, H., Mikami, A., Flockerzi, V., Takahashi, H., Kangawa, K., Kojima, M., Matsuo, H., Hirose, T., and Numa, S. (1987). *Nature* **328:**313.

17. Ellis, S.B., Williams, M.E., Ways, N.R., Brenner, R., Sharp, A.H., Leung, A.T., Campbell, K.P., McKenna, E., Koch, W.J., Hui, A., Schwartz, A., and Harpold, M.M. (1988). *Science* **241:**1661.

18. Ruth, P., Röhrkasten, A., Biel, M., Bosse, E., Regulla, S., Meyer, H.E., Flockerzi, V., and Hofmann, F. (1989). *Science* **245:**1115.

19. Bosse, E., Regulla, S., Biel, M., Ruth, P., Meyer, H.E., Flockerzi, V., and Hofmann, F. (1990). *FEBS Lett.* **267:**153.

20. Jay, S.D., Ellis, S.B., McCue, A.F., Williams, M.E., Vedvick, T.S., Harpold, M.M., and Campbell, K. (1990). *Science* **248:**490.

21. Hofmann, F., Biel, M., Hullin, R., Bosse, E., and Flockerzi, V. (1993). GTPase in biology, in *Handbook of Pharmacology* (Springer, Berlin), in press.

22. Hullin, R., Biel, M., Flockerzi, V., and Hofmann, F. (1993). *Trends Cardiovasc. Med.* **3,** in press.

23. Mikami, A., Imoto, K., Tanabe, T., Niidome, T., Mori, I., Takeshima, H., Narumiya, S., and Numa, S. (1989). *Nature* **340**:230.

24. Biel, M., Ruth, P., Bosse, E., Hullin, R., Stühmer, W., Flockerzi, V., and Hofmann, F. (1990). *FEBS Lett.* **269**:409.

25. Perez-Reyes, E., Wei, X., Castellano, A., and Birnbaumer, L. (1990). *J. Biol. Chem.* **265**:20430.

26. Diebold, R.J., Koch, W.J., Ellinor, P.T., Wang, J.J., Muthuchamy, M., Wieczorek, D.F., and Schwartz, A. (1992). *Proc. Natl. Acad. Sci. U.S.A.* **89**:1497.

27. Biel, M., Hullin, R., Freundner, S., Singer, D., Dascal, N., Flockerzi, V., and Hofmann, F. (1991). *Eur. J. Biochem.* **200**:81:

28. Williams, M.E., Brust, P.F., Feldman, D.H., Patti, S., Simerson, S., Maroufi, A., McCue, A.F., Velicelebi, G., Ellis, S.B., and Harpold, M.M. (1992). *Science* **257**:389.

29. Seino, S., Chen, L., Seino, M., Blondel, O., Takeda, J., Johnson, J.H., and Bell, G.I. (1992). *Proc. Natl. Acad. Sci. U.S.A.* **89**:584.

30. Mori, Y., Friedrich, T., Kim, M-S., Mikami, A., Nakai, J., Ruth, P., Bosse, E., Hofmann, F., Flockerzi, V., Furuichi, T., Mikoshiba, K., Imoto, K., Tanabe, T., and Numa, S. (1991). *Nature* **350**:398.

31. Dubel, S.J., Starr, T.V.B., Hell, J., Ahlijanian, M.A., Enyeart, J.J., Catterall, W.A., and Snutch, T.P. (1992). *Proc. Natl. Acad. Sci. U.S.A.* **89**:5058.

32. Williams, M.E., Feldman, D.H., McCue, A.F., Brenner, R., Velicelebi, G., Ellis, S.B., and Harpold, M.M. (1992). *Neuron* **8**:71.

33. De Jongh, K.S., Warner, C., and Catterall, W.A. (1990). *J. Biol. Chem.* **265**:14738.

34. Jay, S.D., Sharp, A.H., Kahl, St.D., Vedvick, T.S., Harpold, M.M., and Campbell, K.P. (1991). *J. Biol. Chem.* **266**:3287.

35. Norman, R.I., Burgess, A.J., Allen, E., and Harrison, T.M. (1987). *FEBS Lett.* **212**:127.

36. Singer, D., Biel, M., Lotan, I., Flockerzi, V., Hofmann, F., and Dascal, N. (1991). *Science* **253**:1553.

37. Hullin, R., Singer-Lahat, D., Freichel, M., Biel, M., Dascal, N., Hofmann, F., and Flockerzi, V. (1992). *EMBO J.* **11**:885.

38. Pragnell, M., Sakamoto, J., Jay, S.D., and Campbell, K.P. (1991). *FEBS Lett.* **291**:253.

39. Perez-Reyes, E., Castellano, A., Kim, H.S., Bertrand, P., Baggstrom, E., Lacerda, A., Wei, X., and Birnbaumer, L. (1992). *J. Biol. Chem.* **267**:1792.

40. De Jongh, K.S., Merrick, D.K., and Catterall, W.A. (1989). *Proc. Natl. Acad. Sci. U.S.A.* **86**:8585.

41. Bosse, E., Bottlender, R., Kleppisch, T., Hescheler, J., Welling, A., Hofmann, F., and Flockerzi, V. (1992). *EMBO J.* **11**:2033.

42. Welling, A., Bottlender, R., Bosse, E., and Hofmann, F. (1992). *Naunyn-Schmiedeberg's Arch. Pharmacol.* **345**:70.

43. Tanabe, T., Adams, B.A., Numa, S., and Beam, K.G. (1991). *Nature* **352**:800.

44. Nastainczyk, W., Röhrkasten, A., Sieber, M., Rudolph, C., Schächtele, C., Marme, D., and Hofmann, F. (1987). *Eur. J. Biochem.* **169**:137.

45. Röhrkasten, A., Meyer, H.E., Nastainczyk, W., Sieber, M., and Hofmann, F. (1988). *J. Biol. Chem.* **263:**15325.

46. Rotman, E.I., De Jongh, K.S., Florio, V., Lai, Y., and Catterall, W.A. (1992). *J. Biol. Chem.* **267:**16100.

47. Lory, P., and Nargeot, J. (1992). *Biochem. Biophys. Res. Commun.* **182:**1059.

48. Klöckner, U., Itagaki, K., Bodi, I., and Schwartz, A. (1992). *Pflügers Arch.* **420:**413.

49. Singer-Lahat, D., Gershon, E., Lotan, H., Hullin, R., Biel, M., Flockerzi, V., Hofmann, F., and Dascal, N. (1992). *FEBS Lett.* **306:**113.

50. Dascal, N., Lotan, I., Karni, E., and Gigi, A. (1992). *J. Physiol.* **450:**469.

51. Lacerda, A.E., Rampe, D., and Brown, A.M. (1988). *Nature* **335:**249.

52. Snutch, T.P., Leonard, J.P., Gilbert, M.M., Lester, H.A., and Davidson, N. (1990). *Proc. Natl. Acad. Sci. U.S.A.* **87:**3391.

53. Nukada, T., Mishina, M., and Numa, S. (1987). *FEBS Lett.* **211:**5.

PART 5

Molecular Pharmacology

Chapters 13 through 19 have demonstrated how mutational analysis can be used to assign functional properties of ion channels, such as voltage sensing and ion conduction, to structural domains within the protein molecule. A powerful adjunct to this approach is the use of drugs as probes of these structural domains. From a practical point of view, better drugs with greater potency, efficacy and specificity may emerge from developing a new molecular pharmacology which would combine strategies of drug synthesis with mutational analysis. For example, if we know that a drug acts as an open channel blocker and if we know where in the linear sequence of amino acids the pore domain is located, then protein engineering using recombinant DNA methods should enable us to identify the residues that form the receptor in the pore for a particular drug. Armed with this knowledge, the methods of organic chemistry should permit the design of drugs with a range of affinities for this site.

Two necessary preconditions are that we identify classes of drugs specific for different K^+, Na^+ and Ca^{2+} subfamilies of voltage-dependent ion channels and understand the mechanism of action of these drugs. The papers in this Section deal with how these questions can be resolved. In Chapter 20, Dr. Strauss examines the effects of two commonly used K^+ channel blockers, 4-aminopyridine (4-AP) and quinidine, on cardiac K^+ currents. An essential relationship must be kept in mind when drug blockade is being evaluated. The "on" and "off" rates of drug association and disassociation for its receptor site on the channel protein must be related to the rates at which the channel transits between open, closed and inactivated states. This obviously is because access of a drug to its receptor site depends on the state in which the drug finds the channel when it comes in contact with it.

Quinidine blockade of human K^+ channels is highly relevant here. Quinidine is one of the most widely prescribed drugs for the treatment of cardiac arrhythmias and blocks open channels in a voltage-dependent manner. The block and unblock rates are slower than the gating rates for the channel and at faster than normal heart rates the block is cumulative and shows, what is called "use dependence".

The opposite phenomenon in which block becomes less effective at faster rates is called "reverse use dependence" and has been observed for some therapeutic blockers of I_K. An explanation for reverse use dependence is given by Dr. Colatsky in Chapter 21. The explanation utilizes the two components of the delayed rectifier K^+ current described by Dr. Sanguinetti in Chapter 7. Using this framework, the rapid component I_{Kr} is blocked specifically by benzensulfonamides, such as sotalol. However, the slow component I_{Ks} is unaffected by this drug and at high heart rates becomes more prominent than normal. The blocking drug is apparently less effective, but this is only because another channel on which it has no action now comes into play.

For high threshold, L-type cardiac Ca^{2+} channels, the most potent antagonists are the dihydropyridines (DHPs) and these are widely used clinically to suppress conduction through the atria-ventricular node. These compounds are neutral at physiological pH, are markedly hydrophobic and thus are likely to have access to the channel through the lipid phase of the membrane. In Chapter 22, we learn from Dr. Kass that charged DHP's block Ca^{2+} channels when applied extra-, but not intra-cellularly. On the other hand, charged members of another major class of Ca^{2+} channel blockers, the phenylalkylamines block only from the intracellular surface. In addition, this block is influenced by the charge carrier and Ca^{2+} ions seem to stabilize the blocked state. Thus, DHP's can access the DHP receptor via both hydrophobic and hydrophilic pathways. This kind of information should prove pharmacologically useful in the design of Ca^{2+} channel blockers which may act preferentially by dissolution in a membrane or by an aqueous pathway to the pore.

Drug-binding domains can now be localized directly in Ca^{2+} channel proteins by using models of channel structure to design sequence-specific antibodies. Antibodies are then used to immunoprecipitate peptide fragments from channel proteins tagged previously for example, by a photoaffinity label. This approach was taken by Dr. Streissnig in Chapter 23 to localize the phenylalkylamine receptor to a region of the channel thought to be near the inner mouth of the pore. Using similar methods, the DHP receptor was localized to a region thought to be near the outer pore mouth. Finally, a charged derivative of another major class of Ca^{2+} channel blocker, the benzothiazepines, of which diltiazem is the most widely known member, was used to establish that the receptor site for this class of antagonists was near the external mouth of the pore.

The papers in this Part demonstrate very well how functional mechanisms of drug blockade, determined electrophysiologically can be assigned to structural domains of the channel protein. Confirmation can be achieved independently by affinity labelling of the drugs to the channel protein. Such approaches are essential for the drug discovery strategies discussed in the following Section.

Arthur M. Brown & Peter M. Spooner

20

Conformation-Dependent Drug Binding to Cardiac Potassium Channels

Randall L. Rasmusson, Donald L. Campbell,
Yusheng Qu, and Harold C. Strauss

Repolarization of the cardiac action potential is an important but complex and incompletely understood phenomenon. Repolarization modulates the refractory period and, to a lesser extent, tension development. In pathological situations disturbances in repolarization may lead to arrhythmic events such as early after-depolarizations and triggered events (1). In cardiac myocytes different voltage-gated K^{2+}, Ca^{2+}, and Cl^- channels have been hypothesized to be involved importantly in generating currents responsible for controlling and/or modulating (i) rapid-phase 1 repolarization; (ii) the plateau and early-phase 3 repolarization; (iii) frequency-dependent changes in action potential configuration; and (iv) interspecies, intracardiac, and age-dependent differences in action potential configurations (2, 3). Among the voltage-dependent K^+ currents that are thought to contribute to the overall configuration of the action potential and repolarization are the inwardly rectifying K^+ current ("I_{K1}"), a "plateau" K^+ current ("$I_{K,P}$"), the transient outward K^+ current ("I_{TO}"), which in different cardiac myocyte types may be composed of two different components: a voltage-dependent ["$I_{TO,1}$"] and a calcium-mediated component ["$I_{TO,2}$"]), two types of delayed rectifier ("I_{KR}" and "I_{KS}", for "rapid" or "rectifying" and "slow," respectively), as well as neurotransmitter-activated (e.g., "$I_{K,Ach}$") and metabolically regulated channels (e.g., "$I_{K,ATP}$").

Class I antiarrhythmic drugs that demonstrate local anesthetic and Na^+ channel blocking properties typically display "use dependence" (4). The term "use dependence" indicates that the more frequently the channel is activated, the greater is the degree of block. Physiologically, such class I drugs are more effective blockers at increased heart rates. Another class of blocking compounds that prolong action potential duration, the so-called "class III" antiarrhythmic drugs (e.g., amiodarone, sotalol, and clofilium), are believed to do so by blocking K^+ channels (5). Many class III compounds also display use-dependent blocking characteristics. However, recent hypotheses (6) have suggested that some class III compounds produce *less* block of K^+ channels with increased frequency of channel activation. As a result, such drugs may be more effective at blocking K^+ channels at slower heart rates. This behavior is the opposite of conventional use dependence displayed by class I compounds, and has therefore been referred to as "reverse-use dependence."

The phenomenon of use-dependent blockade of Na^+ channels by local anesthetics corresponds closely with "use-dependent" changes in electrophysiological variables, such as action potential upstroke and conduction velocity (7). Presumably because of this correspondence, the term use dependence has been used to describe both changes in action potential upstroke and propagation velocity, as well as I_{Na}. Because K^+ channels contribute to the repolarizing phase of the action potential, use dependence is sometimes inferred from the effects of K^+ channel blockers on repolarization. Although in many cases use dependence at the channel level may translate into use dependence at the repolarization level and vice-versa, the two do not always coincide (8). One reason for this lack of correspondence lies in the complex nature of repolarization, wherein several potassium channels contribute to repolarization, and the fact that these outward currents are also closely balanced by inward currents, such as I_{Ca}, I_{Na}, and $I_{Na/Ca}$. As a result, no one current dominates repolarization (9–11). For these reasons, we will use the term "use dependence" to refer to effects observed at the channel level unless otherwise explicitly stated.

Class I antiarrhythmic drugs typically do not act solely upon Na^+ channels, but also block others such as K^+ (12) and, in some cases, Ca^{2+} channels (13). As is suggested by differences in use-dependent characteristics between class I and III blockers, the mechanisms of action, as well as the specific targets of drug-channel interaction, would appear to be different. In the future, our physical understanding of events generating cardiac arrhythmias, and perhaps our ability to manage such disorders effectively, will rely heavily on compounds with greater channel specificity and with well-defined mechanisms of action. The potential for achieving this goal has been greatly increased by recent advances in previously separate and distinct fields, such as electrophysiology and molecular biology. These advances have shed light not only on mechanisms of arrhythmogenesis, but also have provided detailed information on how channels function. For example, the recent discovery, sequencing and expression of a family of related K^+ channels (14), has provided considerable insight into gating mechanisms and structure of K^+ channels, and begun the reconciliation of channel structure and function at a molecular level. This new information, when considered in conjunction with the variety of distinct K^+ channel types found in cardiac muscle, make K^+ channel blockers fertile ground for the exploration of antiarrhythmic agents, as well as powerful probes for studying channel structure–function relationships.

The molecular biologist might be thought of as working from the sequence to secondary and tertiary structure, and ultimately to channel function. In contrast, cellular electrophysiologists have for many years approached the problem of channel structure–function relationships from virtually the opposite direction, starting with the properties of channel function and directing experimental efforts at deducing what sort of physical and chemical structures are producing the observed behavior. Combining information from these two fields to understand drug-channel interactions for cardiac K^+ channels is in its infancy. In this chapter we will review some aspects of conformation and state-dependent drug blockade of cardiac K^+ channels.

Rather than presenting a comprehensive catalog of known blockers and their putative state-dependent effects on the various K^+ channel types in cardiac muscle, we emphasize herein differences in channel-blocking mechanisms for two established drugs. Chapter 21 discusses the classification of these antiarrhythmic drugs and focuses on some recently developed compounds. We compare two major state-dependent blocking mechanisms (open versus closed) for quinidine and 4-aminopyridine (4-AP) effects on two important cardiac K^+ channel types: the delayed rectifier I_{KS} and the voltage-gated transient outward I_{TO}. We present some of the basic electrophysiological characteristics associated with open-state block of macroscopic I_{KS} by quinidine, versus closed-state block of macroscopic I_{TO} by 4-AP, and discuss how such properties give rise to conventional versus reverse use dependence. We also briefly review some of what is known concerning molecular mechanisms involved in state-dependent block, and how they may relate to various aspects of K^+ channel structure.

Basic Concepts

The conformation of a channel, or of any protein, is the three-dimensional physical arrangement of the chemical bonds and atoms comprising the macromolecule. At physiological temperatures a channel protein embedded in a lipid membrane may have literally millions of possible conformations. As any amino acid side chain shifts or as any hydrogen bond is formed or broken we can say that the channel conformation has changed. The local motions of amino acid side chains, peptide backbones, and tertiary and quaternary protein conformational changes, processes undoubtedly related to gating, can occur in a fraction of a millisecond. Attempting to study a channel protein at such a level of detail is an analytically intractable problem. Fortunately, channels do not appear to open and close in a gradual fashion (e.g., like a sphincter, with conductance being roughly proportional to pore diameter); rather, single-channel recordings indicate that they abruptly transition between conducting and nonconducting conformations. This has lead to a more functional description of channel behavior based on the idea of different kinetic *states*, [i.e., the concept that a group of related channel conformations with similar physical configurations and conductance properties gives rise to the behavior governing channel gating kinetics (activation/deactivation and inactivation/recovery) and conduction].

A kinetic state is a mathematical abstraction that relates the kinetic behavior of the channel to a particular physical conformation. Although attempts have been made to describe channel conformation in terms of diffusional or fractal mechanisms, Markov modeling has been particularly useful for describing the behavior of ion channels and state-dependent drug interactions. In Markovian formalism, changes in conformation are modeled as discrete transitions or jumps between distinct states. Each Markov state is one that satisfies the following three conditions: (i) the amount of time previously spent in a given state has no bearing on the subsequent expected dwell time in that state; (ii) the dwell time of a particular state is independent of how that state was reached; and (iii) the probability of exiting to one state or another is independent of both the direction of entry into the state or the dwell time before transition.

Because of these "memoryless" properties, it can be shown that the expected dwell time of any state must be exponentially distributed. For molecular systems the physical arrangement should also satisfy these "memoryless" Markov properties, because the only physical property associated with past conformations is momentum, which for the masses involved at physiological temperatures should be negligible (15). In keeping with current practice for the remainder of this chapter we use "conformation" when referring to the physical properties of a channel protein and "state" when referring to kinetically distinct behavior as measured electrically.

The salient feature that distinguishes state-dependent blockade of channels from state-independent blockade is that state-dependent blockade not only reduces current magnitude, but also alters current kinetics. State-dependent channel blockade has been observed for many channel types (for recent reviews see refs. 16 and 17). How state-dependent channel blockade is manifested depends on the specific kinetics of the particular drug-channel state interactions. Binding speed and affinity of the compound for particular states determine the kinetic behavior of the macroscopic current in the presence of drug. Based on single-channel kinetic studies, it has been suggested that binding of drugs can be grouped according to interaction rates with the channel (16–18). Briefly, these drug-channel interaction rates are (i) *slow*—Channel-blocking kinetics (i.e., dwell time) are very slow relative to channel open times; (ii) *intermediate*—Channel-blocking kinetics are sufficiently similar to channel open times to permit resolution of blocking kinetics with patch-clamp techniques, resulting in decreased channel open time; and (iii) *fast*—drug-channel binding and unbinding occurs more rapidly than today's techniques resolve, resulting in an apparent reduction in open-channel conductance.

The effects of drugs on macroscopic currents are also distinctly different for these three different forms of block. This has been described elsewhere (16–18) and will not be discussed at length herein. Instead we examine the evidence presented in support of open-state block of cardiac-delayed rectifier-type currents by quinidine, and compare and contrast this with the evidence for closed-state block of Ca^{2+}-insensitive I_{TO} by 4-AP.

Evidence for State-Dependent Blockade: The "Cross-over" Phenomenon

Figure 1 (top) shows a representative recording of the effects of 5 mM 4-AP on I_{TO} in a ferret right ventricular myocyte elicited by an 800 msec voltage-clamp pulse to 50 mV from a holding potential of -70 mV; 5 mM 4-AP reduced I_{TO} appreciably. However, block is more complicated than a simple reduction in current magnitude. 4-AP not only reduces I_{TO}, but also slows down the apparent rates of *both* activation and inactivation of the current waveform recorded in its presence. As a result, there is a *cross-over* of the current waveforms recorded before and after application of 4-AP (19). Figure 1 (bottom) shows the effects of quinidine on guinea pig I_{KS} as a function of time. Quinidine (dotted line) altered the kinetics and magnitude of both the activating current and the deactivating tail. Block was greatest during the early portion of the activating pulse, but because the channel does not inactivate at depolarized potentials, no cross-over was reported (20). However, on stepping to -30 mV, deactivation of tail currents seemed slowed in the presence of quinidine, resulting in a cross-over of the tail current waveforms at -30 mV.

Figure 1 (top and bottom) can be described as demonstrating cross-over in the presence of drug. Both are thought to arise from state-specific drug-channel interactions. However, electrophysiological data described herein indicate that they arise from interactions with completely different states of the channel. The cross-over observed for I_{TO} at 50 mV after application of 4-AP is thought to arise from closed-state binding of the drug. Consider the simplified sequence of events associated with channel opening in response to a depolarizing step. Under ordinary circumstances the applied potential causes the resting closed state, C, to become unstable, resulting in an activation transition to an open and conducting state, O, which is then followed by an inactivation transition to a final absorbing inactive state, I. This can be diagrammed as a series of Markov states as follows:

$$C \rightarrow O \rightarrow I$$

This qualitative behavior gives rise to the transient nature of the I_{TO} current. Channel blockade, which is specific to the closed state of the channel, alters the scheme previously described:

$$B \leftrightarrow C \rightarrow O \rightarrow I$$

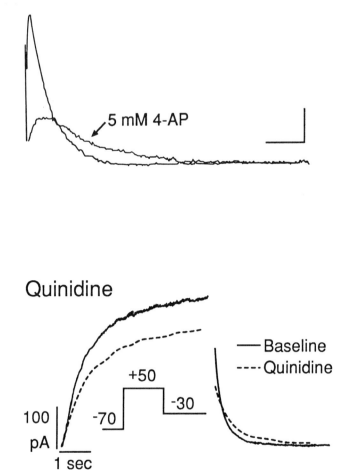

Figure 1. Cross-over of current waveforms. **(Top)** Effect of 4-AP on I_{TO} recorded from isolated ferret right ventricular myocytes. Current traces were recorded in a Na$^+$-free (NMDG replacement) saline in the presence of 50 μM tetrodotoxin and 500 μM Cd by applying 800 msec voltage-clamp pulses to 50 mV (holding potential = −70 mV) and after applying 5 mM 4-AP (calibration: horizontal bar, 100 msec; vertical bar, 100 pA). Note that 4-AP not only reduced the peak amplitude of I_{TO}, but also altered its apparent kinetics in that it slowed activation and the time course of current decay. This resulted in a "cross-over" of the current waveforms. [From Campbell et al. (19).] **(Bottom)** Action of quinidine on I_{KS} in isolated guinea pig ventricular myocytes. Activation of I_K upon depolarization from −70 mV to 50 mV and subsequent deactivation at −30 mV (inset: voltage-clamp protocol). Currents were measured before (solid line) and during (dotted line) application of 10 μM quinidine. Note that quinidine reduced current activation in response to a depolarizing pulse and that, upon deactivation of the current at −30 mV, the initial magnitude of the current in the presence of quinidine is reduced but decays more slowly to initial conditions than control, resulting in a cross-over of the tail current. Experiments were performed in the presence of La^{3+} to isolate the slow component of the delayed rectifier current. [From Balser et al. (20).]

The new state, B, is the drug bound form of channel. This binding scheme can give rise to the cross-over phenomena described for I_{TO} observed experimentally. Before the channel can activate (open) and inactivate, the drug must dissociate from the channel. If drug dissociation is slow compared with the rate for the $C \rightarrow O$ transition, then the onset and peak of the current are delayed. Although peak current is delayed, the kinetics of open-channel inactivation subsequent to drug unbinding are not affected by such a mechanism. Consequently, measured current in the presence of drug is larger at later times, because the opening of channels is delayed by drug unbinding, and the current traces in the presence and absence of drug must "cross over" each other.

Delayed opening is not necessarily dependent on slow kinetics of closed-state channel blockade, but can also be due to delay in delivery of channels into the open state. Consider the situation in which channel binding and unbinding are instantaneous. For concentrations near the K_d, at rest a closed-state blocker will result in a distribution of ~50% in the B state and 50% in the C state. The rate at which channels are delivered to the open state from the closed state is proportional to the number of channels occupying the closed state; drug binding effectively reduces the proportion of channels available for transition from $C \rightarrow O$ by 50%. Under these conditions activation of the channel is slowed by 50%, even though block and unblock of the channel are essentially instantaneous.

Delayed rectifier channels do not show significant inactivation in response to a depolarizing pulse over the time frame shown in Fig. 1 (bottom). Thus, activation of I_K might be described by:

$$C \rightarrow O$$

and open-state blockade by

$$C \rightarrow O \leftrightarrow B$$

that resembles the sequence of states shown for inactivating channels. If drug binding kinetics are appropriate, open-channel blockade can resemble inactivation. Indeed quinidine action on the HK2 delayed rectifier-type current does introduce some transient behavior (see Fig. 2). Similar actions have been described for internally applied quaternary ammonium ions on other K^+ channel types (e.g., squid axon delayed rectifier; refs. 22 and 23). Noninactivating channels do not show cross-over from channel blockade in response to a depolarizing step. However, following a repolarizing step the channel will undergo the transition sequence:

$$B \leftrightarrow O \rightarrow C$$

It is obvious that open-state blockade delays delivery of channels to the open state. As a result, the process of deactivation ($O \rightarrow C$) is delayed. This produces a cross-over of the deactivating tail currents similar to that illustrated in Fig. 1 (bottom). It should be noted that open-channel block-

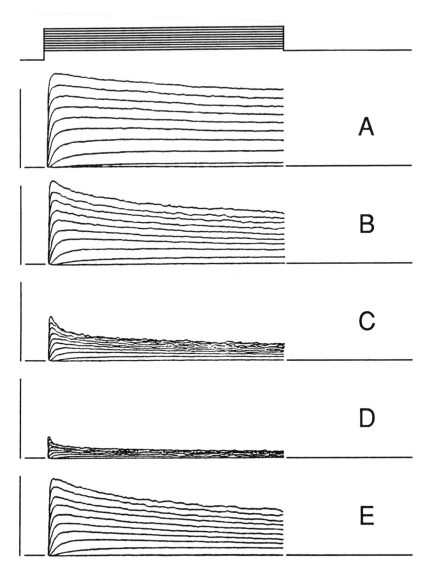

Figure 2. Reduction of magnitude and induction of inactivation-like behavior by quinidine on HK2. Currents are shown for depolarizations from −80 to voltages between −30 and 60 mV in steps of 10 mV; final voltage −50 mV. **(A–E)** Control: 6, 20, and 60 μM quinidine and washout, respectively (calibration: horizontal bar, 100 msec; verticle bar, 2 nA). [From Balser et al. (20)].

ade can also potentially produce a cross-over in response to depolarizing pulses for channels that exhibit inactivation. Consider such a model:

$$B$$
$$\updownarrow$$
$$C \rightarrow O \rightarrow I$$

where binding to the open state is essentially instantaneous and drug concentration is at approximately the K_D for the open state of the channel. Under such conditions the open state can only undergo transition to the inactive state when it is in the unblocked open state. This means that inactivation will proceed at only half its normal rate producing cross-over.

Cross-over is an unambiguous demonstration that drug interactions delay transition to stable nonconducting states. Although cross-over is an indicator of state-dependent binding, it does not necessarily define the mechanism of drug-channel interaction. Furthermore, not all state-dependent drug-channel interactions have kinetics that will produce, or more importantly, allow, experimental observation of cross-over. Demonstration of cross-over is a critical observation nonetheless, because current in the presence of drug "crosses over" the current observed under matched control conditions is actually greater at delayed times. The residual current remaining after drug application cannot be attributed to "unmasking" of a second component of membrane current or a drug-insensitive component. At least part of the current must be due to modification of gating transitions or drug-induced activation of another current.

Closed-State Blockade of Cardiac I$_{TO}$ by 4-AP

4-AP blockade of I_{TO} in ferret ventricle displays a marked dependence on frequency of stimulation (24). One frequently used bench mark of drug affinity is the apparent K_d. The apparent K_d is defined here as the concentration required to produce 1/2 maximal reduction in peak current. As can be seen in Fig. 3 (top) the apparent K_d for 4-AP can be markedly altered by the rate at which the current is activated. For a pulse rate of 1/(10 to 12 sec), the apparent K_d is 1.4 mM, but for a slower stimulation rate [1/(30 to 120 sec) at low concentrations] the apparent K_d is 0.2 mM. Thus, 4-AP clearly displays reverse-use dependence, with more frequent stimulation producing less effective block at any given concentration, consistent with closed-state blockade.

Closed-state blockade may also be manifested by decreased effectiveness of channel blocker with sustained, rather than frequent, depolarization. In direct contrast to the development of block by quinidine with sustained depolarization, 4-AP block of the transient outward current in ferret right ventricle is removed by sustained depolarization (25). This was demonstrated by application of a modified two-pulse protocol in which the duration of the first pulse was allowed to vary and the effect of blockade

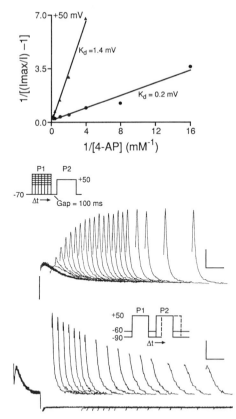

Figure 3. Time- and potential-dependent block of cardiac K$^+$ channels by 4-AP. **(Top)** Frequency dependence of 4-AP apparent affinity for block of peak I$_{TO}$ by 4-AP. The curves were constructed as the mean reduction in control peak I$_{TO}$ following a transition from the holding potential of -70 mV to the test potential of 50 mV as a function of applied 4-AP. Data have been fit with a single binding site equation with the derived apparent K$_D$ values indicated (mean values from N = 5 to 6 myocytes at each 4-AP). Upper trace: stimulation at a rate of 5 to 6/min yields an apparent K$_d$ of $\sim$1.4 mM. Lower trace: stimulation at a rate of 0.5 to 2/min yields an apparent K$_d$ of $\sim$0.2 mM. **(Middle)** Effects of 4-AP on ferret ventricular I$_{TO}$ at depolarized potentials. Voltage-clamp protocol illustrated in the schematic inset (calibration 200 msec, 200 pA). The gap of 100 msec allowed sufficient recovery of I$_{TO}$ to occur with only a minimal amount of 4-AP reassociation. Note that with increasing P1 duration, I$_{TO}$ during P2 progressively increased, indicating that 4-AP was dissociating during P1 with kinetics reflected in the P2 waveform. [From Campbell et al. (19).] **(Bottom)** Effects of 4-AP on ferret ventricular I$_{TO}$ current at hyperpolarized potentials. Representative results obtained using a conventional 500 msec double-pulse recovery protocol (see schematic inset) conducted at holding potential = -60 mV in 10 mM 4-AP (calibration 400 msec, 100 pA). Initially I$_{TO}$ during P2 was greater than that during P1, but with increasing interpulse interval duration the P2 I$_{TO}$ declined back to the control P1 level. Such biphasic recovery behavior is consistent with 4-AP dissociating during P1 and slowly reassociating with the closed states of the I$_{TO}$ channel during the hyperpolarized interpulse interval. [From Campbell et al. (25).]

was assessed by measuring peak current during the second pulse (Fig. 3, middle). In the presence of 10 mM 4-AP, peak I_{TO} during the second pulse progressively increased as the first pulse duration increased, until reaching a final saturating value after several hundred milliseconds.

The kinetics of closed-state binding of cardiac I_{TO} by 4-AP was quantified by a conventional double-pulse P1–P2 recovery protocol in the presence of 4-AP (see schematic inset in Fig. 3, bottom), where the interpulse interval was allowed to vary. As can be seen, the behavior of I_{TO} during P2 in the presence of 4-AP is highly unconventional compared with the recovery curve obtained from myocytes under control conditions (cf. Fig. 8 in ref. 19). At short interpulse intervals (~200 msec) I_{TO} during P2 is *larger* than I_{TO} during P1; however, as P1 and P2 are separated by a progressively increasing time, I_{TO} during P2 slowly declines back to the control P1 level. The data in Fig. 3 are consistent with the hypothesis that 4-AP dissociates from the I_{TO} channel at depolarized potentials (i.e., during the P1 to 50 mV) and then slowly reassociates with the closed I_{TO} channel at hyperpolarized potentials during the interpulse interval. This increased blockade with sustained hyperpolarization is qualitatively dissimilar to the slowed monophasic recovery from inactivation observed for quinidine in rabbit atrium I_{TO} (26) and is also in direct contrast to the effects of quinidine on delayed rectifier-type channels (20, 21).

At physiological pH >98% of the 4-AP exists in the cationic form (4-AP⁺), with the remainder existing as uncharged pyridine. To date, we have not experimentally addressed the issue of which possible form of 4-AP (4-AP⁺ or the uncharged pyridine) produces block of I_{TO} in ferret ventricular myocytes. (For a detailed discussion of these issues in other cell types, see ref. 27.) Furthermore, all of our measurements were conducted using extracellularly applied 4-AP. Nonetheless, our data indicate that 4-AP does not produce any measurable open-channel block, but appears to be interacting exclusively with the closed states of I_{TO} channels. Because the majority of 4-AP exists in cationic form, 4-AP might be expected to display an intrinsic voltage dependence of binding. However, the voltage-dependence of 4-AP block that we have measured indicates that (i) the apparent affinity of the I_{TO} channel for 4-AP decreases with depolarization and (ii) association of 4-AP with its binding sites becomes progressively slower with increasing hyperpolarization (19, 25). These potential-dependent effects are opposite to what would be predicted for a simple membrane field effect on 4-AP⁺ binding to sites on the channel (i.e., either simple electrophoresis or a "Woodhull-type" model is inappropriate; refs. 16, 27–29). In this regard, it is important that a model of 4-AP blockade be able to reproduce quantitatively the major characteristics of 4-AP block without incorporating any voltage-dependent binding terms (i.e., the K_d values for binding to the three closed states are potential-independent).

The following model (19, 25) based on multiple closed states can account for effects we have reported:

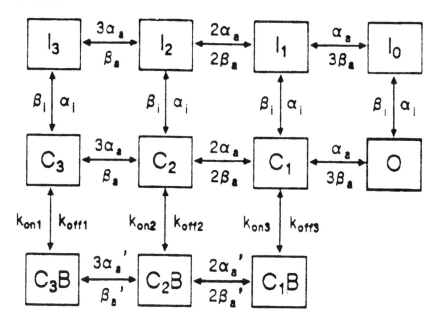

This model has the following properties (see refs. 19 and 25 for numerical details): (i) 4-AP slowly binds to the three closed states (C_{0-2}) of the I_{TO} channel at hyperpolarized potentials with progressively lower affinities and progressively increasing turnover rates; (ii) 4-AP does not bind to either the open (O) or the inactivated states (I_{0-2}); (iii) 4-AP must dissociate from the bound closed states (B_{0-2}) before the channel can enter the open-activated state (O); (iv) 4-AP dissociation from the three bound closed states (B_{0-2}) becomes the overall rate-limiting step in the gating process at depolarized potentials; and (v) 4-AP alters the gating transitions between states [$\alpha'(V)$ and $\beta'(V)$] in a proportional fashion consistent with the constraints of thermodynamic reversibility (c.f. refs. 19, 25, 30–32).

Within this framework, the characteristics of 4-AP block can be success-fully reproduced. Once 4-AP dissociation has occurred from any closed state, the transition to the next state proceeds at its normal rate; however, the kinetics 4-AP dissociation (i.e., K_{on1-3} and K_{off1-3}) are slow compared with normal I_{TO} gating kinetics [i.e., $\alpha(V)$ and $\beta(V)$ values]. Consider the case of the cross-over phenomenon presented in Fig. 1 (top). Upon depolariza-tion, 4-AP dissociation essentially acts as a "bottleneck" in the supply of available closed-channel states that can subsequently enter either the acti-vated state or one of the various inactivated states. This is the basis of the "cross-over" phenomenon. The kinetics of 4-AP dissociation are more rapid at depolarized potentials. As a result, during a fixed-gap, double-pulse P1–P2 protocol, as P1 is made progressively more depolarized, more unbound closed-state channels become available during the interpulse interval at the holding potential. As a depolarizing P1 pulse is progressively increased in duration, 4-AP progressively dissociates, allowing more unbound channels to enter the inactivated state. This progressively growing population of unbound inactivated channels recovers from inactivation with normal kinetics upon hyperpolarization back to the holding potential. As a result, more unbound closed-state channels are activated during the following P2 pulse. This is the basis for the dissociation behavior observed at depolarized potentials.

Upon hyperpolarization following a depolarizing P1 pulse, unblocked inactivated channels rapidly recover at their normal rates (25), whereas 4-AP reassociates with closed channels at a much slower rate. As a result, for brief interpulse intervals (up to ~150 to 200 msec), there are more unblocked channels available for activation during the second P2 pulse than during the control P1 pulse. This is the basis of the biphasic recovery-association phenomenon. In combination, these effects are predicted to produce the "reverse-use dependent" characteristics of I_{TO} block by 4-AP. Thus, the model reproduces the voltage dependence of association and dissociation due to the voltage-dependent kinetics of transitions between the various channel states. In other words, the model emphasizes the importance of *conformational state* of the I_{TO} channel in affecting the characteristics of 4-AP block.

In summary, several criteria and lines of evidence to support and quantitate closed state block of I_{TO} by 4-AP in ferret ventricle have been considered. These include (i) the appearance of the "cross-over phenomena" in which the peak current is delayed in the presence of 4-AP at depolarized potentials; (ii) relief of block at depolarized potentials; and (iii) reassociation of 4-AP at hyperpolarized potentials. At hyperpolarized potentials, 4-AP associates slowly (τ_{assoc} ~800 msec to 1,300 msec in 10 mM 4-AP) with closed states of the channel (apparent $K_d \approx 0.2$ mM); however, at depolarized potentials 4-AP dissociates more rapidly ($\tau_{dissocs}$ ~350 msec to 150 msec). Consequently, the properties of 4-AP binding to the I_{TO} channel undergo a transition in the range of potentials over which channel activation occurs (-30 to 20 mV). Although not presented, several pieces of negative evidence gave indirect support to Campbell et al.'s (25) conclusion that block occurs primarily through a closed-state mechanism. Briefly, measurements of kinetics of recovery and deactivation in the presence of 0.5 to 1.0 mM 4-AP are unaltered compared with control measurements in the absence of drug, indicating that drug binding to open and inactivated states is not an important determinant of channel behavior.

Comparison of 4-AP Block of K⁺ Channels From Other Tissues

The majority of results from studies of 4-AP interaction with cardiac transient outward K⁺ currents indicate that a closed-state blocking mechanism can account for the observed time- and voltage dependence of current inhibition. Simurda et al. (33) first reported relief of 4-AP blockade of the transient outward current in dog ventricular myocytes. Similar results have been subsequently reported by Castle (34) for rat ventricular transient outward K^+ current. The closed-state blocking mechanism of 4-AP on cardiac K^+ channels seems to extend to the delayed rectifier K^+ channel (HK2) cloned and expressed in a mammalian L-cell line (35). Blockade of the HK2 channels is somewhat different from that observed in ferret ventricular cells in that binding does not seem to be maximal at resting or hyperpolarized potentials, but appears to be maximal to a closed state that is at or near the threshold for activation (35). The closed-state block of voltage-activated cardiac K^+ channels seems to be a frequently observed phenomenon.

The action of 4-AP seems also to be strongly dependent on cell type. Although in many cell types closed-state blockade by 4-AP does appear to be described by similar models [e.g., for squid axon delayed rectifier (30), or "$I_K(f)$" in rat melanotrophs (32)]. K^+ channels from many other cell types show evidence of more complicated mechanisms of blockade incorporating various combinations of open, closed, and inactivated channel blockade [e.g., "I_A" in molluscan neurons (31); inactivating I_K in mouse lymphocytes (36) or *Drosophila* (37), suggesting that the presence of the phenomenon depends on the cell type studied and the specific type of K^+ channels present (38)]. This presumably reflects changes in the location of the binding site produced by differences in the channel protein sequence.

Open Channel Block of Cardiac K^+ Currents by Quinidine

Quinidine, the *d*-isomer of quinine, has been long used as an antiarrhythmic agent (for historical review, see ref. 39). Virtually all of the studies involving quinidine block of K^+ channels show some results that are suggestive of state-dependent block. This is consistent with the studies on the actions of quinidine on Na^+ channels. Quinidine is thought to act largely as an open Na^+ channel blocker in its ionic form. Although quinidine may also block closed and inactivated channels, its affinity for those states is so comparatively low that its use-dependent properties result primarily from interactions with the open state (40). Thus, although there is consensus on the general mode of action by quinidine on Na^+ current, there is still debate concerning what state description best describes drug action, and hence which model best represents the conformational aspects of drug association (41–45).

There is less information concerning the mechanism of quinidine block on cardiac K^+ channels. The blocking action of quinidine on human cardiac K^+ currents is probably best characterized for cloned HK2 expressed in a mouse L-cell line (21). The effect of quinidine on HK2, which is a voltage-activated potassium channel with characteristics akin to those of I_{KS}, has been modeled by open-channel block (21). As illustrated in Fig. 1

(bottom), the ionic tail currents associated with this channel show cross-over in response to a repolarizing step. Presumably this delay in deactivation of the current represents open channels unblocking and returning to their resting closed state. In addition, application of quinidine produces inactivation-like behavior (Fig. 2): currents that display only a weak and very slow inactivation show a peak and rapid decrease to a new steady-state level in the presence of quinidine (21). There seemed to be two components to the voltage dependence of quinidine's action on HK2 channels: (i) a steep component that parallels channel activation (or opening); and (ii) a weaker component that appears due to inherent effects of transmembrane potential on quinidine binding kinetics. Snyders et. al. (21) showed that all of these qualitative effects could be reproduced by a simple voltage dependent open-channel blocking mechanism:

$$C \rightarrow C \rightarrow C \rightarrow C \rightarrow O \leftrightarrow B$$

This model differs from the simple model of open-channel block described earlier in only two respects: (i) there are multiple closed states that are necessary to produce the sigmoidal delay in activation of the delayed rectifier; and (ii) the binding of quinidine has an intrinsic voltage dependence. Although binding site location and affinity are largely determined by chemical bonds and steric considerations, this intrinsic voltage dependence has an important physical interpretation. When the channel enters the open conformational state, presumably the binding site for the blocker is revealed. If this site is within the permeation pathway and the blocking compound is charged, then the blocking compound may experience at least part of the membrane potential. For a charged compound that is too large to pass entirely through the channel, we can consider the situation where the compound enters the open channel from one side, moves partially through the channel, and then meets a restriction in the permeation pathway that is too large to allow the compound to pass, thus resulting in channel block. To remove block, the compound must diffuse in the reverse direction and exit the channel from the same side by which it entered. An applied membrane potential can either enhance entry and diminish exit or diminish entry and enhance exit, depending on the charge of the compound, side of the membrane from which entry occurs and polarity of the membrane potential (28). The magnitude of the effect is determined by the charge of the compound, the strength of the applied potential, and the distance (δ) through the transmembrane electrical field at which the restriction site appears. Because the charge or valence (z) of a compound is generally known, the membrane potential (V) is controlled experimentally, and sidedness of application of many compounds is usually known, the voltage dependence of equilibria between and open state and blocked state (expressed as a K_D) can be measured to give an expression of the fractional electrical distance, δ, as follows:

$$\delta = (RT/zFV)\{-\ln (K_D(V)/K_{D,0mv})\}$$

where F, R, and T have their usual meanings, $K_D(V)$ is the observed K_D at a particular voltage (V), and $K_{D,0mv}$ reflects the concentration dependence of equilibrium binding to the open or blocked state for a particular blocking compound at 0 mV, assuming a single binding site model. Rearranged, this equation can be used to calculate the equilibrium binding for a given concentration of open-channel blocker, [B], to an open channel by:

Fraction of open channels blocked $= [B]/([B] + K_{D,0mv}\exp(-\delta FV/RT))$

The equations shown herein are based on equilibrium assumptions, and several reviews deal with the subject of fractional electrical distance and kinetic models (16). Although the electrical distance is frequently thought of as being equivalent to the physical distance through the pore, these two quantities are not necessarily the same. Reconciliation of the physical distance with the electrical distance requires more detailed knowledge of other aspects of pore structure.

The majority of cardiac class I and III antiarrhythmic compounds, including quinidine, exist in both a charged and uncharged form that can partition within, and diffuse across, the lipid bilayer into the intracellular space. With a pK_a of 8.9, quinidine is predominately in the positively charged form at physiological pH. If quinidine acts from an intracellular binding site, it should show increasing block of open channels with membrane depolarization. Snyders et al. (21) have demonstrated such a voltage dependence of open-channel blockade by quinidine with HK2 channels and have assigned the binding site to the intracellular side of the membrane. From the same measurements, they also estimated that the fractional electrical distance was 0.19 [i.e., quinidine moves through ~20% of the transmembrane electrical field to reach its receptor (or restriction site) when blocking the HK2 channel]. This voltage dependence is very similar to that measured for tetraethylammonium (TEA), a compound that is thought to bind to the pore at a site that is also near the intracellular mouth of the pore (64). This similarity has led to a proposal for a putative binding site associated with specific residues in the pore region that are responsible for quinidine binding.

Other cardiac-delayed rectifier K^+ channels also show time-dependent characteristics that are consistent with open-channel blockade. Furukawa et al. (46) showed that quinidine blockade of guinea pig–delayed rectifier develops with time in response to a depolarizing pulse, and slows the decay of the delayed rectifier tail currents. Balser et al. (20) also reported time-dependent effects consistent with open-channel block for the guinea pig–delayed rectifier, including time-dependent relief of block at hyperpolarized potentials (Fig. 4A). The effects of quinidine on other cardiac K^+ channels is less well understood. Quinidine has been demonstrated to block both the steady-state inwardly rectifying K^+ current (I_{K1}) (13) and the transient outward current (26). The quinidine-induced changes in the time course of activation and inactivation of the transient outward current in

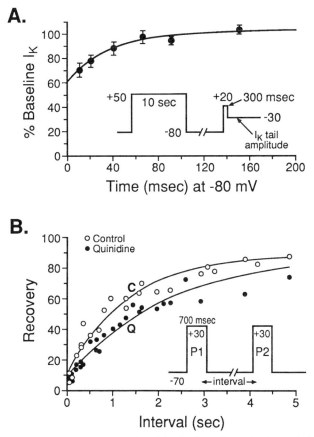

Figure 4. Time- and potential-dependent block of cardiac K⁺ channels by quinidine. **(A)** Time-dependent relief of quinidine block of guinea pig–delayed rectifier tail currents by holding at hyperpolarized (−80 mV) potentials. Using a paired-pulse protocol (inset), the effect of quinidine was assessed as a function of the amount of time spent at −80 mV. Magnitudes of I_K tail amplitudes were shown before (open circles) and after (closed circles) the application of 10 μM quinidine to the bath. Differences between predrug and postdrug measurements are apparent only at early time points and show exponential decay of relief of block. The average time constant for relief of quinidine block by holding at −80 mV was reported to be 38.5 msec. [From Balser et al. (20).] **(B)** Slowed recovery from inactivation produced by quinidine in the transient outward current of rabbit atrial cells. Effect of μM quinidine on the recovery from inactivation kinetics in rabbit atrium. Inset shows the protocol. Identical pulses (P1 and P2) to 30 mV from a holding potential of −70 mV were applied every 15 sec, and in the interval between them the change in time (t) was varied from 0 sec to 5 sec (open circles, control data). Note that after application of 10 μM quinidine (closed circles), the time course of recovery was slowed substantially. Recovery data have been fitted with single exponential functions; the time constant for the control data was 1.3 sec, whereas that for quinidine was 2.3 sec. [From Imaizumi and Giles (26).]

rabbit atrium and ventricle suggest an open-channel blocking mechanism. For example, quinidine slows the recovery from inactivation of this current (Fig. 4B). This slowing of recovery may be due to open-channel blockade, but the possibility that quinidine associates with one or more of the multiple-inactivated states can not be ruled out.

In summary, the effect of quinidine on voltage-activated cardiac K^+ channels is consistent with conventional use dependence. In general the major action of quinidine on cardiac K^+ channels is through an open-channel mechanism. The major criteria used to establish open-channel blockade of delayed rectifier K^+ channels in cardiac cells are (i) time-dependent development of blockade of tail currents during the preceding depolarized pulse; (ii) delay in channel deactivation resulting in cross-over; (iii) measurement of an effective electrical distance; and (iv) appearance of inactivation-like behavior following application of drug. As previously mentioned, the appearance of these phenomena are sensitive to the exact kinetics of blocking compound applied. Consequently, not all of these criteria may be observed for a particular open-channel blocker.

Physical Relationship Between Channel Conformation and State Dependent Block

With the identification, sequencing, and expression of a family of K^+ channels from *Drosophila,* our understanding of the physical nature of K^+ channels has increased dramatically in recent years (14, 47). Because of the very recent nature of much of this new information, relatively little has been published as yet on the relationship between this molecular structural information and drug binding. Therefore, our final section discusses several of the physical considerations that are likely to be important as we bridge the gap between molecular structure and electropharmacology of cardiac K^+ channels in the future.

Magnitude of the Physical Conformational Change

For open-channel blocking compounds at least one gross physical characteristic of the channel is paramount: pore diameter. The physical dimensions of channel pores may be determined directly via x-ray crystallography. However, a high-resolution crystallographic map of voltage-gated K^+ channels has yet to be obtained. Fortunately, we are not without some information concerning the size of the channel pore and how this size may change between transitions between open and closed conformations.

The opening and closing of voltage-dependent ion channels obviously involves significant alterations of channel conformation. Changes in channel conformation are responsive to applied forces initiated experimentally. Manipulation of membrane potential is the most common physical force applied to channel proteins, and it renders data concerning the movement of charge that accompanies the physical conformational changes. Zimmerberg and Parsegian (48) have devised a method in which mechanical force (osmotic pressure) may be applied to the channel and gives us information concerning changes in the physical dimensions of the channel protein.

Zimmerberg and Parsegian (48) used large molecular weight polymers expected to be physically excluded from the pore region to create an osmotic pressure gradient between the open channel and the bulk medium. Using this approach they determined that the polymer inaccessible volume changes associated with opening and closing of voltage-dependent anion channels from rat liver and *Neurospora* were large and corresponded to a change of 2 to 4×10^4 Å^3. Later studies using the osmotic pressure technique on internally perfused squid axon revealed that for the delayed rectifier K$^+$ current, changes in polymer-inaccessible volume associated with channel opening and closing were much smaller, being on the order of 1 to 2×10^3 Å^3 (49). Such changes are somewhat larger than those observed for the Na$^+$ channel of crayfish axons ~800 Å^3 (50), which is thought to have a pore lining region similar in many gross characteristics to the voltage-gated potassium channels. Should the changes in polymer-inaccessible volume changes that have been measured to date extend generally to other voltage-gated potassium channels, they will provide an important constraint when considering physical models of channel conformational change.

Additional information concerning the dimensions of the pore region of the K$^+$ channel can be inferred from the diameter of permeant and impermeant ions and organic compounds. This "cation sieving" indicates that K$^+$ selective channels have a minimum cross-sectional area that appears to be in the range of 9 Å^2 (51). It should be noted that the radius determined by this method is a measure of the minimum radius occluding the permeation pathway. As previously mentioned, methods have been developed using biophysical approaches to determine the location, in terms of fractional electrical distance, of such a restriction within the pore. This fractional electrical distance combined with site-directed mutagenesis and different-sized blocking compounds can be a powerful approach for probing pore structure.

Changes in Charge Distribution

In addition to measurement of some of the mechanical features of the ionic channel, there are changes in the electrostatic conformation of the channel that accompany gating. It is well accepted that voltage-gated channels assume different stable conformations in response to shifts in transmembrane potential. This alteration in stability is equivalent to a change in the relative free energy between the conformations. This free energy change is mediated by the net movement of charge through all or a portion of the membrane. This charge movement may be accomplished through movement of static charge or by a reorientation of dipole moments. Regardless of the mechanism, the minimum effective charge movement can be calculated from the change in the equilibrium between the open and closed states (52). This quantity is called the elementary charge, q, and is related to the voltage dependence of gating from the Boltzmann equation:

$$P_{open}(V)/P_{closed}(V) = K_{0mV} * \exp(-qFV/RT)$$

where F, R, and T have their usual meanings, and K_{0mV} is the equilibrium value when the membrane potential, V, equals 0 mV. Although the form of this equation implies that q traverses the entire membrane field, this may not be the case; a larger amount of charge may traverse a smaller fraction of the transmembrane field to generate an equivalent charge movement. q is a minimum measurement of charge movement per channel, because there may be additional charge movement associated with other portions of the molecule that do not contribute to stabilization of the open state. For some cloned K^+ channels, the charge movement associated with various conformational translations in the activation process can be measured directly (53). "Gating currents" (as these measurements are termed), are our only direct measure of transitions between various nonconducting states.

Changes in charge distribution that accompany state transitions are important, not only as an indicator that may aid in identifying interactions between drugs and various closed states, but also because the charge redistribution that accompanies channel gating may contribute directly to the energetics of drug-channel interaction. Electrostatic effects are thought to play a major role in drug affinity for the channel. As illustrated in Fig. 5 (bottom) the movement of charge from one side of the membrane to the other will result in changes in the electrostatic distribution of charge on the channel. Where binding sites for charged blocking compounds are located on one side of the membrane or the other, electrostatic repulsion or attraction can result from gating charge movement. Such effects may not be limited to changes in a binding site that is within the channel protein itself. Changes in dipole moment can alter electrostatic field effects or image potentials (54) that are external to the channel and can result in concentrations near the mouth of the pore that differ from those in bulk solution.

Structural Elements Deduced from Sequence Information

The amino acid sequence and putative tertiary structure of the functional K^+ channel complex is discussed in detail in other chapters. Herein, we briefly summarize some aspects of the physical picture of K^+ channels likely to be of importance in understanding state-dependent channel block-

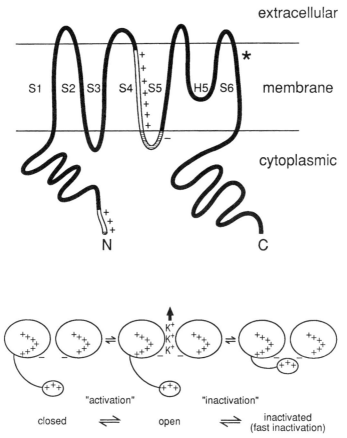

Figure 5. Schematic representation of a K^+ channel. **(Top)** Planar representation model of membrane topology showing a hydrophobic core region and both the amino- and the carboxyl-terminal regions (not to scale) on the cytoplasmic side. The S4 sequence carries basic residues at every third position and is postulated to be the voltage sensor of the channel. The amino-terminal region contains a few basic residues that are involved in fast inactivation, which may mediate electrostatic interactions between the amino terminus ("inactivation ball") and its receptor. The sequence between the S4 and the S5 (the S4–S5 loop) carries an acidic residue (glutamate) and probably functions as part of the receptor for the fast inactivation gate. The S4–S5 loop may form the permeation pathway. [From Jan and Jan (14).] **(Bottom)** Schematic model of K^+ channel function. Channel activation is voltage-dependent and involves movements of charges intrinsic to the channel molecule, tentatively postulated to be the positive charges on the S4 sequence. N-type inactivation generally follows activation and involves a cytoplasmic gate on the amino terminus of the channel subunit. This gate, or ball, carries a net positive charge and interacts with a receptor that is likely to reside in the S4–S5 loop. The channel can also enter a "slow-inactivated state" (C-type), either from the open state or from the fast inactivated state; the mechanism underlying slow inactivation is not yet known. [From Jan and Jan (14).]

ade. Sarcolemmal K^+ channels are thought to be composed of four homologous subunits. One typical subunit is illustrated in Fig. 5 (top). It consists of six putative membrane spanning regions of which S4 is thought to comprise the voltage sensor that activates the channel. The pore lining region is thought to be formed by a small segment of residues that lie between the S5 and S6 membrane spanning regions. So-called "N-type" inactivation (also referred to as "fast inactivation") has been demonstrated to be produced by a small "tethered ball sequence" of ~21 amino acid residues on the amino terminus of the protein (55). Another form of inactivation (referred to as "C-type" and as "slow inactivation") is produced by an as yet unknown mechanism, involving residues located in the S6 subunit and possibly other portions of the protein, including the carboxyl terminus (see discussion in ref. 14).

The pore region of the channel protein is of particular relevance for open-channel blockers. The pore region of voltage-gated K^+ channels is hypothesized to be formed by an eight-stranded antiparallel β-barrel (56, 57) formed by the "loop" between the S5 and S6 regions described and is structurally similar to models of the Na^+ channel (58). A minimum energy description of this putative structure has been reported by Boguz and Busath (56). When filled with water molecules, this pore gives an estimate volume of ~38 water molecules, a value in very close agreement to the value of 40 to 50 molecules calculated for the volume change experimentally measured by Zimmerberg et al. (49). Thus, all available data indicate that the pore region of the voltage-activated K^+ channels is very narrow.

The pore region has been identified and sequenced (along with the rest of the channel protein) for two types of human cardiac K^+ channels (HK1 and HK2; ref. 59). It is highly homologous between the two channel types and with K^+ channels from other species and organs (Fig. 6, bottom). Shown in Fig. 6 (top) is a schematic of the pore lining region of HK2 and a tentatively identified binding site for quinidine. The assignment of a quinidine binding site to this residue was determined from the similarity in effective electrical distance to TEA in other K^+ channel types (e.g., *Drosophila Shaker-B* channels; ref. 60). Hydrophobic residues near the mouth of the pore may be involved in binding the hydrophobic domains of quinidine by a mechanism similar to that for binding of quaternary ammonium compounds with lipophilic side chains. This structural information reveals several insights into the general action of open-channel blocking compounds that act from an intracellular site: (i) the pore region itself is so homologous that it is unlikely that blocking compounds will show much specificity based solely on interactions with the pore region; (ii) physical dimensions of the pore place steric constraints on drug-pore interactions; (iii) channel specificity may be conferred by hydrophobic interactions near the mouth of the pore; and (iv) drug binding near the mouth of the pore suggests that drug binding may interact significantly with N-type inactiva-

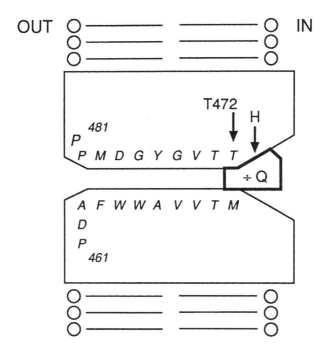

Homology in Pore Region Between Different K⁺ Channel Clones

```
        S5                    |                      |           S6
Sh      YFAEAGSENSFFKSIPDAFWWAVVTMTTVGYGDMTPVGFWGKIVGSLC
RCK1    -----EEAE-H-S------------S---------Y--TIG--------
RCK4    ----DEPTTH-Q--------------------K-IT-G--------
HK1     -----DEPTTH-Q--------------------K-IT-G--------
HK2     -----DNQGTH-S--------------------R-ITVG---------
DRK1    F---KDEDDTK-----AS----TI---------TY-KTLL-----G--
```

Figure 6. Pore lining region and putative binding site for quinidine. **(Top)** Possible binding site for quinidine in the HK2 pore. The sequence of amino acids from the H5 region of one subunit (see Fig. 5, top) is shown. The internal threonine residue (T472) that has been shown to be involved in TEA block in *Shaker* K⁺ channels is shown at ~20% into the membrane. The charged residue (+) on quinidine (Q) is shown binding to this site and occluding the intracellular mouth of the channel pore. Additional hydrophobic interactions may occur with other portions of the quinidine molecule and are denoted by H. [From Synders et al. (21).] **(Bottom)** Similarities of the pore lining region of the HK1, HK2, and various other K⁺ channels. Sequence of the putative pore lining region (proline to proline) of HK1 and HK2 (21, 59, 62–69).

409

tion, which also binds near the same putative site (61), and may also interact with C-type inactivation.

In conclusion, although some insight has been gained into the possible molecular mechanisms underlying quinidine binding to cardiac K^+ channels, to date we do not know of any site-directed mutagenesis experiments involving 4-AP in cardiac K^+ channels. Given the multiplicity of effects on various K^+ channels types, it will be of interest to examine the differences in sequence that give rise to the very different actions of 4-AP. 4-AP and similar compounds have the presently unrecognized potential of becoming extremely powerful tools for gaining insight into the underlying molecular mechanisms governing cardiac K^+ channel gating (47). In channel types in which 4-AP acts by binding preferentially to closed states, the use of 4-AP or similar compounds could potentially allow for testing of specific kinetic models of cardiac K^+ channel gating, give insights into possible mechanisms underlying cardiac K^+ channel neuromodulation, and serve as a probe of the underlying molecular mechanisms governing transitions among the various closed states.

Acknowledgments

This work was supported in part by grants from the American Heart Association, North Carolina Affiliate (NC 91-G-11) to D.L.C., and the National Heart, Lung, and Blood Institute (19216, 41732, and 17670) to H.C.S.

Note added in proof. Since the writing of this chapter mutagenesis experiments have been reported that have localized the site of 4-AP binding to the cytoplasmic domains of S5 and S6 (70). Mutations in other regions which alter 4-AP binding may do so indirectly through alteration of activation properties (70, 71, 72).

References

1. Wit, A.L., and Rosen, M.R. (1992). Afterdepolarizations and triggered activity: Distinction from automaticity as an arrhythmogenic mechanism, in *The Heart and Cardiovascular System* (Raven Press, New York), pp. 2113–2163.

2. Binah, O. (1990). The transient outward current in mammalian heart, in *Cardiac Electrophysiology: A Textbook,* M.R. Rosen, M.J. Janse, and A.L. Wit, Eds. (Futura Publishing Company, Mt. Kisco, NY), pp. 93–106.

3. Cohen, I.S., Datyner, N.B., Gintant, G.A., and Kline, R.P. (1986). Time-dependent outward currents in the heart, in *The Heart and Cardiovascular System. Scientific Foundations,* H.A. Fozzard, E. Haber, R.B. Jennings, A.M. Katz, and H.E. Morgan, Eds. (Raven Press, New York), pp. 637–669.

4. Courtney, K.R. (1975). Mechanism of frequency-dependent inhibition of sodium currents in frog myelinated nerve by the lidocaine derivative GEA 968. *J. Pharmacol. Exp. Ther.* **195:**225–236.

5. Colatsky, T.J., Follmer, C.H., and Starmer, C.F. (1990). Channel specificity in antiarrhythmic drug action: Mechanism of potassium channel block and its role in suppressing and aggravating cardiac arrhythmias. *Circulation* **82:**2235–2242.

6. Hondeghem, L.M., and Snyders, D.J. (1990). Class III antiarrhythmic agents have a lot of potential but a long way to go. Reduced effectiveness and dangers of reverse use dependence. *Circulation* **81**:686–690.

7. Packer, D.L., Grant, A.O., Strauss, H.C., and Starmer, C.F. (1989). Characterization of concentration- and use-dependent effects of quinidine from conduction delay and declining conduction velocity in canine Purkinje fibers. *J. Clin. Invest.* **83**:2109–2119.

8. Jurkiewicz, N.K., and Sanguinetti, M.C. (1993). Rate-dependent prolongation of cardiac action potentials by a methanesulfonanilidine class III antiarrhythmic agent: Specific block of I_{Kr} by dofetilide. *Circ. Res.*, in press.

9. DiFrancesco, D., and Noble, D. (1985). Model of cardiac electrical activity incorporating ionic pumps and concentration changes. *Phil. Trans. Roy. Soc. Lond.* **307**:353–398.

10. Rasmusson, R.L., Clark, J.W., Giles, W.R., Robinson, K., Clark, R.B., Shibata, E.F., and Campbell, D.L. (1990). A mathematical model of electrical activity in the bullfrog atrial cell. *Am. J. Physiol.* **259**:H370–H389.

11. Luo, C.H., and Rudy, Y. (1991). A model of the ventricular cardiac action potential. Depolarization, repolarization, and their interaction. *Circ. Res.* **68**:1502–1526.

12. Colatsky, T.J. (Ed.) (1990). *Potassium Channels: Basic Function and Therapeutic Aspects* (Wiley-Liss, New York).

13. Hiroaka, M., Sawada, K., and Kawano, S. (1986). Effects of quinidine on plateau currents of guinea-pig ventricular myocytes. *J. Mol. Cell. Cardiol.* **18**:1097–1106.

14. Jan, L.Y., and Jan, Y.N. (1992). Structural elements involved in specific K⁺ channel functions. *Ann. Rev. Physiol.* **54**:537–555.

15. Eyring, H. (1935). The activated complex in chemical reactions. *J. Chem. Phys.* **3**:107–115.

16. Hille, B. (1992). *Ionic Channels of Excitable Membranes* (Sinauer Associates, Inc., Sunderland, MA).

17. Snyders, D.J., Bennett, P.B., and Hondeghem, L.M. (1992). Mechanisms of drug-channel interaction, in *The Heart and Cardiovascular System* (Raven Press, New York), pp. 2164–2193.

18. Moczydlowski, E. (1986). Single-channel enzymology, in *Ion Channel Reconstitution* (Plenum, New York), pp. 75–113.

19. Campbell, D.L., Rasmusson, R.L., Qu, Y., and Strauss, H.C. (1993). The calcium-independent transient outward potassium current in isolated ferret right ventricular myocytes. I. Basic characterization and kinetic analysis. *J. Gen. Physiol.*, in press.

20. Balser, J.R., Bennett, P.B., Hondeghem, L.M., and Roden, D.M. (1991). Suppression of time-dependent outward current in guinea pig ventricular myocytes: Actions of quinidine and amiodarone. *Circ. Res.* **69**:519–529.

21. Snyders, D.J., Knoth, K.M., Roberds, S.L., and Tamkun, M.M. (1992). Time-, voltage-, and state-dependent block by quinidine of a cloned human cardiac potassium channel. *Mol. Pharmacol.* **41**:322–330.

22. Armstrong, C.M. (1969). Inactivation of the potassium conductance and related phenomena caused by quaternary ammonium ion injected in squid axons. *J. Gen. Physiol.* **54**:553–575.

23. Armstrong, C.M. (1971). Interaction of tetraethylammonium ion derivatives with the potassium channels of giant axons. *J. Gen. Physiol.* **58**:413–437.

24. Campbell, D.L., Qu, Y., Rasmusson, R.L., and Strauss, H.C. (1991). Interaction of 4-AP with I_{TO} in ferret ventricular myocytes. *Biophys. J.* **59**:A280.

25. Campbell, D.L., Rasmusson, R.L., Qu, Y., and Strauss, H.C. (1993). The calcium-independent transient outward potassium current in isolated ferret right ventricular myocytes. II. Closed state "reverse use-dependent" block by 4-aminopyridine. *J. Gen. Physiol.*, in press.

26. Imaizumi, Y., and Giles, W.R. (1987). Quinidine-induced inhibition of transient outward current in cardiac muscle. *Am. J. Physiol.* **253**:H704–H708.

27. Howe, J.R., and Ritchie, J.M. (1991). On the active form of 4-aminopyridine: Block of K^+ currents in rabbit Schwann cells. *J. Physiol. (Lond.)* **433**:183–205.

28. Woodhull, A.M. (1973). Ionic blockage of sodium channels in nerve. *J. Gen. Physiol.* **61**:687–708.

29. Strichartz, G.R. (1973). The inhibition of sodium currents in myelinated nerve by quaternary derivatives of lidocaine. *J. Gen. Physiol.* **62**:37–57.

30. Yeh, J.Z., Oxford, G.S., Wu, C.H., and Narahashi, T. (1976). Dynamics of aminopyridine block of potassium channels in squid axon membrane. *J. Gen. Physiol.* **68**:519–535.

31. Thompson, S. (1982). Aminopyridine block of transient potassium current. *J. Gen. Physiol.* **80**:1–18.

32. Kehl, S.J. (1990). 4-Aminopyridine causes a voltage-dependent block of the transient outward K^+ current in rat melanotrophs. *J. Physiol. (Lond.)* **431**:515–528.

33. Simurda, J., Simurdova, M., and Christe, G. (1989). Use-dependent effects of 4-aminopyridine on transient outward current in dog ventricular muscle. *Pflügers Arch.* **415**:244–246.

34. Castle, N.A. (1992). Characterization of 4-aminopyridine block of I_{TO} in rat ventricular myocytes. *Biophys. J.* **61**:A307.

35. Snyders, D.J., Po, S.S., Tamkun, M.M., and Bennett, P.B. (1992). High affinity, state-dependent block of a cloned human cardiac K^+ channel by 4-aminopyridine. *Circulation*, in press.

36. Choquet, D., and Korn, H. (1992). Mechanism of 4-aminopyridine action on voltage-gated potassium channels in lymphocytes. *J. Gen. Physiol.* **99**:217–240.

37. Hice, R.E., Swanson, R., Folander, K., and Nelson, D. (1992). Aminopyridines alter inactivation rates of transient potassium channels. *Biophys. J.* **61**:A376.

38. Rudy, B. (1988). Diversity and ubiquity of K^+ channels. *Neuroscience* **25**:729–749.

39. Roden, D.M. (1991). Quinidine, in *Electrophysiology and Pharmacology of the Heart: A Clinical Guide* (Marcel Dekker, New York), pp. 493–516.

40. Snyders, D.J., and Hondeghem, L.M. (1990). Effects of quinidine on the sodium current of ventricular guinea-pig myocytes: Evidence for a drug associated rested state with altered Kinetics. *Circulation Research* **66**: 565–579.

41. Starmer, C.F., Grant, A.O., and Strauss, H.C. (1984). Mechanisms of use-dependent block of sodium channels in excitable membranes by local anesthetics. *Biophys. J.* **46:**15–27.

42. Starmer, C.F., Packer, D.L., and Grant, A.O. (1987). Ligand binding to transiently accessible sites: Mechanism for varying apparent binding rates. *J. Theor. Biol.* **124:**335–341.

43. Starmer, C.F. (1987). Theoretical characterization of ion channel blockade. *Biophys. J.* **52:**405–412.

44. Hondeghem, L.M., and Katzung, B.G. (1984). Antiarrhythmic agents: The modulated receptor mechanism of action of sodium and calcium channel blockers. *Ann. Rev. Pharmacol. Toxicol.* **24:**387–423.

45. Snyders, D.J., and Hondeghem, L.M. (1987). Use-dependent unblocking of quinidine-blocked sodium channels: Slowed activation and inactivation. *Circulation* **76:**150a.

46. Furukawa, T., Tsujimura, Y., Kitamura, K., Tanaka, H., and Habuchi, Y. (1989). Time- and voltage-dependent block of the delayed K⁺ by quinidine in rabbit sinoatrial and ventricular nodes. *J. Pharmacol. Exp. Ther.* **251:**756–763.

47. Miller, C. (1991). 1990: Annus mirabilis of potassium channels. *Science* **252:**1092–1096.

48. Zimmerberg, J., and Parsegian, V.A. (1986). Polymer inaccessible volume changes during opening and closing of a voltage-dependent ionic channel. *Nature (Lond.)* **323:**36.

49. Zimmerberg, J., Bezanilla, F., and Parsegian, V.A. (1990). Solute inaccessible volume changes during opening of the potassium channel of the squid giant axon. *Biophys. J.* **57:**1049.

50. Rayner, M.D., Starkus, J.G., Ruben, P.C., and Alicata, D.A. (1992). Voltage-sensitive and solvent-sensitive processes in ion channel gating: Kinetic effects of hyperosmolar media on inactivation and deactivation of sodium channels. *Biophys. J.* **61:**96–108.

51. Bezanilla, F., and Armstrong, C.M. (1972). Negative conductance caused by entry of sodium and cesium ions into potassium channels of squid axons. *J. Gen. Physiol.* **60:**588–608.

52. Hodgkin, A.L., and Huxley, A.F. (1952). A quantitative description of membrane current and its application to conduction and excitation in nerve. *J. Physiol. (Lond.)* **117:**500–544.

53. Bezanilla, F., Perozo, E., Papazian, D.M., and Stefani, E. (1991). Molecular basis of gating charge immobilization in Shaker potassium channels. *Science* **254:**679–683.

54. Jordan, P.C. (1986). Ion channel electrostatics and the shapes of channel proteins, in *Ion Channel Reconstitution* (Plenum, New York), pp. 37–55.

55. Hoshi, T., Zagotta, W.N., and Aldrich, R.W. (1990). Biophysical and molecular mechanisms of Shaker potassium channel inactivation. *Science* **250:**533–538.

56. Boguz, S., and Busath, D. (1992). Is a β-barrel model of the K⁺ channel energetically feasible? *Biophys. J.* **62:**19–21.

57. Durell, S.R., and Guy, H.R. (1992). Atomic scale structure and functional models of voltage-gated potassium channels. *Biophys. J.* **62:**238–250.

58. Guy, H.R., and Conti, F. (1990). Pursuing the structure and function of voltage-gated channels. *Trends Neurosci.* **13**:201–206.

59. Tamkun, M.M., Knoth, K.M., Walbridge, J.A., Kroemer, H., Roden, D.M., and Glover, D.M. (1991). Molecular cloning and characterization of two voltage-gated K⁺ channel cDNAs expressed in rat heart. *FASEB J.* **5**:331–337.

60. Yellen, G., Jurman, M.E., Abramson, T., and MacKinnon, R. (1991). Mutations affecting internal TEA blockade identify the probable pore forming region of a K⁺ channel. *Science* **251**:939–942.

61. Choi, K.L., Aldrich, R.W., and Yellen, G. (1991). Tetraethylammonium blockade distinguishes two inactivation mechanisms in voltage-activated K⁺ channels. *Proc. Natl. Acad. Sci. U.S.A.* **88**:5092–5095.

62. Stuhmer, W., Ruppersberg, J.P., Schroter, K.H., Sakmann, B., Stocker, M., Giese, K.P., Perschke, A., Baumann, A., and Pongs, O. (1989). Molecular basis of functional diversity of voltage-gated potassium channels in mammalian brain. *EMBO J.* **8**:3235–3244.

63. Tempel, B.L., Papazian, D.M., Schwartz, T.L., Jan, Y.N., and Jan, L.Y. (1987). Sequence of a probable potassium channel component encoded at the *Shaker* locus of *Drosophila*. *Science* **237**:770–775.

64. MacKinnon, R., and Yellen, G. (1990). Mutations affecting TEA blockade and ion permeation in voltage-activated K⁺ channels. *Science* **250**:276–279.

65. Kamb, A., Tseng-Crank, J., and Tanouye, M.A. (1988). Multiple products of the *Drosophila Shaker* gene may contribute to potassium channel diversity. *Neuron* **1**:421–430.

66. Frech, G.C., VanDongen, A.M. J., Schuster, G., Brown, A.M., and Joho, R.H. (1989). A novel potassium channel with delayed rectifier properties isolated from rat brain by expression cloning. *Nature (Lond.)* **340**:642–645.

67. Hartmann, H.A., Kirsch, G.E., Drewe, J.A., Taglialatela, M., Joho, R.H., and Brown, A.M. (1991). Exchange of conduction pathways between two related K⁺ channels. *Science* **251**:942–944.

68. Stuhmer, W. (1991). Structure-function studies of voltage-gated ion channels. *Ann. Rev. Biophys. Biophys. Chem.* **20**:65–78.

69. Catterall, W.A. (1988). Structure and function of voltage-sensitive ion channels. *Science* **242**:50–61.

70. Kirsch, G.E., Shieh, C.C., Drewe, J.A., Vener, D.F. and Brown, A.M. (1993). Segmental exchanges define 4-aminopyridine binding and the inner mouth of K⁺ pores. *Neuron* **11**:503–512.

71. Kirsch, G.E., Vener, D.F., Drewe, J.A., and Brown, A.M. (1993). Modulation of 4-aminopyridine block by mutation of deep pore residues in delayed rectifier K⁺ channels. *Biophys. J.* **64**:A226 (Abstract).

72. Castle, N.A., Logothetis, D.E. and Wang, G.K. (1993). 4-AP block of RCK1 K¹ currents expressed in SOL-8 cells: relationship between block and channel activation. *Biophys. J.* **64**:A197 (Abstract).

21

Block of Myocardial Potassium Channels by Antiarrhythmic Drugs: Dependence on Channel Gating

Thomas J. Colatsky, Walter Spinelli, and
Issam F. Moubarak

Myocardial potassium channels have received increasing attention as important targets for antiarrhythmic drug action. Although some of the newest antiarrhythmic drugs currently under clinical investigation were designed to be potent and highly selective potassium channel blockers (e.g., dofetilide, E-4031), voltage clamp studies have shown that even agents with primary actions on sodium and calcium channels can suppress one or more of the potassium currents underlying repolarization in the heart. In most cases, the presence of potassium channel block is revealed as a prolongation of the cardiac action potential and its electrocardiographic manifestation, the QT interval. However, drugs may produce significant effects on potassium channels even when there are no overt changes in repolarization time course. For example, the class Ic agents, flecainide and encainide, which were used in the Cardiac Arrhythmia Suppression Trial, have been recently shown to block the delayed rectifier potassium current I_K in cat ventricular myocytes at concentrations considered to be therapeutic (1, 2), despite the fact only small and variable effects on repolarization are seen both in animals studies and in man (3).

Although a number of new compounds targeting specific cardiac potassium channels are now available, our understanding of how these agents act at the molecular level remains at a very elementary stage. One particular question about the use of potassium channel blockers as antiarrhythmics is that their efficacy may be diminished at fast heart rates, whereas slow heart rates may exaggerate their actions, leading to a failure of repolarization and the initiation of severe proarrhythmia (torsade de pointes). This property has been termed "reverse use-dependence," because it is opposite the rate-dependent enhancement of block that is typically associated with agents acting on sodium and calcium channels (4). The studies discussed herein address interactions between antiarrhythmic drugs and cardiac potassium channels, including possible molecular mechanisms underlying the "reverse" use-dependence observed with the class III agents.

Specificity of Potassium Channel Block

Until recently, there have been few, if any, agents that could discriminate among various myocardial potassium channel subtypes. With the exception of the class I agents lidocaine and recainam, and the newer class III agents such as E-4031 and dofetilide (UK-68,798), most antiarrhythmic drugs in clinical use today block multiple channels at therapeutic or near-therapeutic concentrations (Table 1). Lidocaine and recainam act principally by blocking the excitatory sodium current, whereas the newer class III agents appear to be highly selective for the rapidly activating component of delayed rectification (I_{Kr}) (5, 6).

Because the ability to block potassium channels is shared by a wide range of chemically diverse compounds, it is somewhat difficult to elucidate a unique and specific pharmacophore associated with this particular activity. At the present time, there is also limited insight into what functional groups are responsible for determining the selectivity of a drug for one potassium channel subtype over another. This remains an important area of research, because an understanding of the structure–activity relationships for block of specific potassium channels may provide information about the chemical structure of the drug binding site for each channel type.

Table 1. Specificity of Antiarrhythmic Drugs for Cardiac Potassium Channels.

Class	Agent	I_{to}	I_K	I_{K1}
1A	Quinidine	Yes	Yes	Yes
	Disopyramide	Yes	Yes	Yes
IB	Lidocaine	No	No	No
IC	Flecainide	?	Yes	No
	Encainide	No	Yes	No
	Recainam	No	No	No
III	Clofilium	Yes	Yes	Yes
	Sotalol	Yes	Yes	Yes
	Amiodarone	No	Yes	?
	Dofetilide	No	Yes	No
	E-4031	No	Yes	No
	Tedisamil	Yes	Yes	No
	RP-58866	No	No	Yes

The presence or absence of block for each is assessed relative to therapeutically relevant concentrations. I_{to}, transient outward current; I_K, delayed rectifier current; I_{K1}, inward rectifier current.

General Properties of Class III Antiarrhythmics

Available clinical evidence suggests that the class III antiarrhythmics will be more effective than conventional class I drugs against supraventricular and life-threatening ventricular arrhythmias, but less effective against low-grade ectopy (7). In addition, they should be better tolerated in patients with ventricular dysfunction, because they do not depress myocardial contractility but may in fact exert a modest positive inotropic effect through their ability to prolong the duration of the cardiac action potential plateau. From the standpoint of preclinical drug discovery, the class III agents are largely ineffective against the kind of experimental arrhythmias that had previously been used to study class I antiarrhythmics, such as the 24 to 48 hr Harris dog and ouabain toxicity models, whereas they are extremely effective in suppressing the reentrant ventricular tachycardias induced by programmed electrical stimulation and in protecting against the onset of ventricular fibrillation in models of secondary infarction.

One remarkable property of the class III antiarrhythmics is that they appear capable of spontaneously restoring sinus rhythm during ventricular fibrillation. One example is shown in Fig. 1 using the investigational class III antiarrhythmic WAY-123,398 (8, 9). In this experiment, a train of stimuli were delivered to the ventricle to produce a run of polymorphic ventricular

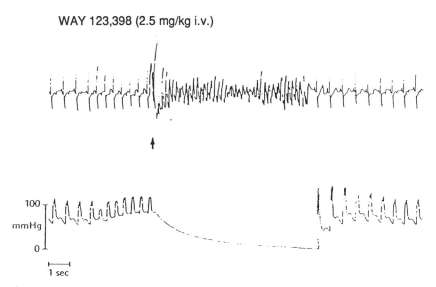

Figure 1. Restoration of sinus rhythm without electrical cardioversion by WAY-123,398 in one open-chest dog. Electrical stimulation of the ventricle during the vulnerable period (marked by arrow) produces ventricular fibrillation with hemodynamic collapse (upper trace: lead II ECG; bottom trace: arterial pressure). Prior administration of WAY-123,398 (2.5 mg/kg) led to the spontaneous termination of ventricular fibrillation after ~0 sec, with restoration of sinus rhythm and recovery of arterial pressure.

417

tachycardia/fibrillation that was not tolerated hemodynamically. During the arrhythmia, no pulse pressure was generated, and arterial pressure rapidly approached zero. After a few seconds, the arrhythmia suddenly reverted to sinus rhythm, with full and immediate recovery of the arterial pulse. This finding was observed in 2 of 6 dogs treated with WAY-123,398 and dofetilide, and 1 of 6 dogs treated with E-4031. No reversion to sinus rhythm without electrical countershock was ever observed in untreated animals, or in animals administered a class I antiarrhythmic agent. Spontaneous reversions of electrically induced ventricular fibrillation to sinus rhythm have also been reported for other class III drugs, including clofilium, bretylium, bethanidine, and d,l-sotalol, and appears to be a general property of this antiarrhythmic drug class.

Mechanisms of Potassium Channel Block

The mechanism by which the permanently charged quaternary ammonium derivative, tetraethylammonium (TEA$^+$), blocks the delayed rectifier current in nerve (10) provides a useful basis for understanding how antiarrhythmic drugs block potassium channels in the heart. Summarized briefly, studies in squid axon have established that: (i) TEA$^+$ blocks most effectively when added to the inside of the cell, rather than to the bathing medium; (ii) analogs of TEA$^+$ with larger hydrophobic substituent groups are more potent blockers than TEA$^+$ itself; (iii) block is not instantaneous, but develops with time after the channels are opened, producing an apparent "inactivation" of the current; and (iv) delayed rectifier tail currents show a blunted peak and a prolonged decay that is consistent with drug dissociating from open channels. These results are consistent with a quaternary ammonium compound blocking site located within the potassium channel pore, accessible only from inside the cell, and only when the channel is open.

Similar results have been obtained for block of myocardial potassium channels by both class I and class III antiarrhythmic drugs. Quinidine in particular has been extensively examined in a variety of preparations, and, except for studies in guinea pig ventricular myocytes (11), appears to show the type of voltage dependence noted for block of neuronal delayed rectifier channels by TEA$^+$ [i.e., block is enhanced by depolarization and relieved by hyperpolarization (12, 13)]. We have recently observed a similar link to channel activation for delayed rectifier block by the class I agents, flecainide and encainide (2). In these experiments, membrane currents were recorded using the single suction pipette voltage-clamp technique with freshly dissociated cat ventricular myocytes. The delayed rectifier current in the cat, unlike guinea pig, appears to be composed of only a single I_{Kr}-like component, as evidenced by the ability of E-4031 to suppress tail currents completely in this preparation (1, 5). When activation curves are constructed by plotting peak tail currents against the associated test potential, both flecainide and encainide appeared to block $I_{K(dr)}$ more effectively at positive potentials, with only negligible changes occurring at more negative potentials. The difference in the degree of block observed at positive and negative potentials suggests that these agents are blocking the delayed rectifier channel in a voltage-dependent manner. If data from these experiments are replotted as fractional block, they can be seen to track the activation curve very closely, suggesting a close link between block and channel opening. Relationships of these type have also been obtained for the class III agents WAY-123,398 and amiodarone, and appear to be a fairly general property of blockers of the cardiac delayed rectifier current.

Interactions of the potassium channel blockers with open channels are also reflected by characteristic changes in the tail current time course (Fig. 2). In the presence of drug, delayed rectifier tail currents exhibit a distinct rising phase that is associated with a delayed time to peak and a slowed rate of decay at later times. These changes in time course are similar to those reported for block of I_K by quaternary ammonium ions in nerve (10) and would be expected if drug-blocked open channels released drug upon repolarization, and became available to conduct outward current transiently before deactivating. Cross-over and blunting of tail currents have also been reported to occur with quinidine block of rabbit (12) and human (13) delayed rectifier channels.

"Reverse-use Dependence" and K⁺ Channel Block

The drug-channel interaction found for the class I and class III agents [i.e., increasing block with depolarization and removal of block upon repolarization] resembles the conventional type of use and voltage dependence associated with sodium channel blockade. However, it is well known that the ability of the class III agents to prolong cardiac action potential duration is diminished at fast heart rates and accentuated at slow heart rates (4). This is opposite to the use-dependent behavior of class I agents, which show enhanced pharmacologic activity (i.e., conduction slowing) at fast heart rates and reduced efficacy at slow heart rates.

Experiments were performed to determine whether repetitive depolarizations could reduce the amount of block seen with class III drugs. For

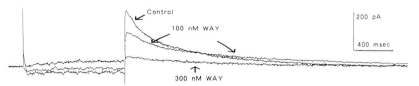

Figure 2. Whole-cell membrane currents recorded from isolated cat ventricular myocytes. Currents were elicited by 1-sec step depolarizations to 50 mV from a holding potential of −40 mV. The observed "cross-over" of the tail currents recorded in the presence and absence of drug reflects unblocking of open channels. WAY-123,398 was added to the bath at final concentrations of 100 and 300 nM.

these experiments (Fig. 3), we used voltage steps that corresponded to the voltage range of the cardiac action potential: from a holding voltage of −90 mV, myocytes were depolarized to 30 mV for 250 msec, then repolarized back to −90 mV and held at this voltage until the beginning of the next cycle. After repeating this conditioning protocol for 19 cycles, the myocytes were finally repolarized to −55 mV and the amplitude of the tail current measured. Fast heart rates were simulated by shortening the time spent at −90 mV between successive depolarizations. Under predrug conditions, the amplitude of the tail current was stable over a wide range of

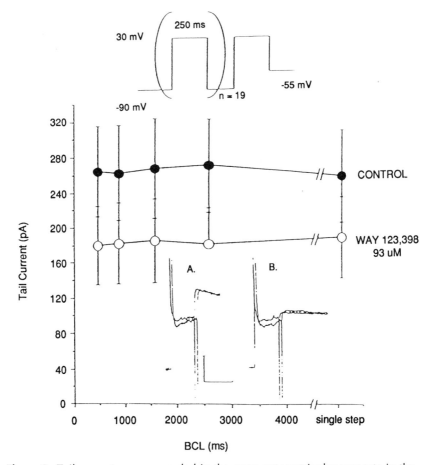

Figure 3. Tail currents were recorded in the same cat ventricular myocyte in the absence of conditioning protocol and after conditioning at interpulse intervals of 400, 800, 1,500, and 2,500 msec, before and after addition of 300 nM WAY-123,398. I_{Na} and I_{Ca-L} were blocked by adding tetradotoxin (30 μM) and nisoldipine (300 nM), respectively, to the bathing medium. Data are the averages of currents measured in six separate experiments (±SEM).

cycle lengths, indicating a lack of residual activation between depolarizing steps, even at the shortest cycle length. After superfusion with 0.3 μM WAY-123,398, the tail amplitude was decreased by the same amount (80 pA) at every cycle length. Thus, these results did not show any evidence of decreased block of I_K at shorter cycle lengths. Similar results have also recently been reported with dofetilide (14).

It has been proposed that the progressive shortening of the cardiac action potential at faster rates of stimulation occurs because delayed rectifier current does not deactivate completely during diastole, but accumulates from beat to beat (15). Under this hypothesis, one would expect selective blockers of I_K to be even more effective at faster rates of pacing, because the contribution of I_K to the total repolarizing current should be increased under these conditions. However, the opposite is found, suggesting that other sources of repolarizing current (e.g., currents generated by ion exchange mechanisms) may become more prominent at short cycle lengths. Considering these results, it seems reasonable to suggest that the decrease in efficacy of the class III agents at a faster rate of beating might be explained by a concomitant increase of other repolarizing currents and not by an intrinsic "reverse use-dependence" as has been reported for quinidine.

Based on the observation that unblocking appears to occur principally via open channels, one might postulate that use-dependent effects will not be present at holding potentials where deactivation is sufficiently fast to "trap" drug within the channel (i.e., at negative potentials). This presumed mechanism is illustrated in Fig. 4. The results obtained in these studies are consistent with the idea that block occurs rapidly (i.e., during the first pulse) and does not reverse with repolarization to potentials at which the channels deactivate very rapidly. However, use-dependent changes in delayed rectifier tail currents have been noted at intermediate membrane potentials, where the kinetics of deactivation are slow relative to the rate of drug dissociation from its binding site (14).

Conclusions

Sudden cardiac death remains an important clinical problem, particularly in patients with poor ventricular function. However, it is likely that new insights being gained into arrhythmic mechanisms in conjunction with the discovery of specific pharmacologic probes of channel function will help to extend our ability to design and use new antiarrhythmic drugs. Although specific blockers are currently available only for I_{Kr} (e.g., dofetilide, E-4031), $I_{K,ATP}$ (e.g., glyburide and tolbutamide), and I_{K1} (RP 58866), chemical efforts directed toward identifying specific blockers of other K⁺ channels (e.g., I_{Ks}) are still ongoing and may yield compounds of interest in the near future. Although the number of new class III agents entering clinical trials is increasing, sufficient data are not yet available to permit a clear recommendation about which of the various K⁺ channel targets pro-

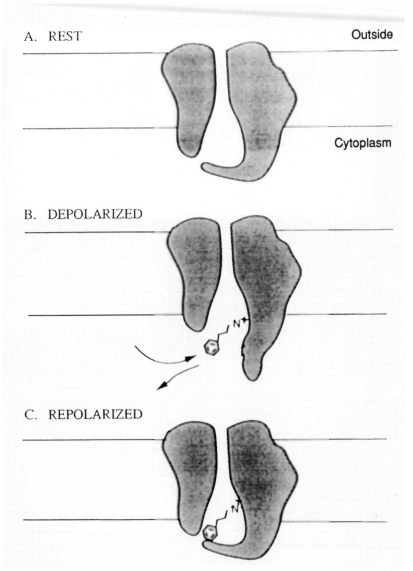

A. REST

Outside

Cytoplasm

B. DEPOLARIZED

C. REPOLARIZED

Figure 4. Possible mechanism underlying the absence of the use-dependent block and unblock of delayed rectifier channels at negative holding potentials.

vides the best therapeutic advantage in terms of safety and efficacy. Further, rigorous evaluation of these newer drugs in both basic studies, as well as in controlled clinical trials, are needed to resolve these important issues.

References

1. Follmer, C.H., and Colatsky, T.J. (1990). Block of the delayed rectifier potassium current I_K by flecainide and E-4031 in cat ventricular myocytes. *Circulation* **82**:289–293.

2. Follmer, C.H., Cullinan, C.A., and Colatsky, T.J. (1992). Differential block of cardiac delayed rectifier current by class Ic antiarrhythmics: Evidence for open channel block and unblock. *Cardiovasc. Res.* **26:**1121–1130.

3. Somberg, J.C., and Tepper, D. (1986). Flecainide: A new antiarrhythmic agent. *Am. Heart. J.* **112:**808–813.

4. Hondeghem, L.M., and Snyders, D.J. (1990). Class III antiarrhythmic agents have a lot of potential but a long way to go. Reduced effectiveness and dangers of reverse use dependence. *Circulation* **81:**686–690.

5. Sanguinetti, M.C., and Jurkiewicz, N.K. (1990). Two components of cardiac delayed rectifier K⁺ current. Differential sensitivity to block by class III antiarrhythmic agents. *J. Gen. Physiol.* **96:**195–215.

6. Colatsky, T.J., Follmer, C.F., and Starmer, C.F. (1990). Channel specificity in antiarrhythmic drug action: Mechanism of potassium channel block and its role in suppressing and aggravating cardiac arrhythmias. *Circulation* **82:**2235–2342.

7. Anderson, J.L. (1990). Clinical implications of new studies in the treatment of benign, potentially malignant, and malignant ventricular arrhythmias. *Am. J. Cardiol.* **65:**36B–42B.

8. Ellingboe, J.W., Spinelli, W., Winkley, M.W., Nguyen, T.T., Parsons, R.W., Moubarak, I.F., Kitzen, J.M., VonEngen, D., and Bagli, J.F. (1992). Class III antiarrhythmic activity of novel substituted [(4-methylsulfonyl)amido]benzamides and sulfonamides. *J. Med. Chem.* **35:**705–716.

9. Spinelli, W., Parsons, R.W., and Colatsky, T.J. (1992). Effects of WAY-123,398, a new class III antiarrhythmic agent, on cardiac refractoriness and ventricular fibrillation threshold in anesthetized dogs: A comparison with UK-69798, E-4031 and dl-sotalol. *J. Cardiovasc. Pharm.* **20:**913–922.

10. Armstrong, C.M. (1971). Interaction of tetraethylammonium ion derivatives with the potassium channels of giant axons. *J. Gen. Physiol.* **58:**413–437.

11. Balser, J.R., Bennett, R.B., Hondeghem, L.M., and Roden, D.M. (1991). Suppression of time-dependent outward current in guinea pig ventricular myocytes. Actions of quinidine and amiodarone. *Circ. Res.* **69:**519–529.

12. Furukawa, T., Tsujimura, Y., Kitamura, K., Tanaka, H., and Habuchi, Y. (1989). Time- and voltage-dependent block of the delayed K⁺ current by quinidine in rabbit sinoatrial and atrioventricular nodes. *J. Pharmacol. Exp. Ther.* **251:**756–763.

13. Snyders, D.J., Knoth, K.M., Roberds, S.L., and Tamkun, M.M. (1992). Time-, voltage-, and state-dependent block by quinidine of a cloned human cardiac potassium channel. *Mol. Pharmacol.* **41:**322–330.

14. Carmeliet, E. (1992). Voltage- and time-dependent block if the delayed rectifier K+ current in cardiac myocytes by dofetilide. *J. Pharmacol. Exp. Ther.* **262:**809–817.

15. Hauswirth, O., Noble, D., and Tsien, R.W. (1972). The dependence of plateau currents in cardiac Purkinje fibers on the interval between action potentials. *J. Physiol.* **222:**27–49.

22

Dihydropyridine Modulation of Cardiovascular L-Type Calcium Channels: Molecular and Cellular Pharmacology

Robert S. Kass

Voltage-dependent calcium channels contribute to the control of diverse cellular activities, including activation of contractile proteins and synaptic transmission, because they regulate the influx of calcium into cells as cell membrane potential changes. In the cardiovascular system, it has been known since the pioneering work of Reuter (1) that calcium entry into the cytoplasm is key to maintenance of cardiac electrical and mechanical activity (2–4). Thus it is not surprising that drugs that modulate the entry of calcium, the channel blockers, have been found to be powerful therapeutic tools in the treatment of a variety of cardiovascular diseases, including hypertension, angina, and some forms of cardiac arrhythmias. More recently, therapeutic applications of these drugs have been expanded to the treatment of congestive heart failure, cardiomyopathy, atherosclerosis, and cerebral and peripheral vascular disorders [reviewed by Triggle (5)]. In addition to the major contributions calcium channel blockers have made to the treatment and management of clinical disorders, these drugs have been equally important to the development of our understanding of the molecular properties of calcium channels. An understanding of the molecular mechanisms of action of this class of drugs will provide basic scientists with information that can be used in the synthesis of drugs designed to target specific tissue and pathophysiological conditions.

Although at least four calcium channel subtypes (P-, T-, N-, and L-) have now been identified based on their pharmacological and/or biophysical properties (6–8), the L-type channel is the target of the most extensively developed calcium channel pharmacology. Of all the chemical compounds that interact with calcium channels, the dihydropyridines (DHPs) have proven to be the most useful in molecular studies of the L-channel, because these drugs bind to the channel with highest affinity and specificity (9).

Calcium channel antagonists in general, and the DHP derivatives in particular, regulate calcium influx by modulating channel gating (10–14). Drug-induced gating changes resemble modes of gating that can occur under drug-free conditions (15, 16) supporting the view that molecular perturbations induced by these compounds promote indigenous conformational changes of the channel proteins. Although it has been shown that the α_1-subunit contains the specific binding sites for all three major classes of calcium channel blockers (17–19), it is very likely that drug-induced conformational changes of the α_1-subunit underlie these gating changes.

Calcium ions play a unique role in the modulatory activity of calcium antagonists in general and the DHPs in particular (20, 21). Divalent ions inhibit the binding of radiolabeled phenylalkylamines to membrane-bound L channels, but high-affinity DHP labeling of L-type channels in brain, cardiac, or smooth muscle membranes depends on the presence of divalent ions (18, 22), as does the binding of DHPs to the purified DHP receptor (23). Binding of calcium also has important regulatory roles in the permeability and gating properties of drug-free native L-type channels. Calcium influx and the high calcium selectivity of skeletal muscle and heart L-type channels. Calcium influx and the high calcium selectivity of skeletal muscle and heart L-type channels are best explained by a multiple (at least two) ion binding model in which ion–ion repulsion is seen as the key to overcoming strong intrapore cation binding (24). Divalent ion binding has been shown to induce protein conformational changes that, in turn, could affect the binding of other ions, notably H^+ (25), and inactivation of cardiac L-channels has also been shown to be influenced by calcium being enhanced with calcium entry (26, 27). Thus, it is very likely that binding of calcium to at least one regulatory site changes the conformation of the α_1-subunit such that DHP-receptor interactions are modified and possibly permeating and/or gating are controlled in the absence of drug binding.

The aim of this chapter is to review recent experiments designed to investigate molecular properties of DHP-sensitive L-type calcium channels by studying functional properties of the channels as they are modulated by specific drugs. Two aspects of channel activity are discussed: (1) the location of the drug binding site for DHPs in cardiac cells and (2) the role of calcium and other divalent ions in stabilizing the drug-channel interaction. An experimental strategy and its results are described that point to an extracellularly located binding site for these important compounds. These basic findings are related to possible clinically relevant properties of amlodipine, a recently synthesized, second-generation calcium channel antagonist.

Strategy

The approach used to provide functional evidence for the location of the high-affinity binding site for DHPs relies upon experiments previously conducted to probe the location of a site in sodium channels to which local anesthetic molecules bind (Fig. 1). Based on ideas and experimental results described by Hille (28) and others (29), it was shown that the ionization state of a drug molecule is a very useful tool in testing for access and binding to a channel-associated receptor. Because the channel is a

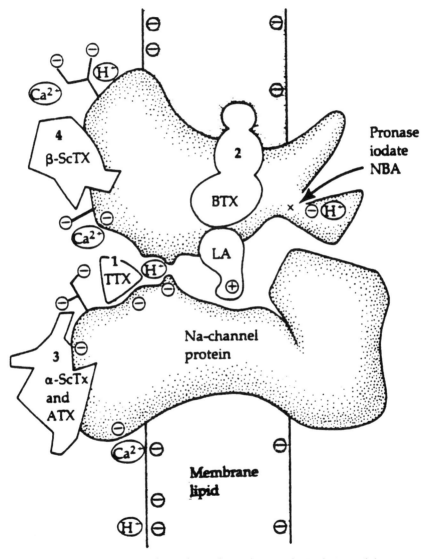

Figure 1. Drug receptors on the sodium channel. Hypothetical view of the sodium channel macromolecule in the membrane. Receptors labeled as follows: (1) tetrodotoxin (TTX), (2) batrachotoxin (BTX), (3) scorpion (α-ScTx) and anemone peptide toxins (ATX), and (4) β-scorpion toxin (β-ScTx).

protein inserted into a lipid bilayer membrane, drugs that are ionized (hydrophilic) are restricted in the pathways by which they can gain access to the drug receptor: they are restricted to hydrophilic pathways. In contrast, un-ionized drugs can follow either hydrophilic (channel pore) or hydrophobic (lipid membrane) pathways. By carefully applying test drugs to either side of the cell membrane and designing voltage protocols that limit or recruit the number of times channels open, it is possible to map the location of the receptor for the test drug with respect to membrane sideness and channel location within the membrane field or channel pore.

This approach was applied very successfully to the nerve sodium channel and provided a biophysical profile of the channel pore for this channel before molecular details of the proteins were known (Fig. 1). However, until recently, the same approach had not been used to study the DHP binding site associated with L-type channels, because almost all previously investigated DHP derivatives were neutral drugs, and thus, not restricted in their access to the DHP binding site (30). More recently (31, 32), a limited number of charged DHPs have been made available for the investigation of ion channel properties.

Channel Block by DHPs

Before experiments could be conducted to determine the location of the DHP binding site relative to the membrane surface, it was first necessary to determine whether charged DHP compounds—such as amlodipine, quaternary amlodipine, and SDZ-207-180—block channels in a characteristic voltage-dependent manner. DHP binding to and modulation of L-type channels is markedly voltage-dependent (10, 14). Channels are inhibited more potently at depolarzied potentials than at negative (resting) potentials (Fig. 2). This voltage dependence can therefore be taken as functional evidence for an interaction between the drug molecule and its receptor. The unique voltage dependence of inhibition (and recovery from inhibition at negative potentials) can therefore be used as a fingerprint by which DHP-channel interactions can be identified. As shown in Fig. 2, neutral DHP derivatives, such as nisoldipine and nitrendipine, have been shown to inhibit reversibly channel activity in this voltage-dependent manner.

The DHP amlodipine was used to probe the modulation of L-type channels in guinea pig ventricular cells by an ionized DHP. Unlike other previously investigated DHP calcium channel blockers, amlodipine is a tertiary compound with $pK_a = 8.6$, and thus at physiological pH, 94% of amlodipine molecules are ionized. At pH 10.0, 96% of amlodipine is neutral. For comparison, previously investigated DHP derivatives—such as nitrendipine, nisoldipine, and PN 200-110—all have pK_a's <3 and are thus virtually 100% neutral over a pH range of 6.0 to 10.0. The strategy of the present experiments was to compare the block and unblock of I_{Ca} by neutral

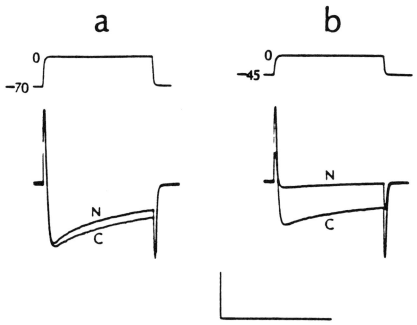

Figure 2. Membrane potential modulates nisoldipine inhibition of calcium channel currents in the Purkinje fiber. Currents measured in the absence (C) and presence (N) of 200 nM nisoldipine from -70 mV **(a)** and -40 mV **(b)** holding potentials. Nisoldipine completely blocks currents recorded from -40 mV but not from -70 mV [see Sanguinetti and Kass (14) for methodology]. Calibration bars: 150 nA, 50 msec.

and charged amlodipine and to use this information to probe the location of the DHP receptor-binding site on the calcium channel protein. Different forms of the drug were selected by changing external pH (pH_0) allowing comparison of the effects of neutral ($pH_0 = 10$) and ionized ($pH_0 \leq 7.4$) drug molecules.

Amlodipine had previously been shown by others (33) to compete with nitrendipine binding sites, and thus it was not surprising that its neutral form (pH_0 10.0) blocked I_{Ca} in a voltage-dependent manner that closely resembled other neutral DHP compounds (Fig. 3). Block was promoted by depolarization and changes in holding potential in the absence of additional pulsing was sufficient to cause block to develop. Most importantly, block by neutral amlodipine was rapidly relieved when membrane potential was returned to negative values in a manner that, again, resembles other previously investigated neutral DHPs. Ionized amlodipine applied externally also blocked I_{Ca} in a voltage-dependent manner, but block onset was slower than the neutral drug form, and the development of block appeared to be influenced by depolarizing pulses. Significant, however, was the finding that recovery from block by ionized amlodipine (pH 7.4) was very slow

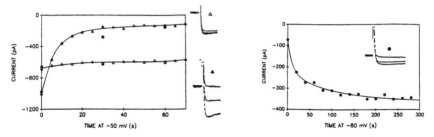

Figure 3. Onset of and recovery from calcium channel block by neutral (pH 10) amlodipine. **(Left)** Peak calcium channel current amplitude is plotted against time after start of depolarizing train protocol in the absence (open) and presence (filled) of 3 μM amlodipine. **(Right)** Recovery of calcium channel current after amlodipine block assayed by a recovery train protocol applied from −80 mV holding potential. The plot shows peak current plotted against time after start of the protocol in the absence and presence of 3μM amlodipine. Note full recovery from block in 30 sec. The pH was 10.0 throughout. Ionic currents in all experiments here were recorded from single cardiac cells of adult guinea pig ventricle (42) with the patch-clamp procedure for the whole-cell configuration (43). Solutions and voltage protocols are described in detail in Kass and Arena (41). Amlodipine and its quaternary derivative were dissolved in water as concentrated stock solutions. Concentrations were chosen as previously described (33, 41, 44). SDZ 207-180 was a gift of Sandoz, Ltd (Basel Switzerland). Nisoldipine was a gift from Miles Laboratories (New Haven, CT). Amlodipine and quaternary amlodipine were gifts from Pfizer Central Research (Sandwich, U.K.).

and very incomplete, suggesting that access to the DHP binding site might be restricted for the ionized, but not neutral form of the drug.

The recovery from block was used as an assay for access of the drug-bound receptor by external H^+. After blocking channels at pH 7.4, recovery from block was promoted by returning the membrane potential to −80 mV. At pH 7.4, recovery was always slow and very incomplete. Then, with membrane potential fixed at −80 mV, external pH was rapidly changed from 7.4 to 10.0, and recovery of current was monitored. It was found that drug-blocked channels rapidly recovered from block when external pH was increased (Fig. 4), showing that drug-bound receptor could be titrated by external pH. The same effects of external pH were observed even if channels had been completely blocked by amlodipine in pH 7.4. Thus, it appeared that open channels are not necessary in order for the drug-bound receptor to be titrated by external H^+.

These results resemble those obtained for local anesthetic block of sodium channels, in that the drug-receptor complex can be titrated by external H^+. It was worth speculating that, like the sodium channel local anesthetic receptor, the DHP receptor-binding site might be accessible to ionized drugs only from an intracellular pathway. In this view, at pH 7.4 externally applied amlodipine accesses the DHP receptor via the small fraction of drug (6%) that is neutral under these conditions.

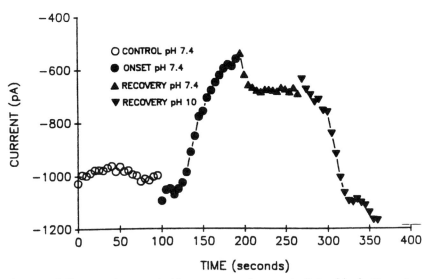

Figure 4. Influence of external pH on recovery from amlodipine block. Current amplitude is plotted against time before (open) and after application of 3 μM amlodipine (filled). Onset of block, measured at pH 7.4, is shown as filled circles. Recovery in pH 7.4 is slow and incomplete (filled, Δ), but rapid and complete when external pH is changed to 10.0 (filled, ∇). [From Kass and Arena (41).]

To test for an intracellular location of the DHP binding site, the sensitivity of calcium channel current to internal and external drug application was measured. Internal application was accomplished by including a high drug concentration in the patch pipette and allowing sufficiently long times for these molecules to diffuse out of the pipette and reach steady-state concentrations in the cell under investigation. Drug-channel interactions were distinguished from channel rundown in the dialysis experiments by the voltage dependence of channel inhibition. Although tertiary amlodipine was an attractive drug to use in this study, because it is 94% ionized at pH 7.4, it was possible that intracellular application of this drug could provide misleading results because the small fraction of neutral molecules that can diffuse across the cell membrane and offset the dialysis of drug into the cell via the patch pipette. Thus, results with tertiary amlodipine were compared with those obtained with the permanently charged compounds, quaternary amlodipine and SDZ-207-180 (31). The ionization groups on the permanently charged molecules restrict these compounds from diffusing out of the cell across the lipid membrane (28).

As controls for internal dialysis, the effects of internally applied D890, a permanently charged phenylalkylamine derivative that has been shown to block I_{Ca} from the inside of cardiac cells, were measured and found, as previously reported (34), to promote pulse-dependent block during pulse-train protocols (31).

In contrast, ionized DHPs had little effect when applied internally to heart cell calcium channels. This can be seen in Fig. 5, which compares pulse-dependent block after 20 min of dialysis with 50 μM intracellular amlodipine, to a 3-min exposure to 10 μM amlodipine applied externally to the same cell (32). Similar results were obtained for intracellularly and extracellularly applied SDZ-207-180 (31) and, more recently, quaternary amlodipine (32).

To be certain of the insensitivity of I_{Ca} to internal application of amlodipine and SDZ 207-180, results obtained in heart cells were compared with experiments conducted in GH_4C_1 pituitary tumor cells. GH_4C_1 cells are small (mean $C_T = 12.65 \pm 1.2$ pF, $N = 12$), and the predicted diffusional time constant for cell dialysis is 40 seconds. As was the case for heart cells, I_{Ca} was not blocked by internal SDZ 207-180 in GH_4C_1 cells, but was

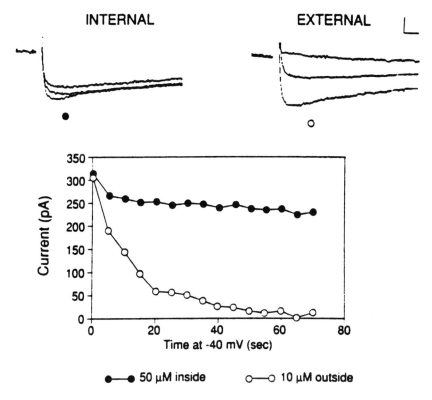

Figure 5. External, but not internal, amlodipine blocks I_{Ca}. Peak inward currents were measured during depolarizing voltage pulse trains after 20-min dialysis with 50 μM amlodipine (filled symbols) and then after an additional 3-min exposure to 10 μM amlodipine applied externally (open symbols). Little indication of voltage-dependent block of I_{Ca} is seen for internally applied drug compared with externally applied drug despite the 5-fold increase in internal drug concentration. Charge carrier is calcium. [From Kass and Kwan (32).]

blocked by external drug application (Fig. 6) (31). From these experiments, it was concluded that ionized drug (amlodipine and SDZ 207-180) access to the DHP receptor is not via the inner surface of the cell membrane.

These functional data therefore were more consistent with the results of studies from Catterall's laboratory (35, 36) than with those of Regulla et al. (37), in which photo-affinity labeling and peptide-specific antibodies were used to identify the DHP binding domain on the isolated skeletal muscle α_1-subunit. These studies are discussed in more detail in other chapters in this volume.

Divalent Ions Interact Preferentially with Charged DHPs

It is well-known that there exists an interrelationship between the blocking activity of calcium channel blockers in general, and the DHPs in particular, with calcium ion concentrations (38). Because of the identification of putative calcium binding domains on the α_1-subunit of the L-type channel (39) and its proximity to possible DHP binding sites (37), there is considerable interest in determining the regulatory role, if any, of calcium in DHP modulation of L-type channel activity. In addition, calcium influx and the high calcium selectivity of skeletal muscle and heart L-type channels are best explained by a multiple (at least two) ion binding model in which ion–ion repulsion is seen as the key to overcome strong intrapore cation binding (24). Lee and Tsien (34) suggested that DHPs do not bind to one of the intrapore, high-affinity calcium-binding sites proposed to underlie the unique selectivity of L-type calcium channels. However, they did test

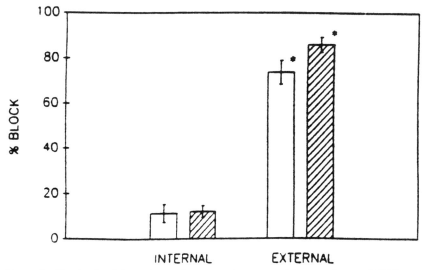

Figure 6. Block of calcium channel currents by external but not internal SDZ 207-180 in heart (open) and GH_4C_1 cells (striped). [From Kass et al. (31).]

for and find a difference in the blocking activity of nitrendipine when barium replaced calcium as the permeant charge species in the L-type channel. This effect was found to be due, in part, to indirect effects of barium and calcium ions on the membrane surface potential of the cardiac cell (3, 4), but the mechanism of the unique drug action on calcium, in contrast to barium, currents was not identified.

More recently, it was shown that charged forms of the DHP compounds amlodipine and SDZ 207-180 share a common sensitivity to calcium that is not shared by the neutral DHPs nisoldipine or nitrendipine (32). The kinetics of the onset of block by the charged compounds, but not nisoldipine, are significantly slower when calcium carries the charge through the channel than under conditions when Ca_0 is buffered by EGTA and when cesium or sodium are the charge carriers. These results suggest that the interaction of DHP compounds with the DHP receptor may depend on the ionic species of the charge carrier and that ionized compounds are more sensitive to this phenomenon than neutral compounds.

Moreover, it was consistently found that different permeant ion species differed in the recovery from channel block, when measured at negative membrane potentials. These observations are summarized in Fig. 7, which plots the percentage of blocked current that was recovered at −80 mV

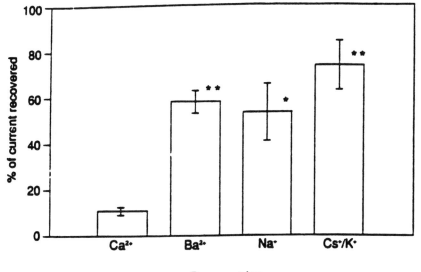

Figure 7. Influence of charge carrier on recovery from block by ionized amlodipine. The bar graphs show the mean percentage of current recovered at − 80 mV after block during onset train protocols for calcium ($N = 8$), barium ($N = 8$), sodium ($N = 5$), and outward currents ($N = 9$). **Significantly greater than calcium, $P \leq 0.005$. *Significantly greater than calcium $p \leq 0.005$ (one-way ANOVA).

current as a function of charge carrier. The recovery of calcium currents is significantly smaller than recovery for the other charge carriers. In order to determine whether neutral and charged DHP compounds share a common sensitivity to the presence of extracellular calcium or to the ionic species carrying the charge through calcium channels, experiments were undertaken with two compounds that were either 100% ionized (SDZ 207-180) or 100% neutral (nisoldipine) at pH 7.4. It was shown that the permanently charged compound SDZ 207-180, but not the neutral drug nisoldipine, exhibited similar charge-carrier sensitivity to amlodipine (31). These results strongly suggest that charged DHPs are much more sensitive to divalent ions either in the extracellular solution, or passing through the calcium channel itself.

Extracellular Access to the DHP Binding Site

Experiments that compared intracellular and extracellular application of ionized amlodipine and SDZ 207-180 in heart and GH_4C_1 cells provided evidence that these two charged DHP compounds cannot reach the DHP receptor via an intracellular pathway. This suggests that the DHP binding site is closer to the extracellular, rather than the intracellular, face of the cell membrane. Because of the long hydrocarbon chain that separates the pyridine ring from the charge group on SDZ 207-180 (31), we can only estimate the location of the DHP binding site within the resolution of the length of this chain; however, our electrophysiological data are consistent with recent binding studies that provide structural evidence for opposite localization of the phenylalkylamine and DHP binding sites (35, 36, 40). Future experiments using different distances between pyridine rings and charge groups in other permanently charged DHP derivatives will improve the resolution of the location of this binding site.

Calcium Ions Stabilize Block by Ionized DHP Derivatives

These results indicate that ionized DHP molecules are more sensitive than the neutral drug molecule to ions permeating the calcium channel. In other experiments at pH 10, a condition in which 96% of amlodipine molecules are neutral (41), recovery from amlodipine block is also not markedly dependent on the species of ion permeating the calcium channel (data not shown). However, the ionized form of amlodipine and the permanently charged compound SDZ 207-180 are very sensitive to the type of ion carrying charge through the channel, and in both cases, the drug-channel interactions (when calcium is the permeating ion) contrast most dramatically with interactions when other ions permeate the channel.

DHP compounds modulate monovalent currents through calcium channels under conditions in which divalent ion concentrations are buffered to micromolar concentrations with either EDTA or EGTA. We find, in addition, that the voltage dependence of DHP channel block remains in the presence of these two chelating agents. Thus, it is not likely that the contrast in recovery from block of monovalent ion and calcium current block is due to an interaction between the calcium chelators and the DHP receptor. Instead, we suggest that, upon return to negative voltages, it is a difference in channel conformation induced by the species of charge carrier, or by the presence of calcium in the extracellular solution that underlies the contrast in recovery from block of calcium and other ionic currents.

In a previous study of the mechanism of organic calcium channel antagonists that included the neutral DHP nitrendipine, the phenylalkylamine D600, and the benzothiazepine diltiazem, Lee and Tsien (34) showed that block by each of these compounds was more difficult to reverse by changes in the extracellular concentration of the permeant ion if calcium rather than barium was the charge carrier. These results could not be explained by differential effects on channel gating caused by barium and calcium ion-induced changes in membrane surface potential (34). Instead, our present results suggest that Ca-induced stabilization of channel conformation may contribute, at least in part, to this observation.

Clinical Relevance: Unique Pharmacokinetic Properties of Amlodipine, a Second Generation Calcium Channel Blocker

Amlodipine is a DHP that has pharmacokinetic properties that distinguish it from previously investigated DHP calcium channel blockers. It has a long elimination half-life and a high volume of distribution, and it is extensively but slowly metabolized by the liver. This profile has been thought to be due to the very slow binding kinetics of amlodipine (33), but the underlying mechanism has resisted explanation. Our results show that the ionized form of amlodipine blocks calcium channel currents in a voltage-dependent manner, but that, in the presence of physiological extracellular calcium, drug-blocked channels remain in a very stable nonconducting state. Channels blocked by neutral amlodipine in the presence of calcium can be unblocked readily at hyperpolarized potentials.

Under physiological conditions, amlodipine exists in both the charged and neutral forms (41). In addition, it is clear that a high concentration of drug partitions into the cell membrane where both charged and neutral forms of the drug are likely to exist (25). The results of these investigations of the cellular properties of this and other charged DHP drugs suggest that the very slow binding kinetics and unique pharmacokinetics of amlodipine are due to the relative contributions of neutral and charged forms of the drug to channel block. Access to the DHP receptor will be different for ionized and neutral forms of the molecule (28), and, clearly, the rate of recovery from block will be markedly different for ionized and neutral molecules. This is particularly relevant for physiological conditions in which the extracellular calcium ion concentration is on the order of 1 to 2 mM. The presence of extracellular calcium at physiological pH stabilizes the drug-bound channel and greatly slows channel unblock. Acidification of the extracellular medium, such as might occur under conditions of ischemia, ionizes a greater fraction of the drug molecules and further impedes channel block and unblock. Future studies are being designed to determine the following under physiological conditions: (1) what fraction of amlodipine block is due to neutral versus ionized molecules; (2) what fraction of amlodipine block is due to membrane-bound versus extracellular drug; and (3) whether the calcium dependence of the block by ionized amlodipine and SDZ 207-180 is related to the unique structures of these drugs, or whether it is a general property of ionized DHP compounds.

The results of this work will be useful in further refining the specificity of these drugs and might be particularly relevant in the design of a calcium channel blocker that is targeted toward inhibiting calcium entry during ischemia or reperfusion.

References

1. Reuter, H. (1967). The dependence of slow inward current in Purkinje fibres on the extracellular calcium-concentration. *J. Physiol.* **192**:479–492.

2. Reuter, H. (1979). Properties of two inward membrane currents in the heart. *Ann. Rev. Physiol.* **41**:413–424.

3. Kass, R.S., and Krafte, D.S. (1987a). Negative surface charge density near heart calcium channels. Relevance to block by dihydropyridines. *J. Gen. Physiol.* **89**: 629–644.

4. Kass, R.S., and Krafte, D.S. (1987b). Electrophysiology of calcium channels in excitable cells: channel types, permeation, gating, and modulation, in *Structure and Physiology of the Slow Inward Calcium Channel* (Alan R. Liss, New York).

5. Triggle, D.J. (1991). Calcium-channel drugs: Structure-function relationships and selectivity of action. *J. Cardiovascular Pharmacol.* **18**:S1–S6.

6. Bean, B.P. (1989). Classes of calcium channels in vertebrate cells. *Ann. Rev. Physiol.* **51**:367–384.

7. Hess, P. (1990). Calcium channels in vertebrate cells. *Ann. Rev. Neurosci.* **13**:337–356.

8. Tsien, R.W., Ellinor, P.T., and Horne, W.A. (1991). Molecular diversity of voltage-dependent Ca channels. *Trends Pharmacol. Sci.* **12**:349–354.

9. Janis, R.A., and Triggle, D.J. (1990). *The Calcium Channel: Its Properties, Function, Regulation and Clinical Relevance* (Telford Press).

10. Bean, B.P. (1984). Nitrendipine block of cardiac calcium channels: High-affinity binding to the inactivated state. *Proc. Natl. Acad. Sci. U.S.A.* **81**:6388–6392.

11. Hess, P., Lansman, J.B., and Tsien, R.W. (1984). Different modes of gating behaviour favoured by dihydropyridine agonists and antagonists. *Nature* **311**:538–544.

12. Kass, R.S. (1987). Voltage-dependent modulation of cardiac calcium channel current by optical isomers of Bay K8644: Implications for channel gating. *Circ. Res.* **61:**I1–I15.

13. Sanguinetti, M.C., Krafte, D.S., and Kass, R.S. (1986). Bay K8644: Voltage-dependent modulation of Ca channel current in heart cells. *J. Gen. Physiol.* **88:**369–392.

14. Sanguinetti, M.C., and Kass, R.S. (1984). Voltage-dependent block of calcium channel current in the calf cardiac Purkinje fiber by dihydropyridine calcium channel antagonists. *Circ. Res.* **55:**336–348.

15. Pietrobon, D., and Hess, P. (1990). Novel mechanism of voltage-dependent gating in L-type calcium channels. *Nature* **346:**651.

16. Artalejo, C.R., Ariano, M.A., Perlman, R.L., and Fox, A.P. (1990). Activation of facilitation calcium channels in chromaffin cells by D1 dopamine receptors through a cAMP/protein kinase A–dependent mechanism. *Nature* **348:**239–242.

17. Catterall, W.A., Seagar, M.J., and Takahashi, M. (1988). Molecular properties of dihydropyridine-sensitive calcium channels in skeletal muscle. *J. Biol. Chem.* **263:**3535–3538.

18. Glossmann, H., and Striessnig, J. (1990). Molecular properties of calcium channels. *Rev. Physiol. Biochem. Pharmacol.* **114:**1–105.

19. Hosey, M.M., and Lazdunski, M. (1988). Calcium channels: Molecular pharmacology, structure and regulation. *J. Membr. Biol.* **104:**81–105.

20. Fleckenstein, A. (1983). *Calcium Antagonism in Heart and Smooth Muscle* (Wiley, New York).

21. Fleckenstein, A. (1977). Specific pharmacology of calcium in myocardium, cardiac pacemakers, and vascular smooth muscle. *Ann. Rev. Pharmacol. Toxicol.* **17:**149–166.

22. Glossmann, H., and Striessnig, J. (1988). Calcium channels. *Vitam. Horm.* **44:**155–328.

23. Flockerzi, V., Oeken, H.J., Hofmann, F., Pelzer, D., Cavalie, A., and Trautwein, W. (1986). Purified dihydropyridine-binding site from skeletal muscle T-tubules is a functional calcium channel. *Nature* **323:**66–68.

24. Tsien, R.W., Hess, P., McCleskey, E.W., and Rosenberg, R.L. (1987). Calcium channels: Mechanisms of selectivity, permeation, and block. *Ann. Rev. Biophys. Biophys. Chem.* **16:**265–290.

25. Mason, R.P., Chester, D.W., Gonye, G.E., and Herbette, L.G. (1988). The effects of drug charge and membrane structure on the partitioning and location of 1,4-dihydropyridines in model and native lipid bilayers. *Biophys. J.* **53:**348a.

26. Kass, R.S., and Sanguinetti, M.C. (1984). Calcium channel inactivation in the cardiac Purkinje fiber. Evidence for voltage- and calcium-mediated mechanisms. *J. Gen. Physiol.* **84:**705–726.

27. Yue, D.T., Backx, P.H., and Imredy, J.P. (1990). Calcium-sensitive inactivation in the gating of single calcium channels. *Science* **21:**1735–1738.

28. Hille, B. (1977). Local anesthetics: Hydrophilic and hydrophobic pathways for the drug-receptor reaction. *J. Gen. Physiol.* **69:**497–515.

29. Hondeghem, L.M., and Katzung, B.G. (1977). Time and voltage dependent interaction of antiarrhythmic drugs with cardiac sodium channels. *Biochim. Biophys. Acta.* **472:**373–398.

30. Rodenkirchen, R., Bayer, R., and Mannhold, R. (1982). Specific and non-specific Ca antagonists: A structure-activity analysis of cardiodepressive drugs. *Prog. Pharmacol.* **5:**9–23.

31. Kass, R.S., Arena, J.P., and Chin, S. (1991). Block of L-type calcium channels by charged dihydropyridines. Sensitivity to side of application and calcium. *J. Gen. Physiol.* **98:**63–75.

32. Kass, R.S., and Kwan, Y.W. (1992). Amlodipine block of heart calcium channels: Mechanisms underlying slow kinetics. *J. Cardiovas. Pharmacol.* **20:**S6–S13.

33. Burges, R.A., Carter, A.J., Gardiner, D.F., and Higgins, A.J. (1985). Amlodipine, a new dihydropyridine calcium channel blocker with slow onset and long duration of action. *Br. J. Pharmacol.* **85:**281P.

34. Lee, K.S., and Tsien, R.W. (1983). Mechanism of calcium channel blockade by verapamil, D600, diltiazem, and nitrendipine in single dialyzed heart cells. *Nature* **302:**790–794.

35. Nakayama, H., Taki, M., Striessnig, J., Glossmann, H., Catterall, W.A., and Kanaoka, Y. (1991). Identification of 1,4-dihydropyridine binding regions within the α_1-subunit of skeletal muscle Ca^{2+} channels by photoaffinity labeling with diazepine. *Proc. Natl. Acad. Sci. U.S.A.* **88:**9203–9207.

36. Striessnig, J., Murphy, B.J., and Catterall, W.A. (1991). Dihydropyridine receptor of L-type Ca channels: Identification of binding domains for H-PN200-110 and H-azidopine within the alpha-1 subunit. *Proc. Natl. Acad. Sci. U.S.A.* **88:**10769–10773.

37. Regulla, S., Schneider, T., Nastainczyk, W., Meer, H.W., and Hofmann, F. (1991). Identification of the site of interaction of the dihydropyridine channel blockers nitrendipine and azidopine with the calcium-channel α_1-subunit. *EMBO J.* **10:**45–49.

38. Fleckenstein, A. (1988). *Calcium Antagonists: Pharmacology and Clinical Research*, P.M. Vanhoutte, R. Paoletti, and S. Govoni, Eds. (Annals of the New York Academy of Sciences, NY), pp. 1–15.

39. Babitch, J. (1990). Channel hands. *Nature* **346:**321–322.

40. Striessnig, J., Glossmann, H., and Catterall, W.A. (1990). Identification of a phenylalkylamine binding region within the α_1 subunit of skeletal muscle Ca^{2+} channels. *Proc. Natl. Acad. Sci. U.S.A.* **87:**9108–9112.

41. Kass, R.S., and Arena, J.P. (1989). Influence of pH_0 on calcium channel block by amlodipine, a charged dihydropyridine compound: Implications for location of the dihydropyridine receptor. *J. Gen. Physiol.* **93:**1109–1127.

42. Mitra, R., and Morad, M. (1985). A uniform enzymatic method for dissociation of myocytes from hearts and stomachs of vertebrates. *Am. J. Physiol.* **249:**H1056–H1060.

43. Hamill, O.P. Marty, A., Neher, E., Sakmann, B., and Sigworth, F.J. (1981). Improved patch-clamp techniques for high-resolution current recording from cells and cell-free membrane patches. *Pflügers Arch.* **391:**85–100.

44. Burges, R.A., Gardiner, D.G., Gwilt, M., Higgins, A.J., Blackburn, K.J., Campbell, S.F., Cross, P.E., and Stubbs, J.K. (1987). Calcium channel blocking properties of amlodipine in vascular smooth muscle and cardiac muscle in vitro: Evidence for voltage modulation of vascular dihydropyridine receptors. *J. Cardiovasc. Pharmacol.* **9:**110–119.

23

Calcium Antagonist Binding Domains of L-Type Calcium Channels

Jörg Striessnig, Steffen Hering, Wolfgang Berger,
William A. Catterall, and Hartmut Glossmann

In 1962 Hass and Hartfelder reported that the coronary vasodilator verapamil possessed negative inotropic and chronotropic effects not seen with other vasodilatatory agents. Subsequently, Fleckenstein and coworkers (1) discovered that this cardiodepression was due to the reduction of depolarization-induced Ca^{2+} influx into cardiac myocytes resulting in inhibition of excitation-contraction coupling and selective block of tetrodotoxin-insensitive, slow action potentials (2). The finding that different chemical classes of drugs ("Ca^{2+} antagonists") selectively interact with one type of high voltage-activated Ca^{2+} channel, so-called L-type Ca^{2+} channels (for review see ref. 3), prompted the development of high-affinity radioligands to reversibly label the channel protein in different tissues (4). Functionally active channels were first purified from skeletal muscle transverse-tubules (4, 5) where they also serve as the voltage sensors for excitation-contraction coupling (6). Ca^{2+} influx through Ca^{2+} antagonist-sensitive L-type Ca^{2+} channels also triggers the contraction of cardiac muscle, controls smooth muscle tone, and mediates neurotransmitter and hormone release (5).

L-type Ca^{2+} Channel Structure

Skeletal muscle Ca^{2+} channels consist of an oligomeric complex of four noncovalently associated subunits (4, 7), termed α_1, α_2/δ, β, and γ. The cDNAs of these subunits have been cloned and sequenced. Cloning and functional expression from different excitable tissues (7, 8) revealed the existence of multiple subunits, isoforms derived either from different genes or by alternative splicing (8). All types of voltage-activated Ca^{2+} channels examined appear to consist of an α_1-subunit that is associated with at least a β- and an α_2/δ-subunit. α_1-Subunits share structural homology to voltage-activated Na^+ and K^+ channels and form the channel pore. The

α_1-associated subunits affect the expression and functional properties of α_1 (7, 8). Their possible physiological roles are discussed elsewhere in this volume.

At least seven different chemical classes of Ca^{2+} antagonists have now been described (4). Their modulatory effects are mediated by the reversible binding to distinct stereoselective domains on the channel protein (Table 1).

Photoaffinity labeling of L-type Ca^{2+} channels in different tissues with domain-selective probes ([³H]azidopine; [³H]diazipine; (+)-[³H]PN200-110 for the dihydropyridine (DHP) binding domain; [³H]LU49888 for the phenylalkylamine (PAA) binding domain; and [³H]azidobutyryl diltiazem and [³H]azidodiltiazem for the benzothiazepine (BTZ) binding domain) revealed that these domains are exclusively located on the α_1-subunit (4, 5, 9, 10). Thus, mammalian cells transfected with α_1-subunits alone were found to express high-affinity DHP binding sites, allosterically modulated by PAAs and BTZs (11).

An Allosteric Model of Drug Binding

Our current view of the allosteric interaction between different Ca^{2+} antagonist binding domains on the α_1-subunit is illustrated in Fig. 1A. It is based on extensive kinetic and equilibrium binding studies of the reversible interaction of domain-selective radioligands with purified and membrane-bound L-type Ca^{2+} channels from different tissues. The original model

Table 1. Ca^{2+} Antagonist Binding Domains on L-type Ca^{2+} Channels

Domain selective for	Typical drugs	References
DHPs	Nifedipine (+)-PN200-110 Azidopine	Glossmann and Striessnig (4)
PAAs	Verapamil Desmethoxyvera-pamil	Glossmann and Striessnig (4)
BTZs Benzazepinones	(+)-cis-Diltiazem SQ32,910 SQ32,428	Glossmann and Striessnig (4) Das et al. (36) Kimball et al. (37)
Benzolactams	HOE 166	Glossmann and Striessnig (4)
Piperidines	Pimozide Fluspirilene	Kaczorowski et al. (this volume) Glossmann and Striessnig (4)
Pyrazines	Amiloride Benzamil	Garcia et al. (42)
Indolizinsulfones	SR33557	Schmid et al. (43)

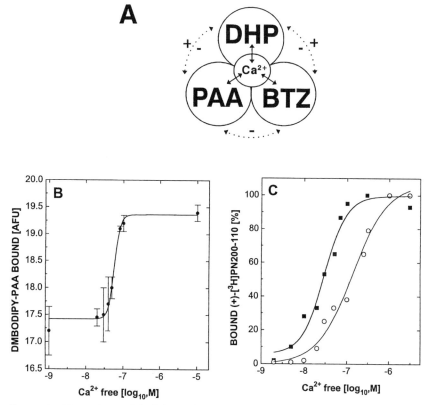

Figure 1. Allosteric model of the Ca²⁺ antagonist binding domain of L-type Ca²⁺ channel α₁-subunits. **(A)** The binding domains selective for DHPs, PAAs, and BTZs are drawn as circles. Arrows symbolize the interdependent binding of the drugs with a high-affinity Ca²⁺ binding domain on the channel. The negative (−) and positive (+) bidirectional allosteric interactions (symbolized by arrows) between the drug-binding domains (four additional domains are omitted for clarity) are at least in part transmitted via drug-induced changes in Ca²⁺ binding. **(B)** Dependence of DMBODIPY-PAA binding on free Ca²⁺ of purified rabbit skeletal muscle L-type Ca²⁺ channel protein (0.019 mg) was incubated with 8.4 nM DMBODIPY-PAA and different concentrations of CaCl₂ buffered with EGTA for 30 min at 22°C. Free Ca²⁺ concentrations were measured by Fura2 fluorescence. EC₅₀: 58.4 ± 3.2 nM. Free Ca²⁺ concentrations (with Ca²⁺ channel present) in the absence of chelators were 5 to 9 µM, determined with 5,5′-dibromo-BAPTA. [Redrawn from Knaus et al., (13).] **(C)** Positive allosteric regulators of DHP binding increase the apparent affinity of Ca²⁺ for the channel. Partially purified skeletal muscle Ca²⁺ channels (0.0098 mg of protein/ml) were incubated with 2.1 nM (+)-[³H]PN200-110 and increasing concentrations of EGTA/CaCl₂ for 60 min at 22°C. The following EC₅₀ and n_H values were obtained by computer fitting: ○, control, EC₅₀ value = 300.1 ± nM, n_H 0.699 ± 0.11; ■, 10 µM (+)-tetrandrine, EC₅₀ value = 30.1 ± 3.4 nM, n_H 1.374 ± 0.3. [Redrawn from Staudinger et al., (24).]

predicted that the binding domains for the different classes of Ca^{2+} antagonists are allosterically coupled to each other and to Ca^{2+} binding sites (12). Detailed analysis of the effects of Ca^{2+} ions on drug binding suggests that at least some of the allosteric effects between the distinct drug-binding domains are transmitted via allosteric conformational changes of one or more Ca^{2+} binding sites on the channel.

This model is based on the observation that Ca^{2+} binding and drug binding are interdependent: occupation of a very high-affinity Ca^{2+} binding site ($K_{0.5}$ = 58 to 300 nM) is required for high-affinity DHP and PAA binding to neuronal and purified skeletal muscle channels (Fig. 1B) (13, 14). Conversely, some Ca^{2+} antagonists can modulate the affinity of Ca^{2+} for this high-affinity binding site, and should therefore affect its binding kinetics. Thus any drug able to modify Ca^{2+} binding has the potential to act as allosteric modulator for other Ca^{2+} antagonists. This has been experimentally confirmed for positive allosteric regulators of DHP binding, like (+) − tetrandrine, (−) − BM20.1140, and (+) − cis-diltiazem. These drugs stimulate DHP binding by increasing the affinity of Ca^{2+} for the channel (Fig. 1C).

Identification of the Ca^{2+} Antagonist Binding Domains

To extend our understanding of interactions of Ca^{2+} antagonists with the channel on a structural level, α_1-subunit regions participating in the formation of different drug binding domains need to be identified. This should provide new insight into Ca^{2+} channel structure, and additional information about the folding and the transmembrane topology of the α_1-subunit.

Different biochemical approaches have been used to localize drug and toxin-binding domains on ion channels and receptor proteins (15, 16). Some of these are based on the isolation of drug-modified peptides released from the photoaffinity-labeled binding domains by proteolytic cleavage. The location of a labeled peptide within the known primary structure of the protein of interest can readily then be determined directly by microsequencing (15) or by immunoprecipitation with sequence-directed antibodies (16). The former approach is feasible only if the photo-labeled proteolytic fragment can be separated from unlabeled peptides and is recovered in picomolar quantities. The antibody approach is the method of choice if hydrophobic peptides are labeled with low yields or if the covalent bond formed between the drug and its binding domain is unstable under the conditions of peptide purification and sequencing (e.g., at acidic pH, see refs. 17 and 18). Sequence-directed antibodies were successfully used to identify the binding regions for α-scorpion toxin on the α-subunit of rat brain voltage-activated Na^+ channels (19). This approach was therefore also used for the localization of the photolabeled binding domains of DHP and PAA Ca^{2+} antagonists on skeletal muscle L-type Ca^{2+}

channels. It should be noted that this is the only L-type Ca^{2+} channel preparation that can be isolated, reconstituted, and labeled secondarily with Ca^{2+} antagonist ligands.

PAA Binding Domain

[³H]LU49888 (see Fig. 2) is the only high-affinity probe currently available to specifically photoaffinity label the PAA binding domain on the α_1-subunit of muscle and brain L-type Ca^{2+} channels (4). Exhaustive

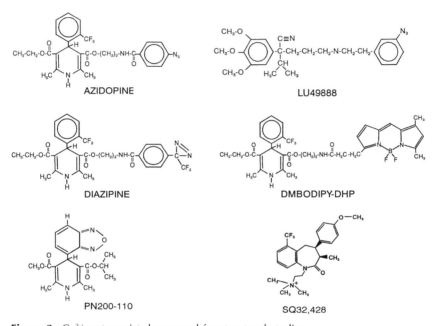

Figure 2. Ca^{2+} antagonist drugs used for structural studies. Azidopine, diazipine, and (+)-PN200-110 specifically photoaffinity label the DHP binding domain on the α_1-subunit of L-type Ca^{2+} channels. Azidopine carries a photoreactive phenylazide group that generates reactive nitrene radicals upon photolysis. The phenyldiazirine group of diazipine forms carbene intermediates. The benzofurazane group of (+)-PN200-110 can also be photoactivated (26). The phenylazide LU49888 specifically photolabels the PAA binding domain on the α_1-subunit. In contrast to the phenyldiazirine, the phenylazides form acid labile covalent bonds with their binding domains (17, 18). (−)-DMBODIPY-DHP is a novel fluorescent probe for L-type Ca^{2+} channels. The (−)-enantiomer binds to purified skeletal muscle L-type Ca^{2+} channels with 2- to 3-fold higher affinity than its optical antipode and is prefered in fluorescent binding assays. SQ32,428 is a novel benzazepine Ca^{2+} antagonist that is permanently charged (quaternary amine). It is considered membrane-impermeable and suitable to study the "sidedness" of the benzazepine binding domain. SQ32,428 binds to the (+)-cis-[³H]diltiazem–labeled BTZ binding domain with a K_i value of 1.29 µM. The respective membrane-permeable derivative (with the tertiary amine substituent at $N - 1$) is ~100-fold more potent (K_i = 8.9 nM).

treatment of photolabeled skeletal muscle α_1-subunits with TPCK-trypsin generates a small tryptic fragment of 9.5 kDa that contains two-thirds of the specific labeling associated with the intact α_1-subunit (20). This fragment is specifically immunoprecipitated by two sequence-directed antibodies against the extracellular (anti–CP1339-1354) and intracellular (anti–CP1382-1400) sides of segment S6, in domain IV, of α_1 (for nomenclature, see Fig. 3). The 9.5 kDa fragment is further cleaved to a labeled

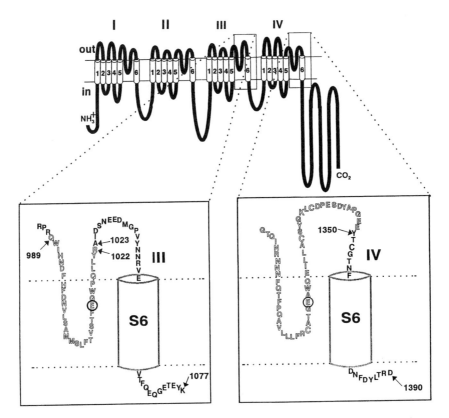

Figure 3. Proteolytic fragments of the skeletal muscle α_1 subunit photolabeled with DHP and PAA-Ca^{2+} antagonists. The α_1-subunit of all voltage-activated Ca^{2+} channels cloned so far is homologous to the pore-forming subunits of voltage-activated Na^+ and K^+ channels. It contains four homologous domains (I–IV), each consisting of six transmembrane segments S1–S6. Portions of the connecting loop between S5 and S6 fold back into the membrane as extended antiparallel β-helical structures (29). These regions form an 8-stranded β-barrel in the folded conformation of α_1 that participates in the lining of the channel pore. The amino acid sequence is shown for the proteolytic peptides specifically photoaffinity labeled with several radioactive DHPs and the PAA [^{3}H]LU49888. The numbers indicate the position of the respective residues in the rabbit skeletal muscle α_1-subunit according to Tanabe et al., (40). The circles highlight acidic residues on the C-terminal region of the antiparallel β-strands that could participate in the formation of a Ca^{2+} binding site (41).

446

fragment of ~5 kDa by V8 protease, which is still bound by anti–CP1382-1400, but not by anti–CP1339-1354. This restricts the site of photolabeling to a 41 amino acid residue extending from Tyr-1350 to Asp-1390. This region includes the transmembrane segment IV-S6 and adjacent extracellular and intracellular amino acid residues (Fig. 3). Functional studies have shown that a quaternary membrane impermeable verapamil analog reaches its binding domain only after application to the cytoplasmic side (21). Therefore, the intracellular end of segment IV-S6 and/or adjacent intracellular amino acid residues must contribute to the formation of the PAA binding domain (20).

DHP Binding Domain

In contrast to the PAA binding domain, several photoligands are available to specifically photolabel the DHP binding domain in muscle and brain. [³H]azidopine, [³H]diazipine (22), and (+)-[³H]PN200-110 possess distinct photoreactive groups positioned at different distances from the DHP ring (Fig. 2). The phenylazide [³H]azidopine and the phenyldiazirine [³H]diazipine were used in racemic form. As shown for [³H]azidopine (23), the less active (+)-enantiomers of these DHPs still bind with nanomolar affinity to the skeletal muscle α_1-subunit and are expected to contribute to specific photolabeling at higher ligand and channel concentrations used for preparative photolabeling (17, 24). Their photoreactive groups, located on the long side chain of the C-3 substituent, can extend up to 14 Å from the DHP ring (25) and are oriented toward opposite sides in the two enantiomers. It is expected that these ligands also label peripheral regions of the DHP binding domain that may interact with the long side chains.

In contrast, the photoreactive benzofurazane group (26) of the optically pure (+)-[³H]PN200-110 is located next to the DHP ring, which comprises the drug's binding center (Fig. 2). (+)-[³H]PN200-110 should therefore mainly label the core of the domain. Tryptic cleavage of skeletal muscle α_1-subunits specifically photolabeled with [³H]azidopine, [³H]diazipine, and (+)-[³H]PN200-110 generates three proteolytic photolabeled peptides derived from different regions of α_1 (Fig. 3). The distribution of labeling in these peptides is different for the three ligands. [³H]diazipine labels a 3.0 kDa fragment (4.4 kDa after incomplete cleavage), which is recognized by antibody anti–CP1011-1026. It comprises amino acid residues Gln-989–Arg-1022 in the connecting loop between segments S5 and S6 in domain III. In addition, [³H]diazipine labels fragment Tyr-1350–Asp-1390 (which is photolabeled by [N-methyl-³H]LU49888 as previously discussed). [³H]azidopine labeling is found in both peptides and in a 7.3 kDa tryptic fragment. This was immunoprecipitated by antibody anti–CP1025-1040 and corresponds to the peptide comprising amino acid residues Ala-1023–Lys-1077 containing transmembrane segment S6 in domain III and adjacent extra- and intracellular amino acids. Photolabeling associated with peptides

Gln-989–Arg-1022 and Ala-1023–Lys-1077 was also immunoprecipitated in a 10.6 kDa fragment produced by cleavage after lysine residues with endoproteinase Lys-C. In contrast to [^{3}H]azidopine and [^{3}H]diazipine, (+)-[^{3}H]PN200-110 almost exclusively labeled Ala-1023–Lys-1077. These data indicate that the core of the DHP binding domain labeled by (+)-[^{3}H]PN200-110 is located close to segment S6 in domain III. More peripheral regions contributing to the binding of the side chains of [^{3}H]azidopine and [^{3}H]diazipine are identified between segments S5 and S6 in domain III and close to segment S6 in domain IV.

Because the DHP binding domain is accessible for membrane-impermeable DHPs only from the extracellular side in intact cells (27, 28), the amino acid residues at the extracellular ends of segments S6 in domains III and IV must participate in the formation of the DHP binding domain (16).

Implications for Channel Folding

These data imply that the extracellular ends of all three photolabeled regions must be located close to each other in the folded structure of α_1. As shown in Figs. 3 and 4, our photolabeling results are consistent with a folding model proposed by Guy and coworkers in which the hydrophobic portions of the connecting loops between segments S5 and S6 in each domain fold back into the membrane in an extended nonhelical conformation, most likely as antiparallel β-sheets (so-called P-element, previously called SS1–SS2 region; ref. 29). These regions are thought to participate in the formation of the channel pore. This model locates the extracellular ends of the S6 segments, and thus the proposed DHP binding domain, close to the extracellular mouth of the ionic pore. DHPs inhibit or activate (e.g. [−]-BayK 8644) L-type Ca^{2+} channels by modifying channel gating and are believed to allosterically interfere with channel function rather than acting as simple pore blockers (30). As previously outlined, this is probably due to conformational changes within one of the Ca^{2+} binding domains. A putative binding site for Ca^{2+} ions is located right next to the DHP binding domain in the C-terminal part of the P-elements in domains III and IV.

Sequence-directed mutagenesis of voltage-dependent Na^+ channels indicates that the highly conserved acidic residues Glu-1014 and Glu-1323 (in domains III and IV; see Fig. 3) are involved in Ca^{2+} binding in the α_1-subunit of voltage-activated Ca^{2+} channels. It is tempting to speculate that the binding of a DHP close to the extracellular channel mouth induces allosteric conformational changes of the adjacent P-elements region, thereby affecting the coordination of Ca^{2+} with these residues. Conversely, removal of Ca^{2+} from this site could cause conformational changes at the extracellular side of segment S6 in domains III and IV, resulting in a loss of high-affinity DHP binding.

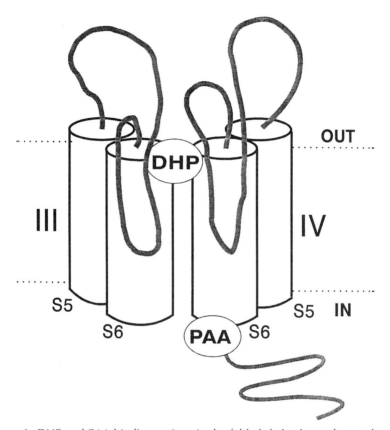

DRUG BINDING REGIONS

Figure 4. DHP and PAA binding regions in the folded skeletal muscle α_1-subunit. A simplified view of the folded structure of the α_1-subunit in the region of the S5 and S6 segments in domains III and IV is shown (side view of one channel half). For a more detailed discussion of the folding models of voltage-dependent ion channels, see Durell and Guy (29). The DHP binding domain is formed by multiple sites in two different extracellular domains of α_1 (27, 28). (+)-[³H]PN200-110 almost exclusively photoaffinity labels the core of the DHP binding domain (peptide Ala-1023–Lys-1077) on the extracellular end of segment III-S6 (see text for details). DHPs with their photoreactive group up to 14 Å away from the binding center of the DHP ring (azidopine and diazipine) also interact and photolabel the antiparallel β-sheet in domain III (peptide Gln-989–Arg-1022) and the extracellular end of S6 in domain IV (in peptide Tyr-1350–Asp-1390). PAA labeling was mapped to peptide Tyr-1350–Asp-1390 and must be localized on the intracellular side of IV-S6 (see text for details).

In contrast to DHPs, PAAs are believed to bind to a site inside the channel pore, which is reached only from the cytoplasmic side upon channel opening (31). Identification of the PAA binding domain near the intracellular end of IV-S6 suggests that this region also forms a part of the ion conducting pathway in good agreement with Guy's model. A consensus sequence for Ca^{2+} binding is located right next to the C-terminal end of the proposed PAA binding domain (32). Therefore, both Ca^{2+} antagonist binding domains appear to be located in regions of the channel protein where Ca^{2+} binding sites could be involved in coordination of Ca^{2+} flux through the ionic pore.

Implications for Heterogeneity of DHP Binding

The fact that DHPs carrying long substituents in position C-3 of the DHP ring interact with α_1 at multiple sites could help explain the heterogeneity of DHP binding recently described for compounds such as the diastereoisomers of sadopine (33) and B847-67/B847-66 (34) (Fig. 5). Both drugs stereoselectively resolve heterogeneous properties of the DHP binding domain uniformly labeled by $(+)$-[^{3}H]PN200-110. $(+)$- and $(-)$-sadopine are both channel blockers and simple competitive inhibitors of $(+)$-[^{3}H]PN200-110 binding with equal affinity. However, they can be distinguished by their completely opposite allosteric effects on PAA and BTZ binding and their kinetic properties. About 10-fold higher association and dissociation rate constants are found for $(+)$-[^{35}S]Sadopine than for the radiolabeled $(-)$-enantiomer (33). Similarly, the diastereomers of a novel basic (pK_a = 8.5) DHP, B847-67, and B847-66 are simple competitive inhibitors of $(+)$-[^{3}H]PN200-110 labeling in the presence of 1 to 10 mM Ca^{2+}. After decreasing Ca^{2+} to micromolar concentrations, B847-67, but not B847-66, clearly discriminates two different populations of $(+)$-[^{3}H]PN200-110 labeled α_1-subunits, as reflected by biphasic displacement curves (34).

These findings are best explained by a model in which competitive interaction of these drugs with $(+)$-[^{3}H]PN200-110 occurs within the core of the DHP binding domain, whereas the stereoselective interaction of the C-3 substituents with the peripheral sites in domains III and IV determines the allosteric and kinetic parameters of sadopine and allows discrimination of two different α_1-subunit populations by B847-67. The strucutral basis for these different populations is yet unknown.

Heterogeneity of Skeletal Muscle α_1-Subunits as Revealed by Förster's Resonance Energy Transfer (FRET)

Heterogeneity is also seen after specific labeling of the DHP binding domain with optically pure fluorescent DHPs in which the fluorophore (e.g., DMBODIPY) is on position C-3. $(-)$-DMBODIPY-DHP competitively

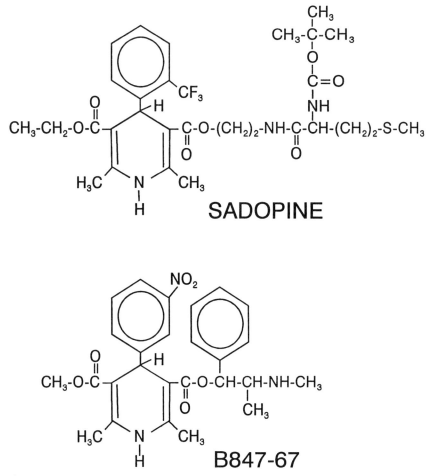

Figure 5. Structure of sadopine and B 847-67. Like azidopine and diazipine, both DHPs carry long substituents in position C-3 of the DHP ring.

inhibits (+)-[³H]PN200-110 binding to different L-type Ca^{2+} channel isoforms (skeletal muscle: K_i = 4.9 nM; brain: 0.9 nM). It was successfully used to label purified L-type Ca^{2+} channels directly by measuring channel-bound fluorescence in a spectrofluorimeter (13) after separation from unbound ligand by charcoal adsorption. We further exploited the fluorescent properties of these ligands to develop a method that allows the direct quantification of channel-bound fluorescence even in the presence of free ligand. This assay is based on the principle of FRET. FRET can theoretically occur between two fluorophores within distances <5 nm, if the absorption spectrum of the energy acceptor overlaps with the emission spectrum of the energy donor (35). For our purposes, tryptophan residues in the α_1-subunit can serve as highly suitable energy donors because their emission spectrum overlaps in the broad wavelength range, between 300 and 400 nm, with the adsorption spectrum of (−)-DMBODIPY-DHP (Fig. 6A).

Because drug binding should bring the DHP within the critical range of 5 nm of one of the 25 tryptophan residues in α_1 (especially those close to the DHP binding domain; see Fig. 3), the possibility of using FRET was investigated. Figure 6B shows the background fluorescence for ligand and protein alone in the range of the emission maximum (517 nm) of (−)-DMBODIPY-DHP, upon excitation of tryptophan residues at 285 nm. At this wavelength the direct excitation of DMBODIPY is expected to be low (Fig. 6A). After rapid mixing of ligand and channel protein, a time-dependent increase of the emission of (−)-DMBODIPY-DHP is observed, which exceeds the background fluorescence. Because the concentrations of ligand and binding sites are kept constant, the change in fluorescence must be due to the formation of ligand-α_1 complexes. This fluorescent signal due to FRET displays properties expected of specific (−)-DMBODIPY-DHP binding. It reversibly decreases after dissociation of the (−)-DMBODIPY-DHP-channel complex following addition of excess nonfluorescent DHP (1 μM (±)-PN200-110), with the half-life expected from conventional assays (13). Analysis of the FRET binding signal in equilibrium studies revealed binding parameters almost identical to those obtained with the conventional assay; (K_d = 11.9 nM, B_{max} = 340 pmol/mg of protein), or by charcoal assay (K_d = 14.2 nM, B_{max} = 355 pmol/mg of protein). These data suggest that this novel binding assay based on FRET can be used to quantify directly DHP binding to the α_1-subunit at a time resolution limited only by the data sampling rate of the spectrofluorimeter. We next exploited this high-time resolution method to obtain a more detailed analysis of the kinetics of (−)-DMBODIPY-DHP binding. The experiment shown in Fig. 6C demonstrates that the dissociation kinetics of (−)-DMBODIPY-DHP are indeed more complex than previously observed with conventional fluorescence and radioligand binding assays (4, 13). Nonlinear curve fitting of the dissociation data revealed the existence of at least 2 time constants for the decay of the channel-DHP complex (see legend to Fig. 6C). This is also evident from the curvilinear semilogarithmic plot (inset). Whether this reflects dissociation of (−)-DMBODIPY-DHP from different channel conformations (e.g., stabilized by Ca^{2+}, channel subunits, or glutamyl transpeptidase-binding proteins) or from structurally different binding domains located on distinct α_1-subunits derived, for example, by alternative splicing (8) is currently under investigation.

BTZ Binding Domain

Although the BTZ binding domain is formed by the α_1-subunit in skeletal muscle, its precise location within the primary structure has not yet been determined. Using the quaternary BTZ analog, the membrane-impermeable Ca^{2+} antagonist, SQ32,428 (36, 37; Fig. 2), we can demon-

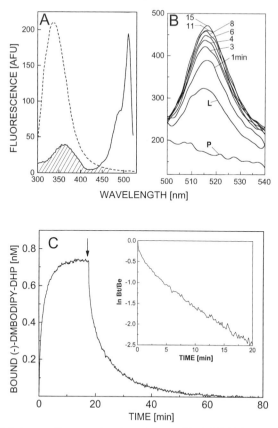

Figure 6. FRET between the α_1-subunit and bound ($-$)-DMBODIPY-DHP.
(A) The spectral overlap (hatched) between the absorption spectrum of ($-$)-DMBODIPY-DHP (____) and the emission spectrum of tryptophan residues after excitation at 285 nM (– – –) is shown. Note that this emission spectrum reflects the ensemble emission spectrum of the tryptophan residues of all channel subunits and contaminating proteins present in the partially purified channel preparation. The efficiency of FRET critically depends on the relative orientation (dipoles) of the two fluorophores, the spectral overlap integral, and decreases with the 6th power of the distance between donor and acceptor (35). **(B)** Time-dependent increase of ($-$)-DMBODIPY-DHP emission between 500 and 540 nm after mixing ($-$)-DMBODIPY-DHP (30 nM) with channel protein (5.25 nM of DHP binding sites). L, spectrum for ligand alone; P, spectrum for protein alone. All measurements were done at 13°C in 1 ml 50 mM Tris-HCl (pH 7.6), 0.1 mg/ml bovine serum albumin, 0.1 % (w/v) digitonin, and containing protease inhibitors (13). **(C)** Time-dependent formation of the DHP-channel complex at 22°C after rapid mixing of 9.5 nM ($-$)-DMBODIPY-DHP and 2.9 nM of DHP binding sites (7.7 µg of protein) measured at 517 nm after excitation at 285 nm. After equilibrium binding was reached (30 min), nonfluorescent ($+$)-PN200-110 was quickly added under constant stirring to induce dissociation. Nonlinear curve fitting demonstrates biexponential dissociation: (site 1: 42%, k_{-1} = 1.23 min⁻¹; site 2: 58%, k_{-2} = 0.115 min⁻¹). A semilogarithmic plot of the dissociation data is shown in the inset. Sampling rate was 1 data point/sec.

strate that the BTZ binding domain is accessible only from the extracellular side. This compound inhibits Ba^{2+} currents through L-type Ca^{2+} channels in skeletal muscle (BC3H1) and in smooth muscle–like cell lines (Fig. 7), following extracellular application, with EC_{50} values of 25 and 21 µM, respectively. In agreement with previous studies (27, 28), no inhibition was found in A7r5 cells with the extracellular quarternary PAA, D575 (Fig. 7), or with D890 (not shown). Control experiments revealed inhibition of Ba^{2+} current by D890 and D575 after intracellular application with BC3H1 or A7r5 cells, whereas SQ32,428 was without effect. These data strongly argue for an extracellular localization of the drug binding domain for BTZ and benzazepine Ca^{2+} antagonists.

Future Prospects

A great deal of our current view of the molecular properties of the α_1-subunit of voltage-activated Ca^{2+} channels is derived from functional

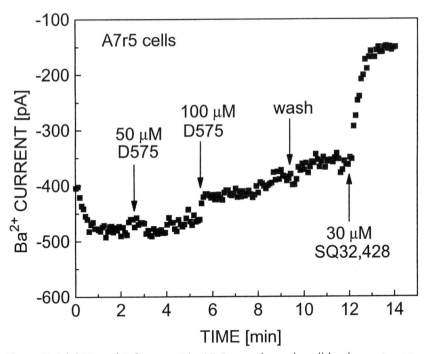

Figure 7. Inhibition of Ba^{2+} current in A7r5 smooth mucle cell by the quaternary benzazepine SQ32,428 after extracellular application. Ba^{2+} inward currents (I_{Ba}) through voltage-activated Ca^{2+} channels in A7r5 cells were measured using the whole-cell configuration of the patch-clamp technique as described previously (33). I_{Ba} was elicited by 0.1 Hz depolarizing pulses (50 msec) from -70 to 0 mV. Quaternary drugs dissolved in dimethylsulfoxide were added directly to the external solution to yield final concentrations as indicated. Currents were normalized with respect to control current at the beginning of the experiment in the absence of drugs. A continuous decrease of current amplitude occurs throughout the experiments and is caused by Ca^{2+} channel run-down.

and structural studies of voltage-activated K^+ and Na^+ channels (29, 38). Expression of mutated and chimeric forms of these channels in *Xenopus* oocytes and mammalian cells has facilitated a detailed analysis of their drug and toxin-binding sites, as well as the identification of physiologically relevant phosphorylation sites (39) and functional domains involved in channel gating (38). Such techniques and other sophisticated approaches will undoubtedly play a key role in further attempts to refine our knowledge of the structure and properties of the binding domains of L-type Ca^{2+} channels.

Acknowledgments

This work was supported by grants from the Bundesministerium für Wissenschaft und Forschung (Austria; to H.G.), the Fonds zur Förderung der Wissenschaftlichen Forschung (S4501 to H.G.; S6602 to J.S.), the Dr. Legerlotz Foundation, a Max–Kade Foundation Fellowship (to J.S.), and National Institutes of Health Grant ROI-NS22625 (to W.A.C.).

We thank Drs. S.D. Kimball and D. Floyd (Bristol-Myers Squibb) for providing tertiary and quaternary benzazepinones and valuable discussions. Work on the fluorescent Ca^{2+} channel ligands was done in collaboration with Drs. H. Kang and R. Haugland (Molecular Probes, Inc.).

References

1. Fleckenstein, A., Kammermeier, H., Doering, H.J., and Freund, H.J. 1967. On the action mechanism of new coronary dilators with simultaneous oxygen-saving myocardial effects, prenylamine and iproveratril. *Zeitschr. Kreislaufforsch.* **56:**716–744.

2. Kohlhardt, M., Bauer, B., Krause, H., and Fleckenstein, A. (1972). Differentiation of the transmembrane Na and Ca channels in mammalian cardiac fibres by the use of specific inhibitors. *Pflügers Arch.* **335:**309–322.

3. Tsien, R.W., Lipscombe, D., Madison, D.V., Bley, K.R., and Fox, A.P. (1988). Multiple types of neuronal calcium channels and their selective modulation. *Trends Neurosci.* **11:**431–438.

4. Glossmann, H., and Striessnig, J. (1990). Molecular properties of calcium channels. *Rev. Physiol. Biochem. Pharmacol.* **114:**1–105.

5. Catterall, W.A., Seagar, M.J., and Takahashi, M. (1988). Molecular properties of dihydropyridine-sensitive calcium channels in skeletal muscle. *J. Biol. Chem.* **263:**3535–3538.

6. Catterall, W.A. (1991a). Excitation-contraction coupling in vertebrate skeletal muscle: A tale of two calcium channels. *Cell* **64:**871–874.

7. Catterall, W.A. (1991b). Functional subunit structure of voltage-gated calcium channels. *Science* **253:**1499–1500.

8. Tsien, R.W., Ellinor, P.T., and Horne, W.A. (1991). Molecular diversity of voltage-dependent calcium channels. *Trends Pharmacol. Sci.* **12:**349–354.

9. Naito, K., McKenna, E., Schwartz, A., and Vaghy, P.L. (1989). Photoaffinity labeling of the purified skeletal muscle calcium antagonist receptor by a novel benzothiazepine, [³H]azidobutyryldiltiazem. *J. Biol. Chem.* **264:**21211–21214.

10. Striessnig, J., Glossmann, H., and Catterall, W.A. (1990). Identification of a phenylalkylamine binding region within the alpha-1 subunit of skeletal muscle Ca^{2+} channels. *Proc. Natl. Acad. Sci. U.S.A.* **87**:9108–9112.

11. Bosse, E., Bottlender, R., Kleppisch, T., Hescheler, J., Welling, A., Hofmann, F., and Flockerzi, V. (1992). Stable and functional expression of the calcium channel α_1-subunit from smooth muscle in somatic cell lines. *EMBO J.* **11**:2033–2038.

12. Glossmann, H., Ferry, D.R., Goll, A., Striessnig, J., and Zernig, G. (1985). Calcium channels and calcium channel drugs: Recent biochemical and biophysical findings. *Drug Res.* **35**:1917–1935.

13. Knaus, H.G., Moshammer, T., Friedrich, K., Kang, H.C., Haugland, R.P., and Glossmann, H. (1992). In vivo labeling of L-type Ca^{2+}-channels by fluorescent dihydropyridines. *Proc. Natl. Acad. Sci. U.S.A.* **89**:3586–3590.

14. Staudinger, R., Knaus, H.G., and Glossmann, H. (1991). Positive heterotropic allosteric regulators of dihydropyridine binding increase the Ca^{2+} affinity of the L-type calcium channel. *J. Biol. Chem.* **266**:10787–10795.

15. Dennis, M., Giraudat, J., Kotzyba-Hibert, F., Goeldner, M., Hirth, C., Chang, J.-Y., Lazure, C., Chrétien, M., and Changeux, J.-P. (1988). Amino acids of the torpedo marmorata acetylcholine receptor alpha subunit labeled by a photoaffinity ligand for the acetylcholine binding site. *Biochemistry* **27**:2346–2357.

16. Catterall, W.A., and Striessnig, J. (1992). Receptor sites for Ca^{2+}-antagonists. *Trends Pharmacol. Sci.* **13**:256–262.

17. Nakayama, H., Taki, M., Striessnig, J., Glossmann, H., Catterall, W.A., and Kanaoka, Y. (1991). Identification of 1,4-dihydropyridine binding regions within the alpha-1 subunit of skeletal muscle calcium channels by photoaffinity labeling. *Proc. Natl. Acad. Sci. U.S.A.* **88**:9203–9207.

18. Regulla, S., Schneider, T., Nastainczyk, W., Meyer, H.E., and Hofmann, F. (1991). Identification of the site of interaction of the dihydropyridine channel blockers nitrendipine and azidopine with the calcium-channel alpha-1 subunit. *EMBO J.* **10**:45–49.

19. Tejedor, F.J., and Catterall, W.A. (1988). Site of covalent attachment of alpha-scorpion toxin derivatives in domain I of the sodium channel alpha subunit. *Proc. Natl. Acad. Sci. U.S.A.* **85**:8742–8746.

20. Striessnig, J., Scheffauer, F., Mitterdorfer, J., Schirmer, M., and Glossmann, H. (1990). Identification of the benzothiazepine-binding polypeptide of skeletal muscle calcium channels with (+)-cis-azidodiltiazem and anti-ligand antibodies. *J. Biol. Chem.* **265**:363–370.

21. Hescheler, J., Pelzer, D., Trube, G., and Trautwein, W. (1982). Does the organic calcium channel blocker D600 act from inside or outside on the cardiac cell membrane. *Pflügers Arch.* **393**:287–291.

22. Taki, M., Kuniyasu, A., Nakayama, H., and Kanaoka, Y. (1991). Synthesis of diazipine and [^{3}H]diazipine: Novel dihydropyridines as photoaffinity probes of calcium channels. *Chem. Pharm. Bull.* **39**:1860–1862.

23. Striessnig, J., Moosburger, K., Goll, A., Ferry, D.R., and Glossmann, H. (1986). Stereoselective photoaffinity labeling of the purified 1,4-dihydropyridine receptor of the voltage-dependent calcium channel. *Eur. J. Biochem.* **161**:603–609.

24. Striessnig, J., Murphy, B.J., and Catterall, W.A. (1991). Dihydropyridine receptor of L-type Ca^{2+} channels: Identification of binding domains for [^{3}H](+)-PN200-110 and [^{3}H]azidopine within the alpha-1 subunit. *Proc. Natl. Acad. Sci. U.S.A.* **88:**10769–10773.

25. Ferry, D.R., Kämpf, K., Goll, A., and Glossmann, H. (1985). Subunit composition of skeletal muscle transverse tubule calcium channels evaluated with the 1,4-dihydropyridine photoaffinity probe, [^{3}H]azidopine. *EMBO J.* **4:**1933–1940.

26. Heinzelmann, W., and Gilgen, P. (1976). Mechanistic studies on photochemical reactions of benzofurazan. *Helv. Chim. Acta* **59:**2727–2737.

27. Kass, R.S., and Arena, J.P. (1989). Influence of pH on calcium channel block by amlodipine, a charged dihydropyridine compound. *J. Gen. Physiol.* **93:**1109–1127.

28. Kass, R.S., Arena, J.P., and Chin, S. (1991). Block of L-type calcium channels by charged dihydropyridines. *J. Gen. Physiol.* **98:**63–75.

29. Durell, S.R., and Guy, H.R. (1992). Atomic scale structure and functional models of voltage-gated potassium channels. *Biophys. J.* **62:**238–250.

30. Hess, P. (1990). Calcium channels in vertebrate cells. *Annu. Rev. Neurosci.* **13:**337–356.

31. Lee, K.S., and Tsien, R.W. (1983). Mechanism of calcium channel blockade by verapamil, D600, diltiazem and nitrendipine in single dialysed heart cells. *Nature* **302:**790–794.

32. Babitch, J.A. (1990). Channel hands. *Nature* **346:**321–322 (Letter).

33. Knaus, H.G., Striessnig, J., Hering, S., Marrer, S., Schwenner, E., Höltje, H.-D., and Glossmann, H. (1992). [^{35}S]Sadopine, a novel high affinity, high specific activity, L-type Ca^{2+} channel probe: Characterization of two equipotent diastereomers with opposite allosteric properties. *Mol. Pharmacol.* **41:**298–307.

34. Lakitsch, M., Knaus, H.G., Topar, G., Romanin, C., Boer, R., Flockerzi, D., Striessnig, J., Hoeltje, H.D., and Glossmann, H. (1993). Heterogeneity of L-type calcium channel α_1-subunits: Stereoselective discrimination of different populations by the novel 1,4 dihydropyridine B874–67. *Mol. Pharmacol.,* in press.

35. Stryer, L. (1978). Fluorescence energy transfer as a spectroscopic ruler. *Ann. Rev. Biochem.* **47:**819–846.

36. Das, J., Floyd, D.M., Kimball, S.D., Duff, K.J., Vu, T.C., Lago, M.W., Moquin, R.V., Lee, V.G., Gougoutas, J.Z., Malley, M.F., Moreland, S., Brittain, R.J., Hedberg, S.A., and Cucinotta, G.G. (1992). Benzazepinone calcium channel blockers. 3. synthesis and structure-activity studies of 3-alkylbenzazepinones. *J. Med. Chem.* **35:**773–780.

37. Kimball, S.D., Floyd, D.M., Das, J., Hunt, J.T., Krapcho, J., Rovnyak, G., Duff, K.J., Lee, V.G., Moquin, R.V., Turk, Ch.F., Hedberg, S.A., Moreland, S., Brittain, R.J., McMullen, D.M., Normandin, D.E., and Cucinotta, G.G. (1992). Benzazepinone calcium channel blockers. 4. structure-activity overview and intracellular binding site. *J. Med. Chem.* **35:**780–793.

38. Miller, C. (1991). (1990): Annus mirabilis of potassium channels. *Science* **252:**1092–1096.

39. West, J.W., Numann, R., Murphy, B.J., Scheuer, T., and Catterall, W.A. (1991). A phosphorylation site in the Na$^+$ channel required for modulation by protein kinase C. *Science* **254**:866–868.

40. Tanabe, T., Takeshima, H., Mikami, A., Flockerzi, V., Takahashi, H., Kangawa, K., Kojima, M., Matsuo, H., Hirose, T., and Numa, S. (1987). Primary structure of the receptor for calcium channel blocker from skeletal muscle. *Nature* **328**:313–318.

41. Heinemann, S.H., Terlau, H., Stühmer, W., Imoto, K., and Numa, S. (1992). Calcium channel characteristics conferred on the sodium channel by single mutations. *Nature* **356**:441–443.

42. Garcia, M.L., King, V.F., Shevell, J.L., Slaughter, R.S., Suarez-Kurtz, G., Winquist, R.J., and Kaczorowski, G.J. (1990). Amiloride analogs inhibit L-type calcium channels and display calcium entry blocker activity. *J. Biol. Chem.* **265**:3763–3771.

43. Schmid, A., Romey, G., Barhanin, J., and Lazdunski, M. (1989). SR33557, an indolizinsulfone blocker of Ca^{2+} channels: Identification of receptor sites and analysis of its mode of action. *Mol. Pharmacol.* **35**:766–773.

PART SIX

Drug Discovery

Papers in the preceding Part relate major advances in understanding the molecular pharmacology of Ca^{2+}, Na^+ and K^+ channels. These channels are especially attractive as targets for antiarrhythmic drug therapy and much progress in understanding has been achieved by the use of drugs which bind to specific sites on the channel proteins. Allosteric interactions between these sites have been demonstrated with binding studies and with current measurements.

This approach is amplified in the first three papers in the following Part as a means to discover better antiarrhythmic drugs. Here drugs specific for Ca^{2+} or K^+ channels are used to identify new drug targets and to reveal features of channel topology. Such information is critical for a rational synthesis of channel modulators with high efficacy and minimal secondary activities. The concluding chapter reviews issues relating to animal testing of potentially effective antiarrhythmic agents. It addresses the corollary problems of developing appropriate drug screening criteria, identifying valid surrogate markers, and correlating measured responses with predictive therapeutic end points in humans. Together these papers illustrate the pragmatic approach prevalent in drug discovery efforts in pharmaceutical and academic laboratories today.

Three chemically different classes of compounds, dihydropyridines, benzothiazepines and aralkylamines have been shown to inhibit the transport function of the L-type Ca^{2+} channel. Each class binds to a distinct channel site and these sites interact allosterically. In the case of the L-type Ca^{2+} channel, at least four additional pharmacological sites have been discovered.

The success achieved to date with Ca^{2+} channel antagonists testifies well to the value of this approach and receives more detailed consideration in the first chapter of this Section by Dr. Kaczorowski. He reviews how strategies developed for targeting voltage-gated Na^+ channels have been extended to multisite analysis of Ca^{2+} channels. Given the close structural relationships between Ca^{2+} and Na^+ channel proteins (see Chapters 5 and 16), this work provides insight into how new classes of channel reagents may be discovered. He also discusses methods which can be used to identify separate structural determinants in multi-step pathways. For example, those involving G-proteins as part of an effector cascade. He extends this approach to the high conductance, Ca^{2+}-activated K^+ channel (Maxi-K^+ channel) important in vascular smooth muscle. This work illustrates general strategies for developing new probes to as yet chemically or structurally undefined sites.

In Chapter 25, Dr. Kimball extends this analysis to further explore structure-activity relationships of the L-type Ca^{2+} channel. He describes an elegant chemical dissection of the diltiazem (a benzothiazapene) binding site and shows how careful analysis can be used to discern the fine structure of the site on the drug which binds to the channel. He shows how a whole new series of channel blockers can be designed whose properties and characteristics are "... limited only by the imagination."

Dr. Lumma in Chapter 26 directs attention to the application of structure-activity relationships to the parallel, probably more complex problem of discovering K^+ channel blockers. His analysis reveals enormous differences among the drugs that comprise this group and illustrates the need to develop more basic information about K^+ channel isoforms in normal and diseased tissue. It becomes apparent from this consideration that many of the physiological factors identified in the first Section of this volume as being important in the epidemiology of arrhythmias (i.e., degree of ischemia, degree of substrate tissue scarring or damage, and autonomic tone), have a major bearing on the effectiveness of drugs directed towards K^+ channel blockade. Given this complexity, Dr. Lumma's expectation is that multiple types of K^+ channel blockers with an array of activities are likely to become useful in dealing with different types of clinical arrhythmias.

Chapter 27, by Dr. Lucchesi, addresses issues of drug efficacy, safety, and selection endpoints. This chapter brings us back full circle to the challenge of antiarrhythmic drug therapy posed in Chapters 1 and 2 by Drs. Strauss and Myerberg. Dr. Lucchesi discusses the dog arrhythmia model pioneered in his laboratory. Choice of paradigm and model he cautions are critical because clinical trials notwithstanding, to date it appears there is no proven pharmacological approach which actually decreases sudden death in susceptible patients. Nor is it apparent that there has emerged an acceptable surrogate marker that can reliably direct such therapy. Dr. Lucchesi addresses these fundamental problems in light of three complicating factors usually associated with arrhythmia development: 1) alterations in concentrations and cell metabolites and ions; 2) alterations in substrate conducting pathways due to tissue scarring; and 3) transient autonomic events that directly affect action potential generation and propagation. He argues that rather than focussing primarily on channels normally involved in genesis of the action potential, equivalent attention should be paid to specific currents, particularly the ATP-sensitive K^+ channel, and the conditions which predominate in pathological or damaged myocardium.

The last chapter, "Report of the Research Recommendations Committee" highlights the lack of basic information on arrhythmic mechanisms and focusses on the need for interdisciplinary studies which apply basic and clinical approaches to the problem. If channel-directed drug therapy is to re-emerge as an effective alternative to surgical ablation or implantation of anti-fibrillatory devices, it seems essential to respond to Dr. Katz's challenge that a great deal of bridge building will need to be done at the interface between basic and clinical science. The report focuses on specific recommendations to accomplish this goal as envisioned by an interdisciplinary group of experts working at the forefront of the field.

Peter M. Spooner & Arthur M. Brown

24

Strategies to Discover Novel Ion Channel Modulators

Gregory J. Kaczorowski, Robert S. Slaughter, and Maria L. Garcia

$\mathbf{A}$ variety of ion channels have been shown to act as multidrug receptors. Ligand binding experiments with known channel modulators demonstrate that discrete high-affinity sites are often localized on channel proteins for many of the different agents that possess either channel agonist or antagonist activities. In addition, these drug binding sites are usually linked to each other via allosteric interactions that are manifested in either negative or positive heterotropic coupling. The voltage-dependent Na^+ channel present in neuronal tissue is a prime example of these concepts. This channel is well characterized because of its rich pharmacology (1). Channel modulators have been identified that interact at seven distinct sites on neuronal Na^+ channels, and many of these receptors display unique allosteric coupling patterns between sites. Although agents that bind to the pore of Na^+ channels (e.g., tetrodotoxin and saxitoxin) do not occupy a site that is strongly coupled to the other drug receptors, the lipid-soluble toxin activators (e.g., veratridine and batrachotoxin), lipid-soluble insecticides (e.g., DDT), peptide channel activators of A and B types (i.e., the α- and β-scorpion toxins, respectively), dinoflagelate toxins (e.g., brevetoxin), and various lower affinity local anesthetics do recognize individual receptors on the channel, all of which are linked by defined patterns. Determination of the effects of test compounds on the binding patterns of Na^+ channel modulators has been used diagnostically to elucidate the sites at which newly discovered agents interact with this channel. Although such an approach is useful for identifying novel classes of ion channel modulators, as well as for developing the molecular pharmacology of previously uncharacterized channels, it does not predict how newly derived molecules will affect channel activity. Functional characterization of the resulting activities by electrophysiological and pharmacological techniques is required for these determinations.

In this chapter, some of the fundamental ideas concerning the discovery of novel ion channel modulators that were originally pioneered with

Na$^+$ channels will be outlined. Two examples will be used for the purpose of illustration: an ion channel with existing pharmacology, the L-type Ca^{2+} channel, and an ion channel whose molecular pharmacology is currently evolving—the high conductance Ca^{2+}-activated K$^+$ (Maxi-K) channel. The principles to be discussed are readily applicable to many other types of voltage- and ligand-gated ion channels as well.

Pharmacology of the L-Type Ca^{2+} Channel

Voltage-gated Ca^{2+} channels are present in both electrically active and inactive cells. These channels are involved in regulating a number of different cellular processes, including excitation-response coupling and electrical excitability. They are controlled by membrane potential and open as the membrane is depolarized. The members of the voltage-gated Ca^{2+} channel family have been subclassified according to their voltage dependence of activation, their inactivation kinetics, and their pharmacological properties. At least four types of channels have been characterized (L-, N-, T-, and P-types). Channel subtypes also exist within this broad classification, and it is conceivable that distinct types of Ca^{2+} channels will still be identified. The L-type Ca^{2+} channel is the most common Ca^{2+} channel, being present in muscle, neuronal, and endocrine tissue. It is activated at relatively depolarized membrane potentials, slowly inactivates after opening, and is blocked by the therapeutically useful classes of organic Ca^{2+} entry blockers.

Indeed, an extensive pharmacology is associated with this system and a wide variety of small organic molecules and peptides have been described that will interact with the L-type Ca^{2+} channel in a potent fashion (2). Several of these organic molecules were originally classified as Ca^{2+} entry blockers based on pharmacological data, but have now been shown to bind with high affinity to distinct receptors that are associated with the α_1-subunit of the L-type Ca^{2+} channel protein complex (3–5). Among the structural classes of these channel modulators are both agonists and antagonists, and these molecules have been indispensable for determining the physiological role of L-type Ca^{2+} channels in target tissues of interest.

It is apparent that a great deal of similarity exists between the L-type Ca^{2+} channel and the neuronal Na$^+$ channel, in terms of the multidrug receptor nature of these proteins. Therefore, in analogy with work done on Na$^+$ channels, it should be possible to extend the molecular pharmacology of L-type Ca^{2+} channels through ligand binding studies with existing channel modulators. In this way, structurally novel agents that interact at defined binding sites on the channel may be discovered, and new drug receptors which could be of utility in basic research applications or therapeutic development may be identified. Originally, three high-affinity drug receptor sites were found to be associated with the L-type Ca^{2+} channel present in plasma membrane vesicles isolated from skeletal, cardiac and brain tissue (for reviews, see refs. 6–8). These binding sites recognize members of the dihydropyridine, aralkylamine, and benzothiazepine Ca^{2+} entry blocker structural classes.

Using [^{3}H]ligands representing each of these classes (e.g., [^{3}H]nitrendipine, [^{3}H]methoxyverapamil (D-600), and [^{3}H]diltiazem, respectively), it was demonstrated that distinct receptors are present on Ca^{2+} channels for each Ca^{2+} entry blocker structural class and that these sites exist in a complex, the members of which are linked allosterically through characteristic interactions. From such investigations, a model was proposed that describes the heterotropic coupling between sites in the Ca^{2+} entry blocker receptor complex present in purified cardiac sarcolemmal membranes (9, 10). More recently, a fourth high-affinity binding site for a distinct structural class of Ca^{2+} entry blocker, substituted diphenylbutylpiperidines such as fluspirilene (Fig. 1), has been identified and demonstrated to have unique properties (11). These data have been incorporated into a model describing the allosteric coupling between drug-binding sites on the cardiac L-type Ca^{2+} channel as illustrated by the scheme shown in Fig. 2. By investigating these interactions through competition binding studies with well-characterized ligands, analysis of ligand binding inhibition patterns using saturation

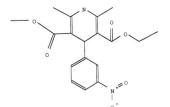

Nitrendipine
(Dihydropyridine)

D-600
(Aralkylamine)

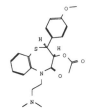

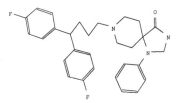

Diltiazem
(Benzothiazepine)

Fluspirilene
(Diphenylbutylpiperidine)

Figure 1. Organic Ca^{2+} entry blockers. Four structural classes of L-type Ca^{2+} channel modulators are shown. Representative [^{3}H]ligands from each of these classes are available for binding studies with L-type Ca^{2+} channels.

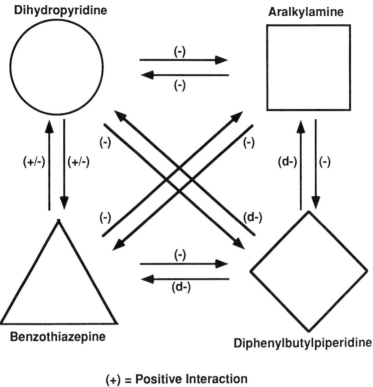

Dihydropyridine

Aralkylamine

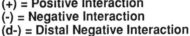

Benzothiazepine

Diphenylbutylpiperidine

(+) = Positive Interaction
(-) = Negative Interaction
(d-) = Distal Negative Interaction

Figure 2. Coupling between Ca^{2+} entry blocker drug-binding sites on the cardiac L-type Ca^{2+} channel. The model illustrated has been developed from binding data presented in refs. 9–11 and 19.

binding techniques, and a kinetic analysis of ligand binding inhibition, novel Ca^{2+} channel modulators have been discovered and their mechanisms of interaction with the L-type Ca^{2+} channel have been elucidated.

In cataloging the number of molecules that bind at each of the four sites in the cardiac Ca^{2+} entry blocker receptor complex, it is clear that there are numerous examples of compounds that compete at either the dihydropyridine, aralkylamine, or diphenylbutylpiperidine receptors. However, only diltiazem and several closely related diltiazem analogs are known to bind at the benzothiazepine receptor on the channel. In order to search for novel molecules that would recognize this site, natural product screening was initiated using [^{3}H]diltiazem binding to cardiac sarcolemmal membrane vesicles as a primary assay. An activity that blocked binding was detected in extracts of the Chinese medicinal herb, *Stefania tetrandra.* This material was subjected to purification, the activity isolated, and shown to correlate with the alkaloid tetrandrine.

Tetrandrine is a dimer of two benzylisoquinoline subunits condensed in a head-to-head, tail-to-tail fashion with α–β stereochemistry at the two chiral isoquinoline carbons. This alkaloid is used in China for the treatment of angina and hypertensive crisis (12). The pharmacological properties of tetrandrine include negative inotropic effects in in vitro cardiac preparations (13), shortening of cardiac action potentials (14), relaxation of smooth muscle contracted by elevated K^+ concentrations (15), hypotensive activity in various normotensive and hypertensive rat models (16), and blood pressure reduction in the dog (17). This profile suggests that tetrandrine possesses functional Ca^{2+} entry blocker activity, but its mechanism had never been characterized at the level of the L-type Ca^{2+} channel. Because tetrandrine is structurally unique from other known chemical classes of Ca^{2+} entry blockers, it is not readily apparent how this agent should be classified. In addition, because the benzothiazepine site is directly coupled to three other sites in the Ca^{2+} entry blocker receptor complex, an effect of tetrandrine on [^{3}H]diltiazem binding does not indicate a priori at which receptor this agent binds.

To demonstrate that tetrandrine interacts directly with the cardiac Ca^{2+} entry blocker receptor complex, and to elucidate its mode of action, the effects of this compound were characterized on three different ligand binding reactions in competition experiments using cardiac membranes (18). In the temperature range 25° to 37°C, tetrandrine completely blocks [^{3}H]diltiazem binding, partially inhibits [^{3}H]D-600 binding, and markedly enhances [^{3}H]nitrendipine binding, with greatest stimulation occurring at 37°C. This preliminary profile resembles that of a benzothiazepine Ca^{2+} entry blocker, because diltiazem elicits the exact same profile. The potency of tetrandrine is increased ~10-fold as temperature is raised from 25° to 37°C (i.e., the K_i against [^{3}H]diltiazem is 500 and 50 nM at these two temperatures, respectively). Scatchard analyses demonstrate that at saturation, inhibition of [^{3}H]diltiazem binding and stimulation of [^{3}H]nitrendipine binding result from either a decrease or increase in the respective ligand affinities, whereas inhibition of [^{3}H]D-600 binding is due to a mixed effect on ligand affinity and maximal receptor site density. Kinetic studies of ligand dissociation indicate that tetrandrine increases the rate of [^{3}H]D-600 loss from its receptor, decreases the off-rate of [^{3}H]nitrendipine, but has absolutely no effect whatsoever on [^{3}H]diltiazem dissociation kinetics. In studies where L-type Ca^{2+} currents were isolated in a GH_3 rat anterior pituitary cell line using patch-clamp techniques, tetrandrine reversibly inhibited channel activity indicating that this compound has functional Ca^{2+} entry blocker activity. Taken together, these data suggest that tetrandrine binds directly at the benzothiazepine receptor in the cardiac Ca^{2+} entry blocker receptor complex, despite the fact it is structurally dissimilar from diltiazem, although it allosterically modulates ligand interactions at other sites in this complex in an identical fashion to diltiazem, itself. Moreover, these findings illustrate the feasibility of discovering novel structural classes of ion channel modulators that will interact at previously characterized ligand binding sites. The data also provide a rationale basis for tetrandrine's therapeutic effectiveness as a Ca^{2+} entry blocker.

In an effort to develop the structure–activity relationship for tetrandrine's interaction at the benzothiazepine receptor, other *bis*-benzylisoquinoline alkaloids that differ in substitutions about the basic ring structure and in stereochemistry at the two chiral isoquinoline carbons (Fig. 3) were explored (19). These compounds represent four conformational classes of analogs possessing either α–β, β–α, α–α or β–β stereochemistry. Individual alkaloid representatives were characterized based on their effects on the binding of ligands at each of the four sites in the cardiac Ca^{2+} entry blocker receptor complex, and their ability to inhibit L-type Ca^{2+} channels in GH_3 cells. These *bis*-benzylisoquinoline structures modulate binding of dihydropyridines, aralkylamines, benzothiazepines, and diphenylbutylpiperidines in cardiac sarcolemma in an interesting fashion. All the analogs completely inhibit [³H]diltiazem binding, but many cause only partial inhibition of [³H]D-600 and [³H]fluspirilene binding. Strikingly, these compounds elicit either stimulation, inhibition, or have no effect on [³H]nitrendipine binding. This profile is not the one predicted for a structural class that binds directly at the benzothiazepine receptor (c.f. diltiazem and tetrandrine). Scatchard analyses demonstrate that modulation of benzothiazepine, aralkylamine, and dihydropyridine binding by the tetrandrine analogs results primarily from effects on ligand K_d values. However, by themselves, such profiles do not indicate at which receptor on the L-type Ca^{2+} channel these compounds interact. Rather, ligand dissociation experiments in the presence of test compounds are more revealing in this regard. Representative members from each conformational class do not effect [³H]diltiazem dissociation rates, but alter dissociation kinetics of [³H]ligands that bind at the other three sites in the Ca^{2+} entry blocker receptor complex. These latter data suggest that despite their atypical effects on dihydropyridine binding, all tetrandrine analogs appear to bind competitively at the benzothiazepine receptor.

As another way of demonstrating the validity of this hypothesis, correlations were sought between the ability of the *bis*-benzylisoquinoline alkaloids to inhibit various Ca^{2+} entry blocker binding reactions and to block voltage-gated Ca^{2+} channels. L-type Ca^{2+} channel activity was conveniently assayed by monitoring depolarization-induced $^{45}Ca^{2+}$ uptake into GH_3 cells. This influx pathway has been shown to be strictly related to opening of the L-type Ca^{2+} channel because: (i) flux rates depend on plasma membrane potential; (ii) many different structural classes of organic Ca^{2+} entry blockers inhibit this flux; (iii) L-type Ca^{2+} channel agonists stimulate Ca^{2+} influx, especially at polarized cell membrane potentials (19). The tetrandrine analogs inhibit depolarization-induced $^{45}Ca^{2+}$ uptake with a defined struc-

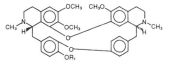

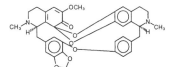

Group Ia, R$_1$ = CH$_3$: Tetrandrine ($\alpha\beta$)
Pheanthine ($\beta\alpha$), Isotetrandrine ($\beta\beta$)

Repanduline ($\beta\beta$)

Group Ib, R$_1$ = H: Berbamine ($\beta\beta$)

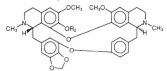

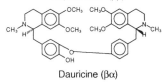

Dauricine ($\beta\alpha$)

Group Ic, R$_2$ = CH$_3$:
(+)Tenuipine ($\alpha\beta$), (-)Tenuipine ($\beta\alpha$)

Group Id, R$_2$ = H:
(+)Nortenuipine ($\alpha\beta$), (-)Nortenuipine ($\beta\alpha$)

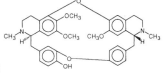

Nemuarine ($\beta\alpha$)

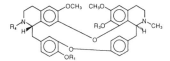

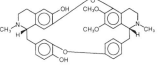

Group IIa, R$_1$ = H, R$_3$, R$_4$ = CH$_3$:
Repandine ($\alpha\beta$), Oxyacanthine ($\beta\beta$)

Dryadodaphnine ($\alpha\alpha$)

Group IIb, R$_1$ = CH$_3$, R$_3$, R$_4$ = CH$_3$:
O-Methylrepandine ($\alpha\beta$)

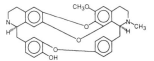

Group IIc, R$_1$, R$_3$ = H:
R$_4$ = H: Daphnoline ($\beta\beta$)
R$_4$ = CH$_2$CH$_3$: N-Ethyldaphnoline ($\beta\beta$)
R$_4$ = COCH$_2$: N-Acetyldaphnoline ($\beta\beta$)

Apateline ($\beta\beta$), Micranthine ($\beta\alpha$)

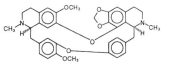

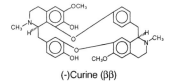

Cepharanthine ($\beta\beta$)

(-)Curine ($\beta\beta$)

Figure 3. Analogs of tetrandrine with Ca^{2+} entry blocker activity. Interaction of various *bis*-benzylisoquinoline alkaloids at the benzothiazepine site of the Ca^{2+} entry blocker receptor complex is described in refs. 18 and 19.

ture–activity relationship. When correlations are made between inhibition of [^{3}H]diltiazem, [^{3}H]D-600, or [^{3}H]fluspirilene binding and block of Ca^{2+} uptake through the L-type Ca^{2+} channel, a linear relationship exists only with the inhibition of diltiazem binding. Importantly, data obtained with diltiazem also fit this correlation. Therefore, these results indicate that a variety of *bis*-benzylisoquinoline congeners will inhibit the L-type Ca^{2+} channel by binding competitively at the benzothiazepine site in the Ca^{2+} entry blocker receptor complex. The unique patterns exhibited by tetrandrine analogs in affecting the allosteric coupling between the benzothiazepine receptor and the other ligand binding sites in the Ca^{2+} entry blocker receptor complex define a new structural class of L-type Ca^{2+} channel modulator that is competitive with diltiazem, but which possesses binding characteristics distinct from those of benzothiazepines.

In independent studies (20, 21), two structurally distinct compounds, KB944 and MDL12330A (Fig. 4) that display the typical pharmacological profile of a Ca^{2+} entry blocker were postulated to be diltiazem-like agents based on their ability to stimulate dihydropyridine binding. Indeed, these compounds display diltiazem-like behavior in competition binding experiments; both completely inhibit [^{3}H]diltiazem binding, are partial inhibitors of [^{3}H]D-600 binding, and produce a concentration and temperature-dependent stimulation of [^{3}H]nitrendipine binding in cardiac sarcolemmal membranes (22). Scatchard analyses of ligand binding at saturation reveal

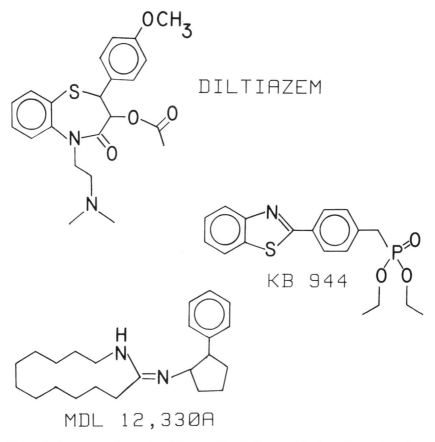

Figure 4. Structures of putative diltiazem-like Ca^{2+} entry blockers. Properties of these compounds that define their site of interaction on the L-type Ca^{2+} channel are described in refs. 20–22.

that these agents inhibit [³H]diltiazem binding by decreasing ligand affinity, whereas inhibition of [³H]D-600 binding results from either a lowering of affinity (KB944) or a decrease in receptor site density (MDL12330A). On the other hand, [³H]nitrendipine is stimulated by each molecule through an increase in receptor affinity, just as is the case with diltiazem. This profile is consistent with both compounds binding at the benzothiazepine receptor in the Ca^{2+} entry blocker receptor complex, despite their structural uniqueness from other compounds known to compete at that site.

However, KB944 and MDL12330A alter the rates of [³H]diltiazem, [³H]D-600, and [³H]nitrendipine dissociation from their respective receptors in kinetic experiments. These data rule out the possibility that a competitive interaction occurs at the benzothiazepine receptor for either KB944 or MDL12330A. Rather, these compounds are likely to bind at a unique site on the L-type Ca^{2+} channel. Therefore, measuring a stimulation in dihydropyridine binding is not strictly a diagnostic test for a diltiazem-like agent. One of the most critical tests for a true competitive agent acting at the benzothiazepine receptor, or at any site in the Ca^{2+} entry blocker receptor complex, is whether or not the test compound affects ligand dissociation kinetics at the receptor in question.

There are other allosteric coupling patterns between sites in the cardiac Ca^{2+} entry blocker receptor complex that are unique and that can be used for diagnostic purposes. One of these involves the substituted diphenylbutylpiperidine receptor where [³H]fluspirilene binds in a very potent fashion with a K_d of 0.6 nM (11). This site exists at a density that is in a 1:1 stoichiometry with the other three Ca^{2+} entry blocker receptors, but it is linked through weak interactions with these sites (Fig. 2). However, a unique feature of the diphenylbutylpiperidine site is that it is also coupled to the pore structure of the L-type Ca^{2+} channel. For example, metal ions that inhibit Ca^{2+} channel activity by binding in the mouth of the pore, such as La^{3+}, Co^{2+}, Cd^{2+}, Ni^{2+}, and Mn^{2+} stimulate binding of [³H]fluspirilene in a concentration-dependent fashion. Cd^{2+} causes the most pronounced stimulatory effect on binding, whereas La^{3+}, the most effective of these cations in inhibiting L-type Ca^{2+} channel activity, is the most potent stimulator of binding. In contrast, the L-type Ca^{2+} channel substrates Ca^{2+}, Ba^{2+}, and Sr^{2+} inhibit [³H]fluspirilene binding. Binding stimulation brought about by metal ions such as Cd^{2+} is due to a maximal increase in the affinity of [³H]fluspirilene from 0.6 to 0.1 nM, as well as to a slight increase in the site density of the receptor. Inhibition of ligand binding activity by Ca^{2+} appears due to an increase in K_d, although it is technically difficult to study this phenomenon given the high nonspecific binding levels that can occur with this ligand. These are particularly noteworthy findings, because binding of other classes of Ca^{2+} entry blockers in heart is not modulated in such a unique fashion by inorganic cations.

The effect of stimulatory cations such as Cd^{2+} on [³H]fluspirilene binding can be used as a diagnostic test to determine whether or not an agent with an unknown mechanism of action competes at the diphenylbutyl-piperidine site. It has been demonstrated that dihydropyridines, aralkylam-ines, and benzothiazepines inhibit binding of [³H]fluspirilene, with K_i val-ues that mimic binding affinities of these ligands at their respective recep-tors. When competition binding experiments are repeated in the presence of Cd^{2+}, each class of Ca^{2+} entry blocker continues to inhibit the interaction of [³H]fluspirilene, but their efficacy in doing so is shifted to lower potency. In marked contrast, agents that compete directly at the substituted diphenyl-butylpiperidine site, such as penfluridol and pimozide, inhibit [³H]fluspiri-lene binding with K_i values in the absence of Cd^{2+} that shift to higher affinity in the presence of the divalent cation. Therefore, [³H]fluspirilene binding cannot only be used to detect agents that interact in or near the external mouth of the L-type Ca^{2+} channel, but also can be applied as a test in the presence of Cd^{2+}, to identify those previously uncharacterized compounds that bind directly at the substituted diphenylbutylpiperidine receptor. It is noteworthy that agents that bind at this site do not display the classic cardiovascular profile typically associated with Ca^{2+} entry blockers (23). This finding suggests that some structural classes may modulate L-type Ca^{2+} channel activity in a unique fashion, and such profiles might be exploited in the development of drugs for novel therapeutic applications.

Analogs of the pyrazine-containing acylguanidine diuretic, amiloride, have been shown to interfere with the activity of a wide variety of cation transporting systems (24). During the in vitro pharmacological characteriza-tion of amiloride derivatives that were known to inhibit cardiac sarcolemmal Na-Ca exchange activity, it was observed that some of these molecules possess potent negative inotropic activity. To determine if this property is the result of blocking Ca^{2+} influx into cardiac muscle through Na-Ca exchange or through the L-type Ca^{2+} channel, the effects of selected amilor-ide analogs were determined on the binding of Ca^{2+} entry blocker ligands (Fig. 5). It was noted that these compounds inhibit the interaction of [³H]nitrendipine, [³H]D-600, [³H]diltiazem, and [³H]fluspirilene at the four sites in the cardiac Ca^{2+} entry blocker receptor complex with a defined rank order of potency (25).

Moreover, the structure–activity relationship observed for these com-pounds in affecting Ca^{2+} entry blocker binding mirrors that found for block of L-type Ca^{2+} channel currents in GH_3 cells using patch-clamp or $^{45}Ca^{2+}$ flux protocols (25, 26). Together, these data imply that amiloride analogs modulate L-type Ca^{2+} channel activity in a direct fashion. Scatchard analyses of ligand binding at equilibrium indicate that the amiloride deriva-tives primarily cause inhibition of ligand binding by decreasing the affinity of [³H]nitrendipine, [³H]D-600, and [³H]diltiazem for their respective receptors. That these compounds do not bind competitively at any of the four well-described sites in the cardiac Ca^{2+} entry blocker receptor complex is demonstrated by their ability to alter the dissociation kinetics of ligands

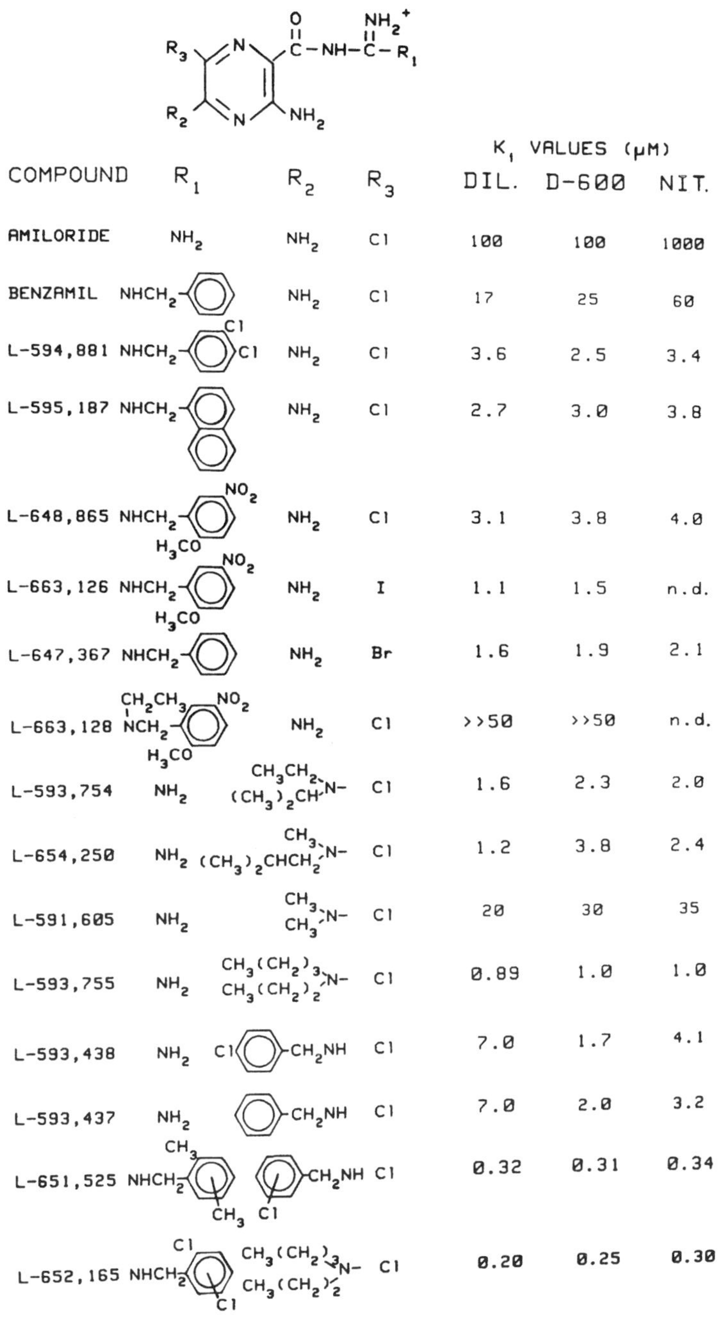

The structure at top: pyrazine ring with substituents R_3, R_2, and the acylguanidine side chain $C(=O)-NH-C(NH_2^+)-R_1$, plus NH_2 on ring.

COMPOUND	R_1	R_2	R_3	K_1 VALUES (µM) DIL.	D-600	NIT.
AMILORIDE	NH_2	NH_2	Cl	100	100	1000
BENZAMIL	NHCH_2-⬡	NH_2	Cl	17	25	60
L-594,881	NHCH_2-⬡(Cl)(Cl)	NH_2	Cl	3.6	2.5	3.4
L-595,187	NHCH_2-⬡⬡ (naphthyl)	NH_2	Cl	2.7	3.0	3.8
L-648,865	NHCH_2-⬡(NO_2)(H_3CO)	NH_2	Cl	3.1	3.8	4.0
L-663,126	NHCH_2-⬡(NO_2)(H_3CO)	NH_2	I	1.1	1.5	n.d.
L-647,367	NHCH_2-⬡	NH_2	Br	1.6	1.9	2.1
L-663,128	NCH_2-⬡(NO_2)(H_3CO) with CH_2CH_3	NH_2	Cl	>>50	>>50	n.d.
L-593,754	NH_2	CH_3CH_2 / (CH_3)_2CH–N–	Cl	1.6	2.3	2.0
L-654,250	NH_2	CH_3 / (CH_3)_2CHCH_2–N–	Cl	1.2	3.8	2.4
L-591,605	NH_2	CH_3 / CH_3–N–	Cl	20	30	35
L-593,755	NH_2	CH_3(CH_2)_3 / CH_3(CH_2)_2–N–	Cl	0.89	1.0	1.0
L-593,438	NH_2	Cl-⬡-CH_2NH	Cl	7.0	1.7	4.1
L-593,437	NH_2	⬡-CH_2NH	Cl	7.0	2.0	3.2
L-651,525	NHCH_2-⬡(CH_3)(CH_3)	⬡(Cl)-CH_2NH	Cl	0.32	0.31	0.34
L-652,165	NHCH_2-⬡(Cl)(Cl)	CH_3(CH_2)_3 / CH_3(CH_2)_2–N–	Cl	0.20	0.25	0.30

Figure 5. Structures of amiloride analogs with Ca^{2+} entry blocker activity. Interaction of various amiloride derivatives with the L-type Ca^{2+} channel is described in refs. 25 and 26.

representing the dihydropyridine, aralkylamine, benzothiazepine, and diphenylbutylpiperidine structural classes.

Some clue into the mechanism of action of the amiloride series has been obtained by monitoring the effects of these compounds on one particular Ca^{2+} entry blocker binding reaction. As previously outlined, Cd^{2+}, a molecule interacting in the pore of the L-type Ca^{2+} channel, stimulates [^{3}H]fluspirilene binding in cardiac sarcolemma. Repetition of this experiment in the presence of amiloride analogs demonstrates that these compounds reduce the potency of Cd^{2+} in a concentration-dependent fashion, but that they do not change the pattern of binding stimulation that occurs with Cd^{2+}. An equilibrium analysis of [^{3}H]fluspirilene binding under these conditions indicates that these amiloride derivatives apparently compete with Cd^{2+} for the same site on the channel. Thus, amiloride derivatives are postulated to act as pore blockers by occluding the ion conduction pathway of the L-type Ca^{2+} channel. This is consistent with independent mechanistic data obtained through electrophysiological analysis of L-type Ca^{2+} channel inhibition (26). Also consistent with this scheme is the finding that inorganic Ca^{2+} entry blockers such as Cd^{2+} inhibit [^{3}H]nitrendipine, [^{3}H]D-600, and [^{3}H]diltiazem binding by increasing ligand K_d values much in the same way as occurs with amiloride analogs. It is curious, however, that amiloride inhibits rather than stimulates [^{3}H]fluspirilene binding as do the metal ion pore blockers. Perhaps, the binding sites for inorganic cations and the protonated acylguanidinium group of amiloride overlap, but the allosteric coupling to the diphenylbutylpiperidine receptor for each of these agents is manifested through different heterotropic interactions.

Because amiloride derivatives with potent Ca^{2+} entry blocker activity possess very hydrophobic properties, it is possible that they might inhibit L-type Ca^{2+} channel activity nonselectively by significantly partitioning into the membrane and disrupting the lipid environment surrounding the channel protein. To confirm that amiloride analogs function in a specific fashion, two different photoactivatable derivatives of amiloride were synthesized; 6-bromobenzylamiloride and 2'-methoxy-5'-nitrobenzylamiloride. Both of these molecules elicit reversible inhibition of Ca^{2+} entry blocker ligand binding reactions in the dark (c.f. Fig. 5). However, when cardiac sarcolemmal membranes are treated with these compounds under illumination, inhibition of ligand binding becomes irreversible. Although the photochemistry of these two amiloride analogs is different (Fig. 6), both will yield reactive moieties upon illumination (27, 28), and this should result in covalent modification of the L-type Ca^{2+} channel after reaction with protein nucleophiles located in proximity to the amiloride binding site.

Irradiation of membranes with monochromatic light at 365 nm in the presence of 6-bromobenzylamiloride, or with monochromatic light at 310 nm in the presence of 2'-methoxy-5'-nitrobenzylamiloride causes time- and concentration-dependent inhibition of [^{3}H]nitrendipine, [^{3}H]D-600, and [^{3}H]diltiazem binding (25). The kinetics of photoinactivation of ligand

PROPOSED MECHANISM OF PHOTOINDUCED REACTIONS

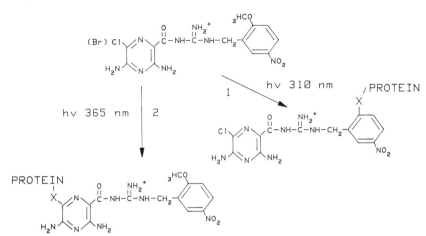

Figure 6. Amiloride photoaffinity probes of the L-type Ca^{2+} channel. Photochemistry and biochemical characteristics of the two amiloride analogs that were used to label the L-type Ca^{2+} channel are described in ref. 25.

binding are first order in each case. Inhibition of $[^{3}H]$D-600 binding is most sensitive to photolysis. Two important characteristics of these photoreactions are that loss of ligand binding does not occur upon illumination of membranes in the absence of photolabel, and that when photolysis is performed in the presence of excess verapamil or diltiazem, the time course of photoinactivation of Ca^{2+} entry blocker binding is dramatically slowed. The fact that Ca^{2+} entry blockers will protect the L-type Ca^{2+} channel from covalent modification by amiloride photoprobes is a strong indication that amiloride analogs interact in a specific fashion with this channel protein at a site allosterically linked to the Ca^{2+} entry blocker receptor complex. Therefore, the two amiloride photoaffinity labels might be useful probes of the pore structure of the L-type Ca^{2+} channel. Unfortunately, these molecules are not selective inhibitors of this channel. Rather, they inhibit a number of different voltage-gated Ca^{2+} channels and various other cation-transporting systems as well. This cross-reactivity renders them useless when used with isolated plasma membrane vesicles. However, because the L-type Ca^{2+} channel has been purified to homogeneity, this preparation provides a much better system for photolabeling studies. Preliminary findings indicate that $[^{3}H]$-6-bromobenzylamiloride can be covalently incorporated into the channel protein isolated from skeletal muscle in a specific fashion (Knauss and Glossman, unpublished observations). Perhaps peptide mapping studies will be useful for identifying those amino acid residues that line the pore structure of the L-type Ca^{2+} channel.

A number of other structural classes of organic Ca^{2+} entry blockers have been described in the literature. Some of these molecules have been investigated using the strategies outlined above. Of particular interest is a series of substituted benzhydrylpiperazines, of which cinnarizine, its analog, flunarizine, and DPI 201-106 are examples (Fig. 7).

The latter compound is also an agonist of the cardiac Na^+ channel and has been shown to possess positive inotropic activity. The mechanism by which these compounds interact with the L-type Ca^{2+} channel was elucidated through binding studies (29). Both cinnarizine and DPI 201-106 inhibit the binding of [³H]nitrendipine, [³H]D-600, and [³H]diltiazem to

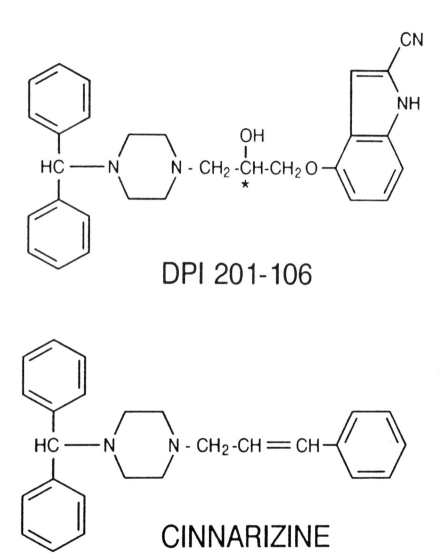

DPI 201-106

CINNARIZINE

Figure 7. Structures of benzhydrylpiperazine Ca^{2+} entry blockers. The Ca^{2+} entry blocker properties of cinnarizine and DPI 201-106 are described in ref. 29.

cardiac sarcolemmal membranes. Previous studies have shown that DPI 201-106 interacts with cardiac Na^+ channels in a stereospecific fashion. However, no stereoselectivity is demonstrated for the interaction of DPI 201-106 with cardiac L-type Ca^{2+} channels, suggesting that dissimilar binding sites exist for this molecule on the two channel types. Analyses of ligand binding inhibition at equilibrium indicate that both cinnarizine and DPI 201-106 inhibit the interaction of Ca^{2+} entry blocker ligands in a mixed fashion (i.e., both K_d and B_{max} effects are manifested). Furthermore, both molecules alter the dissociation kinetics of [³H]nitrendipine, [³H]D-600, and [³H]diltiazem from their respective sites on the cardiac Ca^{2+} entry blocker receptor complex. Given this profile, and the electrophysiological characteristics associated with cinnarizine and DPI 201-106 block of L-type Ca^{2+} channel activity, it would appear that substituted benzhydrylpiperazines interact at a unique, low-affinity, local anesthetic-like site on this protein. Taken together with the data previously outlined, these findings illustrate the idea that the cardiac L-type Ca^{2+} channel is a multidrug receptor with a rich molecular pharmacology.

The cardiac L-type Ca^{2+} channel clearly possess many different binding sites for channel modulators, sites that are coupled by defined allosteric interactions. Using the diagnostic capability of a model that conceptually describes these interactions as illustrated in Fig. 2, it has been possible to discover new structural classes of L-type Ca^{2+} channel effectors by screening at known ligand binding sites. Furthermore, it has been feasible to combine binding data along with functional studies using flux or electrophysiological protocols to elucidate the mechanism of action of novel L-type Ca^{2+} channel modulators. To date, at least seven different drug receptors have been identified on the L-type Ca^{2+} channel, and it is likely that additional sites will be discovered. These data support the view that similarities exist between the L-type Ca^{2+} channel and voltage-gated Na^+ channels in terms of the multidrug binding site nature of the two proteins, and the variety of allosterically linked receptors observed with both systems.

Pharmacology of the Maxi-K Channel

Using the work with Na^+ and Ca^{2+} channels as a paradigm, it should be feasible to develop the molecular pharmacology of ion channels that have not previously been exploited in this fashion. The high-conductance Ca^{2+}-activated K^+ (Maxi-K) channel is an example where this approach has been successful. This channel has a very large conductance (200 to 300 pS) and is activated by both membrane depolarization and intracellular Ca^{2+}. Binding of multiple (i.e., 2 to 6) Ca^{2+} ions to the internal face of the channel shifts the voltage dependency of gating and allows channel openings at more negative membrane potentials. Maxi-K channels are present in neurons, striated and smooth muscle, endocrine tissue, kidney tubules, and the choride plexus. Several smaller conductance Ca^{2+}-activated K^+ channels are also present in these tissues, as well as in blood cells such as platelets and B- and T-lymphocytes. Because only one type of Ca^{2+}-activated K^+ channel has been cloned (30, 31), it is presently not known how many classes of these proteins exist, and if multiple families are responsible for the variety of single channel conductances observed. Maxi-K channels are particularly abundant in many types of smooth muscle, including vascular, airways, gastrointestinal, bladder, and uterine tissue. These channels are not found in cardiac myocytes.

Because one of the physiological roles of the Maxi-K channel is thought to be cell repolarization following membrane depolarization and elevation of intracellular Ca^{2+}, these channels have been implicated in the regulation of muscle contractility, in the control of neuroendocrine secretion, in the movement of ions across epithelial tissues, and in certain cellular signal transduction mechanisms. Given these putative roles, it has been hypothesized that modulators of the Maxi-K channel might have therapeutic utility (e.g., an agonist may yield smooth muscle relaxation, whereas an antagonist may promote neurotransmitter release). However, it has been difficult to test these potential utilities because the pharmacology of the Maxi-K channel is relatively undeveloped due to the paucity of selective high-affinity probes for this protein. However, with the discovery that crude venom of the scorpion *Leiurus quinquestriatus* will inhibit this channel (32), it has been possible to identify and purify a number of unique, high-affinity, peptidyl Maxi-K channel modulators and use these probes to develop the molecular pharmacology of this target. These agents have also been instrumental in characterizing in vitro the biochemical, pharmacological, and physiological properties of this channel.

Leiurus quinquestriatus var. *hebraeus* venom contains many different peptides that modulate Na^+ and K^+ channel behavior. The active component of the venom that inhibits Maxi-K channel activity has been termed charybdotoxin (ChTX; ref. 32). This peptide inhibits channel activity by binding reversibly in the external mouth of the protein through a simple bimolecular reaction, and thereby blocks the ion conduction pathway. This inhibitor does not affect channel gating processes. ChTX has been purified to homogeneity by several different laboratories using a combination of ion exchange and reversed-phase chromatographies (33–37). The complete 37 amino acid primary sequence of this peptide has been elucidated by Edman degradation techniques (33), and later confirmed in three independent studies (35–37). ChTX has been produced by synthetic methodologies (38, 39), and this material possesses the same biological activity as native toxin in terms of potency of Maxi-K channel block and channel selectivity. Synthetic ChTX was used to assign the disulfide bridging pattern of this peptide after proteolytic digestion, and these data suggest that ChTX is a highly compact structure (Fig. 8).

This hypothesis was later confirmed when the solution structure of ChTX was determined by NMR techniques (39, 40). ChTX is a highly basic

Disulfide Bonding Pattern of ChTX

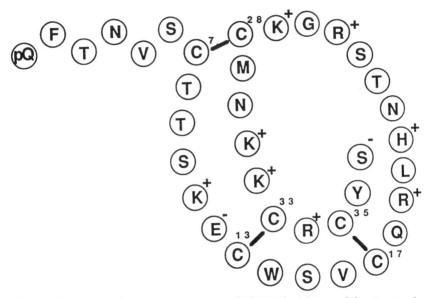

Figure 8. Primary and secondary structure of ChTX. Elucidation of the structural properties of this K$^+$ channel inhibitory peptide is described in refs. 33 and 38.

peptide with an overall net charge of +5 at physiological pH. This property results from the presence of four lysine, three arginine, and one histidine residue, with only a single glutamic acid functionality present in the peptide. These basic residues play an important role in the mechanism by which ChTX blocks Maxi-K channels, and this has been the subject of intense study (41–44).

In order to use ChTX as a biochemical probe of the Maxi-K channel, the peptide must be radiolabeled in biologically active form. ChTX contains a single tyrosine residue penultimate from its C-terminus, and this is a potential site for iodination. Using standard iodination protocols, it has been possible to radiolabel ChTX with Na^{125}I to high specific activity and separate the monoiodotyrosine adduct from the other products of the reaction mixture by reversed-phase HPLC (45). This modified peptide blocks Maxi-K channels in cultured bovine aortic smooth muscle cells by a similar mechanism to that of ChTX, but its potency is reduced ~10-fold from native toxin, and low ionic strength media are required for channel block (45). This property makes it difficult to analyze toxin binding to cells or isolated membrane vesicles in physiological saline solutions. However, under reduced ionic strength conditions, binding studies have been feasible. Because smooth muscle is a rich source of Maxi-K channels, characterization of the interaction between [^{125}I]ChTX and this channel has been facilitated by the isolation of a highly purified sarcolemmal membrane preparation from bovine aorta (46a). These vesicles are enriched in many plasma membrane marker activities, such as the L-type Ca^{2+} channel and Na-Ca exchange, and contain Maxi-K channel activity as demonstrated by reconstitution studies in which channels from these membranes were incorporated into planar lipid bilayers.

When aortic sarcolemma are incubated with [^{125}I]ChTX, specific binding of peptide occurs in a concentration- and time-dependent fashion to a single class of receptors (45). The affinity and density of these binding sites as measured at low ionic strength are 100 pM and 0.5 pmol/mg protein, respectively. The B_{max} of toxin binding can be increased by a factor of 2 by permeabilizing vesicles with detergent, consistent with the notion that ChTX binds solely in the external pore of Maxi-K channels, and that aortic sarcolemmal membranes are a 50:50 mixture of outside-out and inside-out vesicles. [^{125}I]ChTX binding is a reversible bimolecular reaction displaying k_1 and k_{-1} values similar to those determined in electrophysiological experiments. Other ChTX binding properties are also characteristic of those expected if the binding site is associated with Maxi-K channels. Thus, the binding reaction is sensitive to metal ions that are known to interact at various loci along the ion conduction pathway of the channel, as well as to ionic strength. Moreover, the only previously described small molecule inhibitor of the Maxi-K channel, tetraethylammonium ion, inhibits ChTX binding in a competitive fashion, whereas other K^+ channel inhibitory peptides, which have no effect on Maxi-K activity (e.g., noxiustoxin; α-dendrotoxin), do not affect [^{125}I]ChTX binding in smooth muscle. Similar data have been obtained with tracheal sarcolemmal membranes (46b). These results are summarized in Table 1, and, together, strongly suggest that ChTX receptors in smooth muscle are associated with Maxi-K channels.

Table 1. Properties of [^{125}I]ChTX Binding to Maxi-K Channels.

K_d ([^{125}I]ChTX)	100 pM
K_i (K^+)	17 μM
K_i (Ba^{2+})	12 μM
K_i (Cs^+)	100 μM
K_i (Na^+)	20 mM
K_i (TEA)	100 μM
K_i (TBA)	No effect
K_i (ChTX)	10–20 pM
K_i (IbTX)	250 pM
K_i (NxTX)	No effect
K_i (α-DaTX)	No effect

The binding properties of radiolabeled ChTX were determined using purified bovine aortic sarcolemmal membrane vesicles as described in ref. 45. TEA, tetraethylammonium; TBA, ■; NxTx, noxiustoxin; α-DaTx, α-dendrotoxin.

Therefore, [^{125}I]ChTX can be used as a biochemical monitor of the Maxi-K channel, and it should be useful in developing the molecular pharmacology of this target in smooth muscle.

Natural product screening with [^{125}I]ChTX binding in smooth muscle has revealed several interesting activities, two of which can be used to illustrate the utility of this assay. In an attempt to identify a more selective inhibitor of the Maxi-K channel, a large number of venoms from different sources (e.g., scorpion, snake, and spider species) were assayed for their ability to modulate [^{125}I]ChTX binding in aortic sarcolemma. Many activities were identified, but venom from the scorpion *Buthus tamulus* was particularly noteworthy. This extract potently inhibits the [^{125}I]ChTX binding reaction in smooth muscle membranes (47). The venom was fractionated by combined ion exchange and reversed-phase chromatography, and inhibitory activity was detected in two widely separated regions. The less basic component possessing inhibitory activity was purified to homogeneity and shown to be a 4.3 kDa peptide. The primary amino acid sequence of this material, termed iberiotoxin (IbTX), has been determined (Fig. 9). IbTX is 68% homologous with ChTX, but it has four more acidic and one less basic residue than ChTX, giving the peptide an overall net charge of +1 at physiological pH. In addition, there are many significant differences between the properties of IbTX and ChTX. IbTX does not behave as a strictly competitive inhibitor of [^{125}I]ChTX binding in sarcolemmal membranes (47).

The Maxi-K channel blocking properties of this peptide are different from those of ChTX (48) the association rate constant for IbTX (k_1) is slower than for ChTX, channel inhibition is long lasting due to a decreased k_{-1} value, and the ionic strength dependency for channel block is not as pronounced as that for ChTX. Moreover, and most importantly, IbTX is a highly selective inhibitor of the Maxi-K channel. In addition to not having an effect on a wide variety of ion channels (e.g., Na$^+$ channels, L- and T-type Ca^{2+} channels, A-type K$^+$ channels, ATP-dependent K$^+$ channels in β cells, and the *Shaker* H4 K$^+$ channel expressed in oocytes), IbTX does not block other ChTX-sensitive K$^+$ channels. These latter pathways include the ChTX-sensitive voltage-gated K$^+$ channel in human T-lymphocytes (K$_V$1.3; ref. 49) and rat brain (K$_V$1.3; ref. 50), three different small conductance Ca^{2+}-activated K$^+$ channels in human T-lymphocytes (49) and the Ca^{2+}-

ChTX

IbTX

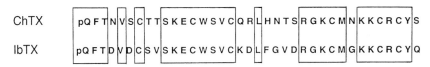

Figure 9. Homology between ChTX and IbTX. Properties of IbTX, a potent and highly selective inhibitor of the Maxi-K channel, are characterized in refs. 47 and 48. Homologous amino acid residues of ChTX and IbTX are enclosed.

activated K$^+$ channel (Gardos Channel) in human red blood cells (J. Hoffman, personal communication). To date, the Maxi-K channel is the only target identified for IbTX. This property is remarkable in light of the fact that the tertiary structure of IbTX as deduced by NMR techniques is virtually identical to that of ChTX (51). These data indicate that the selective inhibitory activity of IbTX for the Maxi-K channel correlates with specific amino acid residues in the primary structure of IbTX (52).

The discovery of IbTX provides a unique tool with which to investigate the pharmacology of the Maxi-K channel in various tissues. For example, this peptide was used to show that the role of the channel in controlling tension development of various quiescent or myogenically active smooth muscles is tissue- and species-dependent (53–55). Furthermore, experiments with IbTX reveal that various classes of K$^+$ channel agonists (e.g., cromakalim and pinacidil) do not relax smooth muscle by activating Maxi-K channels (54, 55). These data confirm findings obtained with ChTX that was also observed not to suppress the activity of a number of different K$^+$ channel agonists (56, 57). However, other mechanisms that promote smooth muscle relaxation appear to involve the Maxi-K channel. In guinea pig trachea contracted by carbachol, IbTX inhibits tissue relaxation induced by β-agonists in a concentration-dependent fashion, whereas glyburide, a blocker of ATP-dependent K$^+$ channels and an antagonist of the currently available K$^+$ channel agonists, is without effect (55). The concentration-response curves for both the β-agonists isoproterenol and salbutamol are shifted in a noncompetitive fashion by IbTX and ChTX, whereas the relaxation provoked by other agents that elevate cAMP (e.g., phosphodiesterase inhibitors, membrane permeant forms of cAMP) are competitively antagonized by these peptides (55, 57). Such data correlate with other recent findings indicating that the Maxi-K channel in airways smooth muscle is regulated by a combination of protein kinase A (58) and glutamyl transpeptidase-binding protein (59) regulatory pathways. It is noteworthy that angiotensin II receptors also appear to be coupled to Maxi-K channels in coronary artery (60), perhaps also through G-protein interactions. Together, data obtained in airways smooth muscle suggest that activation of Maxi-K channels may be associated with the clinical efficacy of β-agonists as antiasthmatic agents. Perhaps a direct-acting Maxi-K agonist would have therapeutic benefit in asthma as well.

During screening of natural products using the [^{125}I]ChTX binding assay in smooth muscle membranes, it was observed that certain fatty acids interfere with the binding reaction. When these compounds were tested in a functional assay using excised membrane patches from bovine aortic smooth muscle cells to record Maxi-K channel activity with patch-clamp techniques, it was noted that one compound with a positive effect (linoleic acid) enhanced channel activity at nM concentrations (61). In inside-out patch experiments, linoleic acid produced a marked concentration-dependent increase in the open time of Maxi-K channels with an ED$_{50}$ of ~40 nM, and this effect was fully reversible upon washout of the fatty acid. With excised outside-out membrane patches, relatively high concentrations of linoleic acid (1 to 10 μM) were required to elicit the same magnitude of agonist effect, indicating a membrane sidedness to the action of the fatty acid. The ability of this structural class to enhance Maxi-K channel activity displays a defined structure–activity relationship in that many fatty acids (e.g., stearic and palmitic), and fatty acid esters (e.g., linoleic methyl ester and linoleic propyl ester) are inactive at a test concentration of 10 μM. Unfortunately, the fatty acids that are active also affect other ion channels in the same concentration range, where they are agonists of the Maxi-K channel. For example, both Na^+ and L- and T-type Ca^{2+} channels are inhibited by 1 μM linoleic acid. These findings indicate that Maxi-K channel activity may be regulated by endogenous fatty acid or lipid constituents of the sarcolemmal membrane. In addition, they demonstrate the feasibility of using ChTX binding to detect molecules with Maxi-K channel agonist activity. However, the present agents do not display the selectivity required for the development of specific small molecule channel modulators. Screening with [^{125}I]ChTX binding in smooth muscle has continued, however, in order to identify novel selective drug-binding sites on the Maxi-K channel that may be exploited for therapeutic drug development.

Using the kind of investigations described in this chapter as a paradigm, the molecular pharmacology of any ion channel that has not previously been characterized can be developed. By identifying a single high-affinity ligand that interacts with the channel of interest, it is possible to detect molecules that bind competitively at the first site and to discover compounds that bind at other allosterically coupled sites. In this fashion, one can uncover novel structural classes of small organic molecules that alter channel activity by unique mechanisms. Such approaches can form the basis for the rationale discovery or design of therapeutically important ion channel modulators.

References

1. Catterall, W.A. (1988). Structure and function of voltage-sensitive ion channels. *Science* **242**:50–61.

2. Bean, B.P. (1989). Classes of calcium channels in vertebrate cells. *Ann. Rev. Physiol.* **51**:367–387.

3. Striessnig, J., Glossman, H., and Catterall, W.A. (1990). Identification of a phenylalkylamine binding region within the α_1-subunit of skeletal muscle calcium channels. *Proc. Natl. Acad. Sci. U.S.A.* **87**:9108–9112.

4. Nakayama, H., Taki, M., Striessnig, J., Glossman, H., Catterall, W.A., and Kanaoka, Y. (1991). Identification of 1,4-dihydropyridine binding regions within the α_1-subunit of skeletal muscle Ca^{2+} channels by photoaffinity labeling with diazipine. *Proc. Natl. Acad. Sci. U.S.A.* **88**:9203–9207.

5. Striessnig, J., Murphy, B.J., and Catterall, W.A. (1991). Dihydropyridine receptor of L-type Ca^{2+} channels: Identification of binding domains for

[^{3}H] (+)-PN200-110 and [^{3}H]azidopine within the α_1 subunit. *Proc. Natl. Acad. Sci. U.S.A.* **88**:10769–10773.

6. Triggle, D.J., and Janis, R.A. (1987). Calcium channel ligands. *Ann. Rev. Pharmacol. and Toxicol.* **28**:347–369.

7. Schwartz, A. (1989). Calcium antagonists: Review and perspective on mechanism of action. *Am. J. Cardiol.* **64**:3–91.

8. Glossmann, H., and Striessnig, J. (1990). Molecular properties of calcium channels. *Rev. Physiol. Biochem. Pharmacol.* **114**:1–105.

9. Garcia, M.L., Trumble, M.J., Reuben, J.P., and Kaczorowski, G.J. (1984). Characterization of verapamil binding sites in cardiac membrane vesicles. *J. Biol. Chem.* **259**:15013–15016.

10. Garcia, M.L., King, V.F., Siegl, P.K.S., Reuben, J.P., and Kaczorowski, G. (1986). Binding of Ca^{2+} entry blockers to cardiac sarcolemmal membrane vesicles. *J. Biol. Chem.* **261**:8146–8157.

11. King, V.F., Garcia, M.L., Shevell, J.L., Slaughter, R.S., and Kaczorowski, G.J. (1989). Substituted diphenylbutylpiperidines bind to a unique high affinity site on the L-type calcium channel. Evidence for a fourth site in the cardiac calcium entry blocker receptor complex. *J. Biol. Chem.* **264**:5633–5641.

12. Wuhan Medical College and Health Department, Wuhan Textile Factory (1979). A clinical study of the antihypertensive effect of tetrandrine. *Chin. Med. J.* **92**:193.

13. Fang, D.C., and Jiang, M.X. (1986). Studies on tetrandrine calcium antagonistic action. *Chin. Med. J.* **99**:638–644.

14. Zong, X.G., Jin, M.W., Xia, G.J., Fang, D.C., and Jiang, M.X. (1983). Effects of tetrandrine on action potential and contraction of isolated guinea pig papillary muscle. *Acta Pharmacol. Sin.* **4**:258–261.

15. Hu, W.S., Pang, X.B., Wang, Y., Hu, C.J., and Lu, F.H. (1983). Mode of action of tetrandrine on vascular smooth muscle. *J. Tradit. Chin. Med.* **3**:7–12.

16. Qian, J.Q., Thoolen, M.J.M.C., van Meel, J.C.A., Timmermans, P.B.M.W.M., and Zwieten, P.A. (1983). Hypotensive activity of tetrandrine in rats. Investigation into its mode of action. *Pharmacology* **26**:187–197.

17. Zeng, D., Shaw, D.H., Jr., and Ogilvie, R.I. (1985). Kinetic disposition and hemodynamic effects of tetrandrine in anesthetized dogs. *J. Cardiovasc. Pharmacol.* **7**:1034–1039.

18. King, V.F., Garcia, M.L., Himmel, D., Reuben, J.P., Pan, J.-X., Lam, Y.K.-K., Han, G.Q., and Kaczorowski, G.J. (1988). Interaction of tetrandrine with slowly inactivating calcium channels. Characterization of cacium channel modulation by an alkaloid of Chinese medicinal herb origin. *J. Biol. Chem.* **263**:2238–2244.

19. Felix, J.P., King, V.F., Shevell, J.L., Garcia, M.L., Kaczorowski, G.J., Bick, I.R.C., and Slaughter, R.S. (1992). Bis-benzylisoquinoline analogs of tetrandrine block L-type calcium channels; evidence for interaction at the diltiazem binding site. *Biochemistry* **31**:11793–11800.

20. Holck, H., Fischli, W., and Hengartner, U. (1984). Effects of temperature and allosteric modulators on [^{3}H] nitrendipine binding: Methods for detecting potential Ca^{2+} channel blockers. *J. Recept. Res.* **4**:557–569.

21. Rampe, D., Triggle, D.J., and Brown, A.M. (1987). Electrophysiologic and biochemical studies on the putative Ca^{2+} channel blocker MDL 12,330A in an endocrine cell. *J. Pharmacol. Exp. Ther.* **243:**402–407.

22. Garcia, M.L., King, V.F., and Kaczorowski, G.J. (1987). Interaction of KB-944 and MDL-12330A with the calcium entry blocker receptor complex in cardiac sarcolemmal membrane vesicles. *Fed. Proc.* **46:**345a.

24. Kleyman, T.R., and Cragoe, E.J., Jr. (1988). Amiloride and its analogs as tools in the study of ion transport. *J. Memb. Biol.* **105:**1–21.

25. Fraser, S., Kenny, B.A., Kilpatrick, A.T., and Spedding, M. (1988). Is fluspiriline a potential ligand for the site of action of class III calcium-antagonists. *Br. J. Pharmacol.* **94:**463P.

25. Garcia, M.L., King, V.F., Shevell, J.L., Slaughter, R.S., Suarez-Kurtz, G., Winquist, R.J., and Kaczorowski, G.J. (1990). Amiloride analogs inhibit L-type calcium channels and display calcium entry blocker activity. *J. Biol. Chem.* **265:**3763–3771.

26. Suarez-Kurtz, G., and Kaczorowski, G.J. (1989). Effects of dichlorobenzamil on calcium currents in clonal GH_3 pituitary cells. *J. Pharmacol. Exp. Ther.* **247:**248–253.

27. Kleyman, T.R., Yulo, T., Ashbaugh, C., Landry, D., Cragoe, E., Jr., Karlin, A., and Al-Awqati, Q. (1986). Photoaffinity labeling of the epithelial sodium channel. *J. Biol. Chem.* **261:**2839–2843.

28. Kleyman, T.R., Cragoe, E.J., Jr., and Kraehenbuhl, J.P. (1989). The cellular pool of Na^+ channels in the amphibian cell line A6 is not altered by mineralocorticoids. Analysis using a new photoactive amiloride analog in combination with anti-amiloride antibodies. *J. Biol. Chem.* **264:**1995–2000.

29. Siegl, P.K.S., Garcia, M.L., King, V.F., Scott, A.L., Morgan, G., and Kaczorowski, G.J. (1988). Interactions of DPI 201-106, a novel cardiotonic agent, with cardiac calcium channels. *Naunyn-Schmiedeberg's Arch. Pharmacol.* **338:**684–691.

30. Atkinson, N.S., Robertson, G.A., and Ganetzky, B. (1991). A component of calcium-activated potassium channels encoded by the *Drosophila* slo locus. *Science* **253:**551–555.

31. Adelman, J.P., Shen, K.Z., Kavanaugh, M.P., Warren, R.A., Wu, Y.N., Lagrutta, A., Bond, C.T., and North, R. (1992). Calcium-activated potassium channels expressed from cloned complementary DNAs. *Neuron* **9:**209–216.

32. Miller, C., Moczydlowski, E., Latorre, R., and Phillips, M. (1985). Charybdotoxin, a protein inhibitor of single Ca^{2+}-activated K^+ channels from mammalian skeletal muscle. *Nature* **313:**316–318.

33. Gimenez-Gallego, G., Navia, M.A., Reuben, J.P., Katz, G.M., Kaczorowski, G.J., and Garcia, M.L. (1988). Purification, sequence, and model structure of charybdotoxin, a potent selective inhibitor of calcium-activated potassium channels. *Proc. Natl. Acad. Sci. U.S.A.* **85:**3329–3333.

34. Valdivia, H.H., Smith, J.S., Martin, B.M., Coronado, R., and Possani, L.D. (1988). Charybdotoxin and noxiustoxin, two homologous peptide inhibitors of the K^+ (Ca^{2+}) channel. *FEBS Lett.* **226:**280–284.

35. Luchesi, K., Ravindran, A., Young, H., and Moczydlowski, E. (1989). Analysis of the blocking activity of charybdotoxin homologs and iodinated derivatives against Ca^{2+}-activated K^+ channels. *J. Membr. Biol.* **109:**269–281.

36. Strong, P.N., Weir, S.N., Beech, D.J., Heistand, P., and Kochner, H.P. (1989). Effects of potassium channel toxins from *Leiurus quinquestriatus hebraeus* venom on responses to cromakalim in rabbit blood vessels. *Br. J. Pharmacol.* **98**:817–826.

37. Schweitz, H., Bidard, J.N., Maes, P., and Lazdunski, M. (1989). Charybdotoxin is a new member of the K^+ channel toxin family that includes dendrotoxin I and mast cell degranulating peptide. *Biochemistry* **28**:9708–9714.

38. Sugg, E.E., Garcia, M.L., Reuben, J.P., Patchett, A.A., and Kaczorowski, G.J. (1990). Synthesis and structural characterization of charybdotoxin, a potent peptidyl inhibitor of the high conductance Ca^{2+}-activated K^+ channel. *J. Biol. Chem.* **265**:18745–18748.

39. Lambert, P., Kuroda, M., Chino, N., Watanabe, T.X., Kimura, T., and Sakakibara, S. (1990). Solution synthesis of charybdotoxin (ChTX), a K^+ channel blocker. *Biochem. Biophys. Res. Commun.* **170**:684–690.

40. Bontems, F., Roumestand, C., Boyot, P., Gilquin, B., Doljansky, Y., Menez, A., and Toma, F. (1991). Three-dimensional structure of natural charybdotoxin in aqueous solution by ^{1}H-NMR. Charybdotoxin possesses a structural motif found in other scorpion toxins. *Eur. J. Biochem.* **196**:19–28.

41. Anderson, C.S., MacKinnon, R., Smith, C., and Miller, C. (1988). Charybdotoxin block of single Ca^{2+}-activated K^+ channels. Effects of channel gating, voltage, and ionic strength. *J. Gen. Physiol.* **91**:317–333.

42. Miller, C. (1988). Competition for block of a Ca^{2+}-activated K^+ channel by charybdotoxin and tetraethylammonium. *Neuron* **1**:1003–1006.

43. MacKinnon, R., and Miller, C. (1988). Mechanism of charybdotoxin block of the high-conductance, Ca^{2+}-activated K^+ channels. *J. Gen. Physiol.* **91**:335–349.

44. MacKinnon, R., and Miller, C. (1989). Functional modification of a Ca^{2+}-activated K^+ channel by trimethyloxonium. *Biochemistry* **28**:8087–8092.

45. Vazquez, J., Feigenbaum, P., Katz, G.M., King, V.F., Reuben, J.P., Roy-Contancin, L., Slaughter, R.S., Kaczorowski, G.J., and Garcia, M.L. (1989). Characterization of high affinity binding sites for charybdotoxin in sarcolemmal membranes from bovine aortic smooth muscle. Evidence for a direct association with the high conductance calcium-activated potassium channel. *J. Biol. Chem.* **264**:20902–20909.

46a. Slaughter, R.S., Shevell, J.L., Felix, J.P., Garcia, M.L., and Kaczorowski, G.J. (1989). High levels of sodium-calcium exchange in vascular smooth muscle sarcolemmal membrane vesicles. *Biochemistry* **28**:3995–4002.

46b. Slaughter, R.S., Kaczorowski, G.J., and Garcia, M.L. (1988). Charybdotoxin binds with high affinity to a single class of sites in bovine tracheal smooth muscle sarcolemmal membrane vesicles. *J. Cell Biol.* **107**:143a.

47. Galvez, A., Gimenez-Gallego, G., Reuben, J.P., Roy-Contancin, L., Feigenbaum, P., Kaczorowski, G.J., and Garcia, M.L. (1990). Purification and characterization of a unique, potent, peptidyl probe for the high conductance calcium-activated potassium channel from venom of the scorpion *Buthus tamulus*. *J. Biol. Chem.* **265**:11083–11090.

48. Giangiacomo, K., Garcia, M.L., and McManus, O.B. (1992). Mechanism of iberiotoxin block of the large-conductance calcium-activated potassium channel from bovine aortic smooth muscle. *Biochemistry* **31**:6719–6727.

49. Leonard, R.J., Garcia, M.L., Slaughter, R.S., and Reuben, J.P. (1992). Selective blockers of voltage-gated K[+] channels depolarize human T lymphocytes: Mechanism of the antiproliferative effect of charybdotoxin. *Proc. Natl. Acad. Sci. U.S.A.* **89**:10094–10098.

50. Vazquez, J., Feigenbaum, P., King, V.F., Kaczorowski, G.J., and Garcia, M.L. (1990). Characterization of high affinity binding sites for charybdotoxin in synaptic plasma membranes from rat brain. Evidence for a direct association with an inactivating, voltage-dependent, potassium channel. *J. Biol. Chem.* **265**:15564–15571.

51. Johnson, B., and Sugg, E.E. (1992). Determination of the three-dimensional structure of iberiotoxin in solution by ^{1}H nuclear magnetic resonance spectroscopy. *Biochemistry* **35**:8151–8159.

52. Giangiacomo, K., Sugg, E.E., Garcia-Calvo, M., Leonard, R.J., McManus, O.B., Kaczorowski, G.J., and Garcia, M.L. (1993). Synthetic charybdotoxin-iberiotoxin chimeric peptides define toxin binding sites on calcium-activated and voltage-dependent potassium channels. *Biochemistry*, in press.

53. Suarez-Kurtz, G., Garcia, M.L., and Kaczorowski, G. (1991). Effects of charybdotoxin and iberiotoxin on the spontaneous motility and tonus of different guinea pig smooth muscle tissues. *J. Pharmacol. Exp. Ther.* **259**:439–443.

54. Grant, T.L., and Zuzack, J.S. (1991). Effects of K[+] channel blockers and cromakalim (BRL34915) on the mechanical activity of guinea pig detrusor smooth muscle. *J. Pharmacol. Exp. Ther.* **259**:1158–1164.

55. Jones, T.R., Charette, L., Garcia, M.L., and Kaczorowski, G.J. (1993). Interaction of iberiotoxin with β adrenoceptor agonists and sodium nitroprusside on guinea pig trachea. *J. Applied Physiol.*, in press.

56. Winquist, R.J., Heaney, L.A., Wallace, A.A., Baskin, E.P., Stein, R.B., Garcia, M.L., and Kaczorowski, G.J. (1989). Glyburide blocks the relaxation response to BRL34915 (cromakalim), minoxidil sulfate and diazoxide in vascular smooth muscle. *J. Pharmacol. Exp. Ther.* **248**:149–156.

57. Jones, T.R., Charette, L., Garcia, M.L., and Kaczorowski, G.J. (1990). Selective inhibition of relaxation of guinea-pig trachea by charybdotoxin, a potent Ca^{2+}-activated K[+] channel inhibitor. *J. Pharmacol. Exp. Ther.* **255**:697–706.

58. Kume, H., Takai, A., Tokuno, H., and Tomita, T. (1989). Regulation of Ca^{2+}-dependent K[+]-channel activity in tracheal myocytes by phosphorylation. *Nature* **341**:152-154.

59. Kume, H., Graziano, M.P., and Kotlikoff, M.I. (1992). Stimulatory and inhibitory regulation of calcium-activated potassium channels by guanine nucleotide binding proteins. *Proc. Natl. Acad. Sci. U.S.A.* **89**:11051–11055.

60. Toro, L., Amador, M., and Stefani, E. (1990). ANG II inhibits calcium-activated potassium channels from coronary smooth muscle in lipid bilayers. *Am. J. Physiol.* **258**:H912–H915.

61. Katz, G., Roy-Contancin, L., Bale, T., and Reuben, J.P. (1990). Arachidonic, linoleic, and other unsaturated fatty acids enhance K[+] and depress Na[+] and Ca^{2+} channel activity. *Biophys. J.* **57**:506a.

25

The Design of New Calcium Antagonists

S. David Kimball, Joel C. Barrish, John T. Hunt,
David M. Floyd, Jack Z. Gougoutas, and Wan F. Lau

At the time we began our medicinal chemistry research program in the 1980s, diltiazem (structure 1) was becoming increasingly popular among physicians for the treatment of angina and hypertension. The popularity of this drug was due in large part to a relative lack of side effects in patients taking this calcium channel blocker. However, the therapeutic profile of diltiazem is still far from ideal (1). It lacks potency both as an antihypertensive agent and as a calcium channel blocker in vitro, particularly when compared with the dihydropyridine class of calcium channel blockers. Importantly, diltiazem is rapidly and extensively metabolized to a number of products in man, all of which are less potent calcium channel blockers (2, 3).

We believed that the combination of safety and efficacy in the clinic made diltiazem an attractive target for improvement and set as a goal the development of potent diltiazem-like antihypertensives that are sufficiently metabolically stable to be allowed administration once a day. In order to discover and develop a new agent fitting these requirements, we had to understand the structure–activity relationships of diltiazem (i.e., determine which parts of its relatively complex structure are important to activity) and how these are arranged in space. Unfortunately, almost no information of this kind was available; very few benzothiazepinone analogs of diltiazem had every been synthesized. A major reason for this lack relates to idiosyncracies of the synthetic chemistry involved. The chemistry used in the preparation of diltiazem cannot be used to prepare benzothiazepinone analogs necessary to establish coherent structure–activity relationships. This was our first challenge: to discover a novel series of compounds that bind to the same site on the calcium channel as diltiazem. It was also important that analogs of these diltiazem-like compounds could be easily synthesized.

The approach we used to discover and develop calcium channel blockers that bind like diltiazem is illustrated in Fig. 1. When the sulfur atom of diltiazem (in box) is replaced by carbon, a new series of compounds

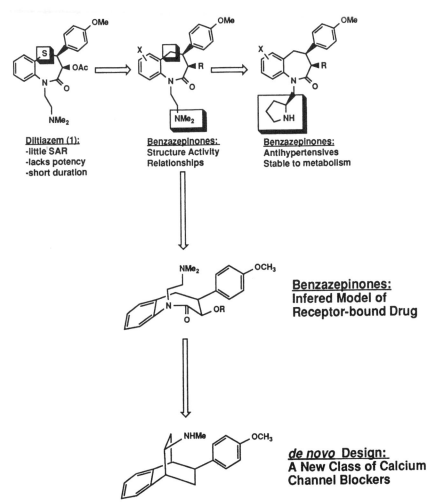

Figure 1. Research strategy. SAR, structure–activity relationship.

analogous to diltiazem is obtained. These benzazepinones were unknown compounds, and we had to work out their synthesis from scratch. Key to the success of the work that followed was the fact that *unlike diltiazem, the synthesis of benzazepinones is general.* Once we had worked out the synthetic chemistry, we could prepare analogs at will. This enabled us to elaborate the structure–activity relationships of benzazepinones; this information was then used to develop benzazepinone analogs of diltiazem that fit our requirements. The discovery of the benzazepine CCBs, their synthesis, and their structure–activity relationships have been described in detail (4, 5).

Figure 1 also illustrates a different, nonclassical approach to drug discovery that confronts the question that is the focus of this chapter: *how does one design a drug to a receptor of unknown structure?* This approach starts from the body of structure–activity relationships that has been obtained from the benzazepinone series. Assuming that the closely related series of benzazepinones bind to the channel receptor protein in the same fashion, we first define the critical pharmacophores and stereochemistry of the molecule that are required for activity. Then, we prepare a series of constrained analogs that help us to define and test hypotheses regarding the receptor-bound conformation of these drugs. Eventually, this process should provide enough information for us to design structurally novel calcium channel blockers that bind to the same site on the calcium channel.

Summarizing our approach (Fig. 1), we mapped out a 2-fold strategy for the discovery of diltiazem-like calcium channel blockers. The first goal was to discover a potent, antihypertensive benzazepine that is stable to metabolism (4). Second, we hoped to use the structure–activity information obtained in achieving the first goal to infer a model of the receptor-bound conformation of the drugs.

From the hypotheses that we generated, we designed structurally distinct diltiazem mimics of comparable potency (6, 7). The binding model that we have established also provides insight into the interaction of desmethoxyverapamil with the calcium channel.

Structure–Activity Relationship Overview

Before proceeding with the receptor-binding model and the design of new molecules, we needed to gain a general understanding of benzazepinone structure–activity relationships (Fig. 2). Our goal here was to distill out only those structural features of diltiazem essential to its activity as a calcium channel blocker. We found that the stereochemistry at C3 and C4 is important to calcium channel blocking activity, and is analogous to the preferred stereochemistry of diltiazem (8). The benzazepinones competi-

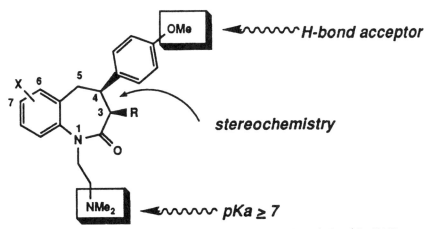

Figure 2. Key features of benzazepinone structure–activity relationship (SAR).

tively displace radiolabeled diltiazem from cardiac and skeletal muscle preparations in vitro; by this criteria they mimic diltiazem exactly.

Figure 2 also highlights (boxes) the two crucial requirements for calcium channel blocking activity. Deletion of either of these pharmacophores ablates activity in vitro and in vivo. First, a basic amino substituent with a $pK_a \geq 7$ must be appended to the N1 nitrogen of the benzazepinone ring. The optimal distance from N1 to the basic amino group is two carbon atoms. Second, the aryl methyl ether is required for activity. From analog studies, it appears that this substituent functions as a hydrogen bond acceptor at the receptor binding site. Analogs in which the hydrogen bond acceptor capability is reduced show diminished activity as calcium channel blockers, and any substantial modification of this substituent leads to a loss of activity.

Once the structural criteria shown in Fig. 2 are satisfied, a wide variety of benzazepinone modifications provide analogs that possess good calcium channel blocking activity. In analyzing the data, we found that the ability of a benzazepinone to relax aortic strips in vitro was highly correlated with the lipophilicity of the compound. Figure 3 shows the relationship derived for a large number of substituents at C3, C6, and C7: activity in vitro is highly dependent on the partition coefficient (P) of the compound. Our interpretation of this result is that the binding site for the benzazepinones

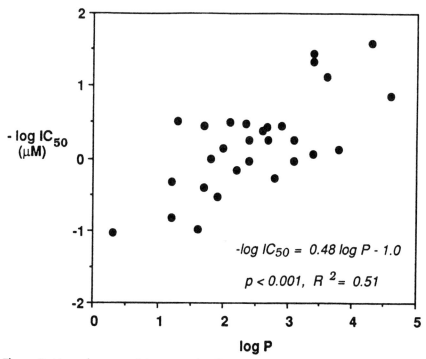

Figure 3. Vasorelaxant activity versus log P.

(and by inference, diltiazem) requires that the molecule partition into the cell membrane. If this is true, then greater partitioning of these drugs into the membrane (increased log P) should translate directly into increased activity in vitro. By enhancing the lipophilicity (log P) of a benzazepinone we can increase its concentration in the lipid membrane phase where the calcium channel is located, and thereby increase its activity. From this type of modification to structure, we concluded that substitution of R and X (Fig. 2) primarily affects delivery of the drug to its target. A detailed overview of these structure–activity relationships has been published (5).

At this point, the structure–activity studies resulted in a greatly simplified picture of diltiazem binding. It appears that only two functional groups on the molecule are essential for calcium channel blocking activity: the hydrogen bond acceptor and a basic nitrogen. The rest of this relatively complicated molecule may thus serve primarily as scaffolding, holding the two simple pharmacophores in the proper spatial arrangement. As we shall see, this has important implications for de novo design.

Receptor Binding Model

Statement of the Problem

Understanding that the benzazepinones require two pharmacophores to express calcium channel blocking activity is not enough for design purposes. Figure 4 shows a prototypical benzazepinone that has all the struc-

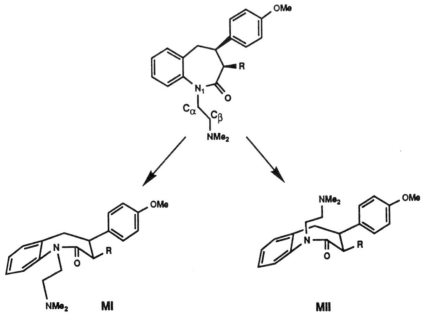

Figure 4. Possible binding modes.

tural prerequisites for activity. However, the exact position of the basic nitrogen pharmacophore relative to the methyl ether hydrogen bond acceptor has not been defined. Free rotation about the N_1—C_α and C_α—C_β bonds allows the two pharmacophores to be oriented in two quite distinct binding modes: MI and MII. In the MI conformation, the dimethylamino group is extended as far from the methoxyphenyl pharmacophore as possible, and lies underneath the plane formed by the benzazepinone amide group. An alternative conformation, MII, has the basic dimethylamino group over the benzazepinone ring and quite close to the methoxyphenyl pharmacophore. In order to arrive at a point where we can design new calcium channel blockers related to the benzazepinones and benzothiazepinones, we first needed to determine which binding mode best describes receptor-bound structure.

Both MI and MII have favorable low-energy conformations. X-ray crystallography has determined that benzazepinones and benzothiazepinones crystallize in both conformations. Figure 5 compares the x-ray crystal structure of compounds in both the MI and MII conformations. On the left is the structure of diltiazem, as determined in our laboratories. The sulfur atom in the benzothiazepine ring is yellow, and the blue nitrogen atom is below the plane of the amide and extended away from the ring. This MI conformation is contrasted with a 3-ethyl substituted benzazepinone (structure 2) in which the pharmacophores are oriented in the MII binding mode (Fig. 5, structure on right). In the MII conformation, the basic nitrogen (blue) can clearly be seen to lie above the plane of the benzazepine amide and near the methoxyphenyl pharmacophore.

Figures 6 to 8 further illustrate the ambiguous spatial relationship between the basic nitrogen and methyl ether pharmacophores. Figure 6 shows the crystal structure of a 3-methyl substituted benzazepinone (structure 3) that crystallizes in the MI conformation. In Figure 7 we have used molecular modeling to map out all possible positions of the basic nitrogen group, when free rotation is allowed around the $N1$—C_α and C_α—C_β bonds of the side chain. The possible positions of the nitrogen sweep out a surface, which describes all conceivable loci of the basic nitrogen atom. However, we can simplify this picture, because many of these locations are very high-energy conformations due to steric crowding between neighboring atoms. Figure 8 shows the nitrogen loci that correspond to the available low-energy conformations of the basic nitrogen, as determined by molecular modeling. The set of points shown in Fig. 8 approximate the conformations of structure 3 that probably exist in solution. As illustrated in Fig. 4, these positions of the basic nitrogen correspond to MI- and MII-type conformations.

The Solution: Preparation of Conformationally Constrained Analogs

In order to solve this problem we have to limit the conformations occupied by the basic nitrogen and correlate these with activity. By synthesiz-

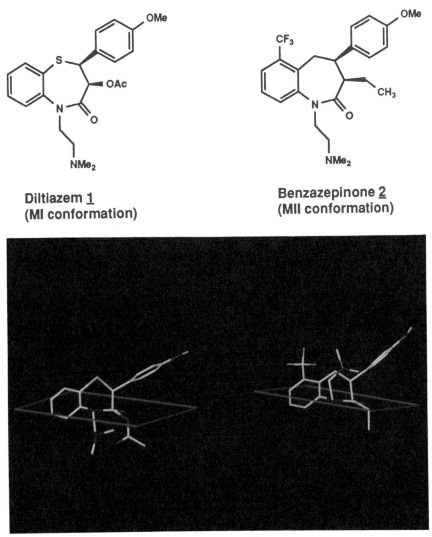

Diltiazem 1
(MI conformation)

Benzazepinone 2
(MII conformation)

Figure 5. X-ray structures illustrating MI and MII conformations.

ing a series of molecules that constrain the nitrogen pharmacophore to a few orientations in space, we hoped to eventually pin down the preferred receptor-bound conformation for all benzazepinones. Scheme 1 shows the preparation of one such benzazepinone (structure **4**) in which the dimethylamino group is appended to a six-membered ring. This compound is active as a calcium channel blocker. Therefore, it must be able to access a conformation adequate for binding to the receptor.

Figures 9 to 11 show the allowed conformations of this compound (structure **4**). The x-ray crystal structure of *trans* cyclohexyl benzazepinone

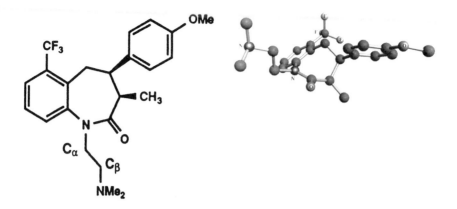

Benzazepinone 3

Figure 6. X-ray structure of **3**.

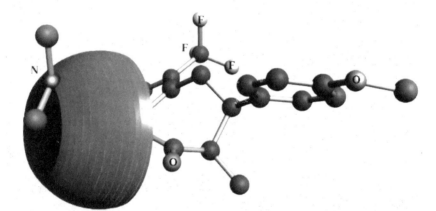

Figure 7. Possible loci of basic nitrogen—benzazepinone **3**.

is shown in Fig. 9. The *trans* substitution on the cyclohexyl ring places both substituents in an equatorial orientation; relative to each other they are *gauche*. It is structurally impossible for the basic amine to be oriented in the MI conformation shown by diltiazem (Fig. 5), because the substituents would then have to be *trans* diaxial to each other. The fact that this compound is a potent calcium channel blocker eliminates the extended MI conformation as a possibility for the receptor-bound conformation. Rotation about the N_1—C_α bond (Fig. 10) generates a torus of possible loci for the amine relative to the methyl ether pharmacophore. As in the previous example, only a subset of these loci are energetically allowable, due to steric crowding. These low-energy conformations are shown in Fig. 11. The active receptor-bound structure of these benzazepinones must be defined by this small subset of conformations. Thus, the preparation of a single

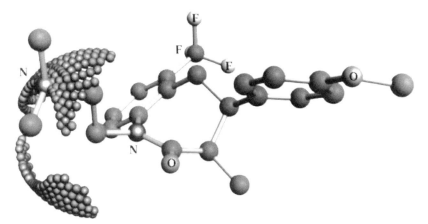

Figure 8. Energetically favorable loci of basic nitrogen—benzazepinone **3**.

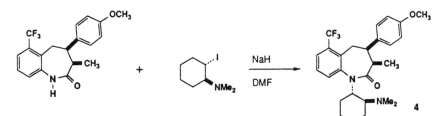

Scheme 1. Synthesis of racemic 3-methyl benzazepinone.

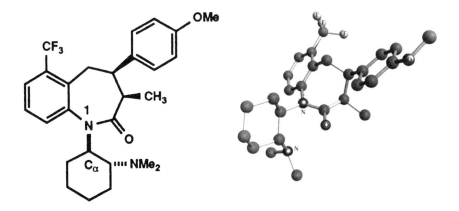

Benzazepinone 4

Figure 9. Conformationally locked cyclohexyl analog **4**.

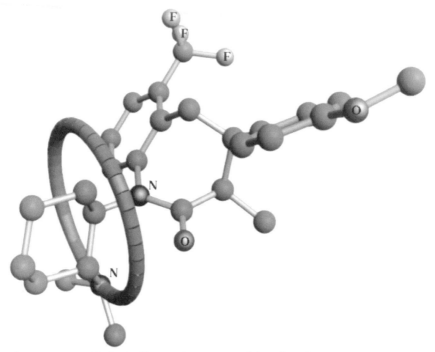

Figure 10. Possible loci of basic nitrogen—cyclohexyl analog **4.**

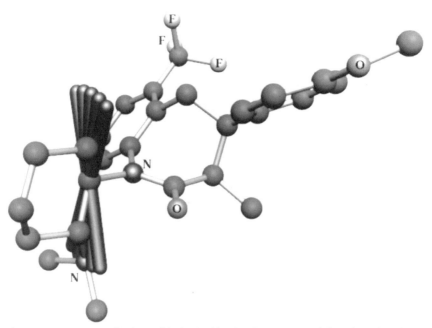

Figure 11. Energetically favorable loci of basic nitrogen—cyclohexyl analog **4.**

analog has simplified the picture enormously; most of the energetically possible conformations of Fig. 8 have now been eliminated from contention as possible active conformations of diltiazem.

We continued to apply this approach by preparing constrained benzazepinone analogs. Some of these compounds, along with their synthesis, are shown in Scheme 2.

The constraints introduced by comparison of structures **5** and **6** is instructive (Fig. 12). The top structure shows the more active analog, compound **5**. ($IC_{50} = 0.32$ μM), in its most favorable (lowest energy by modeling) MII conformation. The nitrogen atom of the pyrrolidinyl ring (purple) is colored in blue. We have drawn a plane through the three atoms that comprise the amide bond. Compound **6** is relatively inactive ($IC_{50} = 3.8$ μM). When compound **6** is oriented with its basic nitrogen in the same MII conformation as compound **5** (Fig. 12, bottom), it corresponds to an unfavorable high-energy conformation. This is because the carbon adjacent to the basic nitrogen is in the plane of the benzazepinone amide. The

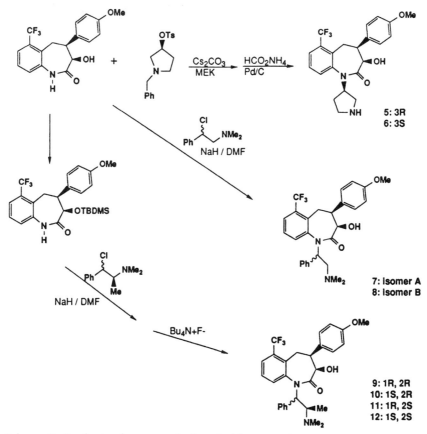

Scheme 2. Synthesis of nonracemic 3-methyl benzazepinone.

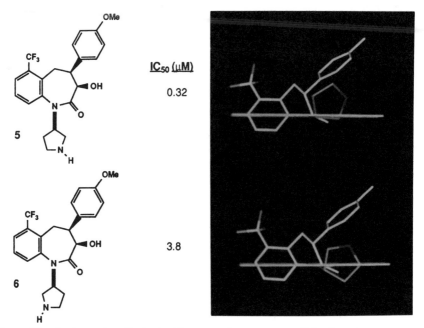

IC$_{50}$ (µM)

0.32

3.8

Figure 12. Conformationally locked benzazepinones—pyrrolidinyl analogs.

subsequent steric crowding makes the MII conformation for structure **6** highly unfavorable. Because the active compound **5** can exist in the MII conformation, but inactive compound **6** cannot, we conclude that the conformation of structure **5** represents something close to the receptor-bound orientation of benzazepinones.

Table 1 shows substitutions of additional compounds we synthesized in a constraint analysis of the position of basic nitrogen. Without going into extensive detail, we can state that all of the active benzazepinones we prepared are able to access the MII binding mode in a low-energy conformation by molecular modeling (manuscript in preparation). Conversely, compounds that cannot access the MII conformation (by modeling) due to steric constraints are relatively inactive. All of our structural and computational studies are therefore consistent with this conclusion: *MII is a close approximation to the receptor-bound conformation of benzazepinones and benzothiazepinones.* In Fig. 13, we illustrate this putative receptor-bound conformation of the diltiazem mimics. The red dot surface represents the van der Waals radius of the methyl ether oxygen atom (hydrogen bond acceptor), whereas the blue dot surface illustrates that of the basic nitrogen pharmacophore. The picture that it presents of the two key pharmacophores, closely juxtaposed and pointing in the same direction, also fits our intuitive sense of how the binding site might be organized. This model is also consistent with the structure–activity relationships we obtained through analysis of a large series of analogs: the key pharmacophores point in one

Table 1. Activity of N1-substituted Benzazepinones In Vitro and In Vivo.

Compound	R₁	R₂	log P (estimated)*	IC₅₀ (μM)†	Kd (μM)‡
3 (±)	Me	[NMe₂]	3.6	0.076 (0.041–0.14)	0.075 ± 0.043
4 (±)	Me	[cyclohexyl NMe₂]	4.5	0.38 (0.22–0.67)	0.39§
5	OH	[pyrrolidinyl NH]	0.93	0.32 (0.19–0.5)	0.24 ± 0.14
6	OH	[pyrrolidinyl NH]	0.93	3.8 (2.2–6.4)	1.8 ± 0.38
7 (isomer A)	OH	[Ph NMe₂]	6.2	0.48 (0.34–0.68)	1.1§
8 (isomer B)	OH	[Ph NMe₂]	4.3	0.34 (0.24–0.50)	0.24§
9	OH	[Me Ph NMe₂]	3.8	0.18 (0.12–0.26)	0.037§
10	OH	[Me Ph NMe₂]	3.0	0.34 (0.23–0.52)	0.17§
11	OH	[Ph Me NMe₂]	—	0.43 (0.27–0.67)	0.50 ± 0.23
12	OH	[Me Ph NMe₂]	4.0	0.51 0.24–1.1)	0.25 ± 0.018

*Log P estimated by reverse-phase high-performance liquid chromatography as described in ref 4.

†IC₅₀ in rabbit aorta strips contracted with KCl (95% confidence interval).

‡Kd determined by displacement of radiolabeled diltiazem in guinea pig–striated muscle (±SEM).

§Based on concentration-effect curve using one animal.

direction toward the receptor, while the scaffolding of the benzazepinone ring is pointed away from these binding interactions. Further, we recall that a variety of substitutions on the scaffolding portion (the benzazepinone ring) have no effect on binding affinity per se, but only affect delivery of the molecule to its receptor.

This simple spatial relationship between these two pharmacophores is clearly not obvious from inspection of the structure of diltiazem. The

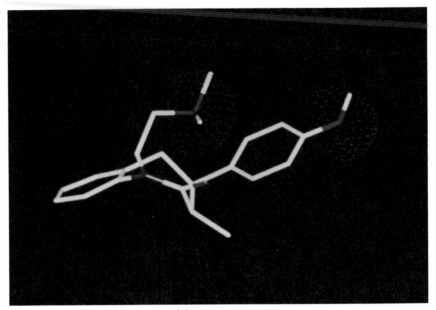

Figure 13. Receptor binding model MII.

orientation of the basic nitrogen and the methyl aryl ether is identical to that of 3-methoxy phenylethylamine. Thus, our conclusion regarding the receptor-bound conformation of diltiazem and its benzazepinone analogs is as follows: *these compounds are nothing more than structurally complex mimics of 3-methoxy phenylethylamine!*

De Novo Design of Novel Diltiazem Mimics

Figure 14 illustrates the route we have traveled. Beginning with benzazepinone structure–activity studies, we have deduced that the receptor-bound conformation of these molecules corresponds to the MII binding mode, and mimics the structure of 3-methoxy phenylethylamine. The next step in testing the binding hypothesis was the preparation of molecules that are locked into the MII conformation by virtue of their carbon skeleton. Compounds with a constrained structure, such as structures **13** and **14** (Fig. 14), represent tests of the MII binding mode hypothesis.

The x-ray crystal structure of compound **14** (Fig. 15) shows how it is physically constrained in the MII conformation. Figure 15 also depicts structure **14** overlaid on the MII receptor-bound conformation model. The exact alignment of the pharmacophores is easily seen in this comparison. The series of compounds related to structure **14** were designed to minimize structural differences with the benzazepinones, to "freeze out" the desired pharmacophore relationship. This makes it easier to relate experimentally determined activity solely to the presence of the MII conformation.

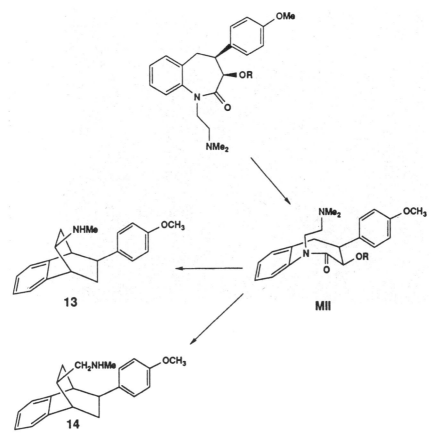

Figure 14. Mimics of dilitiazem—de novo design.

The activity in vitro of two of the series of novel diltiazem mimics is presented in Table 2. Based on K_d and IC_{50} values, these compounds are equipotent to unsubstituted benzazepinones or diltiazem in vitro. These compounds also show activity superior to diltiazem in a Langendorff model of ischemia (manuscript in preparation).

The structure–activity relationships governing activity of diltiazem-like compounds have been worked out earlier, so we expect that they could be applied directly to this series. Most immediately, we should be able to enhance activity significantly by increasing the lipophilicity (log P) of these novel compounds.

Relationship Between Diltiazem and Desmethoxyverapamil

Figure 16 illustrates the allosteric interactions between the three calcium channel blockers that have been studied in the greatest detail. Diltiazem and the benzazepinones bind uniquely to the DTZ site, which is alloste-

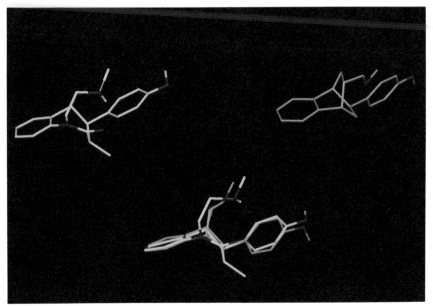

Figure 15. Fit of compound **14** to receptor binding model MII.

rically coupled to both the phenylalkylamine (PAA) and dihydropyridine (DHP) sites. Desmethoxyverapamil has been extensively studied as the prototype PAA ligand. Although the allosteric interactions between the three binding sites are complex, there are unique characteristics that allow one to differentiate between compounds that bind to each of them.

In spite of the fact that desmethoxyverapamil is taken as the prototype PAA ligand, it remains somewhat of a curiosity. Several studies have described the potentiation of DHP binding by desmethoxyverapamil (9, 10), a characteristic otherwise attributable only to ligands that bind at the diltiazem site. Other work has shown that desmethoxyverapamil behaves as a typical PAA ligand, having a negative heterotropic allosteric effect on DHP binding (11). This ambiguity led us to wonder for a long time whether there might be some structural similarity between desmethoxyverapamil and diltiazem. Figure 17 shows how the receptor-bound conformation of diltiazem (MII conformation) mimics a substructure of desmethoxyverapamil, namely 3-methoxy phenylethylamine. Figure 18 further shows how desmethoxyverapamil (as modified from the x-ray structure of verapamil) fits our receptor-binding model for diltiazem. From this compelling structural analogy, it is a short step to postulate that desmethoxyverapamil might actually bind to *both* the PAA site and the DTZ site on the calcium channel. This could explain the anomalous binding results noted previously.

From our knowledge of benzazepinone structure–activity relationships, we further postulate that desmethoxyverapamil should be the *only* PAA that can bind to the DTZ site. We have established (5) that the

Table 2. Novel Diltiazem Mimics: Activity In Vitro

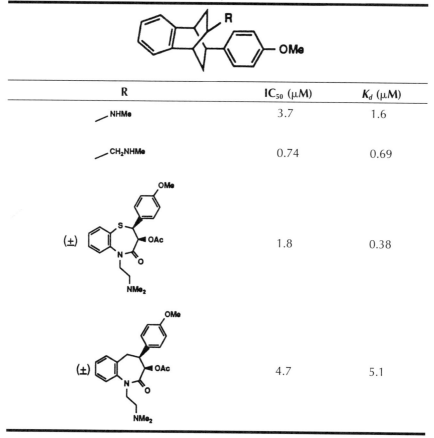

R	IC$_{50}$ (μM)	K$_d$ (μM)
NHMe	3.7	1.6
CH$_2$NHMe	0.74	0.69
($\pm$) [benzothiazepinone structure]	1.8	0.38
($\pm$) [benzazepinone structure]	4.7	5.1

3′,4′-dimethoxy substituted benzazepinone, which would be analogous to verapamil (3,4-dimethoxy substitution), is completely inactive as a calcium channel blocker. Therefore, the two other popular PAA ligands—verapamil and its 3,4,5-trimethoxy analog (D-600)—could not bind to the DTZ site. As luck would have it, desmethoxyverapamil is unique in this respect. We now have evidence (see chapter 23) that the DTZ binding site is accessible from the outside of the cell. This distinguishes it from the PAA binding site, which is believed to be intracellular. The different locations of these two binding sites allows for an experimental test of this hypothesis, which is now in progress.

Summary

In this chapter, we show that it is possible to use structure–activity relationships of benzazepinones to discover structurally novel series of

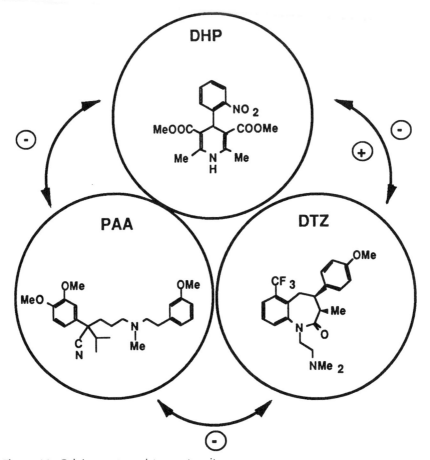

Figure 16. Calcium antagonist receptor sites.

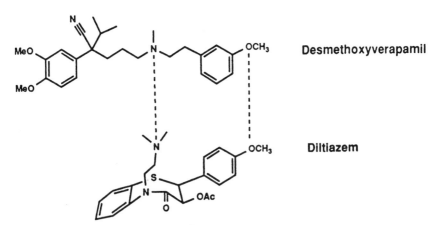

Desmethoxyverapamil

Diltiazem

Figure 17. A common binding mode?

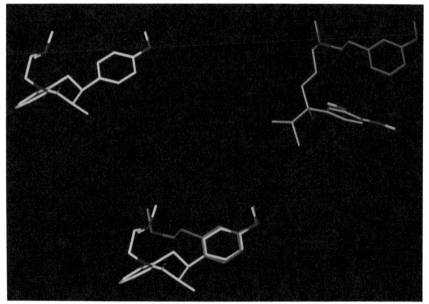

Figure 18. Fit of desmethoxyverapamil to receptor binding model MII.

calcium antagonists By determining the key pharmacophores responsible for activity of the benzazepinones and constraining them in space, we have developed a receptor-binding model for diltiazem-like drugs. This model has been successfully used to design a new series of rigid calcium channel blockers. The design of further series of compounds, based on the receptor-binding model, is limited only by the imagination.

Acknowledgments

The synthesis of constrained benzazepinone calcium channel blockers was conducted in part by V.G. Lee. The preparation of the novel constrained benzazepinone mimics was conducted by S. Spergel. X-ray crystallographic studies were conducted by M. Malley in the lab of Dr. J. Gougoutas. Dr. J.Z. Gougoutas also developed much of the computational and graphical software that was used in this work.

References

1. Buckley, M., Grant, S., Goa, K., McTavish, D., and Sorkin, E. (1990). Diltiazem: A Reappraisal of its pharmacological properties and therapeutic use. *Drugs* **39:**757–806.

2. Schoemaker, H., Hicks, P., and Langer, S. (1987). Calcium channel receptor binding studies for diltiazem and its major metabolites: Functional correlation to inhibition of portal vein myogenic activity. *J. Cardiovasc. Pharm.* **9:**173–180.

3. Sugihara, J., Sugawara, Y., Ando, H., Harigaya, S., Etoh, A., and Kohno, K. (1984). Studies on the metabolism of diltiazem in man. *J. Pharm. Dyn.* **7:**24–32.

4. Floyd, D., Kimball, S.D., Krapcho, J., Das, J., Turk, C., Moquin, R., Lago, M., Duff, K., Lee, V., White, R., Ridgewell, R., Moreland, S., Brittain, R., Normandin, D., Hedberg, A., and Cucinotta, G. (1992). Benzazepinone calcium channel blockers. 2. Structure–activity and drug metabolism studies leading to potent antihypertensive agents. Comparison with benzo-thiazepinones. *J. Med. Chem.* **35:**756–772.

5. Kimball, S.D., Floyd, D., Das, J., Hunt, J., Krapcho, J., Rovnyak, G., Duff, K., Lee, V., Moquin, R., Turk, C., Hedberg, A., Moreland, S., Brittain, R., McMullen, D., Normandin, D., and Cucinotta, G. (1992). Benzazepinone calcium channel blockers. 4. Structure–activity overview and intracellular binding site. *J. Med. Chem.* **35:**780–793.

6. Barrish, J., Spergel, S., Moreland, S., and Hedberg, A. (1992). The synthesis of a conformationally rigid calcium channel blocker. *Bioorg. Med. Chem. Lett.* **2:**95–98.

7. Kimball, S.D., Floyd, D., Barrish, J., Das, J., Hunt, J., Krapcho, J., Rovnyak, G., Duff, K., Lago, M., Lee, V., Moquin, R., Spergel, S., Gougoutas, J., Malley, M., Pudzianowski, A., Flaim, S., Moreland, S., Hedberg, A., and White, R. (1992). *Structure Activity Studies and Receptor Binding Model of 1-Benzazepin-2-one Calcium Antagonists. Trends Med. Chem. '90.* (Blackwell, Oxford), pp. 271–276.

8. Nagao, T., Sato, M., Nakajima, H., and Kiyomoto, A. (1972). Studies on a new 1,5-benzothiazepine derivative (CRD-401). II. Vasodilator actions. *Japan. J. Pharmacol.* **22:**1–10.

9. Reynolds, I., Snowman, A., and Snyder, S. (1986). (–)-^{3}[H] Desmethoxyverapamil labels multiple calcium channel modulator receptors in brain and skeletal muscle membranes: Differentiation by temperature and dihydropyridines. *J. Pharm. Exp. Ther.* **237:**731–738.

10. Striessnig, J., Goll, A., Moosburger, K., and Glossmann, H. (1986). Purified calcium channels have three allosterically coupled drug receptors. *FEBS Lett.* **197:**204–210.

11. Ruth, P., Flockerzi, V., Von Nettelbladt, E., Oeken, J., and Hofmann, F. (1985). Characterization of the binding sites for nimodipine and (–)-desmethoxyverapamil in bovine cardiac sarcolemma. *Eur. J. Biochem.* **150:**313–322.

26

Inhibitors of Cardiac-Delayed Rectifying Potassium Currents as Potential Novel Antiarrhythmic Agents

William C. Lumma, Jr.

Cardiac-delayed rectifier K^+ currents (I_K) play a major role in repolarization following the depolarizing action potential. In vitro blockade of these currents is manifest as an increase in action potential duration (APD) of single-cell recordings of conducting tissue (Purkinje fiber), or atrial and ventricular myocytes (VMs). This effect is usually measured as a particular degree (percentage) of repolarization (e.g., APD_{95}). Selective I_K blockade does not affect maximum upstroke velocity ($\dot{V}_{max}$). Extracellular recordings during premature stimulation reflect an increase in the effective refractory period (ERP) and functional refractory period (FRP). In vivo, I_K blockers prolong the QT interval of the surface electrocardiogram. These effects may be antiarrhythmic by blocking premature stimulation of cardiac tissue by reentrant beats caused by circulating wavefronts around functional (ischemic) or anatomical obstacles. They may also be proarrhythmic by extensively prolonging repolarization, which can lead to early after-depolarizations, or triggered arrhythmias.

K^+-Delayed Rectifier Channels

The delayed rectifier current has been shown to be a sum of slowly activating I_{KS} and rapidly activating (I_{KR}) currents in guinea pig atrial and VMs (1). Most class III antiarrhythmic agents (AAs), defined as agents that increase APD, have been shown to block primarily I_{KR}. The role of I_{KS} in human myocardium has not been established. The channel responsible for I_{KS} is believed to be a relatively small [human, 129 amino acids (2)] protein that has a long time constant (>7.5 sec in guinea pig atria). The potential for selective blockers of I_{KS} to limit tachycardia without causing bradycardia in normal sinus rhythm is an important topic for further research.

K$^+$ channel-blocking effects of experimental Vaughan Williams class III AAs have been reviewed (3). Efficacy of these agents in preclinical models of reentrant arrhythmias has also been reviewed (4). General chemical structure of class III AAs is shown in Fig. 1.

The major factors in development of a safe and effective K$^+$ channel blocking agent for treatment of arrhythmias are:

1. High affinity for cardiac K$^+$ channels.
2. Efficient uptake into cardiac tissues.
3. Balanced effects in normal and diseased cardiac tissues to normalize dispersion of refractoriness.
4. Efficacy in reentrant arrhythmia models.
5. Low incidence of proarrhythmia in models of changing and stable rates of premature ventricular contractions (PVCs).
6. Proper choice of models (species) to represent the role of K$^+$ channels correctly in repolarization of human myocardium.
7. Lack of side effects caused by actions on K$^+$ channels in other tissues and/or control of physicochemical properties to exclude compound from noncardiac tissues (e.g., central nervous system).
8. Oral bioavailability with constant plasma levels.

Physicochemical properties such as basicity (pK$_a$), lipophilicity(log P), and serum albumin binding can be correlated with parameters measured to

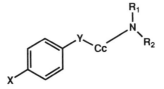

X = <u>CLASS III Pharmacophore</u> ; e.g. : CH$_3$SO$_2$NH - , -NO$_2$; -CN ;

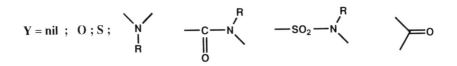

Cc = 2 - 4 ATOM <u>Connecting Chain</u> (Optionally part of a ring)

R1 , R2 = SUBSTITUENTS which control Physicochemical Properties

Figure 1. General structure of class III AAs.

establish trends to optimize potential therapeutic profile, but there exists no report of such a systematic study.

The general structure of many class III AAs is similar to that of class I agents (see Fig. 1). Procainamide, structure **1**, is a class I agent (Na$^+$ channel blocker) that is reversibly acetylated in rapid acetylator phenotype patients to the class III AA acecainide, structure **2**. This fact was the basis for design of the class III AA sematilide, structure **3**, which has no effect on maximum upstroke velocity (Na$^+$ channel) of action potentials in cardiac tissue, no conduction blocking effects, and no efficacy in models of spontaneous arrhythmia [Harris dog (5)]. The apparent efficacy of sematilide in man to reduce PVC frequency (6) probably reflects the fact that a fraction of PVCs (e.g., coupled beats) are actually reentrant arrhythmias (Fig. 2).

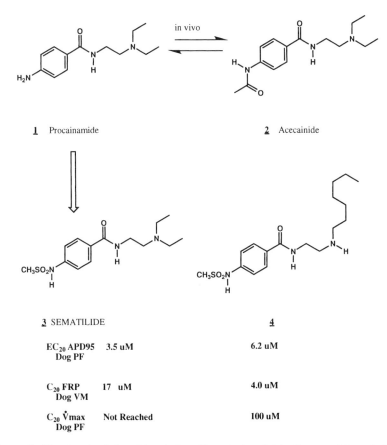

Figure 2. Structural relationship of class III and class I AAs (benzamide series). PF, Purkinje fiber.

Patients susceptible to reentrant arrhythmias are diagnosed during cardiac catheterization using electrodes to deliver premature stimuli that induce tachycardia [i.e., programmed electrical stimulation (PES)]. Pretreatment with a drug that blocks this response indicates potentially effective therapy. In 101 patients with symptomatic monomorphic, ventricular tachycardia (VT) treated orally with sematilide (75 to 150 mg t.i.d.), 25% (25 patients) were noninducible after the first PES protocol, and 7 of 35 nonresponders were successfully treated after a second PES protocol at 125 to 150 mg (total responders 32 of 101 patients). Three patients died of documented proarrhythmia and two of undetermined causes (7); a high degree of treatment failure was also noted.

Structural features of class III and class I AAs are closely related, as further illustrated by the fact that the N-heptyl analog of sematilide, structure 4, has class I activity at higher doses. Introduction of a 1-naphthyl moiety onto the α–C of the connecting chain of sematilide gives structure 5a, which elicited potent class I effects at higher concentrations and weak class III effects at low concentrations, using Purkinje fibers (8). Compound 5a was more efficacious than quinidine in the Harris dog model and approximately equieffective in the PES model (Table 1). Moving the naphthyl substituent to the amide N gives structure 5c, which has a class III profile in Purkinje fibers, but is only moderately efficacious in the PES model and ineffective in the Harris model. Compound 5b with the naphthyl substituent on the β–C of the connecting chain has a pure class III profile in Purkinje fibers. The K^+ channel effects of these compounds have not been reported, but conformational analysis suggests that class I efficacy is associated with a *trans* relationship of the ethanediamine moiety, whereas a class III profile in Purkinje fibers is associated with a gauche conformation in compounds 5b and 5c, and other benzamides. The observed pharmacological differences in this series are not likely caused by dependence of ion channel blocking specificity on physicochemical properties, which are comparable for structures 5a to 5c. Because the efficacy in the PES dog for compound 5c is less than expected from Purkinje fiber data, compounds 5a to 5c, which are >2 orders of magnitude more lipophilic than sematilide ($P = 0.104$, pH 7.4, 10 µM), may not distribute in canine cardiac tissues for optimal class III efficacy in vivo. Ibutilide, structure 6 (scheme 1), has also been reported to show this dichotomy of class III and class I actions (9).

Hondeghem and Snyders (10) have proposed the modulated receptor model to explain "reverse" use dependence of blockade of K^+ channels by selective I_K blockers. Most class III AAs discovered thus far prolong APD to a greater extent at slow heart rates than during tachycardia. This phenomenon has been explained by assuming selective binding of the drug to the closed state of the K^+ channel. The model assumes that resting state blockade is favored for lipophilic drugs, whereas open-state blockade involves a hydrophilic pathway. Agents that appear to block Na^+ channels at high concentration and K^+ channels at low concentration, such as quini-

Table 1. Structural Features Contributing to Antiarrhythmic Class Selectivity of Benzamide Antiarrhythmic Drugs.

	In Vitro		In Vivo			
			No. Protected/Tested			
	Change (conc. uM) decrease		HARRIS	PES Dog		
	%APD^{95}	% Vmax	(dose mg/Kg, I.V.)		Class I	Class III
3 sematilide	33 +/- 2 10 uM	nil			0/10 (10)	5/6 (1)
5a	10 +/- 3 (1) −14 +/- 4(10)	−20 +/-5(1) −74+/-1 (10)			3/3 (2-4)	4/7 (1-6)
5b	29 +/-7 (1)	nil (0.1-100)			-----	-----
5c	51+/-10 (1) 64 +/- (10)	−5 +/-4 (1) −3 +/-4 (10)			0/4 (10)	2/4 (1-3)

Structure labels: 3 sematilide (CH₃SO₂N–benzamide, α, β, NEt₂); 5a (Napth, NEt₂ trans); 5b (Napth gauche, NEt₂); 5c (Napth, NEt₂ trans or gauche).

Napth, naphthyl; NE, norepinephrine.

dine and structures **4** and **5a,** may also be understood by this model if one assumes that K⁺ channel blockade indirectly affects recovery of Na⁺ channels. Alternatively, lipophilic K⁺ channel blockers may be inherently less selective and cause Na⁺ channel blockade. This model does not consider contributions from changes in sympathetic drive that increase with rate and counteract increases in APD and ERP, resulting from I_K channel blockade (vide infra). Other explanations for reverse use dependence

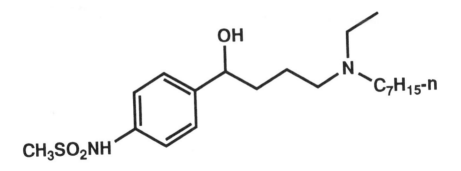

6 Ibutilide

Scheme 1.

include the possibility that I_K plays a lesser role in repolarization at faster rates. The situation is further complicated by differing sensitivities of different tissues in the reentrant pathway in vivo. Thus, models that measure specific effects in specific tissues have limited utility in predicting in vivo results.

Changes in extracellular K^+ concentration and ionic imbalances created by faster heart rates will also affect repolarization (11). Most class III agents, especially I_{KR} blockers, elicit a positive inotropic effect that is probably caused by enhanced Ca^{2+} entry via Ca^{2+} channels and Na^+/Ca^{2+} exchange. Net higher intracellular Ca^{2+} concentration could also alter Ca^{2+} dependent K^+ currents. During ischemia, intracellular K^+ is rapidly depleted and extracellular K^+ increases.

The *m*-isomer [structure **7** (scheme 2)] of sematilide is inactive (5). Incorporation of the ethylene-connecting chain of structure **3** into a cyclo-

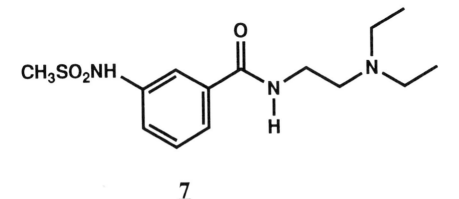

_7_

Scheme 2.

hexane ring *(trans)* results in selectivity for Purkinje fiber over ventricular muscle. The $(-)$-stereoisomer (structure **9**) appears to be more potent in Purkinje fiber than VMs and shows superior potency efficacy in PES models. The K⁺ channel blocking activity and selectivity of structures **8** and **9** (scheme 3) has not been reported, and further data correlating selectivity for K⁺ channels and different cardiac tissues with efficacy against reentrant arrhythmias in different types of infarct would be most useful.

A direct comparison of different class III pharmacophores (see Fig. 1) has been reported for the oxyethylamine series (Y—C = OCH_2CH_2—, Table 2) (4). The *p*-NO_2 group (X) confers several-fold greater class III potency in Purkinje fiber than other class III pharmacophores. In the case of X = 1-imidazolyl, the K⁺ channel selectivity may be different than for X = CH_3SO_2NH—, because the *meta*- and *para*-imidazoles are highly potent in compounds in the benzamide series [**vis**. structures **14** vs. **15** (scheme 4)] (12). Furthermore, potent class III agents without a basic amine moiety may be achieved with this pharmacophore (e.g., structure **16**, Table 3), and the normally preferred *para*-CH_3SO_2NH— pharmacophore is not equivalent (structure **16b**) (13).

Research at Berlex Laboratories (14) and Pfizer, Ltd. (15) established that the basic *N* of the general structure in Fig. 1 may be substituted with two class III pharmacophores [e.g., structures **17** and **18** (schemes 5 and 6)]. These *bis*-pharmacophore designs result in increased class III potency. Compound **18** (dofetilide), which is currently in phase III clinical trials, prolongs APD in guinea pig papillary muscle by 22% at 50 nM in vitro and is a potent I_{KR} blocker (16). Dofetilide may also block K_{ATP} in guinea pig papillary muscle (or functionally antagonize ischemia-induced APD shortening), an effect that has not yet been demonstrated in human tissue (17).

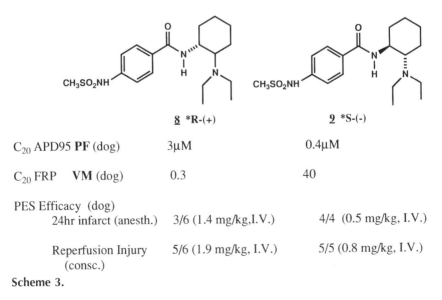

	8 *R-(+)	**9** *S-(-)
C_{20} APD95 **PF** (dog)	3μM	0.4μM
C_{20} FRP **VM** (dog)	0.3	40
PES Efficacy (dog)		
24hr infarct (anesth.)	3/6 (1.4 mg/kg,I.V.)	4/4 (0.5 mg/kg, I.V.)
Reperfusion Injury (consc.)	5/6 (1.9 mg/kg, I.V.)	5/5 (0.8 mg/kg, I.V.)

Scheme 3.

Table 2. Effect of the Phenyl Substituent on Class III Electrophysiological Activity in Canine Cardiac Purkinje Fibers.[a]

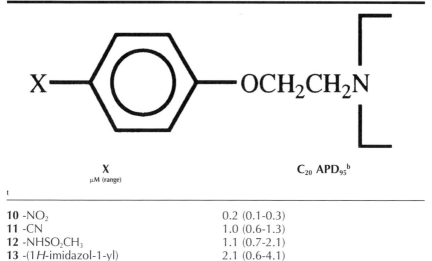

X	
μM (range)	C_{20} APD_{95}[b]

10 -NO_2	0.2 (0.1-0.3)
11 -CN	1.0 (0.6-1.3)
12 -NHSO_2CH_3	1.1 (0.7-2.1)
13 -(1H-imidazol-1-yl)	2.1 (0.6-4.1)

[a]From Morgan and Sullivan 1992
[b]$C_{20}APD_{95}$ = concentration of drug which caused a 20% increase in action potential duration at 95% repolarization (APD_{95}). Reported is the log mean average of 4 determinations with the lowest and highest values given in parentheses

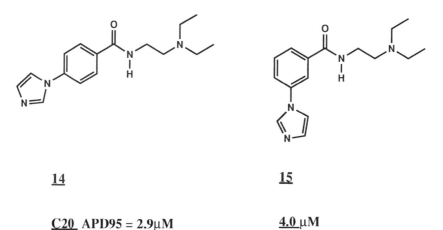

14

15

C20 APD95 = 2.9μM   **4.0 μM**

Scheme 4.

In circumstances of high sympathetic tone, refractoriness of cardiac tissue is reduced. Such conditions arise immediately following cardiac infarct and under anesthesia, such as in norepinephrine-treated, halothane-anesthetized dogs (18). The mechanism of decreased refractoriness has been shown to be augmented I_{KS} current and instantaneous outward (Cl⁻)

Table 3. Nonbasic Class III AA Side Chains.

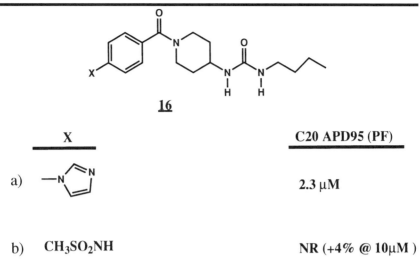

16

	X	C20 APD95 (PF)
a)	(imidazol-1-yl)	2.3 μM
b)	CH₃SO₂NH	NR (+4% @ 10μM)

PF, Purkinje fibers; NR, norepinephrine.

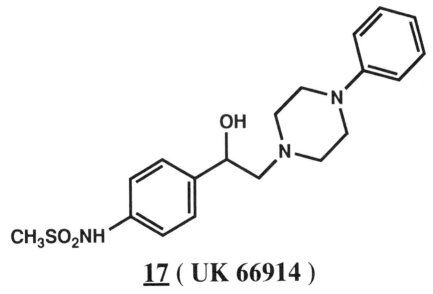

CH₃SO₂NH

17 (UK 66914)

Scheme 5.

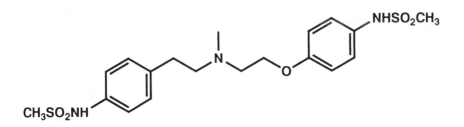

<u>18</u> (UK 68798, dofetilide)

Scheme 6.

current in studies with isoproterenol (β-agonist) in guinea pig papillary muscle (19). The antifibrillatory effects and efficacy against sudden cardiac death of β-adrenergic blockers (e.g., sotalol, compound **19**) may relate to their blockade of these effects, although this hypothesis remains to be verified in human tissues.

As shown in Table 4, sotalol, which is racemic, is more potent as a β-adrenergic blocker than as a class III agent in vitro. The (+)- and (−)-enantiomers of sotalol are equipotent as class III antifibrillatory agents (20), but (−)-sotalol, compound **19b,** is the more potent β-blocker (21). The fact that the class III potency of sotalol enantiomers is intermediate between the β-blocking potencies of impure samples of these enantiomers explains the clinical β-blocking effects of (+)-sotalol at doses used for class III effects.

By combining pharmacophores for known cardioselective β-blockers and class III AAs, scientists at Berlex Laboratories designed a potential class III/II AA with an improved balance of potencies and reduced cardiac and hemodynamic depressive actions in dog models. CK4000 (structure **20**) showed the expected stereoselectivity for potency at the β-receptor and was more than 50 times more selective for β_1- over β_2-receptors in canine cardiac and lung tissues, respectively (12, 14). Compound **20** reduced cardiac output in anesthetized dogs significantly less than sotalol at the high dose of 30 mg/kg, i.v. This compound is a promising candidate for testing as a drug for reduction of postinfarct sudden death. The potency of compound **20** in blocking cardiac K^+ channels has not been reported.

Utilizing the novel β-adrenergic blocking template of 1-arylpiperazines, compound **21** was derived from the class III template of sematilide. Both compounds **20** and **21** were efficacious in the modified halothane-norepinephrine model of PES-induced sustained VT and ventricular fibrillation (22).

Merck scientists succeeded in developing potent, long-acting class III agents based on the spirobenzopyran-2,4′-piperidine (SBPP) nucleus (Table 5). The prototypical compound, L-691,121 (structure **22**) was entered into clinical trials to determine its efficacy and potential for once

Table 4. Class III/II AAs.

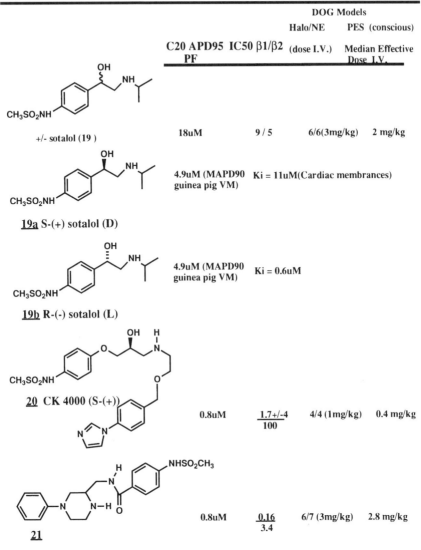

	C20 APD95 PF	IC50 β1/β2	DOG Models	
			Halo/NE (dose I.V.)	PES (conscious) Median Effective Dose I.V.
+/- sotalol (19)	18uM	9 / 5	6/6(3mg/kg)	2 mg/kg
19a S-(+) sotalol (D)	4.9uM (MAPD90 guinea pig VM)	Ki = 11uM(Cardiac membrances)		
19b R-(-) sotalol (L)	4.9uM (MAPD90 guinea pig VM)	Ki = 0.6uM		
20 CK 4000 (S-(+))	0.8uM	1.7+/-4 / 100	4/4 (1mg/kg)	0.4 mg/kg
21	0.8uM	0.16 / 3.4	6/7 (3mg/kg)	2.8 mg/kg

Halo, halothane; NE, norepinephrine; PF, Purkinje fibers

or twice a day dosing (23). Structure–activity studies on the 2-pyridylethyl analogs, structures **23 a–d**, established that moving the CH_3SO_2NH pharmacophore to positions 7 and 8 of the SBPP nucleus reduce potency >15-fold, whereas deletion of this substituent (e.g., structure **23a**) resulted in only a 5-fold reduction in potency for prolonging the ERP in ferret papillary muscle in vitro (24). A 50-fold reduction of potency (ED_{20}) for prolongation of relative refractory period was seen in chloralose anesthe-

Table 5. SBPPs.

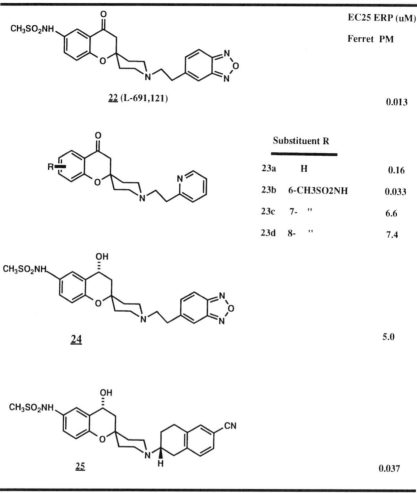

	Substituent R	EC25 ERP (uM) Ferret PM
22 (L-691,121)		0.013
23a	H	0.16
23b	6-CH3SO2NH	0.033
23c	7- "	6.6
23d	8- "	7.4
24		5.0
25		0.037

tized dogs with compound **23a,** relative to compound **23b,** which may be caused by a combination of factors, including intrinsic potency, effect of anesthesia, and tissue distribution (e.g., plasma protein binding).

Concerns that compound **22a** may be metabolized in man, as in dog, to less active metabolites (e.g., compound **24**) led to synthesis of the active diastereomer compound **25**, a potent, selective I_{KR} blocker currently in clinical studies (25). Structure–activity relationships in this series indicate that the SBPP nucleus itself is a class III pharmacophore.

ATP-dependent K⁺ Channels

ATP-dependent K⁺ current (I_{KATP}) is inactive in the presence of ATP and becomes active when intracellular ATP levels decrease. I_{KATP} is also blocked by sulfonylureas, such as glyburide and tolbutamide, and can be activated by specific agonists (PCO), such as cromakalim and pinacidil. By reversing blockade of I_{KATP}, these agonists can be proarrhythmic, especially in ischemic myocardium (26). The importance of I_{KATP} in vascular smooth muscle, including prevalent hypotensive effects of PCOs adds the complication of hemodynamic effects to the study of these agents in arrhythmias.

Mochida is developing *S*-sodium-5-hydroxydecanoate [structure **26**, (scheme 7)] as an AA (selective K_{ATP} blocker) (27). The compound, a natural constituent of human milk, reverses the iodoacetate-induced shortening of APD in guinea pig VMs with no effect on I_{Ki} (inwardly rectifying K⁺ current). Doses of 30 mg/kg, i.v. decreased PES-induced VT 5 to 14 days after coronary artery ligation in dogs (28). The contribution of K_{ATP} currents to arrhythmias under conditions of ischemia and the effects of I_{KR} blockers under these conditions needs to be further investigated (26).

Other K⁺ Channels

No selective blocker of the transient outward K⁺ current (I_{to}) has been reported. The bradycardic agent tedisamil, structure **28** (29), but not the close structural analog ambasilide, compound **29** (30), blocks I_{to}, I_K, and the fast inward Na⁺ current (scheme **8**). Ambasilide appears to block selectively I_K. The rigid structure of compound **28**, and two basic N atoms may contribute to its affinity for the I_{to} K⁺ channel.

Acetylcholine (ACh) activates a cardiac K⁺ channel by G-protein–linked muscarinic receptors (31). Such channels are not fully characterized, but may contribute to the balance between vagal (bradycardic) and adrenergic (tachycardic) tone in the control of cardiac rhythm (32) following coronary occlusion and myocardial infarction (MI). Vagal tone appears to be important in compensatory bradycardia in the human heart (33). Such effects are mediated by parasympathetic innervation of atrial

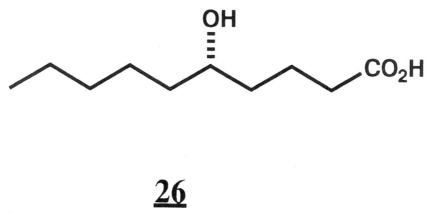

$\underline{26}$

Scheme 7.

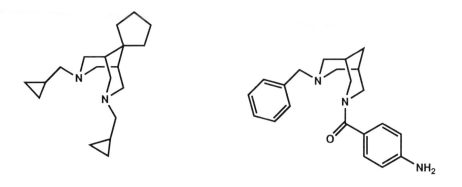

28 Tedisamil

29 Ambasilide

Scheme 8.

pacemakers and the anterior ventricular Purkinje fibers. Thus, the effect on cardiac rhythm depends on involvement of this cardiac region in the arrhythmia substrate. Stimulation of these nerve fibers releases ACh, decreasing phase IV depolarization (by activating outward K^+ currents), which may contribute to an antiarrhythmic response. The exact nature of this response in ischemic and nonischemic tissue is not currently understood. Clearly, class III AAs (I_{KR}) should be investigated in animal models of vagus-induced ventricular fibrillation during acute and late postischemia (34, 35).

The cholinergic drug, edrophonium, increases the frequency of coupled premature beats and VT in patients during the first 2 to 7 hr following MI (36). Atropine exerts primarily an AA effect during the acute postinfarction period (antibradycardic effect), but may be proarrhythmic in an inferior MI, or in later (>5 to 7 hr post-MI) periods, characterized by high levels of automaticity. The possible deleterious effect of I_{KR} blockers under conditions of enhanced vagal tone (bradyarrhythmias) has not been adequately studied.

Regional Effects of Class III AAs on Myocardial Tissues

In patients with stable angina, dofetilide (structure **18**) exhibited class III activity (prolonged QT intervals) at plasma levels of 2.9 ± 0.9 ng/ml and 4.2 ± 0.9 ng/ml by 10% and 13%, respectively (37). Atrial FRP, but not ventricular FRP, showed significantly greater prolongation at the higher dose, compared with the lower dose (basic cycle lengths of 450 and 600 msec). At the lower dose, all refractory periods were significantly increased relative to placebo at both cycle length. No conduction or proarrhythmic effects were noted. The results suggest that atrial effects of the drug are more pronounced than ventricular actions and that electrophysiological changes may not be well correlated with plasma levels in man. Earlier studies in anesthetized dogs showed that dofetilide produced twice the effect on atrial, compared with ventricular, refractory periods (17). Greater effects were seen on Purkinje fibers than on ventricular muscle in the dog.

Almokalant [structure **27** (scheme 9)], a selective I_K blocker in rabbit myocytes (38), increased APD_{90} and APD_{75} by 62.2 ± 9.84 and 61.0 ± 9.24% at 1 μM in isolated human ventricular muscle at a basic cycle length of 1,000 msec (39). No effects on action potential amplitude or $\dot{V}_{max}$ were observed. In addition to delaying repolarization, the drug also increased force of contraction and rate of increase in force with minimal effects on relaxation rate. These results suggest a potentially beneficial cardiotonic effect for almokalant. Previous studies had demonstrated balanced increases in atrial and ventricular refractory periods in man (40). Almokalant did not show b-blocking actions, but b-agonist or norepinephrine releasing actions were not ruled out.

The choice of animal models for assessing contribution of K⁺ currents to repolarization in man is hampered by lack of clinical data. For example, Furukawa et al. (41) showed that activation and deactivation of I_{to} differ in endo- and epicardial myocytes of cats (41). The amplitude of I_{to}, fully activated, was significantly greater in epicardial cells (102 ± 47.7 pA/pF) than in endocardial cells (3.3 ± 3.3 pA/pF). A slower activation and more rapid deactivation were noted for I_{to} in endocardial cells. Fedida and Giles (42) concluded that the transient outward current explains the difference in action potentials in rabbit epicardial versus endocardial tissues. I_{to} channel density varies within the myocardium with estimates 1,495, 1,175 and 895 channels per cell in epicardium, endocardium, and papillary muscle, respectively. I_{to} is a significant repolarizing current in human atrial tissue, but its role in normal vs. ischemic ventricular tissue is unclear. Quinidine may owe some of its antiarrhythmic efficacy to blockade of I_{to}.

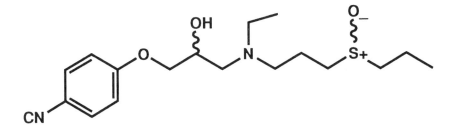

<u>27</u> Almokalant

Scheme 9.

Thus, the therapeutic potential for selective I_K blockers as class III AAs is not clear, because dispersion of refractoriness may actually be increased in an arrhythmic substrate by such an intervention. Argentieri et al. (43) showed that sematilide increased the APD and spontaneous cycle length of rabbit sinoatrial and atrioventral nodal tissues in vitro with equivalent potencies. These effects were attributed to inhibition of I_K. In isolated canine cardiac tissues with ischemic and normal zones, Argentieri et al. (43) showed that bretylium, a nonspecific K^+ channel blocker, caused less increase in dispersion of refractoriness across the border zone in injured subendocardial tissue using Purkinje fiber recordings than sematilide (44). In endocardial to epicardial ventricular muscle, bretylium decreased dispersion of refractoriness, whereas sotalol and clofilium increased it. Further studies in cardiac tissue from animals with inducible reentrant arrhythmias are needed to understand these observations in light of the proven efficacy of I_K blockers, especially in canine models.

Conclusions

This review illustrates the fact that I_{KR} blockers are efficacious in animal models of reentrant arrhythmias and in early clinical studies. However, available data do not indicate universal efficacy of such agents in patients with reentrant arrhythmia. In view of the complex dependence of arrhythmias on changing substrates, on the degree of cardiac ischemia, and adrenergic and muscarinic tone, as well as changes in ion concentrations that can exist in diseased myocardium, several types of AAs may be required to control arrhythmias (45). Single drugs with more than one AA action may also be useful in reducing sudden cardiac death. Areas for further research on K^+ channel blockers are outlined in Table 6.

Table 6. Points for Further Research: Class III Agents as Antiarrhythmics.

1. Distribution of K^+ channels in cardiac tissues (normal/ischemic).
2. Relative responsiveness of different cardiac tissues to K^+ channel blockers— dispersion of refractoriness/ normal/ischemic tissue.
3. In vivo distribution of K^+ channel blockers (e.g., cardiac/plasma); antiarrhythmic/proarrhythmic plasma concentrations and Q_T prolongation.
4. EAD's and K^+ channel blockade.
5. K^+ channel blockade in atrial and conductive tissues—bradyarrhythmias.
6. Isolation of K^+ channel proteins; measurement of binding affinity and off-rates of K^+ channel blockers.
7. Interaction of I_K blockers with balance between sympathetic and parasympathetic tone.

References

1. Sanguinetti, M.C., and Jurkiewicz, N.K. (1991). Delayed rectifier outward K^+ current is composed of two currents in guinea pig atrial cells. *Am. J. Physiol.* **260**:H393–H399.

2. Murai, T., Kakizuka, A., Takumi, T., Ohkubo, H., and Nakanishi, S. (1989). Molecular cloning and sequence analysis of human genomic DNA encoding a novel membrane protein which exhibits a slowly activating potassium channel activity. *Biochem. Biophys. Res. Commun.* **161**:176–181.

3. Colatsky, T.J. (1990). Modulation of cardiac repolarization currents by antiarrhythmic drugs, in *Cardiac Electrophysiology: A Textbook*, M.R. Rosen, M.J. Janse, and A.L. Wit, Eds. (Futura Publishing Co., Mount Kisco, NY), pp. 1–20.

4. Morgan, T.K., Jr., and Sullivan, M.E. (1992). An overview of class III electrophysiological agents: A new generation of antiarrhythmic therapy, in *Program in Medical Chemistry*, Ellis and West, Eds. (Elsevier, London), vol. 29, pp. 65–108.

5. Lumma, W.C., Jr., Wohl, R.A., Davey, D.D., Argentieri, T.M., DeVita, R.J., Gomez, R.P., Jain, V.K., Marisca, A.J., Morgan, Jr., T.K., Reiser, H.J., Sullivan, M.E., Wiggins, J., and Wong, S.S. (1987). Rational design of 4-[(methylsulfonyl)amino]benzamides as class III antiarrhythmic agents. *J. Med. Chem.* **30**:755–758.

6. Wong, W., Pavlou, H.N., Birgersdotter, U.M., Hilleman, D.E., Mohiuddin, S.M., and Roden, D.M. (1992). Pharmacology of the class III antiarrhythmic agent sematilide in patients with arrhythmias. *Am. J. Cardiol.* **69**:206–212.

7. Argentieri, T.M. (1992). Sematilide. *Cardiovas. Drug Rev.* **10**:182–198.

8. Phillips, G.B., Morgan, Jr., T.K., Nickisch, K., Lind, J.M., Gomez, R.P., Wohl, R.A., Argentieri, T.M., and Sullivan, M.E. (1990). Synthesis and cardiac electrophysiological activity of aryl-substituted derivatives of the class III antiarrhythmic agent sematilide. Potential class I/III agents. *J. Med. Chem.* **33**:627–633.

9. Hester, J.B., Gibson, J.K., Cimini, M.G., Emmert, D.E., Locker, P.K., Perrcicone, S.C., Skaletsky, L.L., Sykes, J.K., and West, B.E. (1991). N-[(ω-amino-1-hydroxyalkyl)phenyl]methanesulfonamide derivatives with class III antiarrhythmic activity. *J. Med. Chem.* **34**:308–309.

10. Hondeghem, L.M., and Synders, D.J. (1990). Class III antiarrhythmic agents have a lot of potential but a long way to go. *Circulation* **81**:686–690.

11. Noble, D. (1992). Ionic mechanisms determining the timing of ventricular repolarization: Significance for cardiac arrhythmias. *Ann. N.Y. Acad. Sci.* **644**:1–22.

12. Morgan, T.K., Jr., Lis, R., Lumma, Jr., W.C., Nickisch, K., Wohl, R.A., Phillips, G.B., Gomez, R.P., Lampe, J.W., Di Meo, S.V., Marisca, A.J., and Forst, J. (1990). Synthesis and cardiac electrophysiological activity of N-substituted-4-(1*H*-imidazol-1-yl)benzamides—New selective class III agents. *J. Med. Chem.* **33**:1091–1097.

13. Lampe, J.W., Di Meo, S.V., Morgan, Jr., T.K., Lumma, Jr., W.C., Chou, Y.-L., Erhardt, P.W., Hagedorn III, A.A., Argentieri, T.M., and Wiggins, J.R. (1992). Synthesis and cardiac electrophysiological activity of 4-substituted-N-aroylpiperidines. Abstracts of the American Chemical Society Meeting, San Francisco, CA.

14. Morgan, T.K., Jr., Lis, R., Lumma, Jr., W.C., Wohl, R.A., Nickisch, K., Phillips, G.B., Lind, J.M., Lampe, J.W., Di Meo, S.V., Reiser, H.J., Argentieri, T.M., Sullivan, M.E., and Cantor, E. (1990). Synthesis and pharmacological

studies of N-[4-[2-hydroxy-3-[[2-[4-(1*H*-imidazol-1-yl)phenoxy]ethyl]amino]propoxy]phenyl]methanesulfonamide, a novel antiarrhythmic agent with class II and class III activities. *J. Med. Chem.* **33**:1087–1090.

15. Cross, P.E., Arrowsmith, J.E., Thomas, G.N., Gwilt, M., Burges, R.A., and Higgins, A.J. (1990). Selective class III antiarrhythmic agents. 1. Bis(arylalkyl)amines. *J. Med. Chem.* **33**:1151–1155.

16. Sanguinetti, M.C. (1992). Modulation of potassium channels by antiarrhythmic and antihypertensive drugs. *Hypertension* **19**:228–236.

17. Gwilt, M., Arrowsmith, J.E., Blackburn, K.J., Burges, R.A., Cross, P.E., Dalrymple, H.W., and Higgins, A.J. (1991). UK-68,798: A novel, potent and highly selective class III antiarrhythmic agent which blocks potassium channels in cardiac cells. *J. Pharmacol. Exp. Ther.* **256**:318–324.

18. Mitsuhashi, H., Akiyama, K., and Hashimoto, K. (1987). Effects of betaxolol, a new beta 1 selective blocker, on canine ventricular arrhythmias. *Japan. J. Pharmacol.* **43**:179–185.

19. Sanguinetti, M.C., Jurkiewicz, N.K., Scott, A., and Siegl, P.K.S. (1991). Isoproterenol antagonizes prolongation of refractory period by the class III antiarrhythmic agent E-4031 in guinea pig myocytes. *Circ. Res.* **68**:77–84.

20. Lynch, J.J., Wilber, D.J., Montgomery, D.G., Hsieh, T.M., Patterson, E., and Lucchesi, B.R. (1984). Antiarrhythmic and antifibrillatory actions of the levo- and dextrorotatory isomers of sotalol. *J. Cardiovas. Pharmacol.* **6**:1132–1141.

21. Reid, J., Duker, G., Almgren, O., and Nerme, V. (1990). (+)-Sotalol causes significant occupation of β-adrenoceptors at concentrations that prolong cardiac repolarization. *Naunyn-Schmiedeberg's Arch. Pharmacol.* **341**:215–220.

22. Phillips, G.B., Morgan, Jr., T.K., Lumma, Jr., W.C., Gomez, R.P., Lind, J.M., Lis, R., Argentieri, T., and Sullivan, M.E. (1992). Synthesis, cardiac electrophysiology, and β-blocking activity of novel arylpiperazines with potential as class II/III antiarrhythmic agents. *J. Med. Chem.* **35**:743–750.

23. Elliott, J.M., Selnick, H.G., Claremon, D.A., Baldwin, J.J., Buhrow, S.A., Butcher, J.W., Habecker, C.N., King, S.W., Lynch, Jr., J.J., Phillips, B.T., Ponticello, G.S., Radzilowski, E.M., Remy, D.C., Stein, R.B., White, J.I., and Young, M.B. (1992). 4-Oxospiro[benzopyran-2,4'-piperidines] as class III antiarrhythmic agents. Pharmacological studies on 3,4-dihydro-1'-[2-(benzofurazan-5-yl)-ethyl]-6-methanesulfonamidospiro[(2*H*)-1-benzopyran-2,4'-piperidin]-4-one (L-691,121). *J. Med. Chem.* **35**:3973–3976.

24. Claremon, D.A., Baldwin, J.J., Buhrow, S.A., Butcher, J.W., Elliott, J.M., Lynch, Jr., J.J., Ponticello, G.S., Radzilowski, E.M., Remy, D.C., and Selnick, H.G.. (1992). Clinical candidates selected from a series of spriobenzopyran-2,4'-piperinine class III antiarrhythmic agents. Abstract of the American Chemical Society Meeting, San Francisco, CA.

25. Elliott, J.M., Baldwin, J.J., Butcher, J.W., Claremon, D.A., Lynch, J.J., Ponticello, G.S., Remy, D.C., and Selnick, H.G. (1992). Development of the class III antiarrhythmic agent L-706,000. Abstract of the American Chemical Society Meeting, San Francisco, CA.

26. Lynch, J.J., Jr., Sanguinetti, M.C., Kimura, S., and Bassett, A.L. (1992). Therapeutic potential of modulating potassium currents in the diseased myocardium. *FASEB J.* **6**:2952–2960.

27. Notsu, T., Tanaka, I., Takano, M., and Noma, A. (1992). Blockade of the ATP-sensitive K⁺ channel by 5-hydroxydecanoate in guinea pig ventricular myocytes. *J. Pharmacol. Exp. Ther.* **260:**702–708.

28. Niho, T. (1991). Inhibitory effects and mechanism of action of sodium 5-hydroxydecanoate on experimental ischemic ventricular arrhythmia. *Toho Igakkai Zasshi* **38:**176–189.

29. Dukes, I.D., Cleemann, L., and Morad, M. (1990). Tedisamil blocks the transient and delayed rectifier K⁺ currents in mammalian cardiac and glial cells. *J. Pharmacol. Exp. Ther.* **254:**560–569.

30. Zhang, Z.-H., Sarma, J.S.M., Chen, F., and Singh, B.N. (1990). Inhibition of delayed-rectifying potassium current (I_K) by LU-47710 in guinea-pig myocytes. *Circulation* **82:**SIII:527 (Abstract).

31. Kim, D., Lewis, D.L., Graziadei, L., Neer, E.J., Bar-Sagi, D., and Clapham, D.E. (1989). G-protein βγ-subunits activate the cardiac muscarinic K⁺-channel via phospholipase A₂. *Nature* **337:**557–560.

32. Kent, K.M., Epstein, S.E., Cooper, T., and Jacobowitz, D.M. (1974). Cholinergic innervation of the canine and human ventricular conducting system. *Circulation* **50:**948–955.

33. Corr, P.B., and Gillis, R.A. (1978). Autonomic neural influences on the dysrhythmias resulting from myocardial infarction. *Circ. Res.* **43:**1–9.

34. Corr, P.B., and Gillis, R.A. (1974). Role of the vague nerves in the cardiovascular changes induced by coronary occlusion. *Circulation* **49:**86–97.

35. Myers, R.W., Pearlman, A.S., Hyman, R.M., Goldstein, R.A., Kent, K.M., Goldstein, R.E., and Epstein, S.E. (1974). Beneficial effects of vagal stimulation and bradycardia during experimental acute myocardial ischemia. *Circulation* **49:**943–947.

36. Olson, H.G., Miller, R.R., Da Silva, O., Amsterdam, E.A., and Mason, D.T. (1974). Vagal stimulation in patients with acute myocardial infarction: Antiarrhythmic and hemodynamic effects of edrophonium. *Circulation* **50:**SIII–33 (Abstract).

37. Sedgwick, M.L., Rasmussen, H.S., and Cobbe, S.M. (1992). Clinical and electrophysiologic effects of intravenous dofetilide (UK-68,798), a new class III antiarrhythmic drug, in patients with angina pectoris. *Am. J. Cardiol.* **69:**513–517.

38. Carmeliet, E. (1991). Block of the delayed K⁺ current by hassle 234/09 in rabbit cardiac myocytes. *J. Mol. Cell. Cardiol.* **23SV:**S.79 (Abstract).

39. Carlsson, L., Abrahamsson, C., Almgren, O., Lundberg, C., and Duker, G., (1991). Prolonged action potential duration and positive inotropy induced by the novel class III antiarrhythmic agent H 234/09 (Almokalant) in isolated human ventricular muscle. *J. Cardiovas. Pharmacol.* **18:**882–887.

40. Darpo, B., Almgren, O., Bergstrand, R., Gottfridsson, C., Sandstedt, B., and Edvardsson, N. (1991). Class III mode of action of H234/09—A double-blind cross-over study using transoesophageal atrial stimulation in healthy volunteers. *Cardiovas. Drugs Ther.* **5:**S3:364. (Abstract).

41. Furukawa, T., Myerburg, R.J., Furukawa, N., Bassett, A.L., and Kimura, S. (1990). Differences in transient outward currents of feline endocardial and epicardial myocytes. *Circ. Res.* **67:**1287–1291.

42. Fedida, D., and Giles, W.R. (1991). Regional variations in action potentials and transient outward current in myocytes isolated from rabbit left ventricle. *J. Physiol.* **442:**191–209.

43. Argentieri, T.M., Carroll, M.S., and Sullivan, M.E. (1991). Cellular electrophysiological effects of the class III antiarrhythmic agents sematilide and clofilium on rabbit atrial tissues. *J. Cardiovasc. Pharmacol.* **18:**167–174.

44. Argentieri, T.M., Ambelas, E.M., Sullivan, M.E., and Wiggins, J. (1988). The antiarrhythmic and proarrhythmic mechanism of class III agents in infarcted canine myocardium. *FASEB J.* **2:**7317 (Abstract).

45. Singh, B.N., Sarma, J.S.M., Zhang, Z.-H., and Takanaka, C. (1992). Controlling cardiac arrhythmias by lengthening repolarization: Rationale from experimental findings and clinical considerations. *Ann. N.Y. Acad. Sci.* **644:**187–209.

27

Role of Ion Channels in Antiarrhythmic and Antifibrillatory Drug Action

Benedict R. Lucchesi, Liguo Chi, Shawn C. Black,
Andrew C.G. Uprichard, Gregory S. Friedrichs,
Peter J. Manley, and Jeanne Y. Oh

A major cause of mortality in the industrialized world is attributed to sudden cardiac death, a phenomenon most likely to occur in the diseased heart as a result of altered electrophysiology. Sudden cardiac death generally denotes death that is nonviolent, unexpected, witnessed, and instantaneous or occurs within a few minutes of an abrupt change in the previous clinical state (1). Despite a decrease in the number sudden cardiac deaths over the past 20 years, the number of fatalities in the United States exceeds 300,000/year. Approximately 60% of the fatal events occur in individuals without any previous diagnosis of heart disease (2). Clearly a major health issue of our times, accounting for 50% of all cardiovascular deaths (3), the problem of sudden death is compounded by the recent realization that not only has pharmacologic management done little to improve the situation, but it may also have contributed to the onset of the fatal events in susceptible individuals (4). The extent of the problem has made sudden cardiac death one of the nation's most pressing unresolved clinical and public health concerns.

Sudden cardiac death may be considered to involve an interaction between structural derangements of the heart, transient functional disturbances, and the specific electrophysiological events responsible for the fatal arrhythmia (3). Coronary atherosclerosis and its associated influences on the heart constitutes the major pathological finding in the vast majority of persons who succumb to sudden cardiac death. Patients who have experienced a major cardiovascular event are at high risk of sudden cardiac death during the first 6 to 18 months after the index event, suggesting a time dependence of risk and indicating the need for appropriate therapy in the early period (5).

Are There Predictors of Sudden Cardiac Death That Are Targets for Drug Intervention?

The role of drug intervention in the prevention of sudden death is based on the premise of there being treatable factors that might be identified in those at risk. One factor, recognized for many years, is the finding of chronic ventricular ectopy in patients after myocardial infarction (6–11). The assumption was made that premature ventricular complexes (PVCs) appearing in the vulnerable phase of myocardial repolarization were responsible for the initiation of malignant arrhythmias in these individuals. Therefore, it seemed entirely appropriate that an agent capable of suppressing PVCs would be effective in preventing sudden death. Indeed, early studies with lidocaine, an effective agent in suppressing ectopy (12), suggested that its use might be associated with a decreased incidence of ventricular fibrillation (13). After this, however, there appeared a number of reports using several agents that failed to substantiate this claim, and when reviewed in early meta-analysis, these appeared to suggest an adverse trend (14, 15). Nevertheless, the analyses were not without criticism for dissimilarities in study designs and populations, so it was not until the advent of the Cardiac Arrhythmia Suppression Trial (CAST; 16) that the prescribing public was given a clear picture of the issue. CAST was designed specifically to address the question of whether PVC suppression was an appropriate surrogate for mortality in the postmyocardial infarction population. Encainide, flecainide, and moricizine were identified in the Cardiac Arrhythmia Pilot Study (17) as PVC killers and were considered to be the agents of choice for CAST. Despite ironical concern over the ethics of a placebo arm, it was included in a major multicenter study that used elegant dose-titration in a double-blind manner. Preliminary [CAST I (16)] and final [CAST II (18)] results from this study provided the definitive answer that the use of all three agents was associated with significant increases in arrhythmic deaths. Furthermore, these adverse trends were apparent in all identified subgroups and, in view of the diverging curves, were felt to be ongoing throughout the trial.

An alternative clinical model for the testing of antiarrhythmic drugs is the unmasking of malignant reentrant arrhythmias by electrophysiologic (EP) testing. An appropriately timed stimulus, deliverd via an indwelling cardiac catheter, can induce ventricular tachyarrhythmias in patients at risk of life-threatening disturbances in cardiac rhythm (19). Furthermore, the same arrhythmias may be prevented by the use of individualized drug therapy (20, 21). The induction of sustained ventricular arrhythmia is considered an objective endpoint by which to evaluate candidates for antiarrhythmic drug therapy. The rate at which inducible ventricular arrhythmias are suppressed during serial antiarrhythmic drug testing in survivors of sudden cardiac death ranges from 20% to 50% (20–23). However, even when ventricular fibrillation is induced by programmed electrical stimulation in the electrophysiology laboratory, one cannot be sure that the substrate of the arrhythmia thus generated is identical to that pertaining at the time of sudden death, or that pharmacologic prevention of stimulus-induced ventricular fibrillation reflects protection against sudden death. The question remains, therefore, of whether it is the fact that a patient's arrhythmia can be suppressed that is important, or if it is caused by the associated drug therapy; or is suppressibility per se associated with a good prognosis? To answer this would require a placebo-controlled trial in which patients with suppressible arrhythmias were compared with patients whose arrhythmias could not be prevented. Before embarking on this we must first, however, be assured that EP testing is an appropriate surrogate for mortality. The only study to date that addresses this question is the National Institutes of Health–sponsored Electrophysiology Study Versus Electrocardiographic Monitoring (ESVEM) trial (24). ESVEM utilizes mortality in determining the relative usefulness of EP testing and Holter monitoring in assessing several antiarrhythmics, including quinidine, procainamide, mexiletine, propafenone, sotalol, and pirmenol—a class Ia agent no longer being developed. An imipramine group was removed shortly after the trial was initiated. Until this trial reports out in 1993, EP testing cannot be recommended for routine use.

To summarize the clinical situation, whereas certain drugs (e.g., lidocaine, bretylium, and amiodarone) do have an indication for the prevention of recurrent ventricular fibrillation, no pharmacologic intervention has yet been shown to decrease the incidence of sudden cardiac death. Furthermore, there appears to be no relevant surrogate endpoint for the evaluation of potential new therapies. It seems imperative, therefore, to involve new, more appropriate animal models in early preclinical testing, which are based on our understanding of the pathophysiological milieu pertaining at the time of sudden death.

Damaged Myocardium as the Substrate for Reentrant Rhythms and Ventricular Fibrillation

Postmortem studies indicate that, in the majority of cases, ventricular fibrillation is a primary event that is not related to acute myocardial infarction (25, 26). Sudden cardiac death is known to occur most commonly in patients with previous myocardial ischemic injury secondary to advanced coronary artery atherosclerosis (26a–28). Furthermore, the finding in many cases of intracoronary thrombus without acute infarction suggests that ischemia, per se, may be acting as the trigger for the genesis of ventricular fibrillation in a vulnerable, electrically unstable ventricular myocardium. The EP properties of ischemic myocardium, such as increased excitability, shortening of the ventricular refractory period, slowing of conduction velocity, and increased inhomogeneity in recovery may provide the milieu for the emergence of reentrant rhythms in a heart critically deranged by previous infarction. The concept of ischemia in a region remote from the infarct-related artery acting as the trigger for fatal ventricular arrhythmias was addressed by Schuster and Bulkley (29). In a study of two groups of patients with early postinfarction angina, they found that patients with remote ischemia constituted a group of hemodynamically stable patients who faced an unexpectedly high mortality compared with those patients whose angina arose from the peri-infarcted region. Schwartz and coworkers (30, 31) reproduced this phenomenon experimentally when they demonstrated a high incidence of ventricular fibrillation in a chronic model of myocardial infarction where additional ischemia was initiated using a hydraulic coronary artery occluder. Also using a canine model, Kabell and coworkers (32) demonstrated a diminution in infarct collateral blood flow with distant ischemia. Because this was preceded by delayed epicardial activity within the area of preexisting infarction, it suggested that ischemia might be influencing the substrate of an infarcted area of myocardium to render it more suitable for the emergence of lethal arrhythmias.

Coronary vasospasm has been considered as a triggering mechanism for sudden death, especially because patients with atypical angina have demonstrated serious ventricular arrhythmias during episodes of spasm (33). Although the majority of survivors of cardiac arrest give no previous or subsequent history of atypical angina, in one study, sudden death was observed in 17% of 114 patients with coronary vasospasm followed for a mean of 24 months (34).

Another mechanism to be considered in the genesis of lethal arrhythmias is the role of the autonomic nervous system. Alterations in autonomic tone are well recognized in acute myocardial ischemia and may be inherently arrhythmogenic by nature of an increase in myocardial oxygen consumption and alterations in refractories. Inhomogenous adrenergic stimulation has been shown to precipitate arrhythmias in a number of animal models (34a), whereas others have demonstrated a possible role of the sympathetic nervous system when acute ischemia is produced in the setting of previous myocardial infarction (30, 31, 35). Specifically, sympathetic hyperactivity favors the onset of life-threatening cardiac arrhythmias, whereas vagal activation exerts a protective and antifibrillatory effect (35). Direct neural recording of vagal activity to the heart confirmed that vigorous reflex vagal activation during acute myocardial ischemia is associated with protection from ventricular fibrillation (36). Other factors contributing to the precipitating trigger in sudden death include those biochemical alterations (hypokalemia, hypomagnesemia, etc.) that are known to precipitate fatal arrhythmias in individuals at risk. Thus a variety of factors may predispose the individual at risk to the development of lethal ventricular arrhythmias (Fig. 1). Pathophysiologically, sudden cardiac death involves an interaction between structural abnormalities of the heart, transient functional disturbances, and the specific EP events responsible for fatal arrhythmias.

Ischemia Must Be Differentiated from Infarction

There is a period of healing after myocardial infarction in which the necrotic mass of tissue is converted to a dense, fibrous scar. The healed phase of myocardial infarction is characterized by a chronic alteration in myocardial structure, that in itself, is electrically stable. However, the structural abnormality is capable of influencing EP parameters when other events are superimposed on the heart. In contrast, ischemia is a transient event caused by an absolute or relative reduction in regional myocardial blood flow. The influence of ischemia on a structurally normal heart has a more favorable outcome compared with an ischemic event superimposed on a heart previously subjected to myocardial infarction. There is compelling evidence to indicate that regional myocardial ischemia superimposed on the previously damaged heart, in contrast to a normal heart, is more likely to precipitate malignant and potentially lethal ventricular arrhythmia (37–39). Superimposition of an acute nonocclusive thrombus, an imbalance between oxygen supply and demand, metabolic or electrolyte changes,

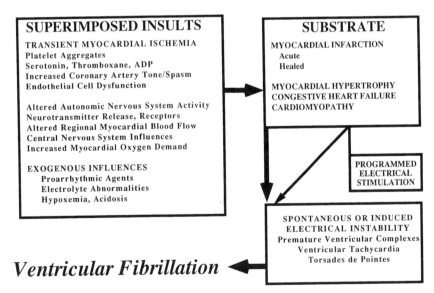

Figure 1. Potential "insults" capable of contributing to the emergence of fatal ventricular arrhythmias in a heart critically deranged from previous myocardial infarction. The use of programmed electrical stimulation in the postinfarction period is capable of unmasking the electrical instability that is ultimately responsible for the terminal arrhythmia.

or neurophysiologic influences may establish the conditions necessary to sustain a reentrant rhythm leading to a lethal arrhythmia. Enhanced coronary artery vasomotor activity, abruptly decreasing myocardial blood flow in a region remote from a region of previous myocardial infarction, may precipitate symptoms of angina, disturbances in rhythm, and sudden cardiac death (34, 40). Platelet aggregation at sites of coronary vessel damage and the release of vasoactive mediators have been implicated as major contributors to the initiation of lethal cardiac arrhythmias (41–44).

Experimental Models for the Preclinical Assessment of Antifibrillatory Drug Efficacy

Until recently, whole animal models for the evaluation of antiarrhythmic activity have relied upon arrhythmogenesis by cardiotoxic agents, electrical stimuli, or arrhythmias associated with coronary artery occlusion, with or without reperfusion (45). Other approaches include arrhythmias induced by catecholamines (46) or electrical stimuli (47, 48) in the subacute phase of myocardial infarction. Although each of these techniques is capable of generating reliable and reproducible arrhythmias, they fail to provide an opportunity to examine the EP environment at the time of ventricular fibrillation, or to study pharmacologic interventions aimed at preventing sudden cardiac death. Table 1 presents a summary of some of the more commonly used experimental methods. The preclinical development of

Table 1. Experimental Methods for Evaluation of Antiarrhythmic Agents

Chemically induced arrhythmias
  Aconitine
  Hydrocarbon-catecholamine
  Barium chloride
  Digitalis glycosides
  Potassium channel openers

Electrically induced arrhythmias
  Ventricular fibrillation/defibrillation threshold
  Repetitive ventricular response
  Programmed electrical stimulation

Neurally induced arrhythmias
  Application of stimuli to the lateral ventricle of the brain
  Elecrical stimulation of the autonomic nervous system
  Emotional- or exercise-induced stress

Ischemia-induced arrhythmias
  Acute interruption of regional coronary artery blood flow (Harris one or two stage)
  Acute interruption of regional coronary artery blood flow followed by reperfusion
  Acute regional ischemia superimposed on a previously infarcted myocardium

antiarrhythmic agents should emphasize the importance of designing animal models to address *ventricular fibrillation,* as it may represent one of the primary rhythm disturbances associated with sudden cardiac death, particularly in the heart altered by coronary artery disease. In light of CAST (16) results, animal models that evaluate a drug's capacity to reduce the number of innocent ventricular premature depolarizations may be of limited value in a new drug development. The ideal drug may be one that is effective against the sustained ventricular tachycardia (VT) and ventricular fibrillation that occur spontaneously in the presence of previous myocardial injury. There may be a clear distinction between antiarrhythmic efficacy and antifibrillatory potential. It may not follow that the latter is simply an extension of the former.

The ventricular fibrillation threshold (VFT) has been considered a reflection of the electrical stability of the whole heart and therefore a measure of its resistance to fibrillate (49). Although used extensively as an indicator of antifibrillatory effectiveness, the model has come under criticism for an inability to correlate alterations in fibrillation thresholds with direct EP actions (50). Despite procedural modifications, such as determinations of VFT under normal and ischemic conditions (51), it appears that, particularly where trains of current are used, there is a release of local stores of epinephrine. The local release of catecholamines would influence outcome by lowering the fibrillation threshold (52). If this is the case, the elevation of fibrillation thresholds seen with the β-adrenoceptor antagonists (53, 54) may relate more to antagonism of the effects of stimulus-induced epinephrine release, than to any direct antifibrillatory phenomenon.

An Experimental Model of VT and Sudden Cardiac Death

Our laboratory described and has made extensive use of a conscious canine model that is susceptible to the initiation of stimulus-induced ventricular arrhythmias in the subacute phase of anterior myocardial infarction (38, 45). Of particular interest in this model was the finding that an additional ischemic insult [initiated by a 150 μA anodal current to the left circumflex coronary artery (LCX)] served as a reliable model for the spontaneous onset of ventricular fibrillation. The same study (38) also demonstrated that previous myocardial damage was a prerequisite for the observed high mortality, because dogs without anterior infarctions exhibited a low risk of ventricular fibrillation. A subsequent study (55) evaluated the model further by looking at the relationship between inducible VT and the subsequent development of ventricular fibrillation. Results suggested that inducible arrhythmias (either sustained or nonsustained) were predictive of spontaneous ventricular fibrillation during posterolateral ischemia. The mass of previously injured myocardium was a critical determinant of both, because animals with inducible arrhythmias (24-hr mortality 93%) had larger infarct sizes (24.7 ± 1.7% of left ventricular mass) than the animals that were noninducible at baseline testing (24-hr mortality 15%; infarct size 5.3 ± 1.1% of left ventricular mass) (Table 2). The use of this model enabled the evaluation of antiarrhythmic activity against arrhythmias thought to share the same reentrant basis as ischemic arrhythmias in man (47, 56). In addition, the model permits one to discriminate between antiarrhythmic activity, as determined with programmed electrical stimulation, versus antifibrillatory activity in the postinfarcted heart subjected to an ischemic event in a region remote from the infarct related artery.

Experimental Procedure for Determining Antifibrillatory Activity

Mongrel dogs of either sex are anesthetized by the intravenous administration of sodium pentobarbital, intubated, and ventilated with room air. Using aseptic technique, the left jugular vein is isolated and cannulated for subsequent drug administration. A left thoracotomy is performed, and the heart exposed and suspended in a pericardial cradle. The left anterior descending coronary artery (LAD) is dissected free at the tip of the left atrial appendage and the LCX isolated ~1 cm from its origin. Anterior wall infarction is achieved by a 2-hr occlusion of the LAD followed by reperfusion in the presence of a critical stenosis. An epicardial bipolar plunge electrode is sutured to the left atrial appendage for subsequent atrial pacing. A bipolar plunge electrode is sutured onto the surface of the heart in the region of the right ventricular outflow tract (RVOT) for the subsequent introduction of extrastimuli during programmed electrical stimulation. In addition, two bipolar plunge electrodes are sutured to the left ventrical wall: one in the distribution of the LAD distal to the site of occlusion [infarct zone (IZ)] and the second in the distribution of the LCX [normal zone (NZ)]. Finally, a 30-gauge electrode is inserted into the

Table 2. Characteristics of the Chronic Canine Model of Sudden Death

Features	Inducible	Noninducible
Anterior infarct size (% left ventricular mass)	24.7 ± 1.7	5.3 ± 1.1*
Time to ischemia (min)	196 ± 39	225 ± 30
Sudden VF† (<1 hr)	11/15	2/15
Delayed VF (<24 hr)	3/15	0/15
Thrombus mass (mg)	7.2 ± 1.81	11.2 ± 2.3
Posterolateral infarct mass	19.0 ± 1.0 (N = 3)	16.7 ± 2.3 (N = 13)

†VF, ventricular fibrillation.
*$P < 0.001$.

lumen of the LCX and secured by suturing to the heart wall. Figure 2 is a schematic representation of the instrumental canine heart, as used in this model of sudden cardiac death.

Programmed electrical stimulation and EP testing is performed in the conscious, unsedated animal, 3 to 5 days after surgical preparation. After determination of the RVOT excitation threshold and refractory period, programmed stimulation continues with the introduction of double (S2, S3) and triple (S2, S3, S4) extrastimuli (4 msec duration at twice RVOT excitation threshold) during sinus rhythm. Previous studies indicated that these stimulation methods will not induce arrhythmias in sham-operated animals (38). EP parameters from normal and infarcted myocardium are determined from the construction of strength-interval curves using data obtained from the NZ and IZ electrodes, respectively. Dogs with sustained or nonsustained VT are allocated randomly to drug or vehicle groups, and electrophysiological testing and programmed stimulation are repeated in full after drug equilibration.

On completion of the post-treatment stimulation protocol, a direct anodal current of 150 μA is applied to the intimal surface of the LCX using a 9 V nickel-cadmium battery and variable resistor. Application of an anodal

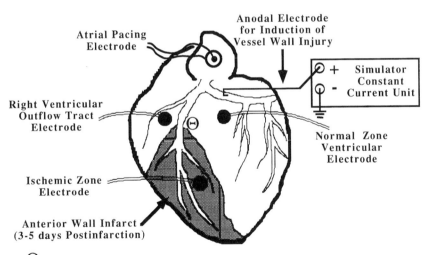

Θ = Site of Occlusion/Reperfusion of the Left Anterior Descending Coronary Artery

Figure 2. Conscious canine model of sudden death (surgical preparation). Anterior myocardial infarction is produced by a 2-hr occlusion of the left anterior descending coronary artery, with subsequent reperfusion in the presence of a critical stenosis. An atrial bipolar epicardial electrode is illustrated, as well as bipolar plunge electrodes in normal myocardium (normal zone), infarcted tissue (infarct zone), and the RVOT. The latter is subsequently used for the introduction of extrastimuli during programmed electrical stimulation, 3 to 5 days after surgery. A silver wire electrode is illustrated within the lumen of the LCX. Ultimate introduction of a 150 μA anodal current results in acute posterolateral ischemia and a high incidence of ventricular fibrillation in the sudden death protocol.

current to the intimal surface of the vessel results in injury and exposure of the underlying collagen matrix. Platelet aggregates form on the denuded surface of the coronary artery accompanied by cyclic variations in blood flow and a high incidence of acute ventricular fibrillation within 1 hr from the onset of ischemia as determined by depression and/or elevation in the ST segment of the electrocardiogram.

Lead II of the ECG is recorded at preset intervals (30 sec every 15 min) by a programmable cardiocassette recorder. After 24 hr of continuous application of the anodal current or the development of ventricular fibrillation, the heart is excised and any thrombus in the LCX is removed and weighed. The heart is sectioned transversely and incubated in a 0.4% solution of triphenyltetrazolium chloride (TTC) for 15 min. Anterior and posterolateral areas of infarction are identified by their inability to reduce TTC enzymatically to a brick-red formazan precipitate. Infarct masses in the myocardial regions are quantified by computer-assisted planimetry and expressed as a percentage of total left ventricular mass. Playback of the cardiocassette provides information regarding the time of onset of ischemia (as assessed by the appearance of ventricular ectopy and/or ST segment changes), the time from ischemia to death, and the percentage change in heart rate before death.

Summary of Experimental Results

When last tabulated, a total of 201 inducible, vehicle-treated dogs had been studied in our laboratory; of these, 188 (94%) had died within 24 hr of posterolateral ischemia in the sudden death protocol (57). An interesting observation in many of the animals that die is the finding of variable periods of sustained monomorphic VT before the onset of ventricular fibrillation. In this respect, the model demonstrates electrocardiographic features not unlike the human clinical situation, where ambulatory monitoring has identified sustained ventricular arrhythmias as the most common terminal mechanism in sudden death (58–60). Pharmacologic protection in this model is apparent when animals survive the arrhythmias associated with the onset of acute posterolateral ischemia and ultimately develop second infarcts in the distribution of the LCX. The results of various pharmacologic interventions in the conscious canine model of sudden death are summarized in Table 3.

What is immediately obvious from Table 3 is the dichotomy of action of many antiarrhythmic agents when tested both against the arrhythmias of programmed electrical stimulation and in their effects against ischemic ventricular fibrillation. In fact, it could be concluded that there is little, if any, value in predicting antifibrillatory efficacy from a drug's effect on stimulus-induced VT. It can be seen that clinically relevant plasma concentrations of the class Ia agent quinidine were capable of preventing the induction of stimulus-induced arrhythmias, but were ineffective in prevent-

Table 3. Drug Efficacy in the Conscious Canine Model of Myocardial Infarction and Sudden Death

Agent	VT Suppression (Programmed Stimulation)	24 Hr Survival (%)
Vehicle	−	6*
Class I		
Quinidine	+	9
Flecainide	−	14
Class II		
Nadolol	−	56–63
Dilevalol	−	20–60
Sotalol	+	63
Celiprolol	−	30
Class III		
d-Sotalol	+	65
Bretylium	+	60
Amiodarone	−	40–80
Clofilium	+	30
CK 3579†	−	70
Sematilide	+	60
E-4031	−	60
UK 68,798	−	42
Class IV		
Diltiazem	−	10
Bepridil	+	30–40
Other		
Alinidine	−	60
Meobentine	−	0
Bethanidine	−	0
Prazosin	−	50
CGS 12970‡	−	30
R 68070§	−	30

Adapted from Lynch and Lucchesi (64).

*Cumulative.
†Class III with β_1-adrenoceptor antagonist properties.
‡Thromboxane synthetase inhibitor.
§Combined thromboxane synthetase inhibitor/receptor antagonist.

ing ventricular fibrillation (61); conversely, if we ignore for the present the confounding issues with sotalol, β-adrenergic receptor blockage appears to be offering some degree of protection in the sudden death model without influencing stimulus-induced VT (62–65), a phenomenon shared by the specific bradycardic agent alinidine (66). Studies with two calcium channel antagonists show bepridil to be antiarrhythmic without affecting mortality (67), whereas diltiazem did not demonstrate any beneficial trends (68). Studies with other agents not covered by the Vaughan–Williams classification offer little additional insight into the antiarrhythmic or antifibrillatory relationship (69–73). Even in the group with the greatest overall effect in the sudden death model, only half of the class III agents tested demonstrated a correlation with antiarrhythmic activity. Thus, it would seem reasonable to conclude that there is little prognostic value from suppression of VT in this model, other than ancillary EP data obtained at the time of testing, which frequently provide an insight into potential antifibrillatory mechanisms.

Clinical Significance of the Conscious Canine Model of Sudden Death

A striking observation from Table 3 is the apparent lack of activity of the class I agents in preventing sudden death in the model. In light of what we have learned from CAST, the study with flecainide was particularly interesting in that 3 of 7 animals—noninducible at baseline and therefore at low risk from posterolateral ischemia—failed to survive the sudden death protocol (74). Thus, potential profibrillatory activity with flecainide had been suggested on the basis of preclinical studies several years before CAST. Class Ic agents are characterized by their ability to slow conduction velocity with only minimal effects on the duration of the refractory period of the ventricular myocardium. Flecainide in particular is of interest in that it increases the ventricular effective refractory period, and to a lesser extent, the action potential duration. On the other hand, in Purkinje fibers, action potential duration is decreased as flecainide concentration increases (75). In contrast to the actions of other antiarrhythmic agents that are sodium channel inhibitors, flecainide, like encainide, exerts a differential effect on repolarization in ventricular muscle and Purkinje fibers, an effect that is likely to aggravate heterogeneity of excitability and refractoriness on the heart and may worsen VTs under certain experimental or clinical situations (75). Depending on the length of the reentrant circuit, slowing of conduction velocity without a coincident lengthening of the refractory period may result in multiple reentrant circuits (76). Quinidine, as well as procainamide, two class Ia antiarrhythmic agents, produce a prolongation of refractoriness and a rate-dependent depression of conduction velocity. The precise role of these EP effects in mediating an antiarrhythmic action is not clear. Studies (77) with procainamide indicate that lesser slowing of conduction velocity and greater prolongation of refractoriness tend to abolish reentry within the reentrant circuit. Drugs that prolong refractoriness appear more likely to be effective against tachycardia caused by reentry than are drugs that produce a slowing of conduction velocity as their major EP effect (78).

The canine model of sudden cardiac death successfully identified the proarrhythmic action of flecainide. The antiarrhythmic and antifibrillatory effects of flecainide acetate during the early postinfarction period were evaluated in the conscious canine model of sudden cardiac death. VT remained inducible early after infarction in 8 of 9 dogs receiving an intravenous loading dose of flecainide (2.0 mg/kg body weight) and 7 of 8 dogs receiving saline vehicle. In both the drug and vehicle groups, there was no significant change in the ventricular refractory period or in the cycle length of the induced VT. With a maintenance intravenous infusion of flecainide, 1.0 mg/kg/hr for 4 hr, the subsequent development of acute posterolateral ischemia resulted in ventricular fibrillation and sudden death in 7 of 8 flecainide-treated and 8 of 8 vehicle-treated dogs. Seven additional postin-farction dogs with noninducible tachycardia during a pretreatment of pro-grammed stimulation [thereby considered to be at low risk for the development of ischemic ventricular fibrillation (55)], were given flecainide in an intravenous loading and maintenance dosing regimen. The subsequent occurrence of posterolateral ischemia resulted in the development of ven-tricular fibrillation in 3 of these 7 dogs. These findings suggest that flecai-nide acetate may not possess pharmacologic properties useful in managing VT or in preventing ischemic ventricular fibrillation in the presence of recent myocardial damage (74, 79).

The only pharmacologic intervention shown to date to have a benefi-cial effect on sudden death is β-adrenergic receptor antagonism. A number of studies on the postmyocardial infarction period have confirmed signifi-cant protection with β-blockade (80–84). In this context there also appears to be a good correlation with the conscious canine model of sudden death, because protection herein has been demonstrated with a number of agents (63–65, 85). The antiarrhythmic and antifibrillatory potential of β-adreno-ceptor antagonism remains, however, unclear, and in particular there is much uncertainty over whether these drugs act by a direct antifibrillatory effect, or via a primary anti-ischemic influence.

Although no individual study with a class III agent has yet demon-strated significant antifibrillatory activity, suggestions of a beneficial trend are apparent in a recent meta-analysis by Teo et al. (86). These authors conducted an overview of randomized controlled trials of classes I and III antiarrhythmic agents and updated earlier overviews on classes II and IV antiarrhythmic drugs. A total of 137 trials involving 96,000 patients made up the study population. It was concluded that mortality was increased significantly with class I antiarrhythmic agents, reduced with classes II and III, and not significantly altered with class IV drugs. Data suggest that amiodarone and β-adrenoceptor blocking agents are the only drugs likely to reduce mortality, whereas other agents may be ineffective or may actually increase the likelihood of a fatal arrhythmia. With the exception of the ESVEM trial (24), most of the major ongoing studies are with amiodarone, with European and Canadian postmyocardial infarction trials and two place-bo-controlled trials in heart failure: the Veterans Administration Congestive Heart Failure Trial of antiarrhythmic therapy and the group study of heart failure survival in Argentina (GESICA).

Drug Protection in the Conscious Canine Model of Sudden Death: Direct or Indirect?

Except where ancillary EP properties are part of a particular agent's pharmacologic profile, the β-adrenergic receptor antagonists, as a group, appear to be devoid of a direct effect on the heart. Despite this, several studies have reported significant antiarrhythmic effects with these drugs, both in clinical (87) and experimental (88, 89) studies. Our laboratory has examined several β-adrenoceptor blocking agents for potential antiarrhythmic and antifibrillatory activity in the canine model of sudden cardiac death. Nadolol, a noncardioselective agent, was studied in the sudden death protocol after pretreatment with 1 ($N = 9$) and 8 ($N = 13$) mg/kg. Respective survival figures were 56% and 63% ($P < 0.01$ vs. placebo) (90). D-nadolol, an optical isomer devoid of β-adrenoceptor blocking properties, was ineffective. An interesting feature in this study was the observation that the majority of nadolol-treated dogs that died did so not from ventricular fibrillation, but as the result of complete heart block, severe bradycardia, and/or pump failure. This phenomenon was also observed in subsequent studies with dilevalol, the R,R-enantiomer of labetalol, where 75% of deaths were consequent on severe bradyarrhythmias (63, 64). The administration of methylscopolamine to postinfarction animals pretreated with dilevalol, however, significantly reduced mortality (40% vs. 100% vehicle-treated, $P < 0.05$), suggesting that dilevalol, like nadolol, was capable of preventing ischemic ventricular fibrillation in this model, but that death was caused by unopposed effects of parasympathetic influences plus the inability of the sinoatrial node to manifest a positive chronotropic action caused by the presence of β-adrenoceptor inhibition.

In a series of experiments with celiprolol, a class II drug with intrinsic stimulant properties, it was of significance that the drug was without effect in preventing sudden cardiac death (65). In particular, ventricular fibrillation was responsible for each of the seven deaths in the drug-treated group. Although the model is not designed specifically to address the question of intrinsic cardiostimulant phenomena, it was noted that resting heart rate did not change after celiprolol administration and it is possible that this feature of the drug attenuated any protection during acute posterolateral ischemia. It has been demonstrated, for example, that the propensity of sympathetic stimulation to induce arrhythmias in the late myocardial infarction period may relate primarily to heart rate (91). Previous studies have shown antagonism of the antiarrhythmic protection afforded by propranolol by overdrive atrial pacing (92). In a recent review of several large prospective double-blind trials with β-adrenoceptor antagonists, Kjekshus (62) demonstrated an almost linear relationship between the reduction in resting heart rate and mortality and noted that drugs with intrinsic sympathomimetic activity produced small reductions in heart rate and lesser effects on mortality. Although it is unclear whether celiprolol's stimulant properties are caused entirely to partial agonism (93), intrinsic sympathomimetic activity is cited as a possible reason why the drug failed to exert a beneficial influence on ventricular arrhythmias in a group of patients with acute myocardial infarction (94).

In an attempt to clarify the role of heart rate in the genesis of sudden death, we evaluated the antifibrillatory effects of alinidine, the *N*-allyl derivative of clonidine. Alinidine is one of a number of agents, the main pharmacological action of which appears to be a reduction in heart rate through a direct action on the sinus node (95, 96). Although capable of attenuating the chronotropic response to isoproterenol, these drugs do not operate by antagonism of β-adrenoceptors (13, 95). Similarly, there is no evidence that the specific bradycardic action involves α-adrenergic or muscarinic receptors, or calcium channels (13, 95, 97). However, studies in isolated tissues have shown a nonvoltage-dependent decrease in the slope of the slow diastolic depolarization, indicating that the drugs' effects may be mediated by restriction of current through anion-selective channels (97). In the canine model of sudden cardiac death, alinidine (1 mg/kg) produced a significant ($P < 0.01$) decrease in resting heart rate and prevented ventricular fibrillation in 6 of 10 animals studied ($P < 0.05$ vs. concurrent placebo group). In a third group of dogs where constant atrial pacing maintained heart rates at predrug values throughout the sudden death protocol, mortality was 100% despite pretreatment with alinidine (66). No changes were observed on parameters of ventricular refractoriness or conduction velocity.

Bradycardic agents, like the β-adrenoceptor antagonists, are capable of increasing perfusion pressure distal to a coronary artery stenosis (98), an effect which, for the bradycardic agents at least, appears to be attenuated by atrial pacing to control (predrug) heart rate values (99). Thus, during posterolateral ischemia, drugs with a negative chronotropic action, may contribute to an enhanced collateral flow in the ischemic bed secondary to slowing of heart rate, prolongation of diastole, and presumed reduction in myocardial oxygen consumption.

An additional property of the β-adrenoceptor antagonists is their ability to attenuate the potentially deleterious influence of enhanced adrenergic stimulation. In this respect, it is interesting to consider results in the sudden death model with the α_1-adrenoceptor antagonist, prazosin. Despite an inability to alter electrocardiographic intervals, ventricular refractories, or the induction of VT by programmed stimulation, pretreatment with 500 μg/kg of drug resulted in a 50% survival rate in the sudden death protocol ($P < 0.05$ vs. placebo) (71). This may be of particular significance in view of the recent suggestion that α-adrenergic responsiveness may be enhanced under conditions of myocardial ischemia (100, 101), and that this is correlated with an increase in α-adrenoceptor concentration (102). Although the relative contributions of α- and β-adrenergic influences in the genesis of ventricular fibrillation remain unclear, it has been suggested that α-mediated prolongation of action potential duration in ischemia areas may combine with β-mediated shortening of action potential duration in nonischemic areas to increase disparity in refractory periods and produce the arrhythmogenic milieu suitable for the emergence of fatal reentrant pathways (103). Antagonism of either adrenergic pathway (by the respective adrenergic antagonist) could, therefore, be seen as an indirect reduction in the EP derangements leading to ventricular fibrillation, and explain the protection afforded by both the β-adrenoceptor antagonists and prazosin in the animal model of sudden cardiac death.

In identifying a common direct EP characteristic to evaluate antifibrillatory efficacy in the experimental model of sudden cardiac death, it becomes apparent that the greatest overall protection has been seen with agents that have as part of their pharmacologic profile, prolongation of the action potential duration (class III activity). Studies with bretylium (104), amiodarone (85), sotalol (105, 106), and a number of experimental agents (107–109) have all demonstrated significant protection in placebo-controlled studies. The effects of clofilium, an alternative class III drug, were less clear (110) and may relate to a failure to provide an appropriate dosing regimen.

Bretylium was introduced into clinical cardiology in the early 1980s and is currently one of the few drugs marketed as an antifibrillatory agent. Its EP properties include direct effects on cardiac action potential duration and indirect effects mediated via its actions on the autonomic nervous system. Early studies with the drug demonstrated suppression of stimulus-induced VT (111, 112), and elevation in ventricular fibrillation thresholds (113). In the sudden cardiac death model, bretylium (10 mg/kg, i.v., 6-hourly) resulted in significant prolongation of ventricular refractoriness and the survival of 6 of the 10 animals studied ($P < 0.05$ vs. placebo). The exact antifibrillatory mechanism of the drug, however, remains obscure; although bretylium has been shown to exert similar electrophysiological effects in the denervated heart (114), the significance of its autonomic effects on the development of ventricular fibrillation are unknown. Furthermore, studies with bethanidine (69) and meobentine (70) failed to prevent ventricular fibrillation and sudden death in the same model, despite similar structural and EP characteristics.

Amiodarone originally was introduced as an antianginal agent, but subsequently was found to have EP features attributable to each of the four Vaughan Williams classes of antiarrhythmic drugs (115–117). In addition, amiodarone reduces the inotropic and chronotropic responses of other agents and has vasodilatory effects on the coronary and systemic vasculature (118). Its outstanding property, however, is prolongation of the cardiac action potential, prompting its identification as a potential antifibrillatory agent. Despite the observation that alterations in action potential duration and ventricular refractoriness are apparent only with chronic dosing, studies in our laboratory have demonstrated significant antifibrillatory protection after long- and short-term oral therapy. Although no differences were observed in plasma or myocardial concentrations of amiodarone between the two dosing regimens, the greater survival in those animals treated for 10 days (80% vs. 60% treated acutely) suggests that long-term therapy may have additional, as yet unidentified actions contributing to greater efficacy.

It is known that the EP effects of amiodarone resemble closely those of hypothyroidism (119, 120); that this is not caused by the iodine moiety of the drug has been shown in experiments where the administration of iodine has had no effect on cardiac action potentials (121). However, the concomitant administration of amiodarone and thyroid hormone has prevented the repolarization changes seen with amiodarone alone, and thyroidectomy can protect postinfarction animals from ischemic ventricular fibrillation in the sudden death protocol (122).

The effects of sotalol and its dextrorotatory enantiomer, *d*-sotalol, have been of particular importance in correlating the antifibrillatory potential of pharmacologic agents with their known EP characteristics. Racemic sotalol is a noncardioselective β-adrenoceptor antagonist that produces a dose-dependent prolongation of action potential duration without associated Vaughan Williams class I (membrane-stabilizing) properties. *d*-Sotalol, however, while retaining the same cardiac EP profile, does not share to the same extent the parent compound's β-adrenoceptor blocking properties. The use of *d*-sotalol allows an assessment of the relative antifibrillatory action of the drug's direct EP effects divorced from the confounding influence of β-adrenoceptor antagonism. Initial studies with racemic sotalol demonstrated a 65% survival in animals treated with the drug and entered into the sudden death protocol (105). The protective effect was associated with significant prolongation of the QT interval (an electrocardiographic parameter of action potential duration) and bridging diastolic electrical activity of the lead II ECG, a phenomenon invariably followed by ventricular fibrillation in vehicle-treated animals. In a subsequent study with the *d*-isomer, Lynch and coworkers (106) demonstrated similar EP and antifibrillatory effects, only without the attenuation of the ischemic increase in heart rate seen with the parent compound. This suggested that the observed antifibrillatory effect of *d*-sotalol was not related to antagonism of the β-adrenoceptor, but stemmed directly from prolongation of action potential duration and the increase in the ventricular refractory period.

More recent studies from this laboratory have reinforced the positive trend seen with agents sharing the ability to prolong ventricular refractoriness. The experimental agents CK-3579 and sematilide (107), E-4031 (108), and UK-68,798 (109) have produced protection in placebo-controlled studies in the canine model of sudden cardiac death.

Class III: One Activity, But Many Mechanisms

The Vaughan Williams classification was the first serious effort to classify antiarrhythmic agents based on what was known regarding common EP characteristics of the available drugs in the early 1970s (123). It is widely recognized, however, that the classification is not without major inadequacies, not least of which being that the system is essentially a hybrid:

classes I and IV represent agents that impair ion channels; class II agents inhibit receptors; and class III agents change an EP variable (the action potential duration) (124). Although actual mechanisms contributing to class III effect were not known 20 years ago, the common feature now appears to be interruption of normal potassium efflux by antagonism of one or more of the potassium channels (125, 126). With the increased understanding of the role of various potassium channels in health and disease has come an explosion of publications on the subject and an ever-increasing number of newly discovered channels in various organ systems (127).

Currently, it is not known which of these several types of potassium channels is responsible for the action of the class III antiarrhythmic agents, but evidence suggests the major effect of these drugs may be directed against the delayed rectifier channel, I_K (128). Blockade of the I_K channel appears to cause the most pronounced prolongation of repolarization in vitro, with the in vivo correlate of global increases in parameters of refractoriness. Blockage of the I_K, however, like any ubiquitous physiological channel, will have effects shared by all cardiac myocytes, normal and abnormal, ischemic and nonischemic. Bearing in mind the basic tenet of arrhythmia generation being a difference in EP characteristics between normal and abnormal myocardium, it can be seen that global increases in any parameter may be antiarrhythmic in one situation while proarrhythmic in another, if inhomogenous prolongation of refractoriness is associated with the emergence of reentrant pathways. Unlike the use-dependence of class I agents, class III drugs appear in many cases to have a reverse-use dependence, with excessive prolongation of action potential duration at slow heart rates. This has been implicated as a possible cause of the reported long QT syndromes (with the associated risks of torsades de pointes and ventricular fibrillation) with these drugs (128).

Potassium Currents that Predominate During Altered Metabolic States

Abnormalities of membrane function arise in response to myocardial ischemia or hypoxia and favor the development of slow conduction and unidirectional block. Both conditions are essential for establishing a reentrant pathway capable of supporting ventricular tachyarrhythmias. Among the EP changes observed in the ischemic or hypoxic tissue is the abrupt increase in extracellular potassium concentration accompanied by intracellular acidosis and a decrease in tissue ATP concentration. In addition, conditions of metabolic inhibition, as with ischemia or hypoxia, lead to the liberation of free fatty acids and a gain in intracellular sodium and calcium ions. The decrease in tissue ATP content, the increase in tissue free fatty acids, and the gain in intracellular sodium and calcium ions each activate separate potassium channels. The single-channel conductance of the potassium channels activated under pathophysiological conditions is greater than that occurring when potassium channels are operative under normal conditions. Conditions of altered myocardial metabolism resulting from hypoxia and/or ischemia, would favor outward rectification so that the outward current predominates over the inward current. Significant outward current would flow during depolarization, resulting in a decrease in the action potential duration. The accumulation of potassium in the extracellular space will depolarize the myocardial cell membrane. The net result of the local ionic events is to decrease conduction velocity and shorten the effective refractory period which, in the presence of a suitable myocardial substrate, has the potential to result in a lethal arrhythmia. The three potassium channels that predominate under pathophysiologic conditions may, thus, act synergistically to favor outward rectification and provide the conditions needed for reentry.

The most widely studied of the three pathophysiologic channels in the heart is the ATP-dependent potassium channel (K_{ATP}). With the discovery that this channel regulates insulin release in pancreatic islet β-cells (129), and their subsequent demonstration in the heart (130), came the realization of a cardiac channel active only in pathological (hypoxic or ischemic) circumstances, where it could potentially play a crucial role in the genesis of fatal reentrant arrhythmias. Furthermore the functional or active K_{ATP} channels would become manifest only in myocardial cells in which intracellular ATP was decreased. The concept was supported by the finding that glibenclamide, a sulfonylurea that (like all members of its class) exerted an antidiabetic effect by promoting the closure of pancreatic K_{ATP} channels, could also reverse the EP consequences of ischemia in isolated myocardial cells (131). At about the same time, independent research had demonstrated that glibenclamide was effective in preventing the development of ventricular fibrillation in isolated heart preparations under conditions of low intracellular ATP, whether the result of ischemia (132, 133) or hypoxia (134). When hearts are made hypoxic or ischemic in the presence of glibenclamide, the potassium loss during the early phase is partially blocked by glibenclamide (135–137). Based on these observations, it appears that part of the potassium loss during hypoxia or ischemia can be attributed to activation of the K_{ATP} channel, although other mechanisms may be involved, such as the sodium-activated and fatty acid-sensitive potassium channels. Arachidonic acid and its metabolites, as well as other unsaturated fatty acids, may thus modulate potassium channel activity by acting on this channel. Understanding the manner in which pharmacologic interventions modulate the several potassium channels in the ventricular myocardium is complicated by the fact that there seems to be an interaction among the activity of potassium channel modulators and tissue metabolites. For example, the effectiveness of glibenclamide to block the K_{ATP} channel depends on the cytosolic concentration of ADP (138), whereas the ability of pinacidil to act as an opener depends on the cytosolic content of ATP

(139, 140). There is no doubt that the tissue content of both ATP and ADP will be altered during intervals of hypoxia and dischemia as well as on reperfusion. Thus, alterations in tissue metabolites will influence the final outcome of any experimental protocol and may account for incongruous results among laboratories, because the content of tissue metabolites may vary according to the particular experimental protocol used.

Our laboratory has confirmed the antifibrillatory effect glybenclamide in the rabbit isolated heart made hypoxic in the presence of pinacidil (141) (Fig. 3). Pinacidil promotes intracellular potassium efflux and significantly reduces action potential duration via an agonist effect on K_{ATP} channels (140, 142). In the normoxic heart during atrial pacing, pinacidil is without discernible effects on cardiac rhythm, despite the fact that a significant decrease in ventricular effective refractory period occurs, presumably caused by opening of the K_{ATP} channel. However, in the presence of pinacidil, but less likely in its absence, ventricular fibrillation occurs in >90% of hearts made hypoxic for 12 min or occurs shortly after the heart is reoxygenated (141). The induction of ventricular fibrillation in the pres-

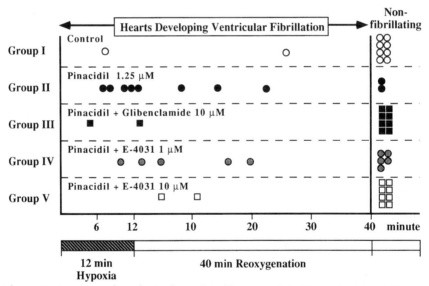

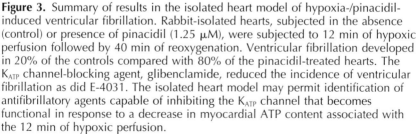

Figure 3. Summary of results in the isolated heart model of hypoxia-/pinacidil-induced ventricular fibrillation. Rabbit-isolated hearts, subjected in the absence (control) or presence of pinacidil (1.25 μM), were subjected to 12 min of hypoxic perfusion followed by 40 min of reoxygenation. Ventricular fibrillation developed in 20% of the controls compared with 80% of the pinacidil-treated hearts. The K_{ATP} channel-blocking agent, glibenclamide, reduced the incidence of ventricular fibrillation as did E-4031. The isolated heart model may permit identification of antifibrillatory agents capable of inhibiting the K_{ATP} channel that becomes functional in response to a decrease in myocardial ATP content associated with the 12 min of hypoxic perfusion.

ence of pinacidil is dependent on a decrease in myocardial cell ATP content, thereby suggesting that the hyocardial K_{ATP} channel shows increased responsiveness to the agonist effects of pinacidil when it is disinhibited as a result of decreased cellular ATP. Glibenclamide, known for its ability to inhibit the K_{ATP} channel, prevents the pinacidil-induced decrease in the effective refractory period and significantly reduces the incidence of ventricular fibrillation in the hypoxic reoxygenated perfused heart (141). The profibrillatory action of pinacidil is unmasked by myocardial hypoxia or ischemia, either of which will decrease myocardial cell ATP content. It is anticipated that a lowering of myocardial ATP will favor opening of the K_{ATP} channel, especially in the presence of the agonist, pinacidil. The two events—lowering of cellular ATP and further opening of the K_{ATP} channel by the agonist, pinacidil—would favor the rapid outward movement of potassium and a marked decrease in the ventricular refractory period.

It is proposed that a special binding site is located on the intracellular side of the membrane by which ATP closes the K_{ATP} channel (143). Opening of the K_{ATP} channel occurs when intracellular ATP content is reduced. Under conditions of reduced intracellular ATP, pinacidil is more likely to facilitate an opening of the K_{ATP} channel, thereby enhancing an effect similar to that of a reduced intracellular ATP concentration. It has been suggested that pinacidil opens the K_{ATP} channel by antagonizing ATP binding or that pinacidil binds to a different site and modulates the affinity of the receptor to ATP by a pseudocompetitive action (144). Consistent with this explanation is the observation that only channels closed by low concentrations of ATP could be opened by potassium channel agonists (140, 145). Therefore, the open probability of the K_{ATP} channel can be significant in the absence of ATP and can be influenced further by the interaction of cofactors formed during ischemia or hypoxia. The possibility must be entertained that during ischemia there may be a finite probability for the channel to open. Half-maximal sensitivity of the channel increases 4-fold by the addition of ADP and GDP in concentrations known to exist during metabolic inhibition or ischemia (146, 147). A significant open probability of the K_{ATP} channel may be expected under appropriate conditions even with millimolar concentrations of ATP (147, 148). The K_{ATP} channel-dependent action potential shortening is likely to occur if ATP concentrations fall below normal levels ($\sim$5 mM), as may happen regionally, or globally, suring myocardial ischemia (149). The known relationship between cellular ATP concentration and the functioning of the K_{ATP} channel would suggest that selective channel agonists should be more effective in the ischemic heart than in normal myocardium. Our observations in the intact postinfarcted canine heart and in the hypoxic perfused heart, would support the conclusion that K_{ATP} channel openers, although of no deleterious consequence during normal oxygenation, become profibrillatory under conditions of metabolic inhibition leading to a decrease in intracellular ATP concentration (133, 141, 150, 151). Confusion arises over whether it is more advantageous to restore an abnormally shortened action potential to a normal action potential by application of a K_{ATP} channel closer (e.g., glibenclamide) or to shorten further the action potential in cardiac cells by administration of a K_{ATP} channel opener (e.g., pinacidil). Studies designed to examine myocardial recovery of contractile function have suggested the later alternative as the desirable course of action to prevent the deleterious effects of ischemia and preserve the viability of cardiac cells and recovery of contractile function (152–156). Future studies must address the issue of whether it is more important to preserve contractile function at the risk of jeopardizing EP properties of the heart subjected to metabolic inhibition. Will inhibitors of the K_{ATP} channel, other than glibenclamide, have the same undesirable effects on recovery of function? To date, class III antiarrhythmic agents known to inhibit the delayed rectifier current, have not been shown to influence ischemic myocardial injury (157), but in contrast, may exhibit a positive inotropic action as assessed by the measurement of dP/dt (158). The class III antiarrhythmic agents differ significantly from glibenclamide with respect to modulating the effects of ischemia on myocardial tissue, because the latter has been reported to have a negative influence on functional recovery and tissue viability after ischemic myocardial injury (152, 159).

Pharmacologic interventions directed at blocking the K_{ATP} channel, thereby preventing a decrease in the ventricular refractory period, may provide a useful approach to the prevention of ventricular fibrillation, without necessarily possessing antifibrillatory activity, as manifest by the reduction or prevention in premature ventricular depolarizations. Based on these observations, it is suggested that inhibition of the K_{ATP} channel, by preventing potassium efflux, will antagonize reductions in the action potential duration and will prevent the shortening of refractoriness in ischemic and ATP-depleted myocardial cells. By so doing, disparity in refractory periods can be avoided and with it the risk of emergent ventricular reentrant arrhythmias.

Using a cohort of small-infarct, noninducible dogs similar to those previously described in the flecainide study, we evaluated the profibrillatory action of pinacidil in the sudden cardiac death model. Compared with a 24-hr mortality in the placebo group of 20% (incidence of ischemic ventricular fibrillation 6.7%), mortality in the pinacidil group was 87% (ischemic fibrillation 60%)—a difference statistically significant at the $P < 0.01$ level. Changes in arterial blood pressure did not reach statistical significance, indicating that the profibrillatory effect could not be explained on the basis of hypotension (150). These studies provide further support for the pivotal role of the K_{ATP} channel in the genesis of fatal cardiac arrhythmias. In the search for the K_{ATP} channel antagonist to be developed as the first potential antifibrillatory agent, the hypoglycemic properties of the sulfonylureas make their evaluation particularly difficult in the intact animal. However, a number of unrelated compounds claim to have K_{ATP}-blocking activity as part of their pharmacologic profile; one in particular, 5-hydroxy-decanoic acid purports to be a pure K_{ATP} channel antagonist and appears to attenuate ischemic ventricular fibrillation in the rat heart (160), and in preliminary studies with the chronic canine model of sudden cardiac death (unpublished observations).

Most of our understanding of the channel-blocking actions of class III antiarrhythmic agents is derived from voltage-clamp studies. Such studies provide a clear demonstration of an hypoxia-induced increase in time-dependent potassium current as being the important factor in shortening of the ventricular action potential. Although the derived information is promising, there remains a void in our knowledge concerning the relationship of the observed EP and ionic changes to the onset of malignant disturbances in cardiac rhythm under conditions that approximate the clinical situation of sudden cardiac death. The use of the canine model of sudden cardiac death has proved valuable in bridging the gap between EP studies and events as they occur in the intact heart under pathophysiologic conditions. The isolated perfused rabbit heart subjected to hypoxia and the K_{ATP} channel opener, pinacidil, represents a valuable addition to the study of class III antifibrillatory agents. In this model, the induction of ventricular fibrillation is dependent on the hypoxia-induced decrease in tissue ATP content, together with the influence of the K_{ATP} channel opener, pinacidil to facilitate the opening of the K_{ATP} channel. The ability of glibenclamide and a number of class III antiarrhythmic agents (E-4031 and 5-hydroxydecanoate) to protect against the development of ventricular fibrillation suggest a role for the K_{ATP} channel in the development of ventricular fibrillation. The antifibrillatory action of these agents may be attributed, in part, to their suppression of potassium release from ischemic hypoxic or ischemic myocardium, perhaps through inhibition of the ATP-regulated potassium channel. In addition to demonstrating antifibrillatory activity for specific interventions, results obtained in the isolated heart support the observations on the intact animal in which profibrillatory events have been uncovered, as was the case with flecainide (74, 161). Class I antiarrhythmic agents—quinidine, aprindine, lidocaine, and flecainide—were selected for study in the isolated heart made hypoxic and treated with pinacidil. Only quinidine prevented the pinacidil-induced ventricular fibrillation. Flecainide in the presence of hypoxia, but in the absence of pinacidil, invariably was associated with the onset of ventricular fibrillation that could be prevented by pretreatment with glibenclamide (161). The observations suggest that ventricular fibrillation can be provoked by the potassium channel agonist, pinacidil, or by flecainide, under conditions that reduce intracellular ATP concentration. Glibenclamide, a selective antagonist of the K_{ATP} channel, prevented the profibrillatory actions of both pinacidil and flecainide.

Conclusions

The lack of effective and safe drugs for the prevention of lethal arrhythmias and sudden cardiac death has served to stimulate renewed interest in the area of drug development and the introduction of several new candidate agents that share a common ability to prolong ventricular refractoriness. Equally important is the recognition that most antiarrhythmic agents have been evaluated with in vitro or in vivo models that have little relevance to the clinical situation of sudden cardiac death. As the recent CAST report (16, 18) has emphasized, the final analysis of a drug's ultimate utility will depend on appropriate clinical testing in patients who are at risk of developing sudden and unexpected life-threatening arrhythmias or ventricular fibrillation. We can no longer afford to use the more expedient and less dependable approach evaluating new agents for their ability to reduce the frequency or complexity of ventricular depolarizations, or their ability to modify the patient's response to programmed electrical stimulation. Despite the formidable task involved in the clinical assessment of an effective therapy for the prevention of ventricular fibrillation, the challenge could be made more readily attainable by preclinical assessment of a candidate drug, based on studies conducted in relevant animal models using meaningful EP endpoints that occur spontaneously. We have used an animal model of sudden cardiac death in which ventricular fibrillation develops within 1 hr from the onset of an ischemic event in myocardial substrate that has been identified, through the use of programmed electrical stimulation, to be capable of supporting an arrhythmic mechanism. The conscious, postinfarcted, canine model has been used by us to confirm antifibrillatory activity of a number of approved antiarrhythmic agents, of several agents at exploratory stages of development, and to warn of profibrillatory dangers with others. A recent publication by Craig Pratt, M.D., Chairman of the Cardiovascular and Renal Drugs Advisory Board of the U.S. Food and Drug Administration, concludes by stating: "Although a number of animal models of sudden death exist, it seems desirable to use the model with previous MI (healed scar) and new induction of ischemia, which may most closely emulate the situation seen in the CAST" (162). The significance of the animal model as a potential solution to a major public health problem becomes particularly important, especially at a time when there is increasing pressure to abandon the physiologic approach to basic research by activists who oppose the biomedical use of animals. The animal model—together with studies conducted at the cellular, biochemical, and molecular levels—will serve as the conduits for understanding the physiopathologic events leading to lethal arrhythmias and developing pharmacologic interventions aimed at preventing sudden cardiac death.

Acknowledgments

This study was supported by the National Institutes of Health–National Heart, Lung, and Blood Institute Merit Award HL-05806-32.

We thank the National Heart, Lung, and Blood Institute for the uninterrupted support of our studies on the analysis of antiarrhythmic agents.

Much of this work would not have been possible without the cooperation of colleagues in the pharmaceutical industry who provided many drugs studied over the past 12 years. We also acknowledge the dedication of the many pre- and postdoctoral fellows and faculty colleagues who participated in our research programs during this period.

References

1. Roberts, W.C. (1986). Sudden cardiac death: Definitions and causes. *Am. J. Cardiol.* **57:**1410.

2. Kannel, W.B., McGee, D.L., and Schatzkin, A. (1984). An epidemiological perspective of sudden death: 26-year follow up in the Framingham Study. *Drugs* **28:**1.

3. Myerburg, R.J., Kessler, K.M., and Castellanos, A. (1992). Sudden cardiac death. Structure, function, and time-dependence of risk. *Circulation* **85:**I-2.

4. Buxton, A.E. (1992). Antiarrhythmic drugs: Good for premature ventricular contractions but bad for patients? *Ann. Intern. Med.* **116:**420.

5. Moss, A.J., DeCamilla, J., and David, H. (1980). Factors associated with cardiac death in the post-hospital phase of myocardial infarction, in *Sudden Death*, H.E. Kulbertus and H.J.J. Wellens, Eds. (Martinus Nihoff Publishing, The Hague, Netherlands), p. 237.

6. The Coronary Drug Project Research Group. (1973). Prognostic importance of premature beats following myocardial infarction. *JAMA* **223:**116.

7. Moss, A.J., et al. (1979). Ventricular ectopic beats and their relation to sudden and nonsudden cardiac death after myocardial infarction. *Circulation* **60:**998.

8. Hinkle, L.E. (1981). The immediate antecedents of sudden death. *Acta Med. Scand.* **651:**207.

9. The Multicenter Postinfarction Research Group. (1983). Risk stratification and survival after myocardial infarction. *N. Engl. J. Med.* **309:**331.

10. Mukharji, J., et al. (1984). Risk factors for sudden death after myocardial infarction: Two-year follow-up. *Am. J. Cardiol.* **54:**31.

11. Bigger, J.T., et al. (1984). The relationships among ventricular arrhythmias, left ventricular dysfunction, and mortality in the 2 years after myocardial infarction. *Circulation* **69:**250.

12. Gianelly, R., et al. (1967). Effect of lidocaine on ventricular arrhythmias in patients with coronary heart disease. *N. Engl. J. Med.* **277:**1215.

13. Lillie, C., and Kobinger, W. (1983). Actions of alinidine and AQ-A 39 on rate and contractility of guinea pig atria during β-adrenoceptor stimulation. *J. Cardiovasc. Pharmacol.* **5:**1048.

14. Furberg, C.D. (1983). Effects of antiarrhythmic drugs on mortality after myocardial infarction. *Am. J. Cardiol.* **52:**32C.

15. May, G.S., et al. (1983). Secondary prevention after myocardial infarction: A review of short-term acute phase trials. *Prog. Cardiovasc. Dis.* **25:**335.

16. CAST Investigators. (1989). Preliminary report: effect of encainide and flecainide on mortality in a randomized trial of arrhythmia suppression after myocardial infarction. *N. Engl. J. Med.* **321**:406.

17. The Cardiac Arrhythmia Pilot Study Investigators. (1986). The Cardiac Arrhythmia Pilot Study. *Am. J. Cardiol.* **57**:91.

18. CAST II Investigators. (1992). Effect of the antiarrhythmic agent morizicine on survival after myocardial infarction. *N. Engl. J. Med.* **327**:227.

19. Wellens, H.J., Schuilenburg, R.M., and Durrer, D. (1972). Electrical stimulation of the heart in patients with ventricular tachycardia. *Circulation* **46**:216.

20. Roy, D., et al. (1983). Clinical characteristics and long-term follow-up in 119 survivors of cardiac arrest: Relation to inducibility at electrophysiologic testing. *Am. J. Cardiol.* **52**:969.

21. Ruskin, J.N. (1992). Role of invasive electrophysiological testing in the evaluation and treatment of patients at high risk for sudden cardiac death. *Circulation* **85**:I-152.

22. Skale, B.T., et al. (1986). Survivors of cardiac arrest: Prevention of recurrence by drug therapy as predicted by electrophysiologic testing or ECG monitoring. *Am. J. Cardiol.* **57**:113.

23. Cupples, L.A., Gagnon, D.R., and Kannel, W.B. (1992). Long- and short-term risk of sudden cardiac death: Population at risk. *Circulation* **85**:I-1.

24. The Electrophysiology Study Versus Electrocardiographic Monitoring (ESVEM) Investigators. (1989). The ESVEM trial: Electrophysiologic study versus electrocardiographic monitoring for selection of antiarrhythmic therapy of ventricular tachyarrhythmias. *Circulation* **79**:1354.

25. Kuller, L., Cooper, M., and Perper, J. (1972). Epidemiology of sudden death. *Arch. Intern. Med.* **129**:714.

26. Baum, R.S., Alvares, H., and Cobb, L.A. (1974). Survival after resuscitation from out-of-hospital ventricular fibrillation. *Circulation* **50**:1231.

26a. Weaver, W.D., et al. (1976). Angiographic findings and prognostic indicators in patients resuscitated from sudden cardiac death. *Circulation* **54**:895.

27. Reichenbach, D.D., Moss, N.S., and Meyer, E. (1977). Pathology of the heart in sudden cardiac death. *Am. J. Cardiol.* **39**:865.

28. Goldstein, S., et al. (1981). Characteristics of the resuscitated out-of-hospital cardiac arrest victim with coronary heart disease. *Circulation* **64**:977.

29. Schuster, E.H., and Bulkley, B.H. (1980). Ischemia at a distant site after myocardial infarction: A cause of early postinfarction angina. *Circulation* **62**:509.

30. Schwartz, P.J., and Stone, H.L. (1980). Left stellectomy in the prevention of ventricular fibrillation caused by acute myocardial ischemia in conscious dogs with anterior myocardial infarction. *Circulation* **62**:1256.

31. Schwartz, P.J., Billman, G.E., and Stone, H.L. (1984). Autonomic mechanism in ventricular fibrillation induced by myocardial ischemia during exercise in dogs with healed myocardial infarction. An experimental preparation for sudden death. *Circulation* **69**:790.

32. Kabell, G., et al. (1984). Mechanisms of ventricular arrhythmias in multivessel coronary disease: The effects of collateral zone ischemia. *Am. Heart J.* **108**:447.

33. Previtali, M., et al. (1983). Ventricular tachyarrhythmias in Prinzmetal's variant angina: Clinical significance and relation to the degree and time course of ST segment elevation. *Am. J. Cardiol.* **52**:19

34. Miller, D.D., et al. (1982). Clinical characteristics associated with sudden death in patients with variant angina. *Circulation* **66**:588.

34a. Malliani, A., Schwartz, P.J., and Zanchetti, A. (1980). Neural mechanisms in life-threatening arrhythmias. *Am. Heart J.* **100**:705.

35. Schwartz, P.J., La Rovere, M.T., and Vanoli, E. (1992). Autonomic nervous system and sudden cardiac death. Experimental basis and clinical observations for post-myocardial infarction risk stratification. *Circulation* **85**:I-77.

36. Schwartz, P.J., et al. (1973). A cardiocardiac sympatho-vagal reflex in the cat. *Circ. Res.* **32**:215.

37. Myerburg, R.J., et al. (1982). Electrophysiological consequences of experimental acute ishchemia superimposed upon healed myocardial infarction in cats. *Am. J. Cardiol.* **49**:323.

38. Patterson, E., et al. (1982). Ventricular fibrillation resulting from ischemia at a site remote from previous myocardial infarction. A conscious canine model of sudden coronary death. *Am. J. Cardiol.* **50**:1412.

39. Garan, H., McComb, J.M., and Ruskin, J.N. (1988). Spontaneous and electrically induced ventricular arrhythmia during acute ischemia superimposed on 2-week-old canine myocardial infarction. *J. Am. Coll. Cardiol.* **11**:603.

40. Maseri, A., et al. (1978). "Variant" angina: One aspect of a continuous spectrum of vasospastic myocardial ischemia. *Am. J. Cardiol.* **42**:1019.

41. Davies, M.J., and Thomas, A. (1984). Thrombosis and acute coronary artery lesions in sudden cardiac ischemic death. *N. Engl. J. Med.* **310**:1137.

42. Haerem, J.W. (1974). Mural platelet microthrombi and major acute lesions of main epicardial arteries in sudden coronary death. *Atherosclerosis* **19**:529.

43. Mehta, J., and Mehta, P. (1981). Role of platelets and prostaglandins in coronary artery disease. *Am. J. Cardiol.* **48**:366.

44. Hammon, J.W., and Oates, J.A. (1986). Interaction of platelets with the vessel wall in the pathophysiology of sudden cardiac death. *Circulation* **73**:224.

45. Lucchesi, B.R., and Lynch, J.J. (1986). Preclinical assessment of antiarrhythmic drugs. *Fed. Proc.* **45**:2197.

46. Maling, H.M., and Moran, N.C. (1957). Ventricular arrhythmias induced by sympathomimetic amines in unanesthetized dogs following coronary artery occlusion. *Circ. Res.* **5**:409.

47. El-Sherif, N., et al. (1977). Re-entrant ventricular arrhythmis in the late myocardial infarction period. 1. Conduction characteristics in the infarction zone. *Circulation* **55**:686.

48. Karagueuzian, H.S., et al. (1979). Protracted ventricular tachycardia induced by premature stimulation of the canine heart after coronary artery occlusion and reperfusion. *Circ. Res.* **44**:833.

49. Moore, E.N., and Spear, J.F. (1975). Ventricular fibrillation threshold. Its physiological and pharmacological importance. *Arch. Intern. Med.* **135:**446.

50. Euler, D.E., and Scanlon, P.J. (1988). Comparative effects of antiarrhythmic drugs on the ventricular fibrillation threshold. *J. Cardiovasc. Pharmacol.* **11:**291.

51. Axelrod, P.J., Verrier, R.L., and Lown, B. (1975). Vulnerability to ventricular fibrillation during acute coronary artery occlusion and release. *Am. J. Cardiol.* **36:**776.

52. Euler, D.E. (1980). Norepinephrine release by ventricular stimulation: Effect on fibrillation thresholds. *Am. J. Physiol.* **238:**H406.

53. Anderson, J.L., Rodier, H.E., and Green, L.S. (1983). Comparative effects of beta-adrenergic blocking drugs on experimental ventricular fibrillation thresholds. *Am. J. Cardiol.* **51:**1196.

54. Patterson, E., and Lucchesi, B.R. (1984). Antifibrillatory properties of the beta-adrenergic receptor antagonists nadolol, sotalol, atenolol and propranolol in the anesthetized dog. *Pharmacology* **28:**121.

55. Wilber, D.J., et al. (1985). Postinfarction sudden death: Significance of inducible ventricular tachycardia and infarct size in a conscious canine model. *Am. Heart J.* **109:**8.

56. Josephson, M.E., et al. (1978). Recurrent sustained ventricular tachycardia. 1. Mechanisms. *Circulation* **57:**431.

57. Uprichard, A.C.G., and Lucchesi, B.R. (1991). Antifibrillatory drugs, in *Basic and Clinical Electrophysiology and Pharmacology of the Heart*, K.H. Dangman and D.S. Miura, Eds. (Marcel Dekker, New York), p. 723.

58. Panidis, J.P., and Morganroth, J. (1983). Sudden death in hospitalized patients: Cardiac rhythm disturbances detected by ambulatory echocardiographic monitoring. *J. Am. Coll. Cardiol.* **2:**798.

59. Kempf, F.C., and Josephson, M.E. (1984). Cardiac arrest recorded on ambulatory electrocardiograms. *Am. J. Cardiol.* **53:**1577.

60. Milner, P.G., et al. (1985). Ambulatory electrocardiographic recordings at the time of fatal cardiac arrest. *Am. J. Cardiol.* **56:**588.

61. Patterson, E., and Lucchesi, B.R. (1983). Quinidine gluconate in chronic myocardial ischemic injury—Differential effects in response to programmed stimulation and acute myocardia ischemia in the dog. *Circulation* **68:**III-155.

62. Kjekshus, J. (1985). Comments—Beta blockers: Heart rate reduction—A mechanism of benefit *Eur. Heart J.* **6:**29.

63. Lynch, J.J., et al. (1987). Antifibrillatory efficacy of concomitant beta adrenergic receptor blockade with dilevalol, the R,R-isomer of labetalol, and muscarinic receptor blockade with methylscopolamine. *J. Pharmacol. Exp. Ther.* **241:**741.

64. Lynch, J.J., and Lucchesi, B.R. (1987). How are animal models best used for the study of antiarrhythmic drugs?, in *Life-Threatening Arrhythmias and Infarction*, D.J. Hearse, A.S. Manning, and M.J. Janse, Eds. (Raven Press, New York), p. 169.

65. Uprichard, A.C.G., Lynch, J.J., and Kitzen, J.M. (1989). Celiprolol, a β1-selective adrenoceptor antagonist with intrinsic stimulant properties does

not protect against ventricular tachycardia or ventricular fibrillation in a conscious canine model of myocardial infarction and sudden death. *J. Pharmacol. Exp. Ther.* **251**:571.

66. Uprichard, A.C.G., et al. (1989). Alinidine protects against ischemic ventricular fibrillation in a conscious canine model: Probable anti-ischemic mode of action. *J. Cardiovasc. Pharmacol.* **14**:475.

67. Lynch, J.J., et al. (1985). Antiarrhythmic and electrophysiologic effects of bepridil in chronically infarcted conscious dogs. *J. Pharmacol. Exp. Ther.* **234**:72.

68. Patterson, E., Eller, B.T., and Lucchesi, B.R. (1983). Effects of diltiazem upon experimental ventricular dysrhythmias. *J. Pharmacol. Exp. Ther.* **225**:224.

69. Patterson, E., Amalfitano, D.J., and Lucchesi, B.R. (1984). Development of ventricular tachyarrhythmias in the conscious canine during the recovery phase of experimental ischemic injury: Effect of bethanidine administration. *J. Cardiovasc. Pharmacol.* **6**:470.

70. Zimmerman, J.M., et al. (1984). Antidysrhythmic actions of meobentine. *Am. Heart J.* **107**:1117.

71. Wilber, D.J., et al. (1987). Alpha-adrenergic influences in canine ischemic sudden death: Effects of alpha1-adrenoceptor blockade with prazosin. *J. Cardiovasc. Pharmacol.* **10**:96.

72. Kitzen, J.M., et al. (1988). Failure of thromboxane synthetase inhibition to protect the postinfarcted heart against the induction of ventricular tachycardia and ventricular fibrillation in a conscious canine model of sudden coronary death. *Pharmacology* **37**:171.

73. Kitzen, J.M., et al. (1990). Effects of combined thromboxane synthetase inhibition/thromboxane receptor antagonism in two models of sudden death in the canine: Limited role for thromboxane. *J. Cardiovasc. Pharmacol.* **16**:68.

74. Kou, W.H., et al. (1987). Effect of flecainide acetate on prevention of electrical induction of ventricular tachycardia and occurence of ischemic ventricular fibrillation during the early postmyocardial periods: Evaluation in a conscious canine model of sudden death. *J. Am. Coll. Cardiol.* **9**:359.

75. Ikeda, N., et al. (1985). Effects of flecainide on the electrophysiologic properties of isolated canine and rabbit myocardial fibers. *J. Am. Coll. Cardiol.* **5**:303.

76. Brugada, J., et al. (1990). Double wave re-entry as a mechanism of acceleration of ventricular tachycardia. *Circulation* **81**:1633.

77. Furukawa, T., et al. (1989). Efficacy of procainamide on ventricular tachycardia: Relation to prolongation of refractoriness and slowing of conduction. *Am. Heart J.* **118**:702.

78. Sasyniuk, B.I., and McQuillan, J. (1983). Mechanisms by which antiarrhythmic drugs influence induction of reentrant responses in subendocardial Purkinje network of 1-day-old infarcted canine ventricle, in *Cardiac Electrophysiology and Arrhythmias*, D.P. Zipes and J. Jalife, Eds. (Grune & Stratton, Orlando), p. 389.

79. Lynch, J.J., et al. (1987). Effects of flecainide acetate on ventricular tachyarrhythmia and fibrillation in dogs with recent myocardial infarction. *Pharmacology* **35**:181.

80. Multicentre International Study. (1975). Improvement in prognosis of myocardial infarction by long-term β-adrenoceptor blockage using practolol. *Br. Med. J.* **3**:735.

81. Norwegian Multicenter Study Group. (1981). Timolol-induced reduction in mortality and reinfarction in patients surviving acute myocardial infarction. *N. Engl. J. Med.* **304**:801.

82. Beta-Blocker Heart Attack Trial Research Group. (1982). A randomized trial of propanolol in patients with acute myocardial infarction. *JAMA* **247**:1707.

83. Yusuf, S., et al. (1985). Beta blockade during and after myocardial infarction: An overview of the randomized trials. *Prog. Cardiovasc. Dis.* **27**:335.

84. The MIAMI Trial Research Group. (1985). Metoprolol in acute myocardial infarction (MIAMI): A randomised placebo-controlled international trial. *Eur. Heart J.* **6**:199.

85. Patterson, E., et al. (1983). Ventricular fibrillation in a conscious canine preparation of sudden coronary death—Prevention by short- and long-term amiodarone administration. *Circulation* **68**:857.

86. Teo, K., Yusuf, S., and Furberg, C. (1992). Effect of prophylactic antiarrhythmic drug therapy on post-myocardial infarction mortality. *Eur. Heart J.*, in press.

87. Rossi, P.R., et al. (1983). Reduction of ventricular arrhythmias by early intravenous atenolol in suspected acute myocardial infarction. *Br. Med. J.* **286**:506.

88. Echt, D.S., et al. (1983). Nature of inducible ventricular arrhythmias in a canine chronic myocardial infarction model. *Am. J. Cardiol.* **52**:1127.

89. Gang, E.S., Bigger, J.T., and Uhl, E.W. (1984). Effects of timolol and propranolol on inducible sustained ventricular tachyarrhythmias in dogs with subacute myocardial infarction. *Am. J. Cardiol.* **53**:275.

90. Patterson, E., and Luccesi, B.R. (1983). Antifibrillatory actions of d,l-nadolol in a conscious canine model of sudden coronary death. *J. Cardiovasc. Pharmacol.* **5**:737.

91. El-Sherif, N. (1978). Re-entrant ventricular arrhythmias in the late myocardial infarction period 6. Effects of the autonomic system. *Circulation* **58**:103.

92. Hope, R.R., et al. (1974). The efficacy of antiarrhythmic agents during acute myocardial ischemia and the role of heart rate. *Circulation* **50**:507.

93. Wolf, P.S., et al. (1985). Celiprolol—pharmacological profile of an unconventional beta-blocker. *Br. J. Clin. Pract.* **39**:5.

94. Payrhuber, K., Kratzer, H., and Kuhn, P. (1986). Celiprolol in acute myocardial infarct. *Wien. Klin. Wochensch.* **98**:171.

95. Kobinger, W., Lillie, C., and Pichler, L. (1979). N-allyl-derative of clonidine, a substance with specific bradycardic action at a cardiac site. *Naunyn-Schmied. Arch. Pharmacol.* **306**:255.

96. Kobinger, W., Lillie, C., and Pichler, L. (1979). Cardiovascular actions of N-allyl-clonidine (ST 567), a substance with specific bradycardiac action. *Eur. J. Pharmacol.* **58**:141.

97. Millar, J.S., and Vaughan Williams, E.M. (1981). Pacemaker selectivity: Influence on rabbit atria of ionic environment and of alinidine, a possible anion antagonist *Cardiovasc. Res.* **15**:335.

98. Gross, G.J., et al. (1984). Effects of three bradycardic drugs on regional myocardial blood flow and function in areas distal to a total or partial coronary occlusion in dogs. *Circulation* **69**:391.

99. Gross, G.J., and Daemmgen, J.W. (1987). Effect of the new specific bradycardic agent AQ-A39 (falipamil) on coronary collateral blood flow in dogs. *J. Cardiovasc. Pharmacol.* **10**:123.

100. Juhasz-Nagy, A., and Aviado, D.M. (1976). Increased role of alpha-adrenoceptors in ischemic myocardial zones. *Physiologist* **19**:245.

101. Sheridan, D.J., et al. (1970). Alpha-adrenergic contributions to dysrhythmia cardiac muscle. *Br. J. Pharmacol.* **39**:657.

102. Corr, P.B., *et al.* (1981). Increased alpha-adrenergic receptors in ischemic cat mycoardium. *J. Clin. Invest.* **67**:1232.

103. Vaughan Williams, E.M. (1985). Cardiac electrophysiological effects of selective adrenoceptor stimulation and their possible roles in arrhythmias. *J. Cardiovasc. Pharmacol.* **7**:S61.

104. Holland, K., Patterson, E., and Lucchesi, B.R. (1983). Prevention of ventricular fibrillation by bretylium in a conscious canine model of sudden coronary death. *Am. Heart J.* **105**:711.

105. Patterson, E., Lynch, J.J., and Lucchesi, B.R. (1984). Antiarrhythmic and antifibrillatory actions of the beta adrenergic receptor antagonist, dl-sotalol. *J. Pharmacol. Exp. Ther.* **230**:519.

106. Lynch, J.J., et al. (1985). Prevention of ventricular fibrillation by dextrorotatory sotalol in a conscious canine model of sudden coronary death. *Am. Heart J.* **109**:949.

107. Chi, L., et al. (1990). Antiarrhythmic and electrophysiologic actions of CK-3579 and sematilide in a conscious canine model of sudden coronary death. *J. Cardiovasc. Pharmacol.* **16**:312.

108. Chi, L., Mu, D.-X., and Lucchesi, B.R. (1991). Electrophysiology and antiarrhythmic actions of E-4031 in the experimental animal model of sudden coronary death. *J. Cardiovasc. Pharmacol.* **17**:285.

109. Black, S.C., et al. (1991). The antifibrillatory actions of UK-68,798, a class III antiarrhythmic agent. *J. Pharmacol. Exp. Ther.* **258**:416.

110. Kopia, G.A., et al. (1985). Antiarrhythmic and electrophysiologic actions of clofilium in experimental canine models. *Eur. J. Pharmacol.* **116**:49.

111. Patterson, E., Gibson, J.K., and Lucchesi, B.R. (1981). Postmyocardial infarction reentrant ventricular arrhythmias in conscious dogs: Suppression by bretylium tosylate. *J. Pharmacol. Exp. Ther.* **216**:453.

112. Patterson, E., Gibson, J.K., and Lucchesi, B.R. (1981). Prevention of chronic canine ventricular arrhythmias with bretylium tosylate. *Circulation* **64**:1045.

113. Anderson, J.L., et al. (1980). Kinetics of antifibrillatory effects of bretylium: Correlation with myocardial drug concentrations. *Am. J. Cardiol.* **46**:583.

114. Namm, D.H., et al. (1975). Effects of bretylium on rat cardiac muscle: The electrophysiological effect and its uptake and binding in normal and immunosympathectomized rat hearts. *J. Pharmacol. Exp. Ther.* **193**:194.

115. Bexton, R.S., and Camm, A.J. (1982). Drugs with a class III antiarrhythmic action. 1. Amiodarone. *Pharmacol. Ther.* **17**:315.

116. Gloor, H.O., Urthaler, F., and James, T.N. (1983). Acute effects of amiodarone upon the canine sinus node and atrioventricular junctional region. *J. Clin. Invest.* **71**:1457.

117. Mason, J.W., Hondeghem, L.M., and Katzung, B.G. (1984). Block of inactivated sodium channels and of depolarization-induced automaticity in guinea pig papillary muscle by amiodarone. *Circ. Res.* **55**:277.

118. Charlier, R. (1970). Cardiac actions in the dog of a new antagonist of adrenergic excitation which does not produce competitive blockade of adrenoceptors. *Br. J. Pharmacol.* **39**:668.

119. Freedberg, A.S., Papp, J.G., and Vaughan Williams, E.M. (1970). The effect of altered thyroid state on atrial intracellular potentials. *J. Physiol.* **207**:357.

120. Johnson, P.N., Freedberg, A.S., and Marshall, J.M. (1973). Action of thyroid hormone on the transmembrane poentials fron sinoatrial node cells and atrial muscle cells in isolated atria of rabbits. *Cardiology* **58**:273.

121. Singh, B.N., and Vaughan Williams, E.M. (1970). The effects of amiodarone, a new anti-anginal drug, on cardiac muscle. *Br. J. Pharmacol.* **39**:657.

122. Venkatesh, N., et al. (1991). Hypothyroidism renders protection against lethal ventricular arrhythmias in a conscious canine model of sudden death. *J. Cardiovasc. Pharmacol.* **18**:703.

123. Vaughan Williams, E.M. (1975). Classification of antidysrhythmic drugs. *Pharmacol. Ther.* **1**:115.

124. Task Force of the Working Group on Arrhythmias of the European Society of Cardiology. (1991). The Sicilian Gambit: A new approach to the classification of antiarrhythmic drugs based on their actions on arrhythmogenic mechanisms. *Circulation* **84**:1831.

125. Colatsky, T.J., and Follmer, C.H. (1980). K^+ channel blockers and activators in cardiac arrhythmias. *Cardiovasc. Drug Rev.* **7**:199.

126. Carmeliet, E. (1992). Potassium channels in cardiac cells. *Cardiovasc. Drugs Ther.* **6**:305.

127. Cook, N.S. (1988). The pharmacology of potassium channels and their therapeutic potential. *Trends Pharmacol. Sci.* **9**:21.

128. Colatsky, T.J., Follmer, C.H., and Starmer, C.F. 1990. Channel specificity in antiarrhythmic drug action: Mechanism of potassium channel block and its role in suppressing and aggravating cardiac arrhythmias. *Circulation* **82**:2235.

129. Noma, A. (1983). ATP-regulated K^+ channels in cardiac muscle. *Nature* **305**:147.

130. Cook, D.L., and Hales, C.N. (1984). Intracellular ATP directly blocks K^+ channels in pancreatic B-cells. *Nature* **311**:271.

131. Fosset, M., et al. (1988). Antidiabetic sulfonlyureas control action potential properties in heart cells via high affinity receptors that are linked to ATP-dependent K channels. *J. Biol. Chem.* **263**:7933.

132. Kantor, P.F., et al. (1987). Effects of glibenclamide on ischemic arrhythmias. *Circulation* **76**:IV-17.

133. Wolloben, C.D., Sanguinetti, M.C., and Siegl, P.K.S. (1989). Influence of ATP-sensitive potassium channel modulators on ischemia-induced fibrillation in isolated rat hearts. *J. Mol. Cell. Cardiol.* **21**:783.

134. Siegl, P.K.S., Scott, A.L., and Sanguinetti, M.C. (1988). Inhibition of anoxia- and BRL 3495–induced shortening of cardiac refractory period by the sulfonylurea, glyburide, in isolated ferret papillary muscle. *J. Mol. Cell. Cardiol.* **20**(suppl III):S32.

135. Kantor, P.F., et al. (1990). Reduction of ischemic K^+ loss and arrhythmias in rat hearts. Effect of glibenclamide, a sulfonylurea. *Circ. Res.* **66**:478.

136. Jiang, C., Crake, T., and Poole-Wilson, P.A. (1991). Inhibition by barium and glibenclamide of the net loss of 86Rb + from rabbit myocardium during hypoxia. *Cardiovasc. Res.* **25**:414.

137. Hicks, M.N., and Cobbe, S.M. (1991). Effect of glibenclamide on extracellular potassium accumulation and the electrophysiological changes during myocardial ischaemia in the arterially perfused interventricular septum of rabbit. *Cardiovasc. Res.* **25**:407.

138. Venkatesh, N., Lamp, S.T., and Weiss, J.N. (1991). Sulfonylureas, ATP-sensitive K^+ channels, and cellular K^+ loss during hypoxia, ischaemia, and metabolic inhibition in mammalian ventricle. *Cir. Res.* **69**:623.

139. Tseng, G.-N., and Hoffman, B.F. (1990). Actions of pinacidil on membrane currents in canine ventricular myocytes and their modulation by intracellular ATP and cAMP. *Pflügers Arch.* **415**:414.

140. Arena, J.P., and Kass, R.S. (1989). Activation of ATP-sensitive K channels in heart cells by pinacidil: Dependence on ATP. *Am. J. Physiol.* **257**:H2092.

141. Chi, L., et al. (1992). Actions of pinacidil at a reduced potassium concentration: A direct cardiac effect possibly involving the ATP-dependent potassium channel. *J. Cardiovasc. Pharmacol.*, in press.

142. Smallwood, J.K., and Steinberg, M.I. (1988). Cardiac electrophysiological effects of pinacidil and related pyridylcyanoguanidines: Relationship to antihypertensive activity. *J. Cardiovasc. Pharmacol.* **12**:102.

143. Ashcroft, F.M. (1988). Adenosine 5'-triphosphate-sensitive potassium channels. *Ann. Rev. Neurosci.* **II**:97.

144. Fan, Z., Nakayama, K., and Hiroaoka, M. (1990). Multiple actions of pinacidil on adenosine triphosphate-sensitive potassium channels in guinea-pig ventricular myocytes. *J. Physiol.* **430**:273.

145. Sauviat, M.-P, et al. (1991). Activation of ATP-sensitive K^+ channels by a K^+ channel opener (SR 44866) and the effect upon electrical and mechanical activity of frog skeletal muscle. *Pflügers Arch.* **418**:261.

146. Nichols, C.G., and Lederer, W.J. (1990). The regulation of ATP-sensitive K^+ channel activity in intact and permeabilized rat ventricular myocytes. *J. Physiol.* **423**:91.

147. Nichols, C.G., and Lederer, W.J. (1991). Adenosine triphosphate-sensitive potassium channels in the cardiovascular system. *Am. J. Physiol.* **261**:H1675.

148. Nichols, C.G., Lederer, W.J., and Cannell, M.B. (1991). ATP dependence of Kₐₜₚ channel kinetics in isolated membrane patches from rat ventricle. *Biophys. J.* **60**:1164.

149. Nichols, C.G., Ripoll, C., and Lederer, W.J. (1991). ATP-sensitive potassium channel modulation of the guinea pig ventricular action potential and contraction. *Circ. Res.* **68**:280.

150. Chi, L., Uprichard, A.C.G., and Lucchesi, B.R. (1990). Profibrillatory actions of pinacidil in a conscious canine model of sudden coronary death. *J. Cardiovasc. Pharmacol.* **15**:452.

151. Antzelevitch, C., and DiDiego, J.M. (1992). Role of K⁺ channel activators in cardiac electrophysiology and arrhythmias. Editorial comment. *Circulation* **85**:1627.

152. McCullough, J.R., et al. (1989). Anti-ischemic effects of the potassium channel activators pinacidil and cromakalim and the reversal of these effects with the potassium channel blocker glyburide. *J. Pharmacol. Exp. Ther.* **251**:98.

153. Grover, G.J., Dzwonczyk, S., and Sleph, P.H. (1990). Reduction of ischemic damage in isolated rat hearts by the potassium channel opener, RP 52891. *Eur. J. Pharmacol.* **191**:11.

154. Auchampach, J.A., et al. (1991). The new K⁺ channel opener Aprikalim (RP 52891) reduces experimental infarct size in dogs in the absence of hemodynamic changes. *J. Pharmacol. Exp. Ther.* **259**:961.

155. Auchampach, J.A., et al. (1992). Pharmacological evidence for a role of ATP-dependent potassium channels in myocardial stunning. *Circulation* **86**:311.

156. Lazdunski, M.P. (1992). Potassium channels: Structure–function relationships, diversity and pharmacology. *Cardiovasc. Drugs Ther.* **6**:313.

157. Holahan, M.A., et al. (1992). Effect of E-4031, a class III antiarrhythmic agent, on experimental infarct size in a canine model of myocardial ischemia-reperfusion injury. *J. Cardiovasc. Pharmacol.* **19**:892.

158. Wallace, A.A., et al. (1991). Cardiac electrophysiologic and inotropic actions of new and potent methanesulfonanilide class III antiarrhythmic agents in anesthetized dogs. *J. Cardiovasc. Pharmacol.* **18**:687.

159. Gross, G.J., and Auchampach, J.A. (1992). Blockade of ATP-sensitive potassium channels prevents myocardial preconditioning in dogs. *Circ. Res.* **70**:223.

160. Niho, T., et al. (1987). Study of mechanism and effect of sodium 5-hydroxydecanoate on experimental ischemic ventricular arrhythmia. *Nippon Yakurigaku Zasshi* **89**:155 (in Japanese).

161. Fagbemi, S.O., Chi, L., and Lucchesi, B.R. (1992). Antifibrillatory and profibrillatory actions of selected class I antiarrhythmic agents. *J. Cardiovasc. Pharmacol.*, in press.

162. Pratt, C.M. (1991). FDA guidelines for antiarrhythmic drug development. *Choices in Cardiology* **5**:44.

PART SEVEN

Research Recommendations

28

Report of the Research Assessment Panel[1] "Ion Channels in the Cardiovascular System"

Arnold M. Katz, Arthur M. Brown, William A. Catterall, Gregory J. Kaczorowski, Harold C. Strauss, August M. Watanabe, Thomas W. Smith, and Peter M. Spooner

Abnormalities in cardiac electrical function constitute a major national health problem on which progress has been particularly slow and difficult. Data published for the year 1989[1,2] indicate approximately 3.4 million Americans had disturbances of cardiac rhythm for which there were more than half a million hospitalizations annually. That year, approximately 45,000 deaths were ascribed to lethal arrhythmias, with an additional 250,000 attributed to sudden cardiac death. Including electrical instabilities associated with heart attacks involving ischemic and coronary disease, rhythmic disturbances contribute to a reported total of about a half million heart disease deaths each year.

The basic molecular components involved in electrical signal generation and conduction to, from, and within the heart are a series of voltage and chemically gated channels for sodium, potassium, calcium and chloride ions. These complex, membrane embedded glycoproteins constitute the major topic addressed at the 1992 NHLBI Ion Channels Conference.

Progress in understanding biochemical and biophysical mechanisms by which channels function has, over the past several years, been quite remarkable. Indeed, the likelihood that this information can now be usefully applied to the development of effective new pharmacologic and biologic therapies relevant to heart disease was a significant motivation in

[1]Recommendations from the panel convened by the NHLBI, September 12–15, 1992, at the Chantilly Virginia Conference on "Ion Channels in the Cardiovascular System"

holding these discussions. Cardiac ion channels, along with a related series of membrane ion pumps and exchangers, constitute one of the most promising and accessible targets for arrhythmia therapeutics. Many channel proteins, including a great many different channel subunits, have recently been isolated, cloned, sequenced and expressed in vitro and their unique and variable characteristics probed at the level of normal, and mutated molecules. Such studies have revealed much about the fundamental nature of ion channels in the cardiovascular system.

Less well represented, but beginning to emerge, is information concerning the identification of channel dysfunctions causally related to arrhythmic disease. This exciting new chapter in molecular medicine is however, beginning to unfold and surely will serve as the topic of future conferences. What the progress at this conference does begin to illuminate is that there is now an enormous new scientific foundation to assist in these efforts, and the underlying potential of the channel approach to provide new, safe, treatments for rhythm disease.

Although efforts to prevent sudden death in high-risk patients with channel directed drugs earlier this decade led to some notable disappointments[3], potentially useful channel-directed drugs continue to be identified and in fact, much has been achieved[4]. Such efforts revealed our earlier expectations—that sodium channel antagonists and inhibitors of depolarization would be effective against lethal arrhythmias—were overly simplistic. Nevertheless this paradigm continues to represent one of the better alternatives to expensive, invasive, surgical treatments. As indicated here, important new leads and compounds have emerged and focus has shifted to "repolarizing" currents and attempts at solving more difficult issues, such as the complexities of manipulating macroscopic currents by modulation of conductances of single channel types, and the extrapolation of clinical information on proarrhythymic properties of early channel drug candidates, into new drug design. Current clinical options appear nonetheless limited, and in fact, one result has been a reversion in treatment patterns away from antiarrhythmics and towards increasing specialization in invasive approaches. This fragmentation in turn has created significant barriers to the development of integrating therapeutic options based on rational drug design. In fact in the opinion of this Panel, ". . .one of the most pressing issues in applied ion channel antiarrhythmic research is that of scientific parochialism and specialization." Basic scientists appear headed in multiple directions, but there is little translation of their findings into medically relevant drug development or clinical evaluation.

To address these concerns from an interdisciplinary perspective, the organizers requested an experienced group of investigators and physician scientists (Roster below) identify programmatic issues and solutions to the challenges as they emerged. This group was asked to provide advise on how work was progressing on basic, clinical and pharmacological research goals and provide suggestions regarding new approaches and opportunities for support. The considerations which follow represent a consensus of the ideas which emerged.

Recommendations For:

Basic Science

Basic studies on sodium, calcium, potassium and chloride channels in many different systems, including those of human cardiovascular origin, are well advanced, and exciting work is progressing rapidly. Much progress has been achieved in providing a comprehensive and detailed biochemical and biophysical analysis of different channel complexes associated with each ion. Drawing from work on other tissues (e.g. neural) and non-mammalian systems (e.g. Drosophila), the primary sequences of many relevant proteins have been determined, cDNA's and mRNA's made or isolated and expressed; and gene regulatory elements explored. Basic channel biology represents one of the most promising areas of contemporary molecular research. As such, it has attracted many talented investigators from diverse fields working in well supported academic, medical and pharmaceutical laboratories. The field appears self driven, with critical questions being rapidly identified and resolved. Many fundamental questions remain however, (e.g. how precisely do voltage and chemical gating domains work ?, how are pores constructed, rectified and regulated at an atomic level ?, etc.), but these are being addressed with notable success. Thus, the Panel does not believe there is a strong case for increased levels of activity here. Rather, members would suggest research workers and funding agencies be cognizant of several more limited recommendations, some of emphasis and others involving development of specific efforts as summarized below.

Recommendation # 1:

New efforts are needed to improve methods of obtaining three- dimensional structures of channel proteins in a native hydrated state within natural and artificial membranes. The ability to readily determine molecular structural features of specific subunits and domains would result in great improvement in our ability to correlate principles of molecular organization with function. Such information would advance our understanding of membrane proteins in general, as well as improve our ability to identify differences in aberrant channels. Identification and comparison of defined structures, with characteristic biochemical and electrophysiological properties, although urgently needed—is at present totally lacking. With knowledge of the number of possible channel subunit structures multiplying rapidly, it is essential to improve the tools required to understand the detailed physical basis of ion current generation.

In contrast to the difficulties encountered in obtaining structural information, progress on channel protein biochemistry has been excellent. Many channel proteins have been sequenced and a variety of isolated and synthetic transcripts expressed in *vitro*. In purified form, these materials constitute a significant resource for future structural analyses—if only such data could be more readily obtained. Besides structural technologies another major obstacle is that the amounts of material available from the in vitro synthetic systems in use are generally insufficient to permit structural determinations using conventional crystallization and X-ray technologies. Structural data, for even a few archetype molecules, would be of theoretical as well as practically benefit. Such information would help explain differences in electrical properties of different channels, isomeric subtypes, tissue and cell variants, malfunctioning channels, and interactions with other related receptors, pumps and transporters.

Recent developments in NMR spectroscopy, optical, electron, atomic force and tunnelling microscopies, along with improvements in X-ray techniques provide improved approaches to resolve and define protein structural domains. Other improvements in computer analysis and in imaging technologies, helpful in defining soluble proteins, could also provide new avenues for the study of membrane proteins. Given that the functional implications of the architecture of specific molecular domains now appear theoretically and technically discernable, the Panel strongly recommends increased support and activity in efforts to stimulate development of membrane structural methodologies and their application to the ion channel field.

Recommendation #2

The Panel believes much has been accomplished in determining electrophysiological and biophysical characteristics of individual ion currents in cardiovascular cells. Much data have been published on current and wavefront propagation in different segments of the heart and its conduction system in disease models and in humans. Information on vascular smooth muscle and endothelial cells is also becoming available. Extension of these studies to correlate specific normal and pathological current characteristics with identifiable channel defects now seems possible. Such studies should proceed vigorously and include greater consideration of alterations in mechanisms of channel biochemical modulation and autonomic control, as well as alterations in expression of appropriate genotypic transcripts. Although we do not yet have concrete examples of "sick channel" molecules underlying arrhythmias (analogous to abnormal chloride channels in cystic fibrosis), this is rapidly being approached (e.g. in long Q-T syndrome). The Panel therefore believes it important to evaluate the possibility single and multi-channel defects are important in different sudden death and arrhythmia syndromes. Because these issues represent an exciting topic in contemporary molecular medicine, it seems probable they will receive ample attention over the ensuing years. For the record, the Panel would like however to emphasize the critical importance of this approach.

Pharmacologic Science

The Panel was impressed with the progress on new strategies to discover agonist and antagonist affinity modulators of channel function and the progress in drug design through improved structural chemistry. Work in understanding "use" and "reverse use" dependance of K^+ channel blockers appears particularly promising in this regard. Nevertheless, it is evident there remain major limitations in our ability to define what domains or even molecules are an appropriate cellular-molecular "target" in antiarrhythmic development. Although recommendation #2 (above) deals with this problem in part, the Panel believes greater information should be obtained to resolve our present lack of data on the distribution of different channels within human cardiovascular tissues of normal, as well as disease origin. Detailed maps of the densities and locations of sodium, potassium and chloride channels within the heart and resistance vessels would be of much value in addressing conductance deficiencies, rhythm and nodal abnormalities. Such explorations should include evaluation of distributions of different channel isoforms in different areas of the heart. For example, at least seven different potassium channels have now been reported within the mammalian myocardium, but their location and exact electrophysiological role, other than in "repolarization", remains largely unknown. Information on sodium channel distributions could similarly provide better information on which receptors to target to elicit changes in "depolarization." The ability to therapeutically target depolarization and repolarization abnormalities at the individual channel level might help resolve the difficult problem of balancing anti- and pro-arrhythmic properties within individual drug molecules.

Recommendation #3

Although the Panel considers pharmaceutical development of high priority, the majority does not believe new funding initiatives, should be required. Instead, it would seem more important to identify and mark for high relevance those projects ongoing or in a planning stage. Panel members believe there is now sufficient activity in various transplantation and clinical research centers to address these questions in humans. The concern is that some opportunities would be lost for lack of adequete interdisciplinary appreciation. Such work can also be undervalued by more traditional peer review procedures used by funding sources by its classification as "descriptive" (as opposed to "mechanistic") and therefore of low priority. The Panel therefore encourages special attention be given to encourage projects in this area.

Clinical Science

Progress in applying basic ion channel information to arrhythmia management has been slow and recently controversial. It is of note for example, that some recent reviews emphasize the view that use of membrane directed antiarrhythmics involves abnormally high risk and should be employed only under controlled conditions[5]. However, alternative approaches, including ablative surgery and implantable defibrillating devices are not of proven benefit in many conditions, although their costs are considerable. The panel believes that while the current paradigm of drug therapy is of uncertain benefit in a number of clinical categories, there are unquestioned advantages to many membrane-directed drugs in regular use whose effectiveness has not been compromised by the negative results of earlier clinical trials. This approach may, in fact, hold the best, potential for, non-invasive, long-term patient management. As a result, pharmaceutical development should be expanded in new directions, rather than diminished as appears to be the case within industry today.

Recommendation #4

Given our limited ability to identify appropriate pharmacologic "targets" for prevention and treatment of arrhythmias and sudden death, the Panel believes support of new antiarrhythmic drug discovery research in basic and clinical laboratories should be a high priority. Since we now believe that older agents effective in suppressing ectopic electrical events in patients may not be of benefit in preventing lethal arrhythmias, better alternatives even to promising new compounds like amiodarone and sotalol, need to be developed. The recent experience with these excellent candidates illustrates the dilemma that we lack the basic knowledge to design effective agents based on a detailed knowledge of underlying arrhythmic mechanisms. Thus, it seems not really surprising that our most promising new compounds are characterized by a variety of still not well understood different mechanisms on the surface of the myocardial cell. It is hoped recent trials of these "less-specific" drugs will provide new clues for new pharmaceutical directions. Formulation and exploration of more mechanistic drug classification schemes (e.g. the "Sicilian Gambit" approach[4]) and focus on specific K^+ channels should also be encouraged. The Panel believes many different approaches should continue to be explored with particular emphasis given to understanding the mechanistic complexity of different arrhythmias as separate disease entities. Continued support for clinically relevant drug evaluation studies is likewise believed important, but recommendations concerning such efforts are beyond the purview of this report.

Concluding Considerations

Overall, the Panel believes one of the most pressing issues in applied ion channel antiarrhythmic research is that of scientific parochialism. At present, specialization has increased to the extent that communication between basic, clinical and pharmacologic investigators is difficult. This in turn has impeded an integrated practical understanding of channel dysfunction in disease. In the combined imagery of several Panel members, "...we appear to have three sophisticated, independent vertical silos of information on different aspects of cardiovascular channels, but only a few narrow bridges between them." Management of patients using channel directed therapy is expected to make slow progress, partly as a result of the CAST Trial and partly for lack of fundamental information. Meanwhile, drug discovery efforts of many pharmaceutical groups appear to be "on hold" until more promising targets are identified. Basic science approaches are, in contrast, flourishing—but often in relative isolation. Concerted efforts to integrate all three approaches may therefore be the most useful means of addressing this growing problem.

References

1. Morbidity and Mortality Chartbook on Cardiovascular, Lung and Blood Diseases, 1992. National Heart, Lung, and Blood Institute, National Institutes of Health, U.S. Department of Health and Human Services, Washington, D.C.
2. 1992 Heart and Stroke Facts, American Heart Association, National Center, Dallas, Texas, 1992.
3. Pratt, C.M., ed. The Cardiac Arrhythmia Suppression Trial—Does It Alter Our Concepts of and Approaches to Ventricular Arrhythmias? Amer. J. Cardiology, *65*, 1–49B, 1990.
4. Task Force of the Working Group on Arrhythmias of the European Society of Cardiology. The Sicilian Gambit: A New Approach to the Classification of Antiarrhythmic Drugs Based on Their Actions on Arrhythmogenic Mechanisms, Circulation *4*, 1831–1851, 1991.
5. Kessler, K.M., Chakko, S. and Myerburg, R.J.: Management of Premature Ventricular Contractions. *Heart Disease and Stroke* 1, 275–280, 1992.

Recommendation and Assessment
Panel Roster

Arnold M. Katz, M.D., Chair
Professor and Head of Cardiology
University of Connecticut
Farmington, CT

Arthur M. Brown, M.D., Ph.D.
Professor and Chairman
Dept. of Molecular Physiology
    and Biophysics
Baylor College of Medicine
Houston, TX

William A. Catterall, Ph.D.
Professor and Chairman
Department of Pharmacology
University of Washington
Seattle, WA

Gregory J. Kaczorowski, Ph.D.
Director, Membrane Biochemistry
    and Biophysics
Merck Research Laboratories
Rahway, NJ

Harold C. Strauss, M.D.
Professor, Department of Medicine
Duke University Medical Center
Durham, NC

August M. Watanabe, M.D.
Group Vice-President
Lilly Research Labs
Eli Lilly & Company
Indianapolis, IN

Thomas W. Smith, M.D.
Chief, Cardiovascular Division
Department of Medicine
Brigham and Women's Hospital
Boston, MA

NHLBI STAFF
    Peter M. Spooner, Ph.D.
    Chief, Cardiac Functions Branch
    Division of Heart and Vascular
    Diseases, NHLBI
    National Institutes of Health
    Bethesda, MD

Index